The Hidden Structure

*To Sara, who was born at
the same time as this book.*

Oxford University Press acknowledges
the generous support of the Policlinico San Matteo
and the University of Pavia in the publication of this book.

The Hidden Structure

A Scientific Biography of Camillo Golgi

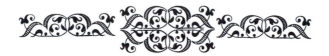

Paolo Mazzarello

Lecturer in History of Medicine, University of Pavia

Translated and edited by
Henry A. Buchtel and Aldo Badiani
University of Michigan and University of Rome 'La Sapienza'

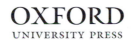

OXFORD

UNIVERSITY PRESS

OXFORD
UNIVERSITY PRESS

Great Clarendon Street, Oxford OX2 6DP

Oxford University Press is a department of the University of Oxford.
It furthers the University's objective of excellence in research, scholarship,
and education by publishing worldwide in

Oxford New York

Athens Auckland Bangkok Bogota Buenos Aires Calcutta
Cape Town Chennai Dar es Salaam Delhi Florence Hong Kong Istanbul
Karachi Kuala Lumpur Madrid Melbourne Mexico City Mumbai
Nairobi Paris São Paulo Singapore Taipei Tokyo Toronto Warsaw

and associated companies in Berlin Ibadan

Oxford is a trade mark of Oxford University Press
in the UK and in certain other countries

Published in the United States
by Oxford University Press, Inc., New York

A catalogue record for this book is available from the British Library

Library of Congress Cataloging in Publication Data
Mazzarello, Paolo.
[Struttura nascosta. English]
The hidden structure : a scientific biography of Camillo Golgi /
Paolo Mazzarello : translated from the Italian by H.A. Buchtel and
Aldo Badiani.
Includes bibliographical references and index.
1. Golgi, Camillo, 1843–1926. 2. Histologists–Italy Biography.
3. Neuroscientists–Italy Biography.   I. Title.
QM16.G65M3913   1999   610'.92–dc21 [B]   99–22934

ISBN 0 19 852444 7

Typeset by Downdell, Oxford
Printed in Great Britain
on acid-free paper by
Bookcraft (Bath) Ltd.
Midsomer Norton, Avon

Foreword

by Gordon M. Shepherd

This is a landmark biography in the history of science. Camillo Golgi has always been considered one of the pioneers of modern biology, but the recognition has been fragmented. Neuroanatomists recognized him for the 'Golgi stain', cytologists for the 'Golgi apparatus', muscle physiologists for the 'Golgi tendon organ', parasitologists for his precise identification of the malarial cycle in humans. Recognition in some cases has been long deferred; witness the varying fortunes of the Golgi stain, the consensus at midcentury that the Golgi apparatus was an artefact just before the electron microscope proved its existence, and the most recent rediscovery of the long forgotten 'perineural net' that he described a century ago. But it was his lost battles over the neuron doctrine that mainly consigned him to the margins of that select group considered to be the giants who contributed to the conceptual development of modern biology.

The process of rehabilitating Golgi reputation began about a decade ago, with a realization that, in his battles against the neuron as a cellular unit, there was much of merit in his concepts, such as in the holistic functions of the brain and the importance of the nutritive substrates for brain function. But what has been needed is a full reassessment, embracing the depth of Golgi's training in medicine and neurology, the milieu within which he made his discoveries, and the motivations he had for the stands he took. It could only be this kind of in depth study, by someone trained in the same traditions, that could give us a full picture of the scientist and his place in the history of biology. In particular, we have sorely needed to understand the reasoning behind his beliefs about what constituted hard-nosed experimental evidence compared with his adversaries, for only with this understanding can we appreciate how he believed he was building his concepts on facts and not speculations.

These needs have been met in this biography by Paolo Mazzarello, an Italian neurologist. Here for the first time we have Golgi's life, previously seen only in brief biographical glimpses, and the different discoveries, viewed only by different disciplines, brought together in a unified whole. We can see how Camillo Golgi was the product of a distinguished scientific tradition, which by itself will open the eyes of modern biologists accustomed to thinking of the rise of experimental biology in the nineteenth century as mainly occurring in central Europe. We gain a new appreciation of Golgi's deep commitment to the experimental method in biology, and how this provided the bedrock for his conceptual contributions, whether or not they ultimately proved to be right or wrong in the light of later studies. The modern biologist with any modicum of modesty will realize that the struggles of Golgi and his contemporaries, in pushing interpretations of their experimental findings to the limit, provide a valuable perspective on our own attempts today with our own methods.

A final benefit of this biography in English is the beautiful narrative, a product of the author and his expert translators, which carries the reader along an absorbing tale of a fascinating life and a momentous series of discoveries. As noted by the author, the association of Golgi's name with the Golgi body alone makes him 'probably the most cited biologist in scientific literature'. It is therefore high time that we give him the attention that he so richly deserves.

Preface

The English edition of this book is not merely a translation of the Italian version of 1996. In many places the book has been rethought, reorganized, and re-elaborated at the end of the dialectical process between author and translators. I have also added new details concerning the life of Camillo Golgi and his laboratory, as well as some references to Italian history that I thought might be useful to help the reader to frame the events surrounding Golgi's life in a larger context. In this I have been greatly helped by the comments and suggestions of the two translators, Drs Henry Buchtel and Aldo Badiani, who also carried out an irreplaceable initial editing of this English edition, and to whom goes all my admiration and gratitude.

The bibliography has been enhanced by the addition of new entries. In particular, Golgi's bibliography should now be virtually complete. In this English version, I have also been able to eliminate a number of imprecisions and some minor errors, which were inevitable in the first edition given the scope of the work and the heterogeneity of the source material. For all these reasons, I have come to regard the present English version as the point of arrival of my systematic research on the life of Camillo Golgi. This research has developed along two main themes: the events in the private life of the scientist (as far as can be discerned from the available material), and the network of contacts with Italian and foreign scientists and intellectuals, concerning which I have explored many dark corners. The life of Golgi the scientist, which I have examined mainly from a chronological perspective, plays a fundamental role in that fascinating chapter in the history of biology represented by the origin of neurosciences, which is still far from being fully investigated. Golgi's story is also central to the history of cytology and the nascent medical microbiology. In writing this book, I followed all avenues of inquiry and have tried not to forgo any details that could have relevance from a biographical point of view. However, if it is true, as maintained by the Russian literary critic Viktor Sklovskij, that it is impossible to write a truly complete biography, this is even more true for a figure such as Golgi, who was a richly multifaceted person but also extremely reserved in private matters. On the other hand, I have tried to minimize the number of conjectures, and in all cases I have indicated them as such. The English edition, like the Italian one, has been made possible by the support of the Policlinico San Matteo and the University of Pavia. In particular, my thanks go to Dr Danilo Morini and Professor Enrico Solcia of the San Matteo, and to Professors Cesare Meloni and Alberto Calligaro of the University of Pavia.

I would also like to thank Professor Giovanni Berlucchi for his encouragement and support in the preparation of both the Italian and English editions. His Pavian roots, added to his personal generosity, might explain the interest he has always exhibited in the completion of this project. I want to express my deep appreciation to Dr Marina Benti-voglio, with whom I have collaborated in the last two years in analyzing a number of important topics in the history of neuroscience, and who has provided many acute obser-vations and suggestions. Thanks are also due to Professor Gunnar Grant, who has given me access to two unpublished manuscripts that have allowed me to clarify some details (and to correct some imprecisions) concerning Golgi and the Nobel Prize.

Many others have helped me in one form or another in writing this book. In particular, I want to thank Ernesto Capanna, Sergio Della Sala, Federico Focher, Marco Fraccaro, Giuseppe Gerzeli, Raffaele Melli, Germana Pareti, Cesare Patrini, Giuseppe Raimondi, Carlo Redi, Carlo Reggiani, Lucio Ricciardi, Gianguido Rindi, Silvano Riva, Alfredo Sellari, Elisa Signori, Silvio Spadari, Lino Stefanini, Vanio Vannini, Flavio Verona, and Bruno Zanobio.

Finally, I would like to thank the Rector of the University of Pavia, Professor Roberto Schmid, and the Executive Committee of the *Centro per la Storia dell'Università di Pavia*, and in particular Professors Faustino Savoldi, Emilio Gabba, and Giulio Guderzo, for their continuous support of this project.

Of course, none of the above cited persons is in any way responsible for any remaining errors of interpretation or shortcomings in the book.

The book was written thanks to the facilities found at the Istituto di Genetica Bio-chimica ed Evoluzionistica (CNR) of Pavia.

Russian names are generally cited using their French translation, which was the form used commonly in the scientific literature of the 1800s. Ramón y Cajal is referred to as Cajal (as is the convention in neurobiological literature).

Golgi's *Opera Omnia* is referred to in the text of *OO*; the works cited are reported by author's name, year of publication (followed by *OO* for those included in the *Opera Omnia*) and page numbers when applicable); page numbers are omitted in references to news-papers and magazines.

Golgi's *Opera Omnia* is comprised of four volumes (Hoepli Editore, Milano); the first three, edited by R. Fusari, G. Marenghi and L. Sala, were published in 1903. The fourth volume, edited by L. Sala, E. Veratti and G. Sala, was added in 1929.

The four volumes gather together the majority of Golgi's scientific publications sub-divided by topic and by year, and are supplemented by 58 plates. The numbering of the pages and the tables is continuous and progressive for the entire work.

Volume I, *Istologia normale*, 1870–1883, pp. 1–396; Volume II, *Istologia normale*, 1883–1902, pp. 397–736; Volume III, *Patologia Generale e Isto-patologia*, 1868–1894, pp. 737–1258; Volume IV, *Scritti su argomenti varii*, 1903–1925, pp. 1259–1566.

The rich documentation of Golgi's scientific life, donated by his heirs to the *Museo per la Storia dell'Università di Pavia*, has been organized and in great part catalogued by his pupil Emilio Veratti. In the citations of unedited documents of the legacy one refers to the Veratti Catalogue, titled *Elenco delle carte lasciate dal Prof. Camillo Golgi senatore del regno*, Pavia, July 1941.

To this material one must add mementoes, diplomas, drawings, and various documents kept in the display cases of the Museum, as well as manuscripts acquired after 1941 and therefore not included in the Catalogue. These are referred to in the text by indicating the nature of the item and the fact that it is in the Museum. Materials already published (in part or in their entirety) will be cited by indicating the publication in which they have been reproduced.

P.M.

Contents

Plates are located between pp. 210–pp. 211

Abbreviations

ALFP	*Archivio del Liceo Foscolo di Pavia*
BUP	*Biblioteca Universitaria di Pavia*
MGA	*Museo Golgiano della 'Pia Casa-Istituto Geriatrico Camillo Golgi' di Abbiate-grasso*
MSUP	*Museo per la Storia dell'Università di Pavia*
MSUP-G-S-N	Veratti's Catalogue of MSUP. G indicates the roman numeral of the group (from I to XXX), S the number of the section of that particular group (when present) and N the number or letter of the subsection.

Exigua est capitis moles, sed
immensa recondit misteria
Giovan Battista Morgagni

I am delighted that I have found a new reaction to demonstrate even to the blind the structure of the interstitial stroma of the cerebral cortex. I let the silver nitrate react with pieces of brain hardened in potassium dichromate. I have already obtained magnificent results and hope to do even better in the future.

– Letter from Camillo Golgi to Nicolò Manfredi, 16 February 1873

1

Introduction: between revolution and conservatism

The scientist bends over the eyepiece of the microscope.

What a fantastic sight! On a yellow, completely transparent background, there appear sparsely scattered black fibres, smooth and small or thick and prickly, as well as black, triangular, star- or rod-shaped bodies! Just like fine India ink drawings on transparent Japanese paper. The scientist gazes upon it in astonishment. He is more accustomed to the chaotic images produced by carminic acid and haematoxylin, which yield one dubious interpretation after another. Here, on the other hand, everything is absolutely clear, without any possibility of confusion. There is nothing more to interpret; one need only observe and note these cells, with their different, ramified extensions, like plants in the morning frost, covering an astonishingly large space in wavy lines; these smooth and uniform extensions which, springing from the cell, cover great distances, before suddenly splitting up into a bunch of innumerable fibres . . . The delighted and astonished gaze cannot tear itself away from this fantastic sight. Methodic wishful thinking has become reality. Metal impregnation has produced a magnificent and unexpected slide.'[1]

This is how the great Spanish histologist Santiago Ramón y Cajal imagined the scene that, one day at the end of 1872 or the beginning of 1873, must have presented itself to the eyes of Camillo Golgi, the young Chief Physician of the 'Pie Case degli Incurabili' (Charitable Home for Incurables)[2] of Abbiategrasso. It is the grand moment of the discovery of the 'reazione nera' (black reaction), a revolutionary method for studying the structure of the nervous system. This discovery contributed, more than 30 years later, to the awarding of the Nobel Prize for Medicine to Golgi.

For every student of medicine or biology, the name Golgi is synonymous with one of the basic structures in the cell: the Golgi apparatus or Golgi complex. But this is only one of the many discoveries and achievements, particularly in the neurosciences, for which Golgi's name deserves to be known by a much wider public than just devotees of biomedical sciences. Unfortunately, his scientific fame lags far behind the historical significance of his discoveries. The historical–critical literature on Golgi is scanty and the appraisal of his scientific work has been negatively affected by the erroneous idea that his discovery of the black reaction was the result of pure chance, and by his refusal to accept the *theory of the neuron*.

The theory of the neuron (definitively confirmed only after the advent of the electron microscope) is an important historical example of a scientific revolution in biology; that is, a new conception that interprets and organizes in a coherent model a collection of observations from a number of different disciplines (in this case, anatomy, histology, embryology, biochemistry, physiology, and pathology). To use the terminology of Thomas S. Kuhn,[3] without necessarily adopting his ideas on the evolution of scientific thought, the theory of the neuron represents the basic 'paradigm' of the neurosciences, in the same sense that atomic–molecular interpretations of matter or the theory of the discrete transmission of hereditary characteristics constitute the basic paradigms of chemistry and genetics, respectively. The concept of neuron (and particularly that of synapses), by virtue of its being the elemental unit of modulation and transmission of information, has also assumed a pre-eminent role in many disciplines associated with the neurosciences, such as informatics and artificial intelligence. The theory of the neuron did not originate from the principles of the cellular theory as an automatic extension to the nervous system, just as quantum mechanics is not simply a consequence of applying classical mechanics to subatomic structures. Given the biophysical characteristics of neurons, the laws of their reciprocal communication, the complexity of their connections, and the extraordinary nature of the activities to which they give rise, it is evident how this theory constitutes the basis of a new area of scientific research that integrates, 'polyphonically', contributions from physics, electrochemistry, informatics, and clinical medicine, and from classical physiology and anatomy–histology. From this perspective, the theory must be considered one of the great intellectual conquests of the nineteenth century.

To the end of his life Golgi remained a fiery opponent of this theory, although, as Golgi himself acknowledged in the acceptance speech for the Nobel Prize, he had contributed materially to its formulation by discovering the black reaction, which allowed the detailed investigation of the morphology of neurons and the architecture of the brain. Just as Luigi Galvani's electrobiological discoveries opened the way to the invention of the first electric battery by Alessandro Volta, and Joseph Priestley's discovery of 'dephlogisticated air' led to the identification of oxygen by Antoine Laurent Lavoisier, so did Golgi's studies provide the indispensable basis for the discoveries of Cajal, which then led to the 'paradigmatic' generalization of the neuron doctrine.

Often in the history of biology (and in scientific discoveries generally), the introduction of a new technique revolutionizes a whole area of research, radically transforming pre-existing disciplines and creating others from scratch. One is reminded of the effect that monoclonal antibodies had on immunology and other branches of biology, or of the impact that the technology of recombinant DNA had on genetics. The black reaction represented, for the histology of the nervous system, a breakthrough of comparable importance, permitting the development of neuroanatomy as an autonomous discipline, and thus contributing to the birth of modern neuroscience. In fact, only after the discovery of the black reaction, and the extraordinary structural descriptions of the nervous tissues obtained with it, did morphological investigations begin to be connected to physiological and functional investigations. Golgi's success also spurred the field to refine new histological techniques for the selective staining of particular structures of cells and nervous tissue.

The results obtained by Golgi and Cajal in neurobiology place them at the highest rank in the history of science: that of the precursors. Golgi's work was at the centre of a revolution that within a few years led to a detailed topographic mapping of the nervous system that was indispensable for a physiological, physiopathological, and clinical analysis of nervous activity.

Golgi's neurophysiology was clearly wrong, but his repeatedly expressed ideas that 'nerve cells work as an ensemble' and that the nervous system exerts 'a unitary action' in carrying out its specific functions, place him at the centre of a holistic tradition still alive in modern neurosciences. Thanks to concepts such as 'parallel information processing' and 'neural network', it is possible to envision the brain as unitary structure in which an enormous number of operations are carried out simultaneously by interconnected neuronal systems. Golgi's work in neurobiology was clearly forward-looking, if one is willing to abandon schematic conceptions based simply on the 'truth' or 'falsity' of a scientific theory, and frame it instead in the more general perspective of the history of ideas.

In addition to his revolutionary work on the nervous system, Golgi also attained significant renown in a sphere that, following Kuhn, we might consider as 'normal science', that is, 'research firmly based upon one or more past achievements, achievements that some particular scientific community acknowledges for a time as supplying the foundation for its further practice'.[4] To the latter kind of achievement belongs the work of Golgi in such areas of biology, cytology, microbiology, and pathology, with contributions that were both basic and rich with therapeutic implications. To him we owe, for example, the discovery of one of the basic constituents of the cell, the 'Golgi apparatus' or 'complex' (because of which he is probably the most cited biologist in scientific literature), the identification and the description of the malarial cycle in the human with an exact description of the correlation between the various forms of the micro-organism and the malarial attack, and the determination of the optimal timing for quinine therapy.

Golgi was always reserved in his private life and there are few testimonials by his pupils or references in letters or documents that can clarify aspects of his character, attitudes, and ideological choices; the few that do exist suggest that he was a man of few words who was dominated by two passions: scientific research, a mission that he pursued with religious fervour, and the University of Pavia, of which he was Rector in two different periods and whose importance and prestige he constantly endeavoured to enhance.

One of Golgi's greatest accomplishments was the creation of an important school of histology and histopathology at the University of Pavia. Pre-eminent figures of this school include: Adelchi Negri, who discovered the bodies that take his name in animals and humans infected with the rabies virus; Emilio Veratti, who described the sarcoplasmic reticulum; Aldo Perroncito, who carried out basic studies on the regeneration of the peripheral nervous system; Carlo Martinotti, whose name is linked to the cells with ascending axons in the cerebral cortex; and many of his pupils who identified in the Golgi complex a universal cellular constituent. A number of other scientists, who later made important discoveries, spent periods of study and specialization in Golgi's laboratory. Among them are Giovanni Battista Grassi, Vittorio Marchi, and Antonio Carini. The first identified the mosquito vector of malaria in the human, the second developed a basic method for the staining of myelin, and the third discovered the micro-organism *Pneumocystis carinii*, which is responsible for recurrent pneumonia in individuals with acquired immunodeficiency. At one time, Golgi's laboratory was also a pole of attraction for foreign scientists, including the Norwegian Fritjof Nansen, the Swiss Rudolf Albert von Kölliker, the American Henry Herbert Donaldson, and the Russian Serge Soukhanoff. For the prestige of its exponent and the far-reaching effects of its scientific legacy, the institute created by Golgi in Pavia has few equals in the panorama of Italian science. One thinks of the group of nuclear physicists led by Enrico Fermi at the Institute of Physics on Via Panisperna in Rome, and of Giuseppe Levi's laboratory in Turin, where Nobel Prize laureates Salvador Luria, Renato Dulbecco, and Rita Levi Montalcini began their work.

One need only open a book of biology or medicine to realize that Golgi is one of the true giants of nineteenth-century science. Despite this, as has been accurately emphasized by Pietro Corsi,[5] Golgi has not become a familiar figure in the Italian cultural panorama, nor has he received the recognition that his role in the development of neuroscience alone should have earned him.

This biography is an attempt to correct, at least partially, this state of affairs.

Notes

1. Cajal (1909, p. 28).
2. The hospital was also known as 'Pio Casa degli Incurabili' or 'Pio Luogo degli Incurabili'.
3. Kuhn (1962).
4. Kuhn (1970, p. 10).
5. Corsi (1986).

2

From the mountains of Valcamonica to the University of Pavia

The family name Golgi can be found in the oldest church records of Pavia, and a 'Torre di Casa Golgi' (Golgi Household's Tower) still dominates Piazza della Posta, one of the City's main squares.

At the beginning of the nineteenth century Golgi's grandfather, the hat-maker Michele Golgi, kept a shop in this Lombard town. In October 1814, Angelica Nicolletti, Michele's wife, gave birth to Alessandro Antonio Nicola Golgi, who was baptized in the ancient church of San Michele.[1] Alessandro Golgi did not follow in his father's steps and, 'wishing to improve his social status', entered the University of Pavia Medical School where he 'followed all lectures very diligently and was a very dedicated student in both theoretical and practical studies', finally graduating in 1838.[2] In that same year Alessandro married his cousin Carolina Golgi, daughter of the carpenter Camillo Golgi[3], and found himself under immediate pressure to obtain a sufficiently well-paid position. Despite the relatively small number of physicians, his job prospects were quite meagre. Medical doctors could expect to make a living in private practice only after long years of free or underpaid work. Positions as hospital doctor were rare and the hopes of an academic career the privilege of an elite. Easier to find were positions as municipal doctors, especially in the most remote areas. This probably explains why Alessandro Golgi accepted a position in Corteno (currently Corteno Golgi), a municipality in the province of Brescia, in the Alps that separate Lombardy from Switzerland.

The village of Corteno was fairly small and its 1900 inhabitants were mostly 'shepherds, mountaineers, and smiths'; many worked most of the year in pork processing factories in Brescia, Mantua, Verona, Vicenza, and Padua.[4] The young doctor performed his duties with great dedication and soon acquired a reputation for competence, conscientiousness, and generosity, drawing clientele from the neighbouring villages.[5] He was also described as a cultivated figure, fond of Latin literature and music. In 1950, asked about Alessandro Golgi, 'some senior citizens of Corteno had vague recollections of him as a good-natured, gentle, and conscientious person'.[6] The social environment of Alessandro and Carolina Golgi was typical of the rural middle class. They befriended the local notables, particularly the pharmacist Pietro Chiodi (sometime mayor, municipal secretary, and Justice of the Peace), Don Bortolino Chiodi, a parish priest, and the Stefanini, Marazzani, and Berneri families.

The Golgis had four children, all born in a house located in Pisogneto in the centre of the municipality of Corteno. The firstborn, Luigi Carlo Angelo Golgi, became Chief Inspector of the State Property Office and lived in Pavia and Brescia, where he died. The second child, Giuseppe Alessandro Golgi, became a pharmacist in Fagnano, close to Busto Arsizio. Bartolomeo Camillo Emilio Golgi, a 'beautiful and strong'[7] baby, was born on 7 July 1843 and baptized in the church of Santa Maria Assunta of Corteno.[8] The fourth child was Maria Teresa, who would marry a pharmacist from Pavia, Siro Campagnoli.

Camillino (diminutive of Camillo) spent the first years of his life in the quiet pastoral environment of Corteno, surrounded by woods and pasture.

The village (though located at an altitude of 825 m) was nothing like Leopardi's *natio borgo selvaggio* (native wild village), being, on the contrary, an agreeable place . . .

. . . around 1843, Corteno must have been just a big alpine village. Camillo Golgi's homeland is, however, a pleasant region in which majestic scenic landscapes and lovely views alternate in the continuously changing nature of the terrain. To the west of the village, emerald green pastures stretch upwards, giving way to larch and aspen woods sprinkled with the white of a rare birch. To the east runs the scenic road connecting Edolo to the Aprica Pass, the latter being less than 8 km from Corteno.

The future Pavian pathologist spent his childhood in a small house, little more than a rural dwelling, located in these peaceful and modest surroundings . . . The young Camillo (his first name Bartolomeo was probably never used) was particularly fond of climbing the road to the Aprica pass. This large and sunny road was the scene of his solitary walks, and during the next fifty years the Aprica Pass remained a favourite walking destination during his sporadic visits to his home town. With the years, however, these visits became more and more rare. After his parents' deaths, Golgi had no relatives or properties left in Corteno, and I have been told that his last visit took place in 1912. However, Golgi kept up a lively correspondence with his father's and his own friends, and often had them as guests in Pavia. He always maintained a tender and affectionate memory of his home town. When visiting Corteno, Golgi used to repeat his walk to the Aprica Pass, and from that wonderful vista on the Valtellina he could enjoy the breathtaking view of the two large valleys below. The Southern valley, with its beautiful lines of masterfully cultivated vineyards, extended as far as Sondrio and Morbegno, whereas the Northern valley reached beyond Tirano. During these walks, he would remain silent most of the time, a resigned listener to the conversation of his companions, and would be completely absorbed in the contemplation of the calm beauty of the mountain vegetation and of the power of human industriousness, which, on the smallest, most insignificant and most rocky terraces, had been able to create the most regular, neat, and beautiful vineyards of the world. And then he descended once again to Corteno.[9]

There is little information about Golgi's childhood. In the words of Ernesto Bertarelli:

I was unable to collect any memorable episode from his childhood and adolescence . . . An introverted personality, he was taciturn and contemplative, and nevertheless his letters reveal a gentle and good-natured side. Those who had known him, either personally in the intimacy of the family environment or through correspondence, concur in this impression of gentle shyness, although they cannot provide information to reconstruct his childhood and adolescence. In

Corteno, I have been told that Golgi loved to observe flowers in their smallest details, and there is no doubt that the developed visual acuteness of the future morphologist was responsible for this attention to shapes.[10]

Around the middle of the nineteenth century, the elementary schools of the part of Northern Italy under Austrian rule (Lombardy and Veneto) were subdivided into a mandatory lower elementary school (two years) and a higher elementary school, the latter for those pupils who would continue their studies. It is very likely that in 1848 the 5-year-old Golgi enrolled in the lower elementary school of Corteno to attend the mandatory two years. Although he could also have attended the first year of the higher elementary school in Corteno, he was sent to Pavia (where he probably lived with some relative) to enrol in the Bishopric school. On 21 August 1851 he was awarded a certificate of 'Excellence' for having distinguished himself 'in the study of the subject matters for the second semester 1851'.[11] It is almost certain that Golgi remained in Pavia for the second year as well, and it is probably there that he passed the exam for the admission to *liceo ginnasio* (grammar school).[12] Golgi attended the first year of *ginnasio* at the Convitto Municipale of Lovere, a school that dated back to the sixteenth century and where his brothers Luigi and Giuseppe also studied. In the school archives one can still find the records of Golgi's performance during the first four years of grammar school (1852–56). They reveal a dedicated student, accustomed to receiving good grades in almost all subjects. In the first semester of the school year 1854–55, for example, his record indicates: 'outstanding' moral conduct, 'intense and consistent' attention, 'serious and consistent' dedication, 'distinguished performance' in Religion, 'outstanding' in Latin, Greek, Italian, History and Geography, and Natural Sciences, 'thoroughly outstanding' in Mathematics, 'handsome' style in writing, no absence from class, and a final rank of 'first with high honours'. His grades were almost identical in all semesters for which there are records, except for German grammar, in which his performance was barely sufficient (first semester 1855–56).[13]

In 1856, Golgi enrolled in the Imperial Regio Ginnasio Liceale (Imperial Royal Grammar School) of Pavia,[14] another school dating back several centuries, where he would complete the remaining four years of grammar school.

In the meantime, Golgi's father, still a municipal doctor in Corteno, was seeking a position that would allow him to stay closer to his family, which had moved to Pavia. In March 1858, owing to the lack of suitable positions in Pavia, he applied for a position of associate physician in the Pie Case degli Incurabili of Abbiategrasso:

I have been a resident of the municipality of Corteno for the past twenty years . . . in my capacity of municipal doctor, and during this period of time I believe I have fulfilled my duties to the satisfaction of the inhabitants of my district as well as that in the surrounding areas. Nevertheless, having moved my family to Pavia to allow my children to attend school, I would like to fill one of the mentioned positions in order to be closer to my family and in a condition to supervise it more effectively. In consideration of this special circumstance, I ask that the prescribed age limit of forty be waived, so that I can participate in the competition even though I am four years over forty.[15]

Alessandro Golgi's application was accepted and in May 1858, he began service in Abbiategrasso.

The years during which Golgi attended elementary school and then grammar school were set in one of the most dramatic periods of Italian history, known as *il Risorgimento* (the Resurgence). In 1848 (the year Golgi enrolled in elementary school) the Italian peninsula was still Metternich's 'geographic expression', with nine independent states and two of its most developed regions, Lombardy (including Pavia) and Veneto, under Austria's rule. In that very year, *il Risorgimento* began with a revolutionary eruption that would spread to the rest of Europe, and that, while doomed to an abysmal failure in the short run, would generate a decade of political, diplomatic, and military convulsions culminating in the unification of Italy. By 1860 (the year Golgi enrolled in the University of Pavia Medical School), following the victorious war waged by Piedmont and France against Austria and the sensational conquest of Southern Italy by Garibaldi's 'Thousand' redshirts, Italy had become a united political entity.

As usual in periods of political turbulence, schools and universities were hotbeds of extreme intransigence and radicalism. Pavian students were no exception and at the end of the 1850s anti-Austrian feelings were running high. According to the accounts of many, the young Golgi, despite his otherwise calm disposition, was an ardent patriot, a trait that would accompany him for the rest of his life. In early December 1858, while a guest of Alessandro Manzoni in Milan, the Italian statesman Bettino Ricasoli wrote in a personal letter: 'Here there is an extreme discontent . . . In Pavia, fifteen students have been arrested and sent here in chains for the trial.' It was ruled, however, 'that there was no case against them and they were released'.[16] According to Luigi Magnaghi, a doctor who probably gathered direct testimony about the events, one of those students was Camillo Golgi, then 15.[17]

Some weeks after this episode, Golgi was involved, out of thoughtlessness rather than deliberately, in an incident that would upset his life as a student. On 4 January 1859, the phrase 'He who studies German is a traitor'[18] appeared on the outside wall and along the two internal staircases of the Imperial Regio Ginnasio Liceale. In that part of Italy, then under Austria's rule, the study of German language and literature was mandatory in grammar school (except for the first year). Golgi's teacher of German was 32-year-old Professor Giuseppe Maschka.[19] When he entered the class that morning at ten, he was probably still upset by the tenor of the graffito attacking his discipline. Maschka noticed immediately a menacing unrest among the students who shortly began to make a noise 'by shuffling their feet'.[20] One of them, Ulderico Doniselli, 'well known as a light-headed'[21] student, began to guffaw and was expelled by Maschka. Doniselli, however, supported by the other students, refused to leave declaring that 'laughing was not a crime'.[20] As soon as the teacher left the class in search of a school porter to whom he could entrust the unruly Doniselli, the uproar began again, even more intensely. Upon his return Maschka found Golgi, who sat beside Doniselli, laughing and 'clapping his hands'. Until that moment Golgi had been 'a model student . . . both in proficiency and conduct'[18] but despite this he was going to be severely punished to serve as an example to his schoolmates. Following a thorough inquiry personally directed by the school principal, Golgi and Doniselli were suspended from school. Doniselli lost the entire year, whereas Golgi was given permission to enrol in another school, the Liceo di Porta Nuova in Milan.[22]

The manifestations of hostility towards Austria continued to grow. In mid-January, eggs were thrown at the emblem of Imperial Austria[23] near the entrance to the school, and Maschka, who was considered a 'German' (although he was Hungarian), began to receive anonymous threatening letters. Particularly disquieting was a letter that he received on 21 January enjoining him not to enter the school and warning that 'many students of this school conspire against his life', and that some 'patriots . . . have sworn on the tip of their daggers . . . to kill him . . . no matter whether in the darkness or in full day light; this being a deed worthy of true Italians and not of assassins'.[24] Maschka notified the school principal and the police; he remained at home for a few days, but then resumed teaching.

For Camillo Golgi, the suspension was a hard blow. Being unable to transfer to Milan, he continued to study privately, hoping for a pardon that would allow him to return to school. On 22 February, Alessandro Golgi sent a first unsuccessful petition on behalf of his son who had committed a 'minor infraction out of thoughtlessness and not because of bad intentions'.[25] Shortly afterwards, he submitted a second petition writing 'I trust that the irreproachable previous conduct of the young man, his contrition . . . which can be confirmed by the very Professor Maschka, against whom he is supposed to have wronged, all should concur in granting him indulgence and forgiveness.'[25]

In April 1859 the process of Italian unification accelerated rapidly with the Austrian invasion of Piedmont. A secret pact between the Piedmontese and the French to provoke Austria into a war and make her look like a villain in the eyes of European public opinion had succeeded. In May of 1859, because of the unfolding military events, the University of Pavia was closed. The French–Piedmontese victories at Magenta and Solferino in early June brought Austria's rule in Lombardy to an end, and on 8 June Vittorio Emanuele II and Napoleon III entered Milan triumphantly. On that very day, the University and the schools of Pavia reopened under the new Piedmontese administration. The poor Maschka, fearing revenge and retribution, resigned his position and left with the retreating Austrian army.

In early August Alessandro Golgi's petition was reconsidered and finally, on 12 August, the pardon was granted.[26] At the eleventh hour, Camillo Golgi was allowed to sit for the entrance examination to the eighth and final year of grammar school. The following year, Alessandro Golgi managed to join his family by obtaining the position of municipal doctor in Cava Manara,[27] a village on the outskirts of Pavia. The Golgis took up residence in the residential area 'Bella Venezia'.[28] Among their new neighbours was Colonel Pizzocaro, who hosted musical gatherings, as was the fashion in those days, for the performance of excerpts from Donizetti's and Verdi's operas, arranged for small ensembles. These small private concerts were attended by Alessandro and Camillo Golgi, the latter being a competent flute-player.[29]

It is all but certain that Golgi entered the University of Pavia Medical School in 1860.[30] The freshman began his medical studies in earnest with the 'only goal of obtaining in due time . . . a medical degree'.[31] Very soon, however, Golgi's interest turned to more scholarly pursuits. It is impossible to understand how this transformation came about without a digression on the cultural environment of the University of Pavia Medical School.

Notes

1. In the parish records of San Michele, one can read (with great difficulty because of indistinct writing) that Alexander Antonius Nicolaus Golgi was baptized on 'Anno D.ni Mill.mo. octing.mo decimo quarto die sexta xbris' (6 December 1814). The civil status record kept in the parish register of Corteno gives 4 October 1814 as Alessandro Golgi's date of birth. The document is reproduced in Bianchi (1973, p. 12) and mentioned also by Goldaniga and Marchetti (1993, p. 12).

2. See the certificate signed by Carlo Cairoli, Professor and Director Emeritus at the Imperial Royal University of Pavia, and released to Alessandro Golgi on 24 December 1845 (MSUP-II-5). At the BUP is kept Alessandro Golgi's thesis (defended on February 1938) on typhoid fever, '*Nonnulla De Febri typhoidea. Dissertatio inauguralis quam annuentibus magnifico domino rectore perillustri facultatis medicae directore spectabili domino decano ac clarissimis d. d. professoribus auspice D. re Aloysio Scarenzio Pharmacologiae et Pathologiae P.O. ad Medicinae Lauream Rite Assequendam in C.R. Archigymnasio Ticinensis Mense Februarii 1838 una cum Thesibus propugnandis publicae disquisitioni submittit Alexander Golgi Ticinensis. Ticini Regii ex Typographia Bizzoni I.R. Universitatis Typograph. 1838*' (Coll. Diss. Med. Ticini T 47 N 19).

3. According to the parish register of Corteno, Golgi's mother was born on 13 December 1813. Additional information can be found in Rondoni (1943, p. 536).

4. Bonomelli (1975).

5. Bianchi (1973, p. 14).

6. Bertarelli (1950, pp. 5ff.).

7. Putelli (1913).

8. In the baptismal record of Santa Maria Assunta in Corteno, one reads 'Pisogneto-Corteno, 12 July 1843, No. 218. Bartolomeo Camillo Emilio, son of Alessandro Golgi and Carolina Golgi, his legitimate wife, was born on 7 July 1843, and baptized by myself, parish priest Stefano Mottinelli, at noon. Godfather was Mr Bartolomeo Zaina, pharmacist in Edolo.' This document is reproduced in Bianchi (1973, pp. 12 et seq.) and mentioned also in Goldaniga and Marchetti (1993, p. 11). According to Bianchi, Golgi was born at noon.

   It appears, therefore, that erroneous birth dates have been given by Sacerdotti (1926), who gave the date as 7 April 1843, Senise (1926), Putelli (1923), the *Gazzetta Medica Lombarda* (1902), pp. 431–40, *Il Popolo-La Provincia Pavese* of 24 January 1926, *Il cittadino di Brescia* of 22 January 1926, and on the commemorative memorial tablet on the house in which Golgi lived in Pavia on Corso Vittorio Emanuele at No. 77 (now Strada Nuova), which reports 9 July 1843. Even the *Encyclopaedia Britannica* continues the uncertainty of Golgi's birth date by giving 9 July 1843, though it mentions the fact that some sources give his birth date as 7 July 1844. The same source identifies Cortona instead of Corteno as the place of his birth. The probable origin of the 9 July 1943 date is a transcription error in one or more certificates (an example from 1877 is currently kept in the MSUP) released by the parish of Santa Maria Assunta di Corteno. Golgi himself, when obtaining his pension, complained about the inexactitude of his date of birth on various certificates in his possession (for the latter I am grateful to Dr Lino Stefanini, who found the reference in a letter from Golgi to his grandfather). The year of birth is reported as 1844 by a number of source, including Medea (1966), Legée (1982), Pagel (1901), *Enciclopedia Treccani* (Istituto dell'Enciclopedia Italiana Editore, 1949), *Biographisches Lexikon der hervorragenden Ärzte aller Zeiten und Völker* (Urban & Schwarzenberg, 1930), and *The Encyclopedia Americana* (Grolier Incorporated, 1988). *The New Encyclopaedia Britannica* (1990) gives the date as '1843 or 1844'.

9. Bertarelli (1950, pp. 3ff).

10. *Ibid.* (p. 9).

11. MSUP-I-I-2. The document is currently kept in the 'Golgiana' showcase of the MSUP. There is no information about attending the school of Corteno because no scholastic records of the epoch can be found.

12. According to Romolo Putelli (1923), Camillo Golgi attended school at Edolo, but no records have been found, either in the parish registry or in the Commune to attest to this attendance. Perhaps it was in this city that the future pathologist passed an admissions exam to the *ginnasio* (grammar school) (Goldaniga and Marchetti 1993, p. 14).

13. See also Goldaniga and Marchetti (1993, pp. 15ff.).

14. The records of the students for that epoch cannot be found in the archives of the school (now called Liceo Ugo Foscolo), but Golgi's attendance is attested to in a document of extension of the school tax for the second trimester of the school year 1856–57. Therefore the statements by Bonomelli (1975) and Fappani (1974–93, p. 14), who asserted that Golgi studied for some time in the Liceo Arnaldo di Brescia, are not supported by the available evidence. Furthermore, Golgi's name is not among the list of students in the school records of the Arnaldo at the time (for this information, I am grateful to Giacomo Goldaniga who checked the school records of the Arnaldo in the Archivio di Stato di Brescia).

15. From the request presented by Alessandro Golgi dated 7 March 1858 to the Director of the Pio Luogo degli Incurabili. Cited also by Riquier (1952, p. 57).

16. *Lettere e documenti del barone Bettino Ricasoli.* (Florence: Successori Le Monnier, 1887, Vol. 2, pp. 461–2.)

17. The testimony is signed on a piece of paper with the heading: 'Dott. Cav. Luigi Magnaghi' (MSUP-I-I-65, attached document).

18. From the report sent by Prof. Giuseppe Maschka to the director of the school on 7 January 1859 (ALFP).

19. The information is taken from the records of service of the professors (ALFP).

20. From the depositions of the students who were witness to the facts (ALFP).

21. The expression recurs in various documents kept at the ALFP, as for example in the report of Maschka of 7 January 1859 to the director of the school.

22. As seen in the copy of a document of 16 April 1859 in which are reported the disciplinary actions in the case of Golgi and Doniselli (ALFP).

23. From a communication of the director of the school to the *Delegazione Provinciale di Pavia*, 17 January 1859 (ALFP).

24. ALFP.

25. MSUP-II-4.

26. Documents concerning Golgi's readmission to school of 1, 7, and 17 August 1859 (ALFP).

27. Alessandro Golgi petitioned to obtain the position of municipal doctor on 14 October 1859 (MSUP-II-6).

28. The official civil status records (*stato di famiglia*) of the Golgi family (kept in the City Hall of Cava Manara) indicate that in January 1860 the family (which no longer included the two older brothers of Alessandro) moved from Abbiategrasso to Cava Manara, in the residential area Bella Venezia. During his training as a medical student at the University of Pavia Golgi lived in 'Corso Garibaldi No. 1480 in the house of the tenant Castagnola Vincenzo' (MSUP; documents not included in 'Veratti's catalogue'). From the municipal records of Pavia it appears that Camillo Golgi and his wife (whom he married in 1877) took up residence in this city in 1880 (even though he had probably already resided there for some years). His sister

Teresa continued to live in Cava Manara until 4 May 1876 and his parents Alessandro and Carolina until 11 November 1878.

29. The Pavian musician Prof. Angelo Rossi possesses two original scores of the romance of the opera *Elisir d'amore* and *Il furioso* of Donizetti 'rescored for two flutes by Golgi Camillo' as one reads on the frontispiece. The transcription preserves the virtuoso cadenzas originally sung by the tenor and soprano, indicating that Golgi must have been a good performer (at least according to the opinion of maestro Bruno Villani, Director of the Civico Istituto Musicale F. Vittadini of Pavia). See Santamaria (1994, pp. 40ff.). This contradicts the opinion referred to in the years just after the outbreak of the First World War, according to which Golgi had learned to play the flute 'not long ago' (Pensa 1991, p. 174).

30. According to Riquier (1952, p. 52), Golgi enrolled in the University at the end of 1859, but from the documents kept in the ALFP it appears that he was admitted to the examinations of the seventh year of grammar school in 1859; in the school year 1859–60 he must therefore have attended the remaining eighth year. I have not been able to verify the date of matriculation at the University because the records for that period are poorly organized, and thus almost unserviceable.

31. The phrase was spoken by Golgi during a speech that he gave on 29 June 1919 to the Fondazione Camillo Golgi-Pro Orfani di Medici (Camillo Golgi Foundation in favour of the orphans of physicians) on the occasion of his retirement celebrations. There is a typewritten copy in the BUP (coll. Misc. 4° T. 1473 n. 27), and another in the Library of the Institute of General Pathology of the University of Pavia. The speech is also reproduced in the album *Fondazione Camillo Golgi pro Orfani di Medici* (MSUP) and previously cited in Belloni (1975, p. 152) and in the collection of his reprints kept by the Società Medico-Chirurgica of Pavia ('Monti' collection No. 7135). It is reproduced *also* in Mazzarello (1993; see p. 334).

3

The University of Pavia Medical School before Golgi

Pavia lies on the river Ticino. In the middle of the nineteenth century, with its towers and medieval churches, it was a tranquil and misty city that could be comfortably and quickly traversed on foot. Pavia did not differ much from other Lombard cities except for the presence of the University, the city's topographic and cultural centre. This institution, whose remote origins can traced back to the year 825,[1] was a powerful cultural magnet for the Lombard bourgeoisie, who sent their sons to study there. The University of Pavia drew students also from other regions of the pre-unified Italy and even from Ticino Canton. They took paid lodgings in private residences, or in two historical institutions, Collegio Ghislieri and Collegio Borromeo, which had been founded in the sixteenth century and were reserved for intellectually endowed but indigent students, although these criteria were not always respected. Far from being simple boarding schools, these were institutions of high learning that hosted lectures, conferences, and a number of other scholarly activities integrated with the University.

The history of the University of Pavia is characterized by long periods of splendour alternating with periods of decadence, a process that mirrored the turbulent political history of Lombardy with its centuries of foreign domination. The University was renowned for the great physicists, mathematicians, writers, and jurists who had studied and taught here, such as Lorenzo Valla, Gerolamo Cardano, Gerolamo Saccheri, Ruggero Boscovich, Cesare Beccaria, Vincenzo Monti, Ugo Foscolo, and Alessandro Volta.[2] According to tradition, Christopher Columbus had also been a student in Pavia.

Above all, however, the glory of the University of Pavia rested on the achievements of its biologists and physicians. In the following overview we shall see how Golgi became heir to a long tradition of morphological and anatomo-pathological studies that stretches back to the early sixteenth century.

The birth of modern anatomy during the Renaissance is closely linked to the Universities of Northern Italy. During the second half of the fifteenth, and the beginning of the sixteenth centuries, the University of Pavia flourished under the munificent rule of the Viscontis and the Sforzas, and was famous throughout Europe. A substantial number of foreign students, particularly Germans, but also French, Spanish, Portuguese, Flemish, and English, attended the University. Indeed, at the end of the fifteenth century, foreign students numbered around 200 and represented a quarter of the total student body.

Around the turn of the fifteenth century Leonardo da Vinci repeatedly visited Pavia to devote himself to the study of 'human anatomy, being helped by and mutually helping' the Veronese anatomist Marcantonio Della Torre, an 'excellent philosopher, who was then lecturing in Pavia and wrote of this matter ... which up to that time had been wrapped in the darkest shadows of ignorance'.[3] The two men were among the first to break the prohibition, which had lasted from the days of ancient Rome, against dissecting bodies for purposes of research. The cadavers that in 1510–11 permitted Leonardo to make substantial progress in the knowledge of the human body, after centuries of dogmatic deference to Galen, came from the San Matteo Hospital of Pavia, which was opened in 1449 (although the act of foundation was granted in 1446).

In 1535 the Duchy of Milan passed into the hands of the Spaniards who ruled Lombardy until 1706, when they were routed by the Austrians. During the two centuries of Spanish domination, particularly in the seventeenth century, there was a progressive decline in the level of cultural and material life of the region. Industrious Milan suffered every kind of taxation and the blockage of exports. Over the span of few decades, the number of munitions factories and textile and mechanical shops declined drastically, as did the population of the metropolitan areas.

Yet during the sixteenth century the University of Pavia, particularly its Medical School, remained at a fair level and, also because of the prestige accumulated over the centuries, continued to attract famous teachers and a large number of students. In 1533, the Senate of Milan decided to build the central university hall near the San Matteo Hospital. The work began the following year and continued during the first period of direct Spanish domination.

Between 1536 and 1562, with some interruptions, the professorship of Medicine was held by Gerolamo Cardano. He was a singular figure, equally learned in medicine, mathematics and astrology (he once even made the horoscope of Christ), whose complex personality embodied the transition from medieval superstition to Renaissance humanism. In the 20 years between 1554 and 1574, anatomy was taught by Gabriele Cuneo, who also directed the construction of the first anatomical theatre in the University. Near the end of the 1500s this discipline was entrusted to a pupil of Fallopius, Giovanni Battista Carcano Leone, who was the first to describe the *foramem ovale* and the *ductus arteriosus* in the fetal heart. Among Leone's students was probably Gaspare Aselli, the discoverer of the lymphatic system, who also taught for a brief period at the University of Pavia.

With the seventeenth century began the decadence of the University, a decay that continued into the first 60 years of Austrian domination. In the second half of the sixteenth century there had been more than 500 students; at the beginning of the eighteenth century there were barely 150. Intellectual stagnation and even regression pervaded all branches of learning. The teaching of philosophy was a compendium of Greek philosophy up to Aristotle; medical students had little notion of the progress made since the Middle Ages because all they were taught was Avicenna's medicine; surgery consisted of purely theoretical lectures.

In parallel with the progressive decline of the University, there developed alternative cultural institutions that, within certain limits, kept the circulation of knowledge alive in Pavia. They were organized around religious orders and professional colleges (Physicians, Theologians, and Jurisconsultants), and in the *Accademie*. The latter were elite institutions, membership of which conferred prestige and social status, so they attracted not only academics and students but also local notables. The most famous, the Accademia degli Affidati (Academy of the Entrusted Ones), was founded in 1562 and had its headquarters in the palace of the Belcredi family. Other important *Accademie* were that of the Chiave d'Oro (Gold Key), hosted by the Malaspina family, that of the Indefessi (Indefatigable Ones), hosted by the Collegio Ghislieri, and that of the Accurati (Accurate Ones), hosted by the Collegio Borromeo.

In the second half of the eighteenth century, the University of Pavia entered a new golden age thanks to the reforms promoted by Empress Maria Theresa of Austria, who, with the 'General Regulation of the Faculty of Medicine', made sure that the University of Pavia would be allocated funds and incomes, 'knowing how important it is to promote the application of science, and convinced that insofar as progress is made in a State, there is a comparable increase in public happiness of its citizens'.[4] These reforms were part of a more general renewal of university institutions throughout most of Europe, a renewal that was made necessary by the need for a new class of efficient and loyal civil servants who could serve the increasingly centralized and bureaucratic State.[5] In the territories subject to the Hapsburgs, reforms were first carried out in Vienna and then extended to the other universities of the Empire. The reforms initiated by Maria Theresa were vigorously continued by her son Joseph II, encouraged in this by his personal surgeon and counsellor Giovanni Alessandro Brambilla, who had done his residency training at the San Matteo Hospital in Pavia.[6] The unique prestige enjoyed by the University of Pavia in the Italian medical establishment throughout the nineteenth century dates back to this period, about which Giovanni Battista Grassi would write:

if then we return a moment to thinking of the glorious University of Pavia, which can be considered the brain of Italian biology during the nineteenth century, in order to trace the origin of the heat that caused so many fruits to mature, that is in order to identify the *genius loci*, it seems to me that one must invoke first of all and especially the exceedingly high esteem in which the professors of the Lombard School were held.[7]

Anatomical studies were given new impetus by Pietro Moscati, Professor of Anatomy, Surgery and Obstetrics from 1763 to 1772, and by Giacomo Rezia, founder of the Anatomical Museum. In the anatomical theatre constructed by Cuneo, Moscati delivered his magisterial lecture 'On the essential corporal differences between animals and humans', in which he introduced evolutionary themes, arguing that humans were originally quadrupeds, and discussed the possible causal relationship between erect posture and the shape of the skull and brain. The text of this lecture was published in 1770, and was reviewed by Immanuel Kant, thus attracting widespread attention in Europe. [8]

The renaissance of the University of Pavia was dominated, however, by the towering figures of Lazzaro Spallanzani and Antonio Scarpa. Abbot Spallanzani, whom Voltaire had called 'the best observer in Europe', and of whom Charles Bonnet said that he had discovered in a few years 'more truths than all Academies combined in half a century',[9] came to the University of Pavia from the University of Modena in 1769 to take over the professorship of Natural History. Spallanzani was already internationally renowned for his formidable attacks on the theory of spontaneous generation and his recruitment was part of the plan to halt the decline of the only university in Austria-ruled Lombardy.

The scope of Spallanzani's work in Pavia is astonishing. Described by his brother Niccolò as a man of 'great stamina',[10] he conducted an impressive series of major studies in a wide variety of different areas of experimental biology. During his first years in Pavia, he continued his microscopic investigation of the 'little animals of the infusions', obtaining results that further undermined the theory of spontaneous generation. In the following years he made important discoveries on the regeneration of tissues, the processes of respiration and digestion, the blind flight of the bat, and artificial insemination. By the 1780s Spallanzani was the most celebrated contemporary European physiologist and there was no honour or distinction that he had not received. In 1768 he was nominated Corresponding Member of the Royal Society of London and in 1767 he was appointed Member of the Academy of Berlin by Frederick the Great, and received a special gold medal from Joseph II.

Spallanzani, however, was an introverted, crusty, and solitary character, and he managed to acquire a number of powerful enemies at the University while leaving no disciples. Much more influential was Scarpa, who created a school of his own and left a permanent mark on the subsequent evolution of morphological studies in Pavia. A disciple of Giovan Battista Morgagni, he had joined the University of Pavia through the good offices of Brambilla, whom he had befriended in Paris. Appointed Professor of Human Anatomy in 1783, Scarpa subsequently held also the professorship of Clinical Surgery.

Scarpa was the greatest Italian anatomist of the period and enjoyed great prestige and international fame for a number of remarkable anatomical discoveries and precise morphological descriptions, including the membranous labyrinth (in which he identified the semicircular canals, the utricle, the saccule and the endolymph), the vestibular ganglion, the nerves of the heart, the olfactory nerve, and the nasopalatine nerve. For the discovery of the innervation of the heart, which he announced in 1794, he received a prize of four thousand gold sequins from the Emperor of Austria. Scarpa also excelled in ophthalmology and in surgery, despite Spallanzani's scathing remarks about his surgical skills.[11] He wrote an extensive treatise on the diseases of the eye, which was later translated into English, French, German, and Dutch. He also studied hernias, congenital deformities of the foot, and aneurysms.

Here is how Achille Monti described Scarpa, reporting memories of his grandparents who had been students in Pavia from 1825 to 1836:

That old man with stern expression and magnetic gaze, who was intimate with no one, who conversed and taught in Latin with great elegance and yet with great imperiousness, who operated at an amazing speed, insensitive to the screams of the patients, was inscrutable as a sphinx, cold as death, and inexorable as Fate. Indeed, he was feared as a mythical figure, as an ancient god, revengeful and cruel.[12]

... the high opinion he had of himself was not inferior to his merits ... endowed with unshakeable will-power, he never allowed his feelings to take over; he knew how to read other people's thoughts and how to subjugate them with his multifaceted and magnetic personality.[13]

Throughout his academic career, Scarpa enjoyed great personal power, owing to his connections with the Austrian Government and to his political opportunism, of which he gave a masterly demonstration during the various political storms that accompanied the Napoleonic adventures in Northern Italy. Indeed, the pre-eminence attained by Scarpa under the Austrians was maintained under the French.

Feeling immune from attacks ... he refused to make an oath of allegiance to the Cisalpine Republic, although he retained, with the approval of the new authorities, his professorship and his role of *éminence grise* behind the scenes. This allowed him to acquire some merits in the eyes of the Austrian court when, in 1799, the Austrian and Russian armies routed the French and closed the University, dismissing or suspending all professors. Indeed, only Scarpa was immediately re-instated, whereas the others, including Volta, had to wait for the victorious return of Bonaparte.[14]

In 1805 Napoleon Bonaparte, visiting the University of Pavia, received the homage of the academic body and, not seeing Scarpa among the professors, demanded to know where he was. He was told that Scarpa had resigned from his position because he had refused to make an oath of allegiance to the new Government. To which the Napoleon allegedly replied: 'oaths and political opinions do not matter ... Dr Scarpa honours the University and my State!' And when Scarpa was finally introduced, Napoleon said to him: 'whatever are your sentiments, I respect them, but I cannot tolerate that you remain separate from an Institute of which you are the ornament. A man like you must, in the guise of a brave soldier, die on the battlefield.'[15] In the same year Scarpa was called back to the professorship of Clinical Surgery and Surgical Operations.

Scarpa's power was put to a good use. Not only did he manage to further the interests of his discipline, by having a new anatomical amphitheatre and a new laboratory built, but with his tireless activism he benefited his colleagues and the entire University.

The University of Pavia owed the prosperity it had then attained to Scarpa. Not only did he exert his influence on the Government and administrators to enlarge and strengthen the University, he also ensured the constant flow of human and material means to make this institution vibrant and productive. To this end, the professors received high salaries, so that they could focus on their research without distractions. Furthermore, they received free lodging, conspicuous funding, and frequent economical incentives.[16]

Scarpa had an important internationalizing influence at the University of Pavia. Financed by his protectors and admirers, such as the Duke of Modena, the Governor of Milan, and the Emperor of Austria, he travelled widely throughout Europe, sometimes in the company of Alessandro Volta, and established contacts with the foremost scientists of his age. In Paris he befriended Feliz Vicq d'Azyr, who offered him the opportunity to study the morphology of the olfactory organ and then to report his results to the Société Royal de Médecine, of which the French scientist was the Permanent Secretary. In London in 1781 he met the brothers William and John Hunter, assisted in Percivall Pott's surgical operations, and learned from William Cruikshank the technique of the injection of mercury, which he later applied to the study of the lymphatic vessels and which was extensively used by his pupil Bartolomeo Panizza. Enriched by the experiences accumulated abroad, Scarpa radically revamped the medical curriculum of the Medical School in Pavia.

Scarpa was the first teacher of consequence who, abandoning the ancient tradition of reading lectures *ex cathedra*, inaugurated experimental teaching by conducting post-mortem examinations before the students in the anatomical amphitheatre and minor surgical operations in the clinical amphitheatre, also before the students. This important innovation, however, was not enough for Scarpa. He also required the students to attend autopsies and clinical examinations in the hospital wards, and to train, taking advantage of the wealth of equipment put at their disposal, in anatomical technique, in surgical medicine, and in the art of surgery under his supervision, so as to acquire first-hand experience, instead of vague theoretical notions. That is, it was Scarpa who made the internship an important feature of medical training, an innovation that represents one of the glories of the University of Pavia.[17]

As interns in a scientific institute, medical students were able to prepare experimental doctoral dissertations and to publish their first scientific papers. In the following decades, this system became the most efficient apprenticeship for research, especially in Golgi's laboratory, where the students were often able to complete important investigations even before graduation.

Scarpa exercised an enormous influence on the growth of anatomical studies at the University of Pavia. He supervised an extensive collection of anatomical specimens in the Museums of Normal Human Anatomy and of Comparative Anatomy, and in the Pathological Collection ('Cabinet'). The feverish collection of anatomical specimens spared no cadaver; anatomical pieces were taken also from the bodies of individuals well known in the City and placed in the Anatomical Museum with the person's full name in view. Only after 1820 were the names removed from the anatomical specimens and, in some instances, from the catalogue of the exhibits. The physicians of the areas around Pavia sent all the pathological specimens that they could collect to the Pathological Cabinet, together with the clinical history and a report on the circumstances of the death, for the benefit of medical students' training. Scarpa's body was no exception. At his death, on 30 October 1832, his remains were distributed to the various anatomical institutions that were 'the apples of his eyes'.[18] Organs with abnormalities were given to the Pathological Cabinet while his head was placed in the Museum of Human Anatomy.[19] Scarpa's head (currently at the Historical Museum of the University of Pavia) attracted the curiosity of numerous visitors, including Joseph Lister, as one can read in his autobiographical notes. In the following decades, Scarpa's cult of the 'beautiful anatomical piece' transmuted, with the introduction of histological techniques, into the cult of the 'beautiful histological piece'.

Despite all his greatness Scarpa was more feared than loved when alive and it is not surprising that he was irreverently jeered after his death. Monti wrote:

But . . . he who does not leave a heritage of love—will not rejoice in the urn: the eulogies contained in the Latin epigraphs, composed by the learned librarian Lanfranchi, did not meet popular approval. Indeed, according to the tradition, a very different kind of epigraph encountered the favour of the common people, an epigraph that, by word of mouth, appeared the day after the funeral at the base of the statue of the Muto dall'accia al collo, which in Pavia at the time served the same function as the statue of Pasquino in Rome, or the *Vomo di Pietra* in Milan.[20]

'Scarpa is dead
I don't give a damn
He lived like a hog,
And died like a dog.'[19]

At the end of the eighteenth century, the University of Pavia Medical School consisted of only five professorships. Students, prior to their doctoral dissertation, had to take comprehensive exams for the various individual courses and the list of all the grades was sent to the Aulic Dicastery in Vienna for record-keeping. Further evidence of the centralized nature of the Austrian administrative apparatus was the procedure for the appointment of professors, who, in addition to the evaluation of their scientific qualifications, had to submit to written and oral examinations, both in Vienna and in the university in which they were candidate. The number of professorships increased to twelve under the French and this number remained stable during the post-Napoleonic restoration of Austrian rule, by means of a series of provisions of 1817, completed in 1825.[21]

The biomedical environment of Pavia during the first half of the eighteenth century was enriched also by influential personalities who operated outside the University. One of the most important of them was Mauro Rusconi.[22] After graduating in Medicine at Pavia in 1806, he worked for several years in Cuvier's laboratory in Paris, at that time a world-renowned centre of anatomical studies. Rusconi, although unsuccessful at obtaining a professorship at the University of Pavia, privately carried out important studies in comparative and embryological anatomy. Among other things, he demonstrated the circulation of blood in the gills of amphibian tadpoles, described the first stages of development in the frog, and discovered the process of reproduction by scission of normal cells. For his research he was awarded the Gold Medal of the Royal Academy of Science of Paris.

Another scientist closely associated with Pavia, although never part of the teaching body of the University, was Agostino Bassi, from Lodi. He had graduated from the University of Pavia Law School, but he attended the lectures of charismatic personalities such as Spallanzani and Scarpa, and his scholarly interests were mainly in biology. Contrary to the prevailing opinion, he demonstrated that the disease ('calcino') of the silkworm was due to a micro-organism. He extended this notion to other contagious diseases, elaborating the theory according to which

all infections, of whatever type, with no exceptions, are products of parasitic beings; that is, by living organisms that enter in other living organisms, in which they find nourishment, that is food that suits them, here they hatch, grow and reproduce themselves.[23]

Thus, Bassi can rightly be considered one of the founders of the study of infectious diseases.[24]

On Scarpa's death, the professorship of Human Anatomy passed to his pupil, Bartolomeo Panizza, who held it from 1815 to 1864.[25] Panizza was among the first to support the spread of microscopic studies in Italy, studies that had already received a great impulse in Germany, France, and England following the invention of the achromatic microscope in 1820 and other technical improvements in optics. He became famous for his research on the anatomy and functions of cranial nerves (in particular the facial, glossopharyngeal, and hypoglossal nerves) and for his confirmation of the Bell–Magendie law on the existence of two major categories of nerves: sensory (in the dorsal roots of the spinal cord) and motor (in the ventral roots). Panizza was also a forerunner of the doctrine of cerebral localization.[26] By carrying out experiments on the effects of the selective destruction of various brain areas and enucleating the eye in order to follow the atrophy of the optic pathways, he was able to localize the visual cortex in the occipital lobes. This discovery anticipated by 6 years the revolutionary studies of Paul Broca on the frontal cortical speech centre and by 15 years those of Theodor Fritsch and Edward Hitzig on the role of the cortex in motor activity. The experimental degeneration (descending degeneration) used by Panizza was rediscovered in 1870 by Bernhard Aloys von Gudden, who systematically applied it to the study of the central nervous system.

Also of great importance were the discoveries on the lymphatic system made by Panizza using injections of mercury, at which he became so adept that after his death it was written that 'To teach Panizza the art of injection was like teaching an eagle the art of flying.'[27] Finally, in his later years, Panizza made interesting observations on the structure of the ovary using a sophisticated and expensive microscope given to him by his friend and colleague the astronomer and histologist Giovanni Battista Amici, a master maker of optical instruments and the inventor of oil-immersion lenses.

Panizza was a modest man who 'didn't want to have anything to do with dedications or portraits, calling them *vanities* and *nonsense*'[28] and who was instead completely dedicated to his research, which he conducted using rigorous experimental methods. To his disciples, who were numerous and important, he recommended 'to guard themselves against *high-falutin' ideas* and theories, and to be sceptical even towards the so-called *facts*.'[29]

His lectures, also attended by Golgi, were described in the following way:

They were not crafted in elegant prose, nor splendid in terms of style, nor models of organization. They were quite removed from the measured eloquence and grandiloquence of Scarpa. Some-times the tone would became casual and sprinkled with vernacular expressions; it was almost kitchen table science. Still, Panizza's lectures were attended by men of every age and class, and among them one could find almost in equal numbers the students of law and of mathematics and those of medicine, and every year the lectures lured some undecided students into medical studies; and though nothing is more arid, cold and sad than the description of bones, muscles, and viscera, these lectures were usually crowned by enthusiastic applause. I will tell you the secret of such a miraculous success.

First of all, Panizza was convinced that anatomy is the basis of medicine and especially of surgery, and he knew how to infuse that persuasion in his audience. 'Listen well', he cried, 'a surgical operation is no more than an anatomical preparation on a living being, or the application of anatomical knowledge. The greatest physicians and surgeons were also great anatomists. Physiology and pathology are reducible to anatomy plus some hypotheses.' These were the refrains with which he was accustomed to hold the attention of even the most sluggish and sleepy students.

In the second place, Panizza always taught from memory, standing, often pacing restlessly before the class; his voice, high and vibrant, resonated to the back of the hall; his manners were dramatic, the methods straightforward, often novel and bizarre, always most effective. His whole body spoke: the face, the gaze, the gesture, the pose. Everything served him as a way to compare and demonstrate and illustrate: the academic gown, the hall, the table, the seat, the handkerchief, the paper. Next, he never asserted anything that he could not persuade himself of and of which he could not immediately provide the material proof, either on a fresh cadaver or on specimens skilfully prepared by himself or under his supervision. For this reason people thronged to his classroom as if they were going to a theatre, and time passed without their realizing it, and that which was learned was never forgotten; and thus one can say that a person who leaves cold from the lessons of Panizza can give up the study of anatomy and medicine.[30]

Panizza was outspoken and coarse 'like an old soldier' and 'He didn't make much use of smiles and compliments. It seemed instead that he was ashamed of appearing good-natured ... and studiously hid all his emotions.'[31] His students reciprocated with the appellation 'gruffy benefactor'. After his return from the disastrous Napoleonic campaign in Russia, in which he participated as 'Assistant Surgeon Major in the ambulance service of the Italian Royal Guard',[32] the 'wrecked survivors of the Russian expedition would remain the source of particular sympathy for him, and it is known that some of them abused this.'[33] He treated his assistants like 'many very dear sons'[34] and tried to help them even after they had left the University.[35]

The two most promising pupils of Panizza were Eusebio Oehl, who would later become Professor of Physiology at the University of Pavia, and Marquis Alfonso Corti, who went on to make important discoveries on the structure of the retina and the internal ear, as indicated by the anatomical structures that still bear his name.

Another important figure at the University of Pavia during the first half of the nineteenth century was Luigi Porta, who can be considered a forerunner of modern vascular surgery. A native of Pavia, Porta held the professorship of Surgery from 1832 to his death in 1875, and his 'Operative' clinic was attended also by Golgi. Beside being a celebrated surgeon Porta was also a great pathologist who had a lasting influence on Pavian pathological studies. He established the Anatomical–Surgical Museum of Pavia and made important contribution to the study of the thyroid gland and of sebaceous tumours.

Despite the presence of Panizza and Porta, medical research at the University of Pavia entered a phase of stagnation around the middle of the nineteenth century, partly as a consequence of the anti-Napoleonic restoration of the preceding decades. Experimental research was seldom performed and theoretical orientations inspired by metaphysical preconceptions, particularly of a vitalistic kind, ran riot.

In the University of Pavia—although there remained an echo of the teaching of Lazzaro Spallanzani, the father of experimental biology, and of the genial intuitions and demonstrations of Agostino Bassi, the ... founder of microbiological theory; and although a scholar of the level of Bartolomeo Panizza held a professorship there—the scientific institutes languished in the most deplorable neglect and the activity of the few who tried to bring medicine back to the traditions of experimental biology encountered the most tenacious resistance.[36]

Disinclined to embrace the principles of focal pathology propounded by Morgagni and then by Scarpa, and which were still followed by Panizza, many in the Pavian medical community became disciples of doctrinal systems that interpreted the multiform clinical expressions of diseases on the basis of a few elementary a priori rules. Given these premises, it was thought completely useless to investigate deeply the causes, pathogenesis, and treatment of individual illnesses, as advocated by Morgagni in his *De sedibus et causis morborum*

of psychiatry and forensic medicine of *fin de siècle* Italy. At the end of 1855, Lombroso enrolled at the University of Vienna Medical School, where he remained for two semesters, attending, among others, courses in pathological anatomy with Rokitansky and clinical medicine with Skoda. Lombroso's eclecticism can be seen in the diversity of his interests. After graduating from the University of Pavia in 1858, with a doctoral dissertation on 'Cretinism in Lombardy', he pursued scholarly studies in psychiatry, hygiene, anthropology, criminology, and forensic medicine.[54] He began his teaching career at the University of Pavia in 1863 with a *corso libero* (that is, an ancillary course for which he received no pay) in Psychiatry and Anthropology. In 1864 he was appointed Adjunct Professor and in 1867 *Professore Straordinario* (that is, non-tenured professor). From 1871 to 1873, Lombroso directed the insane asylum of Pesaro, and after another brief appointment at the University of Pavia he moved as Professor of Forensic Medicine to the University of Turin. In 1865 he published *La medicina legale delle alienazioni mentali studiata con il metodo sperimentale* (Forensic medicine of mental disorders investigated with an experimental methodology), in which he dealt with many of the issues of mental disease that would be taken up again and discussed thoroughly in his later works, *L'uomo delinquente* (The criminal man) (1876) and *Genio e follia* (Genius and madness) (1872). By the end of the century, Lombroso had became a charismatic figure whose influence reached well beyond purely scientific environments. His name was synonymous with the triad madness–genius–criminality, and was mentioned even in literary works, such as Tolstoy's *Resurrection*. In the next chapter we shall see how Lombroso played an important role in Golgi's early scientific career.

Although after Panizza's retirement the Chair of Anatomy passed to Giovanni Zoja, who was interested mainly in macroscopic anatomy, the true heir to Panizza's legacy in morphological studies in Pavia was Eusebio Oehl, who was appointed Professor of Physiology.[55] Oehl was one of the chief Italian anatomists of the nineteenth century and his methodological approach exerted a great influence on the students who trained with him.[56] A steadfast advocate of the experimental method, Oehl was extremely up to date with the new trends in medicine, owing to his post-doctoral specialization studies with Brücke and Hyrtl in Vienna. Even before his appointment to the professorship of Physiology he had a considerable teaching experience. In 1854–56 he taught histology at the Collegio Ghislieri, basing his lectures on his own Italian translation of Kölliker's celebrated *Handbuch*[57] and introducing the students to the 'most precise microscopic techniques', in the words of the Rector of the Collegio.[58] In the academic year 1859–60 he offered a *corso libero* of microscopic and histological anatomy at the University of Pavia. In 1857 he published his important studies on the structure of the skin in the *Annali universali di medicina* which would be translated into German 32 years later by the Hamburg dermatologist Paul Gerson Unna. Oehl introduced two exceptional students to microscopic research: Giulio Bizzozero, about whom we have already heard, and Enrico Sertoli, who carried out important histological research on the structure of the testes, identifying the elongated cells of the seminiferous tubules now called Sertoli's cells.

The resurgence of the University of Pavia was not limited to the arrival of young academics trained in Northern Europe. An important role was also played by Salvatore Tommasi who, despite being from an older generation (he was born in 1813) and having embraced an idealistic philosophical conception of Hegelian mould at the beginning of his career, became an advocate of the new naturalistic and experimental approach. In his treatise of physiology 'avidly sought-after by young scholars',[59] he made an attempt to integrate the physiological–experimental approach of Johannes Müller, the leading exponent of the new German medicine, and the histological approach of Kölliker.[60] A native of Naples, Tommasi was Professor of Applied Medicine (today's 'Medical Pathology') at the University of Naples until he was dismissed and then imprisoned because of his participation in the revolution of 1848. Released from prison and exiled, he went to Paris and London and subsequently settled in Turin where he practised as a physician and lectured in physiology. After the liberation of Lombardy from the Austrians, he was finally appointed Professor of Clinical Medicine and Medical Pathology at the University of Pavia. 'On the eve of national unity, after the annexation of Lombardy by the Kingdom of Sardinia, he began to propound from his Chair of Clinical Medicine at the University of Pavia his ideas for a New Medicine to the young physicians of the new Italy.'[61]

This brief historical overview illustrates how the years in which Golgi began his university studies spanned a period of sweeping changes in medicine and biology.[62] When the experimental and naturalistic approach of the German and Austrian schools collided with more traditional Pavian school, it found fertile soil in the rigorous morphological tradition that had originated with Scarpa and was continued by Panizza. The Pavian school, strictly grounded in experimental data, considered the interpretative moment as a simple corollary, logical and automatic, of the objective findings, and rejected a priori every hypothesis that was not 'totally' supported by 'facts'. Panizza taught his pupils over and over again that 'physiology and pathology are simply anatomy plus some hypotheses' and that 'the thorough and detailed observation of facts is the pillar of science'.

The *disciplinary tradition*[63] of the Pavian school of microscopic anatomy[64] originated with Scarpa and his veneration of the 'beautiful anatomical piece', continued with Panizza and his disciples, and finally percolated into microscopic anatomy. It was an inductive tradition, as opposed to the axiomatic–deductive approaches prevailing in the 1700s, which derived the interpretation of particular facts from a few a priori concepts. Golgi came in contact with this tradition through the teachings of Panizza and Oehl, and especially from Oehl's pupil, Giulio Bizzozero, as we shall see in the next chapter.

Notes

1. The University of Pavia dates back to an act of foundation by Emperor Charles IV who in 1361 designated it as a *generale Studium utrisque juris, videlicet tam canonici quam civilis, nec non philosophie, medicine et artium liberalium* (see Vaccari, 1957, pp. 19–20). There it is prescribed that students, rectors, doctors, and functionaries can be admitted to the same privileges and immunities enjoyed by the students of Paris, Bologna, Oxford, Orléans, and Montpellier, and to them would be extended the protection of the Holy Roman Empire. But an embryo of the future University was established as early as 825 by Emperor Lotario, who with the *Capitulare olonnense ecclesiasticum primum* restructured the higher education of the Kingdom of Italy and established at Pavia a School of Rhetoric and Law that would play an important

role during the High Middle Ages. According to the edict of Lotario, the School of Rhetoric and Law drew students from the vast regions of Liguria, Lombardy, and Piedmont, and thus from the cities of Milan, Brescia, Lodi, Bergamo, Novara, Vercelli, Tortona, Acqui, Genoa, Asti, and Como. The Pavian juridical tradition continued in the successive centuries, and was connected to the philosopher and theologian Lanfranco da Pavia who became prior of the monastery of Le Bec in Normandy in 1045 and Archbishop of Canterbury in 1070 at the request of William the Conqueror.

2. See Corradi (1877–78), Fraccaro (1950), Erba (1976), Gigli Berzolari (1993), Mariani (1900), Spadoni (1925), Vaccari (1957). See also *Pavia e i suoi Istituti Universitari* (Pavia: Tipografia Fratelli Fusi, 1887); *L'Università di Pavia e i suoi istituti* (Pavia: Tipografia Successori Bizzoni, 1925); *Contributi alla storia della Università di Pavia* (Pavia: Tipografia Cooperativa, 1925); and *Discipline e Maestri dell'Ateneo Pavese* (Verona: Arnoldo Mondadori Editore, 1961). Important biographical references on the history of the University of Pavia can be found in Volta (1900).

3. Vasari (1568, pp. 34ff.)

4. Cited in Locatelli (1961, p. 454); the source is Corradi (1877–78).

5. Guderzo (1982, pp. 851ff.).

6. On the figure of Brambilla see Zanobio *et al.* (1980).

7. Grassi (1911, p. 397).

8. Belloni (1961); Lovejoy (1959).

9. Rostand (1951).

10. Castellani (1990, p. 235).

11. *Ibid.* (p. 237). In a letter to Samuel August Tissot, Spallanzani wrote the following of Scarpa: 'After he [Scarpa] arrived in Pavia he made five surgical operations in the hospital, and all five of the people put to the test by him entered happily to the glory of Paradise. If he keeps on like this and if they are chosen souls, with his operations there will be more and more saints in Heaven.'

12. Monti (1927, p. 9).

13. *Ibid.* (p. 41).

14. *Ibid.* (pp. 42ff.).

15. Cited in Grassi (1911, p. 397).

16. Monti (1927, p. 60).

17. *Ibid.* (p. 61).

18. Cited in Monti (1926, p. 11).

19. Monti (1927, p. 54; 1957, p. 104).

20. The 'Mute with wire on his neck' is an ancient statue (which was probably part of a funerary memorial) that at one time was located at the East Gate of Pavia and can now be found in the Civic Museum (Section of Archaeology, Hall IV). The name derives from the physical deterioration of the mouth (hence *Muto*) and from the fact that the toga worn by the statue creates a series of folds around the neck (*collo*) that give the appearance of a skein of coarse wire (*accia*). Like the statue called Pasquino in Rome and the *Man of Stone* in Milan, the *Muto dall'accia al collo* was used by the people as a posting board for anonymous political or personal satire.

21. Locatelli (1961, p. 451); Vaccari (1957, p. 246).

22. On the figure of Rusconi, see Vialli (1961).

23. Cited in Pensa (1961, p. 262).

24. Castiglioni (1948, p. 598).

25. On the figure of Panizza see Pensa (1961) and Verga (1869).

26. Panizza (1855); see also Mazzarello and Della Sala (1993), and Finger (1994, pp. 85–6).

27. Verga (1869, p. 49).

28. *Ibid.* (p. 75).

29. *Ibid.* (p. 72).

30. *Ibid.* (pp. 16ff.).

31. *Ibid.* (p. 77).

32. *Ibid.* (p. 8).

33. *Ibid.* (p. 81).

34. *Ibid.* (p. 76).

35. According to Raggi (1898, pp. 77ff.) one of his assistants, Andrea Verga, while taking care of 'a friend who was a victim of a contagious illness, accidentally contaminated one of his eyes. With immediate treatment and rest he would have been immediately healed, but this was a time of a cholera epidemic . . . and he put the needs of others before his own . . . where it appeared to him that his presence was needed, and by neglecting his own health he ended by losing his eye.' Distressed and fearing that he would no longer be able to assist Panizza, he decided to resign his post and 'get a position as a rural physician'. But Panizza intervened and persuaded Verga to reconsider his decision. 'With only one eye (so he said to him), he would be able to see better and more than many others who make use of both eyes.'

36. Riquier (1952, pp. 51ff.).

37. Cosmacini (1988, p. 258).

38. Guthrie (1958).

39. Golgi (1884, pp. 15ff.).

40. On the figure of Rasori see Bonuzzi (1990); Cosmacini (1982; 1988).

41. Monti (1927); see also Scarpa's correspondence (1938, p. 209).

42. Verga (1869, p. 88).

43. Cited in Grassi (1911, pp. 57ff.).

44. Cited in Gravela (1989, p. 19).

45. Cited in Locatelli (1961, p. 455).

46. Shryock (1936).

47. Pensa (1991, p. 105).

48. *Ibid.* (p. 106).

49. Cited in Locatelli (1961, p. 462).

50. Mantegazza (1859).

51. Cited in Gravela (1989, p. 16).

52. Dianzani (1989).

53. In the yearbook of the University of Pavia for the academic year 1863–64 one finds: 'Lombroso Cesare da Verona, *Libero Docente* of Anthropology and Clinic of Mental Illnesses'. In the year 1864–65 Lombroso became Adjunct Professor of the Clinic of Mental Illnesses and of Anthropology. He would then become a *Professore Straordinario*.

54. On the figure of Lombroso, see Baima Bollone (1992) and Bulferetti (1975).

55. The yearbook of the University of Pavia for the academic year 1859–60 indicates that the Professor of Physiology was the Pavian Angelo Vittadini; Oehl is listed as *Libero Docente* (that is, a non-paid instructor) of Microscopic Anatomy and Histology. In the academic year 1860–61, Oehl (Knight of the Legion of Honour of France) became a *Professore Straordinario*, assistant of Vittadini, and *Libero Docente* of Microscopic Anatomy and Histology. In this academic year, the Laboratory of Experimental Physiology, directed by Vittadini, appears for the first time in the University yearbook. In the year 1863–64 Vittadini became Professor

Emeritus; in the years 1864–65 Oehl is listed as Professor of Physiology. Therefore, it is not entirely correct to attribute to Oehl the foundation of the Institute of Physiology, even though he certainly became its leading exponent.

56. On the figure of Oehl see Golgi (1903) and Grassi (1911, pp. 58ff.).

57. Kölliker (1856).

58. Grassi (1911, p. 59).

59. Foà (1901, p. 376).

60. Gravela (1989, p. 15).

61. Cosmacini (1988, p. 325).

62. Here is how, in 1919, Golgi remembered the university situation in his first years of university study: 'At the end of the eighteenth century, in a period in which, thanks to the names of Malpighi (the founder of microscopic anatomy), Morgagni (the true creator of scientific medicine grounded in pathological anatomy), Spallanzani (who, working with the methods of chemistry and physics, founded experimental biology), Fontana (author of fundamental discoveries on the structure and function of nerves), Galvani (who triumphantly inaugurated electrobiology), Volta (who changed physics), and of many other eminent scientists, the scientific–biological movement in Italy was not inferior to that in other countries and the Italians could withstand comparison with the foreigners, proudly and with head held high. Actually I would rather maintain that the Italians could boast of a supremacy. But unfortunately, for circumstances that cannot be analysed here, around the middle of the last century the conditions of the Italian universities—this assertion is not mine—were in total decline. The University of Pavia was not an exception! In this University, where Spallanzani had made immortal discoveries and created experimental biology, physiology was taught theoretically... without a laboratory! In the field of clinical and pathological medicine, the most abstruse vitalism dominated, and strange to say, it was proclaimed necessary to oppose foreign medicine, which was based on the analytical observation of pathological phenomena, oblivious to the fact that the so-called foreign medicine was born in Italy, and had as its foundation the master Morgagni! It was in such a period of dramatic battles over the direction to take—which, however were seminal for the renewal of our School—that I enrolled in this medical school, with no other aspiration than to acquire my professional diploma in a timely manner. Among the names of my masters, which are vividly engraved in my mind also for the informative influence that they had on my theoretical approach, I mention only those of Salvatore Tommasi, Bartolomeo Panizza, Eusebio Oehl, Paolo Mantegazza, and Giulio Bizzozero'. From the address given on 29 June 1919 at the Fondazione Camillo Golgi-Pro Orfani di Medici . In Mazzarello (1993, pp. 333–5). On the transformation of medicine in Golgi's time, see also Armocida and Zanobio (1994).

63. Following Pancaldi (1983, p. 12) I have used the concept of *disciplinary tradition* to indicate a characteristic manner of transmitting and receiving 'technical' knowledge similar to that of a 'classroom' or 'shop'; that is, the scientist learns the 'art' or 'trade' of his discipline like an artisan. The knowledge acquired in this way carries with it not only the prescription on how to conduct empirical research in a particular local context, but also true 'research strategies that are implicitly shared by those who practise the discipline'.

64. Cimino (1984, p. 297).

4

The morphological choice

At the beginning of 1860 the idea of national unification permeated Italian intellectual circles. It was as if history, long compressed, was expanding under irresistible pressure and all watched in astonishment the precipitous unfolding of events. In March, plebiscites in Parma, Modena, and Tuscany approved annexation to the Kingdom of Sardinia, which until then consisted of Piedmont, Liguria, and Sardinia. In May, Garibaldi's 'Thousand' sailed toward Sicily, and in September they entered Naples. At the end of the year the parliament of the Kingdom of Sardinia was dissolved to allow for the election of a national parliament.

Thus, when Golgi began his studies, the political scene in Pavia reflected the dramatic changes taking place on the national scene and all departments of the University of Pavia were shaken by ideological and power struggles. The entire city was breathing an air of patriotic ferment, excited in anticipation of imminent and extraordinary happenings. The charismatic figure of Giuseppe Garibaldi had fired the hearts of Lombard youths who in the previous year had rushed to enrol in the patriotic militia 'Cacciatori delle Alpi' (Alpine Hunters), fighting at Varese and San Fermo against the Austrians. Public subscriptions, sponsored, among others, by Panizza and other academics, were opened to collect funds for Garibaldi's army. By early April many Pavians had joined Garibaldi to participate in his expedition to Southern Italy. Among them was Benedetto Cairoli who led the 7th Company of the 'Thousand', which included many Pavian students who distinguished themselves in the battles of Calatafimi and Palermo. While the 'Thousand' fought in Sicily, further expeditionary forces were organized in Northern Italy. 'It was without regret, rather with approval, that, in the summer of 1860 he [Panizza] saw his younger son leave for Sicily, enrolled in the [Enrico] Cosenz legion'.[1] Another Cairoli, Luigi, participated in this expedition and died, shortly afterwards, of cholera in Naples.

The intellectual environment of the University of Pavia remained charged with fierce patriotic feelings throughout the 1860s. The ideal unity of 'thought and action', preached by Giuseppe Mazzini, found perfect embodiment in the students and young physicians led by Enrico Cairoli and Edoardo Bassini, who secretly trained in the small courtyard near the Institutes of Anatomy and Pathological Anatomy 'in the use of sword and firearms, even practising on corpses, before the war campaign of 1866 and the expedition of Villa Glori'.[2] Also among those who volunteered to fight with Garibaldi's troops was Edoardo

Porro. The names of some of these young Pavians, such as the brothers Cairoli, would later
be enshrined in the pantheon of Italian *Risorgimento*.

The 17-year-old Golgi witnessed 'the dawn of our *Risorgimento*' with 'intense' patriot-
ism,[3] but the study of medicine was rapidly becoming a burning passion. According to
his father, studying was 'more appropriate to his quiet, thoughtful, methodical, and patient
personality' than action.[4] His life as a student was completely absorbed by long hours of
study, and attending the lectures, the laboratory, autopsies, and, in the last years, the internship in the San Matteo Hospital. During the breaks, he would take his meals in a small
inexpensive café, crowded with students, at the corner of via Carlo Alberto and via Belli,
in front of the Aula Scarpa (Scarpa Hall). Throughout the century, this cafe remained an
institution among the Pavian students. In Golgi's day, it was run by an extremely decent
lady called, in affectionate mockery, '*tettonia*', because of the diminutive size of her breasts
(in Italian *tetta* is a vulgar term for breast). Forty years later, she still remembered proudly
that she had waited upon scientists of the calibre of Golgi and Bizzozero.[5]

During the six years of medical school, Golgi regularly attended several hospital wards,
particularly the Internal Medicine ward directed by Tommasi,[6] and the Psychiatry ward.

Golgi was a student with a reserved personality and a consistently reflective and un-
assuming demeanour. He had enrolled in the University of Pavia Medical School without
particular ambitions beyond becoming a physician. As a young man from a small and
remote alpine village, he must have begun his studies in humbling awe of an academic
environment so rich in tradition. As Antonio Pensa noted:

All who knew him are bound to imagine the feelings of great reverence and anxiety that the
young man must have felt approaching the sciences that had immortalized those who had died
and that crowned with laurel the forehead of the living.[7]

In his social contacts and in conversation, he certainly showed the 'signs of shyness and
introversion that were typical of his character' and that, even after many years, 'marked his
behaviour in a such a way as to make him appear withdrawn and aloof, keeping in awe
those who engaged him in conversation, especially if for the first time.'[8]

Among his fellow students there were brilliant personalities, in whose presence he cut
a modest figure. Many of them would leave their mark on the history of medicine. Beside
Sertoli and Bizzozero, there were Edoardo Bassini, who developed the eponymous
Bassini's operation for the radical cure of hernia, and Edoardo Porro, whose name is linked
to the first hystero-ovariectomy through Caesarean section, carried out in May 1876 in the
San Matteo Hospital. In 1901, the hygienist Giuseppe Sormani, who was one of Golgi's
classmates in Pavia, described the academic environment:

I remember those times, mythical times for us students, with great emotion; also because the most
heroic pages of Italian history were in the making. We attended to our studies in the excitement of
events that were unfolding rapidly in the titanic struggle for our national redemption; and the
University of Pavia, filled at the time with students emigrated from Veneto, was often shaken by
political rumblings. We were full of enthusiasm for our teachers, all of them great scholars shining
like beacons from this Lombard university, which, it must be said with regret, had been kept at
greater heights by the Austrian government than by the present Italian government . . . in the
large lecture halls of the Institute of Clinical Medicine directed by Tommasi, we found ourselves

in the company of Bizzozero, . . . Porro, Golgi, Bassini, Sertoli, and that very Enrico Cairoli who had already been wounded in the head by an enemy bullet and who shortly became the legendary hero of the battle of Monte Parioli.[9]

At the time when Golgi was a student in Pavia, positivistic materialism was penetrating Italian universities and intellectual circles, becoming the prevailing ideology among the progressive intelligentsia. The roots of Italian positivism were quite removed from the ideas of Auguste Comte and were mostly nourished by the dramatic progress in science and technology and the consequent acceleration of urbanization and industrialization. Above all, scientific materialism was fed by the triumphs of German scientists, especially the organic chemists who in the first half of the nineteenth century had obtained astonishing breakthroughs in the analysis and synthesis of organic compounds. As early as 1828 the chemist Friedrich Wöhler had synthesized urea from inorganic reagents, and all subsequent developments in biochemistry suggested the existence of shared physical substrates for the phenomena of life. In 1847 von Helmholtz extended the first law of thermodynamics to living organisms, thus reducing all natural phenomena to matter in motion. The arch-materialist Karl Vogt went so far as to claim that the relationship between brain and thought was similar to that between kidney and urine or between liver and bile.

Italian intellectuals were also particularly receptive to Darwin's theory of evolution,[10] and its implications for 'man's place in nature'. *On the origin of species* was published in 1859, when Golgi was finishing his pre-university studies, and although in that book Darwin had carefully skirted the issue of human origins, others were quick to seize on this question even before the appearance of *The descent of man* in 1871. Huxley's *Man's place in nature* and Vogt's *Vorlesungen über den Menschen* (Lectures on man) were in fact published in 1863, and the *Origine dell'uomo* (Origin of man) by the Italian zoologist Giovanni Canestrini appeared in 1866.

The spread of materialistic positivism in Italy during the 1860s and 1870s was facilitated by the arrival of Dutch and German academics. The first was the Dutch physiologist Jakob Moleschott. In 1852 he had triggered a spirited reaction in the conservative circles of Heidelberg with his book *Der Kreislauf des Lebens* (The circulation of life), in which he claimed that all life processes could be explained by the laws of nature and did not require the intervention of supernatural forces. Even psychic life was simply a particular instance of organization of matter, destined to end and begin again in a cyclical manner under the forces driving chemical reactions. Because of these ideas he was reprimanded by the governing body of the University and accused of materialism and corruption of the youth. At risk of being banned from teaching, and unwilling to renounce his ideas, he chose to expatriate himself to Zürich where he met another exile, the Italian Francesco De Sanctis. De Sanctis was very impressed by Moleschott and when, a few years later, he became Minister of Public Education in Cavour's and Ricasoli's cabinets, he did not forget the Dutch physiologist. Thanks to De Sanctis' good offices, Moleschott was appointed Professor of Physiology at the University of Turin and then at the University of Rome. Moleschott was eventually elected to the Senate of the Kingdom of Italy.

Others foreign scientists followed in Moleschott's steps. In 1863, Moritz Schiff, 'champion of the new experimental physiology based on vivisection, and a standard-bearer of

Darwinism',[11] moved from the University of Frankfurt to Florence, where he held the professorship of Physiology at the Istituto di Studi Superiori until 1876. The following year, Arnaldo Cantani, of Italian descent but born in Hainsbach on the border between Saxony and Bohemia, became Professor of Pharmacology and Toxicology at the University of Pavia. This 'Europeanizing' tradition of the Italian scientific academia would remain alive throughout the 1870s. Franz Christian Boll, who had graduated in medicine at the University of Berlin when barely twenty, became Professor of Physiology at the University of Rome, where he conducted fundamental studies on retinal pigments. Anton Dohrn founded, despite every sort of obstacle, the zoological station of Naples. Nikolai Kleinenberg conducted research in Naples and on the Island of Ischia (where he became popular among the fishermen as 'don Nicola') and energized the study of comparative anatomy and embryology in Sicily. Wilhelm Körner, native of Kassel, taught Chemistry at the Scuola Superiore di Agricoltura in Milan.

The most important role in the penetration of positivism into the Italian universities was played, however, by young physicians who had spent periods of study in Austria and Germany, where the materialistic–mechanistic revolution in biological sciences had rapidly acquired an explicit *medical–naturalistic* connotation. Thus, beginning with the 1860s, Italian medical schools became the strongholds of materialistic positivism and consequently it was almost impossible for medical students not to fall under the spell of the dogmatic system of scientific philosophy. Science was rapidly acquiring the status of a new religion, becoming the organizing force in the lives of many talented youths. This was particularly true at the University of Pavia, which ranked among its faculty some of the most influential Italian positivists, such as Lombroso, Mantegazza, and Tommasi.

In this context, the shy and modest Golgi found himself more and more attracted to scientific research, particularly research on the functioning of the central nervous system in normal and pathological conditions. This was one of the new frontiers where the reductionistic approach of materialistic philosophy, equating psychic phenomena with chemical processes, was being put to the test. Very soon Golgi came under the intellectual influence of Cesare Lombroso and his medical–anthropological entourage, and began to attend the narrow quarters of the Clinic for Mental Disorders, then located in the Palazzo del Maino.[12] It was probably during this period that Golgi became agnostic (or even frankly atheistic), remaining for the rest of his life completely alien to the religious experience. Golgi's nephew, Sandro Golgi, the son of Giuseppe Golgi, related that 'My uncle lived as if God did not exist and this did not trouble him in the least, whereas he was very concerned about the problems of the human condition.' Golgi himself stated on one occasion that 'The religious problem does not exist for me, because I have not even considered it.'[13] Notwithstanding this 'philosophical' position, Golgi was very respectful of religious authority. One of his uncles was a priest, and he had close ties with Romolo Putelli, a priest who sometimes accompanied Golgi on his walks to Aprica during summer vacations. As we shall see in a later chapter, no less of a religious authority than Achille Ratti, the future Pope Pius XI, held Golgi in great esteem.

Lombroso advocated a strictly positivistic epistemology and, in anthropology and psychiatry, he considered as 'scientific' only the conclusions grounded in physical–chemical and anatomical observations, rejecting as unwarranted and 'romantic' all ideas that were based on psychological introspection and empathy. Notwithstanding this methodological premise, Lombroso was inclined to make superficial generalizations and anthropological speculations cloaked in experimental language. Immersed in a cultural environment that reduced psychiatry to neuropathology, Golgi initiated, under Lombroso's supervision, a study of mental illnesses from an anatomical and anthropometric perspective. He received his medical degree on 7 August 1865,[14] defending a doctoral dissertation on the aetiology of mental disorders.[15] Three days later, his friend Enrico Sertoli graduated with a doctoral dissertation on intestinal tuberculosis.

Golgi began his internship at the San Matteo Hospital on 10 August, as a *Medico Secondario aspirante* ('aspirant to the position of Secondary Physician', the lowest ranking and most precarious position in the hospital hierarchy),[16] serving, 'according to the need' in the various medical, surgical, and dermatological (mostly syphilis cases) wards. At the medical examination for military service he was considered unfit for military service[17] (although he later became more robust), but because of the shortage of military physicians, he was temporarily hired by the army.[18] From June 14 to 30, 1866, he served in the 29th battalion of the Guardia Nazionale Mobile (Rapid Deployment National Guard),[19] and then at the Military Hospital of Pavia, where he remained until 1 October when the arrival of two new military physicians 'made the use of civilian physicians unnecessary'.[20] Golgi returned to the wards of the San Matteo to continue his internship.

The following year an epidemic of cholera, one of the recurring health emergencies of the last century, broke out in the region around Pavia. An infectious disease endemic to India for centuries, cholera had begun to spread throughout Europe during the first decades of the nineteenth century in the wake of ever increasing commercial exchanges and long-distance travels. Two important epidemics of cholera had already stricken Pavia in 1835 and 1855, and sporadic cases had occurred in 1849.[21] To fight this new epidemic, the Prefect of Pavia mobilized the local physicians, sending some of them into the surrounding villages where the disease had made its first appearance. Golgi was sent to Zavattarello, a small village in the hills, where he remained from 9 July to 29 August. We have no information about this episode, except that he fulfilled his duties in 'the most praiseworthy manner'.[22] At the time, the causes of cholera were still unknown, although there was an accurate appreciation of the contagious nature of the disease and of the correlation between its incidence and poor hygienic conditions. The freshly graduated Golgi was probably charged with direct care of the patients, who were kept either at home or in special isolation wards, and with the teaching of elementary hygienic precautions to the inhabitants of the area. For his performance during the epidemic Golgi received an official commendation from the Prefect.

When the cholera emergency was over, Golgi returned to his internship at the San Matteo and to the anxious search for a more remunerative and less precarious position. When he learnt that the Ospedale Maggiore della Carità of Novara was looking for a temporary assistant surgeon, he applied for the position and, on 1 March 1868, was hired.[23] After only a few weeks, however, Golgi heard a rumour that the *Medici Secondari aspiranti* of the San Matteo Hospital were up for promotion. Thus, on 26 April he resigned, returning to his old position in Pavia. Two days later, he made an unsuccessful attempt to meet the Director of the San Matteo in order to inquire about the rumoured promotions.

Undeterred, Golgi send to the Director a respectful letter inquiring whether it would be taken into consideration that he had 'greater seniority than Dr Rivella, even taking into account my two months of leave.'[24] Despite his shyness and introversion, Golgi was determined to hold his ground, even if it involved some inelegant elbowing of a colleague. Finally, on 1 July Golgi received the desired promotion to Assistant Physician. This position was still somewhat precarious but it ensured a salary, albeit a modest one. Again, he rotated among the different wards, such as Surgery, directed by Luigi Porta, Dermatology–Venereology, directed by Angelo Scarenzio, and Psychiatry, directed by Lombroso.[25] In 1869, he also served twice as substitute physician in the old Ospedale Santa Corona. An experiment that Golgi conducted on himself at this time is emblematic of the obsessive 'search for the contagion' which pervaded the medical environment at the end of the last century. It appears that Golgi made an attempt 'to solve the problem of the transmissibility of syphilis through the milk of infected women by inoculating himself with infected milk',[26] although no scientific report of this experiment has ever been found.

But Golgi was not content with being a simple physician, and even in the first years after graduation he maintained his link with the University. In 1867–68 he resumed his collaboration with Lombroso. Golgi must have been of great help to Lombroso, because the latter repeatedly mentioned Golgi's work (referring to him as a dedicated collaborator and sometimes as 'friend Golgi') in a number of papers published in 1867 and 1868. These references indicate that Golgi conducted post-mortem histopathological analyses on some of the patients of the psychiatric ward.[27] In addition, Golgi was one of the many individuals (students, friends, and colleagues) who volunteered in Lombroso's experiments on 'electric algometry', that is, the determination of pain sensitivity 'in the normal and insane man' by using graded electric currents.

With Lombroso, Golgi also continued the line of research initiated with his dissertation, exploring the aetiology of mental illness from an experimental and anti-metaphysical point of view. Soon enough, however, the methodological crudities of Lombroso and his propensity to make untestable generalizations, despite a declared allegiance to the experimental method, led to discontentment in Golgi, who was still unsure of which path to follow.[28] Indeed, 'the research strategy suggested by his influential advisor did not satisfy him; the anthropometric, somatic, and purely clinical data only partially satisfied his desire to investigate the fundamental essence of pathological phenomena. On the basis of comments made later by Golgi, it appears that he considered Lombroso an easy prey to unwarranted deductions that did not adhere to the precept, dictated by Lombroso himself, that psychiatry must be a science based on objective observations. Possibly because of this, Golgi escaped Lombroso's orbit, intensifying instead his ties with Bizzozero'.[29] It is indicative of Golgi's feelings toward Lombroso that, in his only autobiographical speech, during the celebrations for his retirement, he never mentioned the latter among the scientists who had influenced his scientific development, despite the close professional and scientific relationship that linked the two men for some years.[30]

In the time that remained after fulfilling his hospital duties, Golgi began to attend the Laboratory of Experimental Pathology directed by Bizzozero, who had fired his passion for histological studies. The two men rapidly became friends. They shared an apartment, property of the Marchioness Luigia Robolini del Majno ('Donna Gina'), which was also a meeting place for Mantegazza, Lombroso (who at one time had lived in the same building), and other young and ambitious academics.[31] It was circle of brilliant personalities who met to discuss the most recent news in science, culture, and politics.

Three years younger than Golgi, Bizzozero was then the rising star of experimental medicine in Pavia.[32] Shortly after enrolling, at 15, in the University of Pavia Medical School, he had joined the newly established Laboratory of Experimental Physiology directed by Oehl. When Bizzozero began to attend the lectures of Paolo Mantegazza, his exceptional scientific talent was immediately noticed by his teacher:

As soon as I discovered him among such a large pool of students, I told myself: here comes a great scientist, and I invited him to join my poor laboratory, which survived on abysmally low funding (400 lire per year) and was equipped with only two chairs, two tables, and a microscope (which was mine). My colleagues and the other students used to say: Mantegazza is an original and is enamoured with Bizzozero and claims that in a few years he will be an Italian glory. Others, with Milanese maliciousness, considered me a madman. It is possible that I am an original, but certainly I am a prophet. In that poor laboratory, where now Golgi makes a new discovery every day, Bizzozero immediately exhibited such exceptional abilities at microscopic observation as to make me understand that my easy prophecy would materialize very soon . . . He was indefatigable, patient, and extremely precise in his observations, and, by the same good fortune, his beautiful little hands could draw, as well as his bright eyes could see. All the drawings that illustrate my works on pathology have been drawn by him, and in what an admirable manner.[33]

Bizzozero graduated in June 1866, aged 20,[34] with a dissertation prepared in Mantegazza's laboratory, and received the Mateucci Prize awarded to the student who obtained the highest grade in all courses. As a student he published six papers on histopathological topics. Immediately after graduation, he travelled abroad to expand his scientific horizon. He visited the laboratory of Frey in Zürich and that of Virchow in Berlin. He came back from this experience propounding the new theoretical and experimental approach of German science and bringing a breath of fresh air into the biomedical environment in Pavia. In August 1865, Mantegazza was elected to the National Parliament for the district of Monza and decided that Bizzozero should substitute for him at the University. On account of the exceedingly young age of the candidate, this appointment was resisted by the other professors, who supported another candidate, an advocate of the old vitalistic school. In the end, however, Bizzozero became Professor of General Pathology at the age of 21, thanks to the pressure that Mantegazza exerted on the Minister for Education, Michele Coppino. This is how Mantegazza remembered the episode at Bizzozero's death:

When my parliamentary duties, entrusted to me by my fellow citizens of Monza, made it impossible for me to discharge my teaching obligations to my satisfaction, I proposed that the freshly graduated Bizzozero be my substitute. The Medical School was up in arms, scandalized, complaining that a youth, even if a genius, could not, must not, be appointed to one of the most prestigious professorships. I learnt of this refusal the very day it was sent to Florence, which at the time was the capital of Italy; I then jumped on a night train, arrived in Florence in the morning, and, at such an inconvenient time, I called on Minister Coppino. He kindly received me, and I declared that if the position is not awarded to Bizzozero I would rather kill myself, by carrying on my parliamentary and professorial duties at the same time, than allow a vitalist to enter my

classroom and cancel from the blackboard what I had written. Coppino, who always loved freedom in politics as well as in science, smiled and showed me the complaint from the University of
Pavia Medical School, a complaint that had travelled with me on the same train. The benevolent
and good-natured smile of the Minister, spoke volumes, and I launched myself in a passionate
defence of Bizzozero's cause, saying, among other things: 'he has only one fault, that both you
and I would like to share with him: he is too young; he has, however, the wisdom of a mature
man and will be soon one of our greatest glories.' Coppino smiled again, more encouragingly, and
shaking my hand said: 'Leave now, leave and return to Pavia, and tell your colleagues that
Bizzozero will be your substitute.'[35]

This is how Ernesto Bertarelli remembered Bizzozero:

Thanks to his eloquence, the discipline he taught acquired an almost geometrical precision: none
of the attributes he used could be changed without diminishing the exactitude of what was being
communicated to the listener. He could have been called a mathematician of pathology. But what
a great mathematician![36]

In an academic environment still dominated by the dogmatic teaching of old-fashioned
theories, and little interested in the most recent discoveries of experimental medicine,
Bizzozero preached that 'science must remove its veil of mystery and authoritarianism:
the teacher should not present science as a series of dogmas supported by the prestige of a
name, but instead expose it in its true condition, with its doubts and its questions.'[37]

If Golgi inherited from Lombroso an interest in neuropsychiatry, it is from Bizzozero
that he got the passion for histological research as the most direct method for penetrating
the mysterious nervous system, 'the thing' with a 'hidden structure' that contained the explanation for all behavioural and psychic phenomena; phenomena that Lombroso insisted
on explaining on the basis of anthropological and philosophical preconceptions. 'As far as
the organs of the central nervous system are concerned, the main task of modern anatomy
is to address the most urgent problems posed by physiology.'[38] During the entire course of
his long career the 'morphological option' remained for Golgi the premise for any well-
defined functional hypothesis. And while his research activity focused in turn on clinical,
therapeutic, and hygienic problems, his preference for morphological studies, which he
often applied to the solution of physiopathological problems having clinical relevance,
was never in doubt.

Indeed, although Golgi always followed with great interest and without preconception
the continuous unfolding of discoveries in bacteriology, immunology, chemistry, and
physical chemistry, and encouraged his pupils to study and apply the latest techniques, he
remained faithful to the morphological approach, convinced that it had not exhausted its
potential; the achievements he attained show that he was right.[39]

In the Laboratory of Experimental Pathology, located in Bizzozero's own offices, that
'still a youth . . . you supervised with the wisdom of a great savant',[40] Golgi completed his
first experimental studies. As he remembered in 1919:

Giulio Bizzozero, who entered the academic arena when still a youth, immediately understood
the nature of the revolutionary changes that were then in progress, and was able to find the
formula that characterized the scientific outlook of the age, indicating the direction to follow to
the other scholars of medicine.

His epoch bears the stamp of his pathbreaking initiatives, of his spurring to research and industriousness an army of disciples, who inspired by his ideas have spread his work throughout Italy.

It was in Bizzozero's laboratory that I did my period of practical training as an aspirant to the position of Assistant Physician and where I learnt the methods of scientific research and received directions for the future.[41]

For Bizzozero the only religion for 'physicians and pathologists should be to observe thoroughly and conscientiously, and to reason only on the basis of facts'[42] and the laboratory training must 'allow the activity of many individuals to be put to the service of science, so that new discoveries, previously the privilege of an elite, are now not infrequently due to the perseverance and well directed activity of a student.'[43]

Bizzozero was at the time a slender and graceful young man, always active and good-humoured, kind and sociable, albeit with a pugnacious side. He had great organizing capabilities, the outlook of a 'strict teacher', and all the hallmarks of a leader.[44] His authority was always accepted but never imposed; this was also due to his impressive scientific competence and to the prestige of an international experience unusual for such a young person. Some of his classmates in the Medical School became interns in his Laboratory of Experimental Pathology (later the Laboratory of General Pathology). And some of the students, who were then beginning their scientific careers under his supervision, such as Golgi, Bassini, Camillo Bozzolo, Domenico Stefanini, and Nicolò Manfredi, were older than he was. Golgi (a physician in Lombroso's Clinic) and Manfredi (an assistant in the Ophthalmology Clinic) worked in Bizzozero's laboratory when not in service. Others were preparing their doctoral dissertations or were post-graduate trainees, such as Pio Foà. Among Bizzozero's pupils, one must also mention Luigi Griffini and especially Carlo Forlanini,[45] who would become internationally renowned for introducing the artificial pneumothorax to treat pulmonary tuberculosis.

This is how the pathologist Benedetto Morpurgo described the atmosphere in Bizzozero's laboratory:

In the small Laboratory in Pavia, individuals came together who were as old or older than the professor: Manfredi, Golgi, Bassini, Bozzolo, and Foà (all of whom would, in turn, become professors in Pisa, Pavia, Padua, and Turin), and who formed around him a cenacle of indefatigable and enthusiastic workers . . . The only trace of youth in such a serious and stern environment was the unceasing activity, the fresh playfulness of productive work.[46]

Bizzozero's enthusiasm for scientific research was instrumental in galvanizing not only his students but also scholars in other disciplines. And it was a multidisciplinary group of scientists that gathered around Bizzozero to found a journal, *Giornale della Società di Scienze Matematiche, Fisiche e Biologiche di Pavia*, of which, however, only a few issues were published (Bizzozero contributed with a paper on tuberculosis). As Golgi wrote later, this project was too advanced for its time.[47] Only ten years later, when Bizzozero had become Professor of General Pathology at the University of Turin, would he succeed in founding the *Archivio per le Scienze Mediche*. The idea of a Pavian scientific society had to wait until much later, when Golgi and others would establish the Società Medico-Chirurgica di Pavia (see Chapter 11).

Problems descended on Bizzozero from a triad of academics of the old guard: Antonio Quaglino, Professor of Ophthalmology; Francesco Orsi, Professor of Internal Medicine; and Sangalli. These individuals, especially Sangalli, openly declared their opposition and 'persisted in their practice of ridiculing the new school'[48] gathered around Bizzozero, because it represented the New and the Future and, therefore, attracted the best students. Of the three, Quaglino was the least hostile and, despite his personal diffidence, he allowed one of his assistants, Manfredi, to work in the Laboratory of Experimental Pathology and to publish a paper with Bizzozero.

Notwithstanding these difficulties, Bizzozero was able to improve the scientific equipment of his laboratory substantially and his group spun out one important study after another. In 1873, immediately after Bizzozero's departure for Turin, Alfonso Corradi, then Rector of the University of Pavia and Professor of Pharmacology, ordered a report on the situation of all university institutes. The following is from the section on Bizzozero's laboratory:

In this Laboratory there is no abundance of scientific instrumentation; nevertheless there are four microscopes available for the researchers and there is no lack of tools for vivisection and other fine research. And a complete chemical bench is now available.

The funds that this Laboratory receives amount to four hundred lira. This scientific institution has already acquired an honourable position among the others . . .

Under Bizzozero as Director, the research in normal and pathological microscopy has made great progress, as indicated by numerous papers on the structure of connective tissue and bone marrow, and by many other pathological and physiological studies conducted by Bizzozero or his pupils. Particularly remarkable among these studies are those of Dr Camillo Golgi on the fine anatomy of nerve centres, and those of Dr Niccolò Manfredi on the retina and on certain pathological secretions.

The permanent Staff of the Laboratory consists of only its Director.[49]

In the years when he was at the helm of the Laboratory of Experimental Pathology, Bizzozero made fundamental discoveries in both physiology and pathology, characterizing the blood-producing function of bone marrow and discovering the phenomenon of phagocytosis many years before Elie Metschnikoff. Among his many scientific contributions while at the University of Turin were his detailed characterization of platelets, which had previously been only vaguely described, and their role in the formation of the 'white clot' and in the process of coagulation in general. He also classified tissues into 'stable, labile, and permanent' and carried out other extremely important studies in pathology, hygiene, and preventive medicine. Another of his achievements was the invention of the chromocytometer, which allowed the quantification of alterations in the content of haemoglobin. His scientific stature can be discerned in this passage from a letter from Victor von Ebner to Kölliker:

I was left very unsatisfied by the enormous literature on clinical haematology, because of the abundance of dogmatic statements that were not supported by facts. The reading of Bizzozero's works has been a relief after all those useless disquisitions, and has convinced me that in this field we do have some precise knowledge, thanks to the learned work of this pre-eminent man.[50]

And Kölliker himself, the most important histologist of the time, wrote to Bizzozero with the tone of a biblical prophet, 'You are the light that makes everything clear!'[50]

Bizzozero's stamp can be found in the most important publications of his disciples in Pavia, such as the first paper by Pio Foà on the pathological anatomy of bone marrow, published in 1872.[51] The influence of Bizzozero was also evident in the early scientific papers of Golgi who, as we shall see in the next chapter, expanded on some of the topics Bizzozero had already investigated.

There is no doubt that Giulio Bizzozero, despite his young age, had became the Master, the Patron and the 'Catalyst in Golgi's mind'.[52]

It appeared as if nature had created them for the sake of contrast: the former being tall, slender, agile, confident, and almost imperious; the latter being stocky, slow, apparently uncertain and subdued. Bizzozero, precocious in maturity and sense of leadership, was appointed, immediately after graduation, to direct a histological laboratory, if this can be said of a poor room equipped with few instruments that were the property of the students who worked there, and among his first disciples he [that is, Bizzozero] found Golgi. Golgi did not give the impression of having a bright future before him. Only Bizzozero perceived immediately that in this quiet, modest, and somewhat awkward son of a municipal physician from Corteno in Valcamonica, there was a deep faith and bold power; the seriousness of intents made it possible for such different souls to understand each other, and favoured a collaboration that would lead to the resurgence of Italian biology.

The investigation of tissues and their pathological alterations had shown the close connection between fine structure and function, and had demonstrated that the natural sciences could no longer be divided between those that investigated morphology and those that speculated on the phenomena of life. The realization of this generated the new approach in biology and its importance was immediately felt by Bizzozero's group and especially by Golgi, who, after being initially inspired by his young Master, very soon manifested his individuality and his marvellous propensity for original research.[53]

A few years after Bizzozero had left for the University of Turin, Golgi became his successor in the professorship of General Pathology in Pavia. The professional and intellectual bonds between the two men would be strengthened by the marriage of Golgi and Giuseppa Evangelina 'Lina' Aletti, daughter of Maddalena Bizzozero and niece of Giulio, who had probably met Golgi during a visit of the latter to the house that the Bizzozeros had in Varese.[54]

In Bizzozero's laboratory, Golgi became a close friend of Nicolò Manfredi. A native of Bosco Marengo, near Alessandria in Piedmont, Manfredi came from an aristocratic family which numbered among its members state officers of the Kingdom of Sardinia, physicians, and members of the church.[55] He had graduated from the University of Turin Medical School in 1860, with a dissertation on 'The therapeutic effects of music',[56] a topic that even today retains a certain interest. Immediately after taking his degree, he won a scholarship to study in Paris, where he did specialized studies in ophthalmology. Back in Italy in 1862, he worked as an Assistant Physician in Turin and published his first paper in 1864. In 1865 he arrived in Pavia to work as an assistant with Antonio Quaglino at the Ophthalmology Clinic, and in time he assisted the meteoric rise of the much younger Bizzozero. The dynamism and ebullience of Bizzozero 'cast a spell on Manfredi, whose feelings for Bizzozero bordered on cult'. The two young men travelled together to Berlin, where Manfredi

attended the Ophthalmology Clinic of the celebrated Albrecht Graefe and, with Bizzozero, Virchow's laboratory.[57] In Berlin, Manfredi acquired his passion for the histological
investigation of the eye, and beginning in 1867 he dedicated his free time to carrying out
research in Bizzozero's laboratory.[58] Working with Manfredi both at the Ophthalmology
Clinic and in the Laboratory of General Pathology, was a dedicated student, Carlo Forlanini, an 'accomplished artist and equally expert in the examination of the eye', who reproduced for Manfredi the appearance of the retinae of some patients 'in true colors'.[59]

Manfredi and Golgi spent long hours together at the microscope, and the fact that
Manfredi's laboratory protocols often mentioned Golgi[60] point to a close scientific collaboration between the two. Golgi and Manfredi also exchanged anatomical specimens from
patients who had died in their respective Clinics. Although his name is now forgotten,
Manfredi was at the time internationally renowned because of a number of important
studies, including a paper in 1868 on the glioma of the retina. Indeed his name can be
found in the most important biographical dictionaries published in Italy and Germany at
the turn of the century.

Occasionally, Golgi and Manfredi spent the weekend together in the beautiful house
of the Manfredis in Bosco Marengo, making music (Manfredi on the violin and Golgi
on the flute) and discussing scientific matters.[61]

In the following years, Golgi's dedication to research began to bear fruit. In 1868, he published his first paper, little more than a clinical exercise, *A case history of non-manic pellagra*,[62]
in which he described the clinical and anatomo-pathological findings in a case of pellagra,
a disease, still common at the time, caused by a corn-based diet deficient in nicotinic acid
and similar vitamins. This topic was very dear to Lombroso who, as early as 1863, had
established a connection between the use of cornbread and the incidence of pellagra in
Lombardy. Beginning in 1868, Lombroso published a series of studies on this problem,
in which he proposed the hypothesis, subsequently proven incorrect, that pellagra was
caused by corn altered by the action of *Penicillum glaucum* or other micro-organisms.
Although Golgi's study on pellagra contained no important data, it foreshadowed Golgi's
scientific style of presenting only objective data: 'the facts'.

In 1869, Golgi published a monograph, *On the aetiology of mental alienations*,[63] which combined the influence of Lombroso with the rigorous experimental approach of Bizzozero.
In this study, Golgi analysed with a broad methodological approach a large number of cases
that he had personally collected in the Mental Hospital of Pavia, reviewing the various
environmental, hereditary, and organismic factors that at the time were considered most
important in the aetiology of 'mental alienations'. Although the topic is the same as that of
his doctoral dissertation, Golgi's monograph contained a great amount of new clinical and
statistical data, mainly from the years 1867–68. A summary of Golgi's work was given by
Lombroso at the 1869 meeting of the Regio Istituto Lombardo di Scienze e Lettere.[63] *On
the aetiology of mental alienations* is a manifesto of the new direction taken by psychiatry under
the influence of positivistic epistemology:

Many alienists, struck by the psychic phenomena of alienation and informed by old-fashioned
pseudo-philosophical systems, a priori assume that the aetiology of alienation must be found in

the psychic sphere, and thus they do not bother with other kinds of investigation. For this reason mental pathology has became an abstract science, so abstract that many do not consider it a science at all.

Nevertheless, although neglected, a new school is now rising in Italy, a school that bears on its flag the motto '*provando e riprovando*' [testing and then testing again] of the old Italian school, and which wants to reduce also this medical discipline to a positive science of observation. Supported by experiments and facts, the new school is making an attempt to test the old hypothesis that madness is a symptom of severe organic alterations, localized either in the nervous centres or in other organs, such as the heart, the lungs, the stomach, etc., etc.

Despite the evidence supporting it, this new approach in psychiatry is stubbornly opposed, unfortunately with some success, by the partisans of the past and especially by the metaphysicists.

To prevail, I used the weapon forged by the new school, that is the experimental method, and therefore I endeavoured to collect objective findings, which when conscientiously gathered without prejudices, always result in some progress.[64]

The stamp of Lombroso is uncanny. In his 1865 book *La medicina legale delle alienazioni mentali studiata con il metodo esperimentale* (Forensic medicine of mental alienations studied with the experimental method), Lombroso wrote:

Disciple of the true Italian school, of the school that has as its insignia the great motto: *provando e riprovando*, I set myself the task of trying to replace all those vague and undetermined, and often controversial, terms, such as human reason, free will, enflamed passions, preponderant instinct, etc., with more concrete terms corresponding to objective facts that could be easily verified. It is only thanks to numbers and precision instruments that science has made those giant steps that we all admire and that play such a great role in our domination of nature. What prevents us from applying this marvellous methodology to psychiatry, from the moment that the alienated is composed not only of spirit but of body as well, and that the changes in psychic force, that is in spirit, must be accompanied by changes in morphology?[65]

Lombroso's influence is also particularly evident in the discussion of the relationship between mental illness and criminality, which foreshadows modern ideas on mental infirmity as a factor to be considered in deciding legal responsibility.

The study of the relationship between mental alienation and crime is becoming more and more important in proportion to the progress made in psychiatry, and presently not only the physicians but also the jurors will realize that often the criminals are only individuals having imperfect conformation, humans afflicted by a special pathological condition, and this realization has already contributed to saving not a few individuals from the infamy of capital punishment.[66]

Golgi then made a timid attempt to distance himself from Lombroso's physiognomic theory of the 'degenerate' by stating that madness does not always manifest itself with unique degenerative stigmata. And, after emphasizing the great importance of hereditary factors in the aetiology of mental diseases, he examined also the role of environmental, infectious (tuberculosis), meteorological, and nutritional (pellagra, alcoholism, and cretinism) factors. Characteristic of the deterministic and positivistic approach to mental disease is Golgi's analysis of psychological and environmental variables, which he refers to as 'moral causes' (religious scruples, domestic problems, love troubles, loss of wealth, shocks, frustrated ambitions, etc.).

We are far from denying the importance of moral causes; on the contrary we agree that strong emotions and sudden violent passions can, like, or more than, a blow dealt to the head or other severe perturbations of the organism, act on the organs of intelligence and cause a disruption in their functions; and these effects will be more easily explained if we accept, in agreement with modern psychophysics, that the mental activity is nothing but a special form of activity of the matter, because in this case moral causes would act like any other physical cause.[67]

Finally, he reported on a number of clinical cases, many of them with a favourable evolution. And with a touch of humour, completely absent in his subsequent scientific and non-scientific writings, he noted that: 'in our mental hospital there are three Napoleons and a certain Italia, who is the wife of the Emperor of Austria'.[68]

In the period between 1865 and 1871 his collaboration with Lombroso is also indicated by forensic-medicine activities as an expert witness in cases of insanity. These reports were later published in the *Annali Universali di Medicina* in a paper co-authored with Lombroso, titled 'Forensic diagnosis carried out with the experimental and anthropological method'.[69] In this paper a number of clinical cases of criminological relevance were described. For each individual undergoing examination, the authors reported the most important physical aspects, the medical history, and, in typical Lombrosian fashion, the anthropometric data; finally, they offered an evaluation of the individual's mental capabilities. There is an abundance of measurements of tactile sensibility (using Weber's aesthesiometer), pain sensibility (using Rühmkorff's coil), and strength (using Broca's dynamometer).

Considerations such as

the principles of morality, even accepting the problematic hypothesis that they are innate in humans, must be rekindled and maintained by attentive and continuous education, without which humans return to those primitive and apish stages in which the moral sensitivity is absolutely nil[70]

foreshadow the notion that 'primitives' represent an 'inferior' form of humanity, a notion that Lombroso would later develop in his 'atavistic' theory, according to which criminals, and to a lesser extent madmen and savages, maintain ancestral characters and represent a regressive, and therefore primitive, form of humanity.

The influence of Bizzozero and his entourage, however, was rapidly having an effect on Golgi. Adopting Virchow's *Die Cellularpathologie* as his bible, Golgi began to experiment with a variety of staining substances and fixatives, and obviously turned his attention to the microscopic investigation of the nervous system. In his first histological study *On the structure and development of psammomas*,[71] published in 1869, he investigated the structure of two meningeal tumours rich in calcareous concretions (from the Greek *psammos* = sand). The first tumour, from a woman with pellagra who had died in the Hospital of Verona, had been sent to Golgi by Lombroso. The second tumour came from a man who had died in the Hospital of Pavia. Under the supervision of Bizzozero, who had already worked on the same problem, Golgi concluded that these tumours, which the great American neurosurgeon Harvey Cushing would later classify as meningiomas, were derived from connective tissue. In this way, Golgi argued against the hypothesis advanced by other scientists that psammomas arose from the endothelium or from the outer layers of the wall of the

blood vessels. In this study is introduced for the first time the term 'endothelioma' to indicate the tumours deriving from the cells that line the serous cavities (currently, and more
appropriately, called mesotheliomas).

Histology was rapidly becoming Golgi's main research interest. In 1869, he participated
in the competition for the Grassi Prize (awarded since 1842 from the bequest of Bernardino
Grassi) for the most distinguished medical essay by a young researcher. In that year there
were only two candidates, and Golgi prevailed over the other with an extensive experimental essay, *On the alterations of the lymphatic vessels of the brain*,[72] in which he extended the
work begun by Bizzozero in 1868.[73] This essay was an ambitious undertaking that indicated the degree of scientific confidence achieved by Golgi and his ability to get to the core
of biological problems. Contrary to what has been written, Golgi never conceived the
detailed description of 'facts' as an end in itself, but only as the path to 'deduce' their
physiological and physiopathological significance with the greatest degree of certainty.
This approach is perfectly illustrated by his study on the lymphatics. He first demonstrated
his thorough knowledge of the international literature with a discussion of the difference
between the lymphatic spaces (or Virchow–Robin spaces, which are tunnel-like spaces
around the blood vessels where they penetrate the brain, limited internally by the vessel
wall and externally by connective tissue) and a more external space, the 'His space' described by Wilhelm His Sr, a putative perivascular space that Golgi would later demonstrate to be artifactual. Then he proceeded to develop, on the basis of precise micrometric
measurements carried out on over two thousand slides, a series of physiopathological
deductions on brain congestion and brain oedema, on the deposition of pus in the
lymphatic spaces during meningitis, and on the route of diffusion of pathological
processes. Finally, he drew the following precise and definitive conclusions:

– The rapid dilation of the blood vessels of the brain (acute cerebral congestion) develops at the
expense of the corresponding perivascular lymphatic spaces, and vice versa the reduction in the
diameter of the blood vessels (cerebral anaemia) results in an increase in the size of the perivascular
spaces. This solves the controversial issue of the possibility of acute cerebral congestion.

– It is possible to have the simultaneous dilation of both the blood vessels and the perivascular
lymphatic spaces; but this happens only in individuals who suffer from chronic cardiac or
pulmonary conditions and are predisposed to congestion and serous transudation. In this case
the volume of the cerebral parenchyma must be reduced to allow for the increase in volume of
the blood vessels and of the lymphatic spaces. In senile atrophy of the brain a remarkable enlargement of the blood vessels is coupled with enormous dilations and varicosities of the perivascular
spaces.

– The localized or generalized oedema of the brain is always associated with an abnormal
dilation of the perivascular lymphatic spaces.[74]

It might be of some interest to notice that Golgi used, in his research on the lymphatic
spaces, the two reagents (potassium dichromate and silver nitrate) that were later used for
the black reaction. In 1870 Bizzozero communicated to the Istituto Lombardo di Scienze
and Lettere (Lombard Institute of Sciences and Literature) a brief note by Golgi summar-
izing his research on the histology of interstitial glia.[75] Golgi would later extend his
findings in the 1871–72 work 'Contribuzione alla fine anatomia degli organi centrali del
sistema nervoso' ('A contribution to fine anatomy of the central organs of the nervous

system'), published in three parts in the *Rivista Clinica*.[76] This is an important study on the structure of the nervous system and Golgi's first important contribution to histology. He demonstrated that both the perivascular space and the epicerebral space (a putative system between the surface of the circumvolutions and the pia mater) described by His, and the pericellular space described by Brücke's disciple Heinrich Obersteiner, were mere artifacts. Obersteiner erroneously thought that the nerve cells were 'suspended', hanging from their processes, in a sort of pouch that was considered to be an intra-parenchymal extension of the perivascular space of His. Another important result by Golgi was to establish conclusively the presence of a direct communication between the Virchow–Robin space and the subarachnoid space, by injecting Berlin blue in the latter.

The paper continued with a detailed analysis of the interstitial stroma, whose nature was subject to contrasting opinions. Since the early nineteenth century it had been hypothesized, especially by Friedrich Arnold, that there existed in the spinal cord an interstitial stroma supporting the nerve cells. It was Virchow, however, who clearly demonstrated, between 1846 and 1853, that throughout the central nervous system there was, in addition to the nerve cells, a 'connective' substance. Virchow described it as a soft, finely granular, amorphous substance, containing a great number of roundish, lenticular cells with large nuclei, and called it 'nervous cement or neuroglia'. These cells were further characterized by another of Virchow's disciples, Otto Friedrich Karl Deiters, who was an extremely productive scientist in his tragically short life. Deiters illustrated the star-like shape of glial cells in an elegant drawing,[77] and in the following years these cells were often referred to as Deiters' cells. In opposition to Virchow's 'connective' theory, Friedrich Gustav Jakob Henle supported the notion that the fine granular substance of the cortex was the 'matrix' on which nerve cells developed. The debate around these two contrasting hypotheses involved the most important histologists of the time, including Kölliker, Joseph von Lenhossék, Franz Leydig, Maximilian (Max) Schultze, Friedrich Siegmund Merkel, Theodor Meynert, Rudolph Wagner, and, obviously, each of them had his own variant. Golgi was finally able to confirm Virchow's and Deiters' hypothesis that neuroglia consists of stellate cells distinct from the nerve cells, by working on pieces of cerebellum, brain, and spinal cord hardened in osmic acid and potassium dichromate, following the methods developed by Heinrich Müller and others. In particular, Golgi demonstrated that the glial cells were roundish, lenticular, or stellate, and that their thin (and often extremely long) processes could end in different ways. In some cases they ended in contact with the processes of other glial cells or the nerve cells; in others, they terminated surrounding blood vessels; and sometimes they vanished without trace. The relationship that the glial cells established with both the nerve cells and the blood vessels led Golgi to hypothesize, years later, that they might play a role in the 'distribution of nutritional material',[78] an idea that seems to foreshadow the concept of blood–brain barrier. Thus, Golgi disputed Henle's hypothesis that the interstitial substance was 'amorphous', 'finely granular', and without cells:

I do not intend with this to deny the existence of an amorphous or finely granular intercellular substance in the specimens I am describing; on the contrary I consistently found it and I had to actively eliminate it with an appropriate preparation of the pieces. It is my conviction, however, that this 'finely granular', or 'reticular', or 'sponge-like', or 'molecular-punctiform', or 'amorphous', or 'gelatinous' substance acquires all the above characteristics either because of cadaveric alterations, or because of the reagents (or other methods) employed. I arrived at this conclusion by noticing the extent to which the amount of this substance varies greatly depending on whether the pieces of brain were more or less fresh at the moment of their immersion in dichromate and on the care I took in preserving them. Whenever I could work on very fresh brains and preserve them accurately, I observed many cells rich in processes with very little granular substance interspersed among these cells and the fibres originating from them. On the contrary, whenever I could not work on very fresh or well preserved brains, I observed a great abundance of finely granular substance, and only with difficulty could I identify the elegant shape of the connective cells. Finally, when different pieces from the same brain were preserved differently, I could obtain a comparable diversity of results. Taken together these findings concur in demonstrating that the interstitial stroma of the cortex consists mostly of connective cells and their processes, whereas the finely granular substance appears, in the standard preparations, in much greater amounts because of a sort of degradation of the fibrillary substance, a degradation that, on the other hand, takes place not only in the processes of the connective cells but also in the finest ramifications of the protoplasmic processes of the nerve cells.[79]

The glial cells appeared to be distributed throughout the central nervous system with different morphological characteristics, depending on whether they were localized in the grey or in the white matter. As he summarized in a later study:

the stroma interspersed among the nerve cells and the fibres, in the brain and in the cerebellum, as well as in the spinal cord, is mostly constituted: in the white matter, by cells having a flat and large body, which continue in a great number of fine, long, and rarely ramified processes; in the grey matter, by cells with an irregular body, which is surrounded by a dense bush of extremely fine processes, not infrequently ramified, sometimes granular, partly homogenous and shiny, processes that play the most important, if not an exclusive, role in forming the interstitial stroma.[80]

Golgi's distinction of two types of stellate glial cells is still valid. Currently, glia are classified into three subtypes: 'true neuroglia' or macroglia (that is, the astrocytes, or stellate cells, to which Golgi's study referred), oligodendroglia (cells that provide an insulating coating of myelin, surrounding the axons in the central nervous system), and the microglia (small scavenger cells that react to nervous system infection or damage). The astrocytes can be subdivided into protoplasmic astrocytes, which have short processes and prevail in the grey matter, and fibrous astrocytes, which have long processes and predominate in the white matter. Thus, Golgi's 1871–72 study might be rightly considered, together with Deiters' 1865 paper, the most important work published in that period on the neuroglia. And all of this was done under conditions of great difficulty, as indicated by Golgi's note communicated by Bizzozero to the Istituto Lombardo. 'Concerning the cerebellum, my observations are still quite incomplete, because of the impossibility of obtaining osmic acid.'[81] The immersion in alcohol, in osmic acid, or in dichromates, was the most efficient means of hardening the tissues before slicing them with a microtome (or knife). The use of alcohol, however, proved to be unsuitable for nervous tissue, because it dissolved the myelin sheath, whereas the osmic acid was very expensive. It is not surprising that Golgi chose to work with potassium dichromate. This choice, born out of necessity, turned out to be instrumental in the discovery of the black reaction.

Golgi's findings on the glia were summarized in 1872 in the *Archivio Italiano per le Malattie Nervose*, by its editor, Andrea Verga, a pre-eminent Italian neuropsychiatrist who had studied anatomy with Panizza. Verga's name is still remembered because of his description of two anatomical structures: Verga's ventricle (a space that is sometimes found between the corpus callosum and the fornix, also called the sixth ventricle) and Verga's lachrymal groove (which runs downwards from the lower opening of the nasal duct). He later became a psychiatrist and the Director of the Mental Hospital of San Celso in Milan, then of the Mental Hospital of Senavra, and finally of the Ospedale Maggiore of Milan. His opinions were, therefore, extremely influential. In his summary of Golgi's study, Verga concluded by suggesting that 'most appropriate topic of investigation for Dr Golgi would be to investigate whether the connective tissue of the central nervous system undergoes modification in cases of mental alienation, and, first of all, whether it is true that it increases in chronic mania and in dementia'.[82] This suggestion was not lost on Golgi, because in 1874 he reported an increase in glial tissue in the basal ganglia and in the fronto-parietal cortex of an individual with chorea and 'mental alienation'.

Golgi's paper on glia received widespread international attention. Summaries in German were prepared by Franz Boll, who regularly summarized in the *Centralblatt für die medicinischen Wissenschaften* the most important studies published in Italian, and by Heinrich H. Hoyer (of Warsaw), in the prestigious *Jahresberichte über die Fortschritte der Anatomie und Physiologie*. Summaries were published also in English and French.[83]

The following year, Franz Boll himself published a massive monograph on the histology and histogenesis of the central nervous system, in which he confirmed, using the chloro-gold method, Golgi's conclusions on the structure of glial tissue and on the artifactual nature of the perivascular and epicerebral spaces of His and of the pericellular spaces of Obersteiner.[84] By the end of 1872, Boll had already sent to Golgi a preprint of his monograph. In the enclosed letter, written in a decent Italian, he expressed his satisfaction for the 'good agreement between my findings and those you have previously published',[85] and then flattered Golgi by stating that the 'Contribuzione alla fine anatomia degli organi centrali del sistema nervoso' was 'the best histological work produced by an Italian laboratory', that he hoped Golgi would follow up with other studies 'on the same subject', and commented that 'in Germany your papers are studied with the greatest interest'.

Golgi could not hide his satisfaction and in his review of Boll's monograph, published in 1873 in the *Rivista di Medicina, Chirurgia e Terapeutica*, he wrote 'It is a great fortune to open the first issue of this *Rivista* with a work so rich in interesting ideas, such as this by Boll, especially because in it I can find confirmation of my recent findings on the histology of the nervous system.'[86]

The findings by Deiters, Golgi, and Boll were, however, challenged by Louis Antoine Ranvier in a study communicated by Claude Bernard to the Académie des Sciences of Paris in 1873.[87] Ranvier, using his own histological method, had reached the conclusion that the glial tissue was not different from common connective tissue, and that the results of the other three were the 'product of mere illusion'. According to him the glia was made of intersecting connective fibres of different lengths and the lamelliform cells positioned at the points of intersection were without processes and, thus, completely independent of these fibres. In the following years Ranvier forcefully reiterated his interpretation.[88]

However, Golgi's ideas on glia were gaining ground even in France. In 1882, J. Renaut of the Laboratory of General Anatomy of the University of Lyon Medical School could write that the cells found in the grey matter of the spinal cord of mammals 'correspond almost perfectly to the description provided by Golgi'.[89]

The description of the glial cells given by Deiters, Golgi, and Boll would later be confirmed by many authors, thanks especially to the black reaction. Golgi himself would use the black reaction in a detailed study of glial cells published in 1885.[90] Although Ranvier's position was briefly revived by Carl Weigert at the turn of the century, the introduction in the following decades of new histological methods based on silver or chloro-gold impregnation conclusively demonstrated the presence of processes emanating from the astrocytes.

Another investigation of the glial cells was carried out by Golgi in a paper co-authored with Manfredi on the histology of the horse retina. The two friends immersed the eyes from a freshly slaughtered horse in potassium dichromate or chromic acid for 10–20 days, following which 'the retina completely loses the rods and cones and almost all the outer layer, and the rest . . . completely dissociates into three layers'.[91] Golgi and Manfredi could then study in detail the structure of the three layers and were able to find glial cells in all three of them. This was an important finding because previous attempts by both Boll and Theodor Leber had failed to locate evidence of glial cells in the retina. In the hope of a review in *Centralblatt*, Golgi immediately sent a reprint of the paper to Boll.[92] The latter appreciated the work and in a letter to Golgi emphasized that it was 'a remarkable discovery' to have found glial cells in the retina.[85] The desired review was published a few months later.[93]

Also connected with his research on glia is the paper 'On the gliomas of the brain' which, although published in 1875 in the *Rivista Sperimentale di Freniatria and Medicina Legale*,[94] reports work done in 1871 under Bizzozero's supervision. The starting point for this research was the rule that neoplasms carry a sort of 'mark' of the tissue from which they derive. This notion provided a major theoretical framework for the research conducted in the Laboratory of Experimental Pathology, and was the theme of a paper in 1872 by Bizzozero: 'On the relationship between the structure of tumours and the characteristics of the tissue from which they originate'.[95] Golgi summarized the idea as follows:

Being now an indisputable axiom in general pathology that the structure of neoformations is modelled on the structure of the tissues from which those same neoformations derive, it is, therefore, obvious to hypothesize that neoformations such as the gliomas, which originate from the interstitial connective tissue of the brain and other parts of the central nervous system, should present a structure analogous to that of the very same connective tissue, that is, that gliomas are substantially made of cells analogous to the normal ones discussed above.[96]

From this starting point, Golgi proceeded to study two samples of glioma, the first from a 24-year-old man, who died in the Psychiatric Clinic following severe epileptic convulsions, the second from a 6-year-old girl who died in the Ophthalmology Clinic (and which he obtained thanks to Manfredi). The structure of the gliomas was analysed after dilaceration of fresh pieces or after immersion in potassium dichromate. Golgi concluded that there was a close relationship between the structure of the glioma and that of the normal glial tissue and established precise histopathological criteria to distinguish between

tumours derived from the astrocytes (true gliomas) and tumours derived from the connective tissue (sarcomas). Similar findings were reported one year before Golgi's work was
published, by Theodor Simon in *Archiv für pathologische Anatomie und Physiologie*.[97]

It is clear, therefore, that Golgi, contrary to what is commonly held, had already attained
international recognition at the beginning of the 1870s with his work on glial cells.
Furthermore, he had joined the editorial board of the prestigious *Rivista Clinica* of
Bologna, for which he reviewed the international literature,[98] and his name had acquired
a certain pre-eminence in the biomedical establishment of Pavia, especially among the
younger academics. Thus, from the scientific point of view he had begun to receive some
personal satisfaction.

His financial situation was, however, far less brilliant. In particular, his hopes for an
academic career were, to his great chagrin, extremely bleak. In 1871 the University of
Pavia Medical School had granted him (probably owing to pressure from Bizzozero and
Lombroso) the privilege of teaching a *corso libero* (Clinical Microscopy)[99]. But that was all.
He was stuck in the mediocrity of an underpaid position as Secondary Physician. It seems
that he may have been 'inhibited at the beginning of his career' by his introverted and shy
personality.[100]

On 1 December 1871, Lombroso left the University to become Director of the Mental
Hospital of Pesaro. On 8 January 1872 Golgi 'was attached to the psychiatric ward and on
12 March he became substitute to the Chief Physician'.[22] Later in that January he added
to his other commitments a collaboration with the Cryptogamic Laboratory[101] (as a paid
trainee from the San Matteo Hospital) to conduct 'cryptogamic research applied to medicine'[26] aimed at verifying what kind of relevance 'plant parasites might have for the human
organism.'

This situation could not be endured for much longer. In the following chapter we shall
see how, under mounting pressure from his father, he had to take the difficult decision to
forgo his academic ambitions and accept a stable, secure, and remunerative position.

Notes

1. Verga (1869, p. 83).
2. Monti (1926, p. 17).
3. Marcora (1927, p. 127).
4. Riquier (1952, p. 52).
5. Pensa (1991, p. 86).
6. In September 1865, Tommasi ranked Golgi as 'one of the most accomplished students I have
   met in the last two years' (recommendation letter dated 23 September 1865; MSUP-I-I-6).
7. Pensa (1926, p. 7).
8. *Ibid.* (p. 75).
9. Cited in Gravela (1989, p. 14).
10. On the spread of Darwinism in Italy see Pancaldi (1983).
11. Cosmacini (1988, p. 329).
12. *L'Università di Pavia e i suoi istituti* (Pavia: Tipografia Successori Bizzoni, 1925, p. 142).

13. *Il Popolo-La Provincia Pavese* (24 January 1926). On the other hand, there is no evidence that Golgi ever received religious education, aside from the class of Religion in school. In the parish records of Corteno of 1851 and 1855, Golgi does not appear among those who received confirmation. (I thank don Giuseppe Pedrazzi, parish priest of Corteno, for this information.)

14. Golgi's diploma, signed by the Rector Giovanni Cantoni, is kept in MSUP.

15. That Golgi graduated in 1865 with a thesis on the aetiology of mental diseases is stated in a number of biographical notes (e.g., Bertarelli, 1950, p.18; Marcora, 1927, p. 117; Perroncito, 1926, p. 12; Riquier, 1952, p. 54; Rondoni, 1943, p. 537; Veratti 1926, p. 1). I could not find a copy of Golgi's dissertation either in the State Archives of Pavia or in the University Archives, currently under reorganization). Thus, there is no support for the claim that Bizzozero introduced Golgi (as his nephew!) to Lombroso in 1866 (Lombroso Ferrero, 1915, p. 98).

16. Certificate released by the San Matteo Hospital on 20 May 1866 (MSUP-I-I-7). Another certificate released by the same hospital on 31 December 1879 states that Golgi began his activity as *Medico Secondario aspirante* on 7 August (MSUP-I-I-30).

17. Certificate released by the Mayor of Corteno on 12 July 1918 (MSUP-I-I-3).

18. Request by the Director of the Ospedale Divisionale Militare of Pavia, dated 14 June 1866 (MSUP-I-I-8).

19. Certificate released by the Commandant of the 29th Battalion of the Guardia Nazionale Mobile on 30 June 1866 (MSUP-I-I-9).

20. Certificate released from the Ospedale Divisionale Militare of Pavia on 24 September 1866 (MSUP-I-I-10).

21. Pasi Testa (1981).

22. Certificate released by the San Matteo Hospital on 31 December 1879 (MSUP-I-I-30).

23. Certificate released by the Ospedale Maggiore of Novara on 26 April 1868 (MSUP-I-I-11).

24. Petition to the Director of the San Matteo, dated 29 April 1868 (MSUP-I-I-12).

25. See Donaggio (1926), Marcora (1927); Morpurgo (1926); Pensa (1926); Perroncito (1926).

26. See *Gazzetta Medica Lombarda* (1902, pp. 431–40) on the occasion of Golgi's academic and marital jubilee.

27. Lombroso (1867, p. 17; 1868, p. 84; 1868a, p. 206; 1868b, p. 302).

28. Bertarelli (1950, p. 20); Pensa (1961, p. 271).

29. Pensa (1961, p. 271).

30. The relationship with Lombroso remained, however, extremely cordial, as indicated by Golgi's handwritten dedication on the reprint of one of his papers (Golgi, 1871–72): 'To Prof. Lombroso, steadfast advocate of Experimental Psychiatry, his disciple Golgi dedicates this histological study'. The front page of this reprint is reproduced in Baima Bollone (1992, Table 3).

31. Lombroso and Lombroso (1906, p. 67).

32. On the figure of Bizzozero see Cappelletti (1968); Golgi (1901; 1905); Gravela (1989); Pogliano (1985).

33. Cited in Gravela (1989, p. 16).

34. The record of Bizzozero's dissertation ('On the process of cicatrization of severed tendons) is kept in the State Archives of Pavia. The written dissertation was presented on 31 May 1866 and approved on the following day with 70 points out of 70. Bizzozero was admitted to the oral dissertation and examined (on a date that cannot be established with certainty because it is indecipherable, probably 4 June 1866) by Professors Vittadini, Cantani, and Lombroso. The transcript of the examination concludes: 'At the end of the exam, without need for

discussion, the Committee granted 70 points out of 70, and therefore the Dean . . . invited the Committee to a new vote, which unanimously deliberated that Mr Giulio Bizzozero had passed the exam with the highest honours, that a special mention of this would be made in the *Gazzetta Ufficiale* [i.e., the official bulletin of the Italian Administration], and that a special silver medal bearing his name would be coined.'

35. Cited in Gravela (1989, p. 18ff.).
36. Bertarelli (1950, p. 22).
37. Golgi (1901, p. 212); the citation is taken (with modifications) from Bizzozero (1873, p. 14).
38. Golgi (1885, p. 3).
39. Veratti (1942–43, p. 101).
40. Dedication to Bizzozero of *Sulla fina anatomia degli organi centrali del sistema nervoso* (Golgi, 1885). The dedication is reproduced at the beginning of the first volume of the *Opera Omnia* (hereafter *OO*).
41. From the speech given on 29 June 1919 at the Fondazione Camillo Golgi Pro-Orfani di Medici. Reproduced in Mazzarello (1993, p. 335).
42. Bizzozero (1873, p. 4).
43. Golgi (1901, p. 212); the citation is taken (with modifications) from Bizzozero (1873, p. 14).
44. Golgi (1905, p. xx); Gravela (1989, p. 20).
45. Grassi (1911, p. 64).
46. Gravela (1989, p. 20).
47. Golgi (1901, p. 206).
48. Grassi (1911, p. 64).
49. Cited in Locatelli (1961, pp. 463ff.).
50. Cited in Golgi (1901, pp. 213ff.).
51. Vanzetti (1926).
52. Bertarelli (1950, p. 22).
53. Morpurgo (1926, p. 32).
54. See Bianchi (1973, p. 16). Bizzozero used to spend the summer and part of the autumn in Varese, where he carried out microscopic studies. He kept up a regular correspondence with Golgi, who informed Bizzozero about his research and the latest news from the Laboratory of General Pathology. Bizzozero invited Golgi to join him in Varese (see, for example, letter of 9 October 1869, MSUP-VII-III-1).
55. Delle Piane (1966).
56. Albertotti (1917, p. 4). A copy of his thesis is kept by the Manfredi family of Bosco Marengo.
57. Alfieri (1916, p. 406).
58. Certificate issued by Bizzozero on 18 January 1872 (kept by the Manfredi family).
59. Albertotti (1917, p. 5).
60. Manfredi's research protocols are kept by the Manfredi family.
61. Personal interview (3 October 1993) with Manfredi's grandson, Nicolò Manfredi.
62. Golgi (1868).
63. *Ibid.* (1869).
64. *Ibid.* (1869; *OO*, pp. 741ff.).
65. Lombroso (1865 p. 7).
66. Golgi (1869; *OO*, p. 753).
67. *Ibid.* (*OO*, p. 763).
68. *Ibid.* (*OO*, p. 765).
69. Lombroso and Golgi (1873).

70. *Ibid.* (p. 252).

71. Golgi (1869a). The work was summarized in German by M. Fränkel in the *Archiv für patho-logische Anatomie und Physiologie und für klinische Medicin* (1870, **51**, pp. 311–12) and by Boll in *Centralblatt für die medicinischen Wissenschaften* (1870, pp. 504–5). Also summarized in Bizzozero (1877) and Perls (1877, p. 373). A recent citation of this work is found in Liberini and Spano (1995, p. 386).

72. Golgi (1870). The work was summarized in German by M. Fränkel in the *Archiv für patho-logische Anatomie und Physiologie und für klinische Medicin* (1870, **51**, pp. 568–70) and by Boll in *Centralblatt für die medicinischen Wissenschaften* (1871, pp. 356–8).

73. Bizzozero (1868).

74. Golgi (1870; *OO*, p. 847ff.).

75. *Ibid.* (1870a). The work was summarized in German by Boll in *Centralblatt für die medicinischen Wissenschaften* (1870, pp. 534–5).

76. Golgi (1871–72).

77. Deiters (1865, Fig. 10).

78. Golgi (1885, p. 154).

79. *Ibid.* (1871–72; *OO*, p. 21).

80. *Ibid.* (1875; *OO*, p. 903).

81. *Ibid.* (1870a; *OO*, p. 4).

82. Verga (1872, p. 357).

83. *Centralblatt für die medicinischen Wissenschaften* (1872, pp. 321–6). *Jahresberichte über die Fortschritte der Anatomie und Physiologie* (Leipzig: F. C. W. Vogel, 1873, Vol. 1, for the literature of 1872, pp. 125 and 141–2). *Quarterly Journal of Microscopical Science* (1873, **13**, p. 96). Gombault (1873).

84. Boll (1873).

85. Letter from Boll to Golgi, from Berlin, 13 December 1872 (MSUP). See Belloni (1980, p. 417).

86. Golgi (1873–75). In particular, see *Rivista di Medicina, Chirurgia e Terapeutica* (1873, **1**, pp. 413–20).

87. Ranvier (1873). Criticisms of Golgi's and Boll's work can be found also in Debove (1873).

88. Ranvier (1882; 1875–86).

89. Renaut (1882, p. 606).

90. Golgi (1885, pp. 129ff.).

91. Golgi and Manfredi (1872; *OO*, p. 71).

92. Letter from Golgi to Manfredi, 19 [month illegible] 1872 (MSUP).

93. *Centralblatt für die medicinischen Wissenschaften* (1872, pp. 69–70). The work was summarized also by Boll in *Jahresberichte über die Fortschritte der Anatomie und Physiologie* (Leipzig: F. C. W. Vogel, 1873, Vol. 1, for the literature of 1872, pp. 218 and 222).

94. Golgi (1875). The work was summarized in *Rivista di Medicina, Chirurgia e Terapeutica* (1875, **1**, pp. 588–90). Also cited in Bizzozero (1877), Perls (1877, p. 361), and Tamburini and Marchi (1883).

95. Bizzozero (1872).

96. Golgi (1875; *OO*, p. 903).

97. Simon (1874).

98. Golgi (1870b).

99. Certificate issued by the Rector of the University of Pavia on 3 August 1875 (MSUP-I-I-26). Golgi lectured from 27 April 1871 'to the end of the academic year' and from 14 April to the end of May 1872.

100. Pensa (1991, p. 75).
101. The Laboratorio Crittogamico (originally Laboratorio di Botanica Crittogamica) was established with Royal Decree 1871, thanks to the efforts of the botanist Santo Garovaglio. Golgi was one of the first employees of the Laboratorio Crittogamico, which was next to the Laboratory of General Pathology. A plate in the courtyard of the Botanical Garden of Pavia commemorates his hiring. More information can be found in Garovaglio (1872).

5

A small circle of Dante

Golgi's precarious economic situation was especially disheartening for his father, who had made many sacrifices to support him through medical studies and was following the vicissitudes of his son's career with trepidation, worried about his future prospects. On 24 May 1871 Alessandro Golgi wrote to his brother-in-law and cousin Giulio Gioacchino Golgi, who was a civil servant at the Central Treasury Office in Florence:

I have been thinking of writing to you for a while . . . I have postponed from day to day in the hope of being finally able to communicate to you that Camillino had found a permanent position; but the hope of getting him an honourable and stable position seems instead to be fading away, and I can write only that he, Camillino, has obtained permission to give a brief series of lectures at our University . . . for which now he fatigues himself immensely without any material advantage.[1]

Alessandro Golgi began to put strong pressure on his son to find a better professional position and to stop fussing about without concrete economic result. Thus, at the age of 28 Golgi felt obliged to find a secure and well-paid position, even if that meant abandoning all hopes of an academic career and scientific research. It was the moment of tough and potentially irreversible decisions about the future.

On 16 January 1872, an announcement for a position of Chief Physician at the Pie Case degli Incurabili of Abbiategrasso was posted. [2] This was the 'honourable and stable' position that Alessandro Golgi had been wishing for his son. Furthermore, this was the same hospital where he had worked as an Assistant Physician with great personal satisfaction, a place that he left only because he wanted to find a post closer to Pavia. If the position of Assistant Physician had been good enough for him, the position of Chief Physician should be all the more so for his son. So he began to bully his son, who in the end, somewhat grudgingly, agreed to participate in the competition. This took place on 12 and 13 March 1872, and included many candidates, all older than Golgi. The candidates were evaluated on the basis of their scientific training and publications, the clinical examination of a patient, two written essays (one on a medical topic and one on surgical topic), and a post-mortem examination.

On 22 March, the President of the Congregazione della Carità (Charitable Congregation) of Milan, which administered the Pie Case, announced that the position had been awarded to Golgi.[3] But the winner was in no hurry to begin his new activity. On 5 April he presented a petition to the President 'to obtain a delay in the taking up of my duties'[4] in order to give the Mental Hospital of Pavia time to find a substitute. Finally on 1 June 1872 he entered into service at Abbiategrasso. His final decision to leave Pavia was due in part to the absence of Lombroso and the prospect of Bizzozero leaving for Turin, about which Golgi would certainly have been aware.

Alessandro Golgi conveyed the news to his brother-in-law Giulio Gioacchino in a letter of 4 August 1872:

Concerning my family, the only news I have to communicate to you is that Camillino has been recently been appointed Chief Physician in the Pie Case degli Incurabili. His salary is 1900 lire per year, which can be increased by 10% after every five years of service;[5] in addition, within a short time, as soon the building is completed, he will have lodgings and fuel. It is a stable job with the right to a pension after ten years of service and little work, the only obligation being one visit to the patients per day, which usually takes less than one hour. The competition was by exam and therefore he had to go to Milan where, at the Ospedale Maggiore, in the presence of a commission of five of the most renowned doctors, he had to sustain a good many exams, that is, written, orally at the bed of a patient, and on a cadaver. There were many participants, but he was selected despite being the youngest.

Camillino, to tell the truth, was not very keen to enter the competition, but I encouraged him to do so because having been myself in [service at the Pie Case degli Incurabili of] Abbiategrasso, I always regretted very much having left it, even though I was only an Assistant Physician and with a much smaller pay; now it seems that he is not discontented with this decision.[6]

The hospital of Abbiategrasso, founded in 1785 by Joseph II, was housed in the Convent of Santa Chiara; in 1811 it was enlarged with the acquisition of an old Franciscan monastery (Monastero dell'Annunciata), two kilometres away, where the male ward was located. When Golgi arrived to take up his duties the two wards were about to be reunited in the Convent of Santa Chiara, so there was intense reconstruction and enlargement work going on. The hospital complex was stately; in 1872 there were 655 chronic patients, some with free treatment and others who paid a daily rate. There were all sorts of patients: epileptics, patients who had mutilations of both hands or feet, paralytics, patients with rickets and severe deformities of the bones, retarded patients, demented patients, psychotics, 'disgusting ones' (patients afflicted by particularly repugnant deformities), 'irredeemably filthy ones owing to the extrophy of the bladder, uncontrollable prolapses of the uterus, of the vagina, and of the rectal intestine with involuntary loss of faeces',[7] etc. There were, in sum, examples of all of the chronic pathologies, including the most loathsome, and some rooms of the Institute would make one think of a small circle of Dante.

Immediately after joining the hospital staff, Golgi was requested to subscribe to the extremely detailed *Istruzioni ed obblighi dei medici delle PP. CC. degli Incurabili in Abbiategrasso* (Regulations and duties of the physicians of the Pie Case degli Incurabili in Abbiategrasso).[8] As a 'Physician I' he was obliged to reside inside the hospital and be on call at night, and to supervise the female wards. On the staff was another physician, Pio Tragella, who as a 'Physician II' was on duty only during the day and was in charge of the male wards. Both had various other tasks: intake examination of the new patients, 'basic surgery, . . . scheduling of the daily diet and of the patients' activities, . . . writing of the medical prescriptions, . . . certification of deaths' etc. They alternated, doing a week at a time, in inspecting the kitchen and verifying the quality and dietetic value of the food. Other duties included discipline, instruction, supervision of the nursing personnel, and, at the request of the Director, they had to make themselves available to verify the state of health of subordinate personnel who absented themselves from work claiming to be sick. Each month the physicians had to prepare a medical report 'on the wards entrusted to them'. Every three months they had to verify, 'after accurate investigations', which patients 'had again become capable of getting back to work', and thus could be discharged. Another of Golgi's duties was to oversee the pharmacy daily, verifying the quality of medicinal preparations. Special mention was made in the 'Instructions' of the need to maintain correctness in the relationships between the two physicians, so as not to offer a negative example to the staff.

Some weeks after his arrival, Golgi complained of 'slight disturbances' that induced in him 'an intellectual torpor so great' as to inhibit 'completely the possibility of working'.[9] By mid-August, however, he had recovered, although for another two months he dragged himself through his work with 'a shameful inertia'.[10]

Everything suggested that, with his arrival in a small town hospital for chronic patients, Golgi's research activity was about to end for good. There was, however, in Article 86 of the 'Instructions' of the Pie Case, salvation in the form of recognition 'as of special merit for physicians to conduct anatomo–pathological studies'. In addition, Article 15 expressly requested that the physicians report on rare and scientifically interesting cases, perform autopsies, and prepare 'those pathological specimens that present extraordinary alterations', to be kept in special cabinets 'for the care of which the Physician I is responsible'.

But Golgi must have quickly sunk into a bitter disappointment. The Pie Case was nearly completely lacking in scientific instruments and furthermore the administrative Director, a myopic and authoritarian person, was contemptuous of Article 86 and forbade the spending of any money for purposes other than those required for the sanitary care and assistance of the patients.[11] The difficulty was overcome by setting up, in the kitchen of Golgi's small quarters, a laboratory consisting of a microscope and a few other instruments. Here, Golgi, away from the grand centres of research but faithful to his vocation and master of histological techniques, stubbornly continued his research.

Having finished taking care of his patients, he retired to the kitchen of his modest lodgings, which had been transformed into a laboratory, thanks more to his private income than to support from the Hospital, and set about the grand task of studying the mystery of the nerves, of the motor and sensory pathways, those pathways that allow our body and mind to live.[12]

In the speech of 1919, which has already been cited, Golgi remembered this period in the following way:

Trained to work with limited means and rich with the sacred fire of scientific work, despite being somewhat isolated, I found no difficulty in continuing my microscopic research in the rudimentary laboratory organized by me in the kitchen of the small apartment that was assigned to me in the Pio Luogo.[13]

Fortunately, he was helped by the influential Milanese neurologist and psychiatrist Serafino Biffi,[14] a member of the Istituto Lombardo di Scienze e Lettere ed Arti (Lombard

Institute of Sciences and Literature and Arts) who supported Golgi's early research at Abbiategrasso:

And it is at Abbiategrasso that, with the support of the illuminated mind of the eminent medical alienist [psychiatrist] Serafino Biffi of Milan, I presented at the Istituto Lombardo my first communications on the results that I obtained working alone.[13]

As a physician Golgi was extremely conscientious and competent. Having attended Porta's surgical ward, he knew how to carry out small surgical operations, and his proficiency in dermatology, acquired with Scarenzio, allowed him to diagnose and cure the dermatological diseases that frequently afflicted the Incurables, such as scabies (he carried out the microscopic identification of 'the acarus that causes it'[15]). But most useful to him was his background in neuropsychiatry. The Pie Case included, in fact, special sections for epileptics, demented patients, and 'maniacs'. Some of the patients were agitated and violent criminals who, after initial isolation, were transferred to a mental hospital. Among the patients of the male ward was the famous bandit Antonio Gasbaroni, called 'Gasparone', who had terrorized the Papal States, targeting 'the rich, priests, and monks' and the poor if they 'betrayed' him. Captured by the pontifical authorities, he had spent many years of prison in the Fortress of Civitavecchia and in the jails of Spoleto and Civita Castellana, before being transferred to Abbiategrasso.[16]

Despite these assorted duties, Golgi had an abundance of free time (as his father had pointed out to his brother-in-law), which he dedicated almost entirely to study and research. His relationship with the Director of the Institute, however, continued to be troubled. During the three years spent in Abbiategrasso, Golgi repeatedly locked horns with the Director in defence of his rights or those of his patients. The first confrontation occurred when the Director, who applied the rules in a rather rigid manner, tried to impose limitations on Golgi's personal freedom of movement:

the condition of being constantly locked-up in a strange state of isolation, and the curfew that you [the Director] rigorously impose on me if I want to take advantage of free lodgings, is of too great moral damage for me to consider their endurance convenient to me and seemingly to the dignity of my position.

And then Golgi threatened the Director that

if you believe it is impossible for you to take any step directed at removing the too grave conditions cited above, I feel obliged to find as soon as possible other lodgings outside the Pia Casa.[17]

In the end, Golgi made good on his threat and moved for a few months to an apartment near the Castle of Abbiategrasso, at a short distance from the Hospital. Obviously, this represented a source of annoyance for the personnel because if his intervention was necessary during the night someone would have to go and call him. The battle lasted for a year, but in the end the Director yielded and in mid-December 1873 Golgi obtained new lodgings and a key for the entry gate.[18]

Another confrontation between Golgi and the Director concerned the diet of the patients. The regulations of the Incurables required the physicians to check the 'Dietary

Table' of the patients' meals. In the spring–summer of 1875 the Director sent Golgi a communication in which he lamented that in some case 'the patients in the infirmary and in the chronic wards were, on medical orders, administered a special diet in excess of their need; therefore, many patients were selling their food.'[19] And this caused 'a major expense unjustified by the real necessity of a better diet'. The Director therefore requested the opinion of the Chief Physician on a proposal to reduce the daily food of the patients. In response, Golgi wrote a report on the dietetic situation in the Institute, emphasizing how

the quantity of food, especially that of the so-called plastic nutrients (meat, eggs, cheese, etc.) fixed for each patient is already at such a low level that instead of supporting the idea of making changes in the direction of a reduction I am rather led to suggest that at least the amount of plastic foods be substantially increased . . .

On the other hand, I care very little about the fact that some patients sometimes have sold bread, wine, or even meat. In my opinion this represents a small inconvenience, in a certain way inherent to the nature of this hospital . . . but certainly it is not as inconvenient as to authorize the physician to propose restrictive measures.[20]

The report was accompanied by comparative data on the quantity of food expected in some European hospitals, which demonstrated how the amounts allowed at Abbiategrasso were already at a minimal level, and made a concrete proposal for balancing the patients' diet better without further burdening the accounts of the Institute.

Whenever possible, Golgi escaped his intellectual and social isolation in Abbiategrasso by taking periods of leave,[21] which he used to bring himself up to date with the international scientific literature and to visit old friends. He also maintained a lively correspondence with Bizzozero, Manfredi, and their common friend and patron Luigia Robolini Del Majno.

His letter to Manfredi and Bizzozero concerned histological problems and news about the laboratory and the University of Pavia. Thanks to Bizzozero, he had been able to maintain for a few months an official appointment at the University as a member of one of the many *commissioni d'esame* (examining panels that assigned grades at the end of each course).[22] Toward the end of 1872, however, the impending departure of Bizzozero for Turin became known. Golgi expressed his regret to Manfredi:

I am greatly distressed by the departure of a friend and a teacher, but I must confess that I am even more saddened by the fact that, with his departure, dies, for the moment, [unreadable] any hope of resurgence for the University of Pavia, to which I am still very attached.[23]

The transition from Pavia to Turin was far from smooth for Bizzozero. Shortly after his arrival he had managed to obtain two rooms where he organized a small laboratory on the model of the one in Pavia. Unfortunately, his young age and his activism very soon triggered hostility, diffidence, and jealousy in a university composed of academics of the old guard, rigidified in a dull and dogmatic style of teaching. And thus, in less than a year, the use of the rooms had been revoked. 'That which I foresaw has happened', wrote Bizzozero to Golgi in November 1873; 'I have just moved my Laboratory, and now I pass the day at my house. For the moment I am a bit crowded.' Bizzozero was wealthy and could afford a private laboratory. He planned to move into a larger apartment where there would be sufficient space to work without problems. He found the idea enticing: 'I am very content with it because I am much more productive when I work in solitude.' And, thinking of how difficult it was for Golgi to conduct research in Abbiategrasso, he tried to encourage him, writing: 'We will hearten each other through our reciprocal letters.'[24]

In 1873, Golgi was called by the authorities to help fight an epidemic of smallpox.[25] During the second half of the 1800s the incidence of this disease had diminished markedly owing to the widespread use of ever improving vaccination, which became mandatory in 1888. But occasional and limited epidemics could always break out where there was a significant concentration of unvaccinated or badly vaccinated people (revaccination was proving to be particularly effective for preventing the disease), in rural areas where public health structures were poorly organized, and where prejudices against the vaccination were strongest. Although Golgi had been called to work only as a physician, his enthusiasm for research led him to carry out scientific work on the disease. He decided to study the pathological anatomy of the bone marrow of the deceased. This research was timely because it continued the work done a few years earlier by Bizzozero, and subsequently Pio Foà, on the blood-producing function of bone marrow. The epidemic, even if not comparable in size to those of the past, was nevertheless not insignificant. Indeed, Golgi carried out autopsies on 25 cases of haemorrhagic smallpox and 20 of pustular smallpox, and wrote anatomo-pathological reports on the specimens of bone marrow and spleen obtained in the two forms, comparing them with those obtained in a case of petechial typhus. He reported his findings in an important paper [26] published in 1873 in the *Rivista Clinica*.[27]

   This episode illustrates the fact that, from the beginning of his career, Golgi's research interests were not limited to the study of the central nervous system, but were already turning toward other topics, in particular to the study of 'contagious' diseases. Golgi's interest in microbiology was spurred not only by Pasteur's revolutionary discoveries, but also the environment of the University of Pavia. Following in the steps of Agostino Bassi, who had foreseen the involvement of living organisms (*quid vivum*), Pavian physicians had in fact played an important role in the search for the causal agents of infectious diseases. The physician and botanist Carlo Vittadini made the first attempts at *in vitro* culture of the micro-organism causing the disease of the silkworm, a parasite that Giuseppe Balsamo Crivelli subsequently called *Botrytis bassiana* in honour of Bassi (today it is called *Beauveria bassiana*). In the middle of the 1870s one of the students of Collegio Ghislieri, Giovanni Battista Grassi, first noticed the presence of the egg of *Ancylostoma duodenale* in the faeces of affected patients, establishing a sure diagnostic procedure for the identification of the parasite in sick individuals. With the intent of clarifying the modality of development of this worm, Grassi went so far as to swallow infested intestinal excretions. He also subjected himself to swallowing ascaridi from a cat, thus demonstrating that this species cannot survive in the human body, and eggs of human ascarids, concluding that intermediate hosts were not necessary.[28] It has been said that because of these experiments 'one delicate young lady cut short any possible feeling of sympathy for the heroic experimenter!'[29]

Notes

1. MSUP-II-7. In citing the last part of this paragraph Riquier also reports the following statement attributed to Alessandro Golgi without mentioning the source: '[Camillo Golgi] graduated almost seven years ago and gets only the meagre salary of a hospital physician; furthermore, he makes great [economical] sacrifices to publish his works; meanwhile I become old and the burden of my duties grows heavier every day that passes! It cannot continue like this!' (1952, pp. 57ff.)

2. The notice of the competition is conserved in the MGA.

3. The decision was taken by secret ballot, as can be read in the minutes of the meeting Council of the Congregazione della Carità of Milan held on 22 March 1972 (*Archivi Storici delle Istituzioni Pubbliche di Assistenza e Beneficenza*, II.PP.A.B.), reproduced in Viviano (1985, p. 52). For further information see letter from the President of the Congregazione della Carità dated 23 March 1872 (MSUP-I-I-21) and document dated 24 March 1872 (MGA, Protocol No. 299). Golgi obtained 45/50 points as can be seen in the certificate that the Congregazione della Carità released to him on 23 December 1879 (MSUP-I-I-29).

4. Petition presented by Golgi to the directors of the Pie Case degli Incurabili on 5 April 1872 (MGA, Protocol No. 342).

5. In reality, Golgi's pay could be increased by 200 lire after ten years of service as indicated by the '*Istruzioni ed obblighi dei medici delle PP. CC. degli Incurabili in Abbiategrasso*', signed by Golgi (MGA).

6. MSUP-II-7. Reproduced with minor changes in Riquier (1952, pp. 58ff.).

7. Concerning the patients admitted to Abbiategrasso see Viviano (1985, pp. 55–6).

8. In taking up their duties, the doctors had to subscribe to these *Istruzioni*. The copy signed by Golgi the day of his assumption of service (1 June 1872) is conserved in the MGA.

9. Letter from Golgi to Manfredi, 4 August 1872 (MSUP). References to Golgi's state of health are found also in the letter that he sent to Manfredi on 7 August 1872 (MSUP).

10. Letter from Golgi to Manfredi, 6 October 1872 (MSUP).

11. Riquier (1952, p. 59).

12. Belfanti (1926, p. 768).

13. From the speech given on 29 June 1919 at the Fondazione Camillo Golgi-Pro Orfani di Medici. Reproduced in Mazzarello (1993, p. 335).

14. On the figure of Biffi, see Zerbi and Trabattoni (1988).

15. Handwritten diagnosis by Golgi (MGA).

16. On the death of Gasbaroni, Golgi endeavoured to have the cranium of the bandit sent to Lombroso: 'I owe to the courtesy of my illustrious colleague Prof. Golgi, to whom fame and doctrine do not lessen the gentleness of the spirit, my possession of the cranium and photograph of Gasparone, who died in Abbiategrasso at 88 years'; Lombroso (1882, p. 269).

17. Letter from Golgi to the Director of the Pie Case, 23 November 1872 (MGA).

18. The receipt for the keys was signed by Golgi on 14 December 1873 (MGA).

19. Cited in a report by Golgi (see Note 20).

20. Report sent to the Director of the Pie Case, dated 15 July 1875. Conserved at the MGA.

21. In the MGA are conserved two requests for vacations by Golgi. The first one of six days, dated '21 July 1872' was motivated by the desire to visit 'some Lombard cities, for the purpose of hygiene and instruction'.

22. Letter from Golgi to Manfredi, 27 June 1872 (MSUP).

23. Letter from Golgi to Manfredi, 4 October 1872 (MSUP).

24. Letter from Bizzozero to Golgi, 22 November 1873 (MSUP-VII-III-I). Bizzozero main-tained his private laboratory until 1876 (obviously his students had to buy with their own money everything required for their research); then he was finally given four rooms in Via Po 18, in the old convent of San Francesco di Paola, where he established the new Laboratory of General Pathology.

25. Perroncito (1926, p. 16).

26. Golgi (1873).

27. The work was promptly summarized in German by Boll in the *Centralblatt für die medicinischen Wissenschaften* (1874, pp. 103–4), reviewed by Bozzolo in the *Rivista di Medicina, Chirurgia e Terapeutica* (1874, **1**, p. 329), and cited by, among others, Raimondi (1880).

28. Corti (1956, pp. 9ff.; 1961, p. 6).

29. *Ibid.* (1956, p. 1).

6

The black silhouette

On 16 February 1873, Golgi wrote to Manfredi:

I have regained the energy that for a few months I had completely lost. I spend long hours at the microscope. I am delighted that I have found a new reaction to demonstrate even to the blind the structure of the interstitial stroma of the cerebral cortex. I let the silver nitrate react with pieces of brain hardened in potassium dichromate. I have obtained magnificent results and hope to do even better in the future.[1]

Thus, Manfredi was probably the first to learn about the revolutionary discovery that would transform the study of the nervous system. The reference to the 'interstitial stroma' seems to indicate that Golgi had identified mainly glial elements. It did not take him long, however, to realize the great advantage of this method for the study of nerve cells.

In the same letter Golgi asked Manfredi to send him, by the end of that same day, 'a few grams of crystalline silver nitrate in crystals and potassium dichromate' and to immerse the 'brain, cerebellum, and spinal cord, preferably taken from a horse that had just been killed' in a 1% solution of 'ammonia dichromate'. And he continued:

The brain and the cerebellum should be cut in small pieces about 2 cm in diameter, with the adhering pia mater in place. The spinal cord should be cut in short transverse segments. If possible, you should repeat the same procedure using a solution of potassium dichromate . . . You could entrust Garibaldi [perhaps 'Gariboldi'] or Carlo with these encumbrances. Please keep a record of all the expenses, including tips, so I can reimburse you. As soon as you have the pieces ready, please send them over through the same courier. Please forgive me for all these troubles and for the indecent form of this letter. I am writing in a rush . . .

Golgi's impatience to continue his investigations using the 'novel reaction' is palpable.

The 'black reaction' appears, therefore, to have come out of nowhere between the end of 1872 and the beginning of the following year. There is, however, some indirect evidence of the path followed by Golgi in making this discovery.

The study of morphology, as Golgi had come to appreciate while working in Pavia with Bizzozero, was severely limited by the complexity of the nervous system and by the lack of appropriate methods for the differential staining of its various components. As he recalled in the early 1880s, when discussing his beginnings in the field of neurohistology:

Since I believed that to move beyond the results obtained with the usual techniques it was necessary to open new paths using special techniques that would match the special and complex structure of the organs studied, my first concern in attacking the study of the anatomy of the central nervous system was to find new methods that, better than the existing ones, would allow me to broaden the field of investigation and to examine the structure of these organs from a different perspective.[2]

And in his earlier writings on the nature of the glia he wrote:

Because among the supporters of these opposite opinions we find the names of the most skilled and experienced investigators, it is clear that these conflicting results must be largely attributed to differences in the reagents and in the protocols used, and that, therefore, the solution of the remaining problems must be found by modifying the techniques and, possibly, by putting to good use the new reagents that continuously enlarge our technical possibilities in microscopy.'[3]

In that study we find in fact the description of various modifications to the histological techniques then in use. Thus, all evidence indicates that Golgi was in search of new histological techniques well before his arrival in Abbiategrasso.[4] Although not stated explicitly, a number of hints scattered in the papers he wrote when still in Pavia suggest that he was looking for something that could reveal the nervous elements by staining them in black. For example, in discussing the glial processes he remarked that 'in successful preparations, they were of a very dark bronze colour and, therefore, they showed up against the grey background of the finely granular intercellular substance'.[5] Again, writing about the osmic acid, he emphasized its ability to stain 'in deep black the fat and the nervous fibres, and in more or less dark brown the other components'.[6]

During his research in Pavia, and, therefore, well before 1873, he had used, in addition to potassium dichromate, silver nitrate for the study of the perivascular lymphatic spaces:

Is the internal side of the perivascular sheets, like that of the lymphatic vessels in other regions of the body, lined by epithelium? A number of observations I made to address this problem, by using the best microscopic technique available for staining the epithelium, that is, by immersing the vessels, taken fresh from the brain, in a weak solution of silver nitrate (0.20–0.50%), consistently gave negative results. In this respect, I want to emphasize that I did not limit my researches to the vessels of the human brain, because, considering the time that elapses between death and autopsy, it is possible to speculate that a structure as fragile as the epithelium might degenerate and that for this reason only the standard reaction with silver nitrate fails to develop; to eliminate such a doubt, I extended my investigation to the brain of freshly killed ox, calf, and dog.'[7]

Silver nitrate had already been used by histologists because it stained the intercellular substance of the epithelium, endothelium, and connective tissue black or brown. Silver nitrate was also contributing to the rapid development of photographic technique.

Therefore, Golgi had used the two chemical reagents for the black reaction a few years before 1873. Only the sequential actions of these two reagents on pieces of nervous tissue, however, allowed the black reaction to occur.

To understand the fundamental importance of Golgi's work it is essential to examine the histological techniques used for the study of the nervous system before the discovery of the black reaction. At that time the most effective procedure consisted of a first phase in which the tissue was fixed in potassium dichromate, followed by staining with carmine. The crucial step in the development of Golgi's method was to use silver nitrate instead of carmine. The 'fixation' (hardening) of the tissue in potassium dichromate was followed by the 'impregnation' of the nervous elements by silver nitrate. The final result is a preparation in which the silhouette of the nerve cell appears in all its morphological complexity, with a well defined outline and all its ramifications, which could be followed and analysed even at a great distance from the cell body. The great advantage of this technique is that, for reasons that still are unknown, silver nitrate selectively impregnates only a few cells (1–5%), which are stained black, and completely spares other cells, allowing individual elements to emerge from the puzzle. The black reaction permitted a detailed description of the different types of nerve cells and ultimately made it possible to develop a precise microscopic neuroanatomy.

The announcement of the discovery of the new technique was made with a brief and reticent report 'On the structure of the grey matter of the brain', published on 2 August 1873, in the *Gazzetta Medica Italiana-Lombardia*.

The article began:

Using a method that I developed and that allows one to stain in black the elements of the brain, a staining procedure that requires the prolonged immersion of the pieces, previously fixed in potassium or ammonia dichromate, in a 0.5–1.0% solution of silver nitrate, I could discover some facts concerning the structure of the grey matter of the brain, that I think are worthy of being reported.[8]

Benedetto Morpurgo, Professor of General Pathology at the University of Turin and Golgi's friend, wrote, quite emphatically, about this breakthrough:

Golgi used to work on small pieces of brain, hardened in dichromate, and, as was his habit, gathered a great amount of material and tested various reagents, either in the course of special investigations, or simply for training or to verify the findings of others. In the process of studying the histological shapes fixed by chromatic fluids and the selective precipitation of metals, especially of silver nitrate, in the connective substance and in certain portions of the nerve fibres, it occurred to him that new results could be obtained by applying the procedure of metallic impregnation to fixed tissues, and, although neither theoretical reasons nor empirical approaches supported his idea, he tried and then tried again with almost single-minded perseverance. After many unsuccessful attempts, traces of silver impregnation appeared in the brain following prolonged fixation in dichromate, and, finally, he obtained the total impregnation of nerve cells with their processes. He saw the light and, understanding the importance of his discovery, perceived an immense new field of research. Muted, as he had been touched by God's grace, he collected himself in religious fervour to reach the coveted goal. Being, since 1872, a physician in the hospital for the incurables of Abbiategrasso, he was allowed by the circumstances to work undisturbed as in a hermitage, to serve his mission.

With great emotion I remember that period of Golgi's life. Alone, without funds for his research, without the support of colleagues or the advice of teachers, with the little treasure of his microscope, spurred by the confidence in the importance of his discovery and delighted by the results that he was obtaining day after day, he worked in silence for an entire year.[9]

It was certainly in the Pie Case per gli Incurabili that Golgi saw for the first time a nerve cell perfectly outlined with all its processes. All the notes on Golgi published after his death by his students and colleagues, as well as the recollections of his relatives[10] concur in dating the final development of his method back to the Abbiategrasso period. The following autobiographical note is also consistent with this: 'It is in Abbiategrasso that I initiated my research on the fine organization of the central organs of the nervous system.'[11] Furthermore, the letter to Manfredi of 16 February is written with the tone of a person who has just made a discovery.

Antonio Pensa and Piera Locatelli emphasize, however, the importance of his earlier work in Pavia,[12] when Golgi used the two reagents of the black reaction in his research on lymphatic vessels. Pensa and Locatelli propose that Golgi had already developed the method (at least in a primitive form) before his arrival in Abbiategrasso. A dedication to Bizzozero written by Golgi[13] for an anthology of important histological papers on the structure of the nervous system, seems to support this alternative conclusion. Golgi wrote (emphasis added):

My dear friend,
I can state that the studies that I am finally able to publish, in the form of disconnected fragments, *were initiated many years ago in the Laboratory of Experimental Pathology of Pavia,* when it was directed by you, still a youth, with the wisdom of an experienced teacher.

Events in my career, various obligations, other research activities in which I found myself engaged, obliged me to interrupt this research repeatedly and for long periods of time. Regularly, however, I have taken it up again, always receiving inspiration from the sober reserve that was characteristic of you as a scientist in the field of biological sciences, and that you have been able to transfuse to your many disciples.

In publishing these studies, now that I am the director of that same laboratory in which *I began them* as an inexperienced student, necessarily I remember who guided my first steps in histology.

I do not know how to express the feelings that such a recollection elicit in me, other than by begging you to accept my dedication of this work to you. With the patronage of your name, I feel that this volume is being published under the most favourable auspices, and I will be grateful to you for this as well.

Your very affectionate
C. Golgi
From the Laboratory of General Pathology
of the University of Pavia, 1 January 1885

As pointed out by Locatelli, Golgi would not have been able to begin those studies if he had not been in possession of the new technique, a technique that, therefore, should be dated back, at least in its preliminary form, to the period before his arrival in Abbiategrasso.

It is possible to speculate that Golgi attempted to study the endothelium *in situ,* that is, in its relationship with the surrounding brain tissue, and that to achieve this he used, besides 'fresh' tissue (as prescribed by the standard histological procedures), some material that had been previously fixed in potassium dichromate, a reagent much more available than osmic acid. Perhaps some incomplete impregnation caught his attention and from there he began to develop the black reaction.

The Swedish histologist Gustaf Magnus Retzius claimed in his autobiography that the discovery of the black reaction evolved from the silver nitrate staining method that he had already employed in his research on the structure of the *membrana limitans retinae* for his doctoral dissertation, defended in 1871. According to Retzius, Golgi impregnated some tissue fixed in potassium dichromate with the intention of staining the pia mater of the brain using silver nitrate and, lacking fresh material, impregnated some tissue that had already been fixed in potassium dichromate. Noticing that the nervous tissue adhering to the pia mater had been stained, Golgi decided to improve on this serendipitous finding.[14] Retzius' reconstruction is not very different from what we have hypothesized above: the use of silver nitrate on tissue previously fixed in dichromate produced the magic reaction.

It has been claimed that the black reaction was the result of completely fortuitous events, and rumours have been spread that it was the mistake of a servant that led to the contact between a piece of brain fixed in potassium dichromate and silver nitrate. There is no evidence, however, of such an occurrence.

We have seen that Golgi was so strongly motivated to find new histological techniques that he financed his research with his own money,[15] struggling to obtain even the most common reagents, and working alone by candlelight[16] well into the night.[17]

At the beginning of the 1870s Golgi's fertile scientific mind was ready for the discovery of the black reaction. Even if there was a certain degree of serendipity in this discovery, it must be remembered that he was prepared to take advantage of this accident and to follow up on it. The same combination of chance and intuition has been responsible for many other scientific discoveries, such as that of penicillin. This was what Pasteur had in mind when he said that in science, chance favours only well prepared minds. Ottorino Rossi, who was one of Golgi's students, wrote:

The marvellous beauty of the black reaction, which allows even the layman to appreciate the images in which the cell silhouette stands out as if it had been drawn by Leonardo and the fibres dissolve in thinner and thinner ramifications, intertwining with the most sophisticated elegance, led someone to remember Golgi as the lucky discoverer of a staining technique for nervous tissue. On the contrary, Golgi was a great scientist who, owing to his unique intuition, made the right choice among the many contrasting approaches in fashion at that time. He choose a novel approach, decided a strategy to penetrate the secrets of the nervous tissue, the most noble and most mysterious tissue, and, to this end, he forged novel and sharp weapons.[18]

And Perroncito:

Concerning the way in which [the black reaction] was discovered, all who were close to Golgi know that he used to repeat the same phrase: that he developed it by studying, through a long series of attempts, the metallic impregnation of pieces that had been fixed following different procedures . . . that's all.[19]

And Veratti:

whoever is familiar with this method is left to wonder what would have happened if others, endowed with less exceptional powers of intuition and tenacity, had hit, let us assume by pure chance, on the early incomplete examples of the silver impregnation of nerve cells. Even though a fertile seed can fall anywhere, following the whims of a gust of wind, it is the fertility of the ground that will decide whether it would develop into a tree rich in leafy fronds and fruits.[20]

In light of the available evidence we must, therefore, conclude that Golgi's method was not the result of an accident, and that 'it did not come out of the blue, as an armoured Minerva from Jupiter's mind'.[21] It was instead the point of arrival, in Abbiategrasso, of repeated attempts, which had already produced some incomplete results in 1868–70, during the period in which he was extending his research on the lymphatic vessels.

In the first report on his new method, Golgi briefly described some preliminary results obtained by applying the black reaction to different nervous tissues (cerebellum, spinal cord, and cerebral cortex). The most important findings of this paper were reported and commented upon by Golgi himself in the *Rivista di Medicina, Chirurgia e Terapeutica*.[22] An abstract of this study appeared in the *Archivio Italiano per le Malattie Nervose*.[23]

Golgi's brief report belongs to that handful of studies that report on a true scientific breakthrough. If a discovery is too far ahead of its time and is not communicated effectively, it can remain buried for many years, and nobody else, meanwhile, will achieve anything similar. On the contrary, the history of science has repeatedly shown that a problem is mature when many scientists, working independently, hit on the same solution more or less at the same time. A scientific study that is truly original often remains ignored for years. Golgi's paper (and the studies that he published in the following years using the same method) did not escape this rule. The method was published in 1873, but it had to wait for about 15 years before being acknowledged internationally by the scientific community. Further evidence of the intrinsic originality of the black reaction is that during the same period no histologist had been able to obtain anything comparable.

It has often been repeated that the main reason for the scarce international interest in Golgi's work was to be found in the limited circulation of the journal in which it was published, although abstracts of the paper appeared in important international journals.[24] Another factor that might have contributed to its limited impact was probably the lack of illustrations.[25] Furthermore, in that period and in the following years, a great number of new histological methods, often unreliable, were being published. Finally, the description of the nerve cell outlined with the black reaction, and its revolutionary implications, was in radical contrast with the theoretical models of the nervous system then prevailing in neurohistology.

A measure of the incredulity met by the black reaction is provided by Boll's reply to a letter that Golgi sent with the reprint of his 1873 paper, a letter that probably contained some additional technical details not included in the paper. Boll did not hide from his Italian colleague that he had read the study with 'the greatest diffidence and if it were not for his other excellent papers, this feeling would have been even stronger'.[26] He added, however, that (evidently referring to the content of Golgi's letter): 'knowing the detail of your method, I cannot deny that your results might be true, at least in part'. Boll expressed his doubts 'with that freedom that I have always used with my friends, and that is the only one worthy of true scientists'.

The attitude of the young German biologist, who was in the best position to appreciate Golgi's findings, is the best evidence of how difficult it was to accept such a revolutionary discovery.

Significant contributions to neuroanatomy had been made in that period by Theodor Meynert, who had described a number of cortical structures and had analysed in detail the hippocampus, septum pellucidum, supraoptic commissure, olfactory bulb, and various corticofugal projection systems. Other important neuroanatomical studies had been conducted by, among others, the Russian Wladimir Aleksandrovitsch Betz (who in 1874 had described the giant cells of motor cortex named after him), the Frenchman Jules Bernard Luys, Kölliker, and Gudden. It was, however, the black reaction that allowed the passage to the descriptive phase, during which the 'hidden structure' of the central nervous system could be systematically investigated. Neurohistology could fully develop only when Golgi's method had allowed the identification and classification of the nerve cell. Even more important was the leap forward made by microscopic neuroanatomy. It finally became possible to map the position of well characterized cellular nuclei and to investigate the reciprocal connections provided by their axons. 'The period between the end of the nineteenth and the beginning of the twentieth centuries was certainly one of the happiest moments for neuroanatomy, since it saw the solution of problems that had defied for centuries the acumen of scientists, and could rightly be named after Golgi because his work and his method have been the starting point and the generating force of this grandiose movement.'[27] Once its importance was understood, the use of the black reaction became universal, and by the 1890s all important neurohistologists had adopted it. The belief that the black reaction had ushered in a new era in the study of the nervous system is attested to by Kölliker, who divided his neurohistological studies between those conducted with Golgi's method and those conducted with other methods.[28] For a young and uninitiated researcher, observing a slide prepared with the black reaction is a fascinating experience. The neurobiologist Karl Spencer Lashley, talking about why he had became fascinated with the labyrinthine complexity of the brain, was fond of recounting the moment when he, then 17 and a laboratory assistant, found in a box of trash some slides of frog brain stained with Golgi's method, and captured by the beauty of these images he decided then and there to devote himself to 'work out all the connections among the cells so that we might know how the frog works . . . I have never escaped from the problem'.[29]

It has been written that, just as Galileo Galilei was able to find new stars by observing with his telescope any sky region, Golgi was able to find new structures by applying his black reaction to any brain region. Finally, the details of the most complex structure in the universe could be characterized. Golgi, with his revolutionary method, gave birth to a new age in the study of the nervous system, which within few years, thanks to the work of Cajal, Retzius, Kölliker, and other histologists and neurophysiologists, particularly Charles Scott Sherrington, would see the rise of modern neuroscience.

Before analysing in detail the work that Golgi conducted in following years, it is necessary to illustrate what was known about the structure and the physiology of the central nervous system during the period in which Golgi discovered the black reaction.

Notes

1. Letter from Golgi to Manfredi, 16 February 1873 (MSUP).
2. Golgi (1882–85; *OO*, pp. 297ff.).
3. *Ibid.* (1871–72; *OO*, pp. 5ff.).
4. Cimino (1984, p. 312); Corsi (1986, p. 6); Zanobio (1963, p. 184).
5. Golgi (1870a; *OO*, p. 2).
6. *Ibid.* (1871–72; *OO*, p. 14).
7. *Ibid.* (1870; *OO*, p. 814).
8. *Ibid.* (1873a; *OO*, p. 91).
9. Morpurgo (1926, pp. 35ff.).
10. Locatelli (1961a, p. 4).
11. See Golgi's speech given on 29 June 1919 at the Fondazione Camillo Golgi-Pro Orfani di Medici (in Mazzarello, 1993, p. 335).
12. Locatelli (1961a); Pensa (1961).
13. In *Sulla fina anatomia degli organi centrali del sistema nervoso* (Golgi 1885, p. 1; 1886, p. 1). See also *OO*.
14. 'I have learnt from one of Golgi's assistants that the so-called Golgi's method had been invented quite unexpectedly while Golgi was trying to replicate an experiment by Key and myself involving the silver staining of the inner layer of the pia mater (which Key and I called intima piae). In using material that had been hardened in potassium dichromate, he fortuitously saw in the neighbouring brain tissue isolated nerve cells stained in dark brown. This led him to develop his method, using silver, and later mercury-silver solutions, on material hardened in dichromate, which allowed him to stain individual nerve cells and their extensions in brown' (Retzius, 1948, p. 145). See also Afzelius (1980, p. 684).
15. Belfanti (1926, p. 768).
16. Veratti (1926, p. 2).
17. *Gazzetta Medica Italiana* (1902, p. 435); Bovero (1926); Chorobski (1936); Da Fano (1926); Ferraro (1953).
18. Rossi (1927, p. 13).
19. Perroncito (1926, p. 14).
20. Veratti (1926, p. 3).
21. Bovero (1926, p. 5).
22. Golgi (1873a).
23. *Archivio Italiano per le Malattie Nervose* (1873, 10, pp. 275–81).
24. Summarized by Boll in *Centralblatt für die medicinischen Wissenschaften* (1873, 51, pp. 806–7); *Jahresberichte über die Fortschritte der Anatomie und Physiologie* (Leipzig: F. C. W. Vogel, 1875, Vol. 2, pp. 55, 59, 135, 144). *Quarterly Journal of Microscopical Science* (1874, **14**, p. 195). See also Majno (1994).
25. Shepherd (1991, p. 90).
26. Letter by Boll (from Neubrandenburg) to Golgi, 4 September 1873 (MSUP) in response to Golgi's letter of 30 August 1873, enclosing a reprint of 'Sulla struttura della sostanza grigia del cervello' (Belloni 1980, pp. 418ff.).
27. Veratti (1942–43, p. 99).
28. Kölliker (1899, pp. 227 and 233).
29. Quoted in Beach *et al.* (1960, p. xvii).

7

Neurohistology and neurophysiology before the 'black reaction'

The notion that vegetables and animals are made of cells is relatively recent. In 1665 Robert Hooke reported the presence of 'cellular' structures in vegetables and soon afterwards Antony van Leeuwenhoek and Marcello Malpighi made analogous but more precise observations in animal and vegetable tissues. For many years, however, the importance of these discoveries was not fully recognized. In 1781 Abbot Felice Fontana glimpsed the internal structures of the cell, the nucleus and nucleolus, but it was Robert Brown, the discoverer of Brownian motion, who in 1831 recognized the nucleus as an essential part of the living cell.

Only in the first half of the nineteenth century were all these findings integrated into the grand 'paradigmatic' generalization of Theodor Schwann and Matthias Jacob Schleiden, the propounders of the cell theory. During a meeting in 1837 they reached the conclusion that the elementary constituents of various animal and vegetable tissues were cells, substantially similar in structure but diverse in form and function. The cell thus came to constitute the fundamental unit of life and the principal factor in its development. The cell theory enunciated in 1839 was further elaborated by Virchow, who also emphasized its relevance to pathological phenomena.

There was, however, one kind of tissue for which an anatomical–functional interpretation based on the cell theory encountered serious problems: nervous tissue. This was due in part to the fact that the study of nervous tissue presented additional problems relative to other tissues. Because of its 'softness' and fragility, nervous tissue was difficult to handle and unsuitable for dissection and slicing, and it was particularly susceptible to deterioration. But the greatest problem of all was its structural complexity, which could not be easily reduced to models derived from the cell theory.

In 1664, the English physician Thomas Willis, to whom we owe the introduction of the term 'neurology', described, in his *Cerebri anatome*, a number of brain structures including the corpus striatum, the mammillary bodies, and the thalamus, and he emphasized the differences between grey and white matter. The structural organization of the nervous tissue remained, however, a mystery.

The first attempt at microscopic investigation of nervous tissue was carried out by Malpighi in 1685. He first dissociated the brain in layers by boiling in hot water, and then stained these layers with ink. He observed artifactual formations consisting of clusters of small spheres and reached the conclusion that the brain was of glandular nature. In 1718, van Leeuwenhoek believed that he had identified a peculiar structure in the nervous tissue, that is, bundles of 'vessels' that made up the nerves. During the entire eighteenth century only a few isolated researchers sporadically engaged in microscopic investigations. One of these was the Abbot Fontana,[1] who studied and characterized nervous fibres and glimpsed axons and the myelin sheath. This paucity of studies was due to a technical problem: the chromatic aberrations typical of the instruments of the time, which at high magnifications prevented satisfactory images. Furthermore, there were no adequate techniques for preparing the tissues, which were simply dissociated in water, compressed between two sheets of glass, and then placed under the microscope. It is not surprising, therefore, that the findings obtained under these conditions were full of artifacts and irreproducible, and that neurohistology could not develop because of the lack of a common ground for scientific comparison and discussion. Microscopic studies of the time abounded in illusory images, 'filamentary−reticular−globular',[2] which did not correspond to any real tissue structure.

This situation changed abruptly in the 20 years after 1820, with the invention of the first achromatic microscope. Rapid technical progress was made in the 1830s and 1840s with the development of appropriate methods for hardening tissue with solutions of chromic acid and its salts. These advances were due especially to the Danish scientist Adolph Hannover, and to Jan Evangelista Purkinje who invented a forerunner of the microtome for cutting thin sections of tissue. In 1842 Benedikt Stilling introduced frozen serial sectioning, done freehand, followed by three-dimensional reconstruction of the spatial relationships of cellular pools (which he called 'nuclei'). At the beginning of 1860s a new microtome was used by Wilhelm His Sr to study the development of an entire embryo, but only in the 1870s and 1880s would several kinds of freezing microtome be introduced. An instrument capable of cutting mechanically guided serial sections had to wait until 1884.[3]

Furthermore, new staining methods based on carmine and chloro-gold allowed, for the first time, the identification of different components of the tissues. Partial nerve cell isolation was obtained by different histologists from macerated nervous tissue blocks. Their procedure involved the immersion of samples in potassium dichromate or chromic acid solutions followed by dissection of single motor nerves using needles under the microscope. This method could be applied only to the largest nerve cells and displayed the cellular bodies and the proximal segments of axons and dendrites. Inevitably, at a certain distance the processes were mechanically broken.

The technical improvements achieved after the 1830s made it possible to conduct meaningful investigations on nervous tissue. The body (soma) of the nerve cell was characterized through the efforts of René Joachim-Henri Dutrochet, Christian Gottfried Ehrenberg (who in 1833 coined the term *Ganglienkugeln*, ganglionic globe), Gabriel Gustav Valentin, and Purkinje. The latter, at a congress of German physicians and naturalists held in Prague in 1837, described the large nerve cells of the cerebellum that carry his name and described the processes that were later called dendrites (the existence of which had been envisioned the year before by Valentin). Purkinje also glimpsed a different type of process but was unable to demonstrate the relationship between it and the nervous fibres in which it continues. The nervous fibres previously studied by Abbot Fontana were further investigated in Purkinje's laboratory by his pupil Joseph F. Rosenthal who in 1839 coined for them the term 'Achsencylinder' ('axis cylinder' or cylindraxis); the term axon was introduced only in 1896 by Kölliker.

Other fundamental studies of the structure of the nervous system were published in those years. Extremely important was the work of Robert Remak who distinguished between myelinated and unmyelinated fibres of the sympathetic nervous system, and demonstrated that fibres of the motor roots of the spinal cord emerge as processes from the nerve cells of the anterior horns. Similar conclusions were reached by Hannover, Wagner, Helmholtz, and Kölliker.

Despite all methodological and technical advances, however, attempts at reconstructing a three-dimensional structure of the nervous tissues were frustrated by the impossibility of determining the exact relationships amongst soma, dendrites, and nervous fibres in the various neuronal populations of the nervous system. That is, the histology of the nervous tissue had been sketched, but there was no microscopic anatomy. The confusion was compounded by Virchow's discovery of the 'nervous cement' or neuroglia, concerning the nature of which, as we have already seen in Chapter 4, there was great disagreement among neurohistologists.

As Golgi would write 20 years later, 'The finest results that could be obtained [in histology] with the means available at the time'[4] were those of the histologist Karl Deiters, published posthumously in 1865, two years after his death from typhus at the age of 29. Deiters had been a student of Virchow and of Max Schultze, under whose direction he had undertaken a thorough histological and anatomical study of the nervous system, using chromic acid and potassium dichromate as fixatives, and carmine as a stain. In addition Deiters dissected individual single motor units from the spinal cord of the ox. At his death he left an unfinished manuscript, later published by Schultze, in which he offered a detailed characterization of the glia and described of a number of brain structures, including the lateral vestibular nucleus, later called Deiters' nucleus. One of the highlights of his book was the description of the nerve cell ('ganglion cell') of which he had personally made beautiful drawings.[5] Deiters maintained that, like the cells of the other tissues, nerve cells were made of protoplasm containing a roundish vesiculated nucleus, which, in turn, contained a nucleolus. Two types of processes originated from the cell body. The first type corresponded to the protoplasmic process (so called because it contained a granular or pigmented extension of the protoplasm; the term 'dendrite' would be introduced only in 1889 by Wilhelm His Sr), which, in most cases, branched dichotomously down to their finest endings and then presumably dissolved in the fundamental intercellular ('porous') substance. The second type of process (of which there was only one per nerve cell) was the nerve process or axis cylinder process (now called axon) which originated from an implantation cone (now called the axon hillock) and which, for Deiters, was never branched. The nerve process also contained granular protoplasm at its origin, but moving away from the cell body it became rigid and hyaline, light-refracting and insensitive to reagents. Its size was proportional to that of the cell body from which it originated, and at a distance approximately equal to the diameter of the soma it first decreased in size and then expanded again, entering a cylindrical medullary sheath (hence the term 'axis cylinder'). In addition to this nerve process, Deiters described another system of

This reticulum represented an essential element of the grey matter and provided a system of anatomical and functional connections among the nerve cells, a protoplasmic *continuum*. Furthermore, from this reticulum nerve fibres would originate.

Not all nerve fibres, however, would have originated in this way. Indeed, Gerlach acknowledged that, as argued by Deiters, in some cases (for example in the cells of the anterior horn of the spinal cord) the nerve process could directly give rise to the cylindraxis. He supposed, therefore, that there were two types of nerve cells. The first type was connected exclusively with the protoplasmic reticulum through its protoplasmic processes, whereas the second type was connected to both the reticulum and a nerve process.

While the second type of cells would provide, at least in the spinal cord, the neurophysiological substrate of reflex actions (because they were directly connected to the muscles), the first type would provide the substrate for automatic actions. With this interpretation Gerlach offered a neuroanatomical model for the physiological explanation of motor mechanisms.[12]

Gerlach summarized his theory in a chapter on the spinal cord written for the celebrated histology treatise edited by Salomon Stricker.[13] Owing to the widespread international success of Stricker's treatise, the theory of protoplasmic reticulum (dendritic reticulum) remained permanently and almost exclusively associated with Gerlach's name, despite the fact that he had only expanded on earlier models (in particular that of Kölliker).[14]

In the early 1870s a number of studies were carried out in an attempt to verify (and possibly reconcile) the different theoretical models of the nervous system.[15] Particularly important was the work of Boll, who substantially confirmed Gerlach's theory[16] and thus contributed to its success, and the work of Victor Butzke, a Muscovite at the Institute of Pathological Anatomy of Bonn, who maintained that the characteristic feature of the nerve cell was the fibrillary nature of the cell body and its processes. These processes, branching out in ever finer ramifications, would finally give rise to extremely slender endings which were the direct continuations of fibrils. The connections among these thin endings was provided by a fine, irregularly distributed reticulum.[17]

While the neuroanatomists were engaged in speculating on the three-dimensional structure of the nervous system, the physiologists were sketching the first diagrams and circuits that could account for the propagation of nerve excitation, which was thought to be electrical in nature.[18] The controversy about 'animal electricity', which had raged at the end of the 1700s between the followers of Galvani and Volta, had concluded with the triumph of Volta's ideas, thanks to his invention of the electric battery. The new discoveries of electrophysiology, however, were lending support to some elements of Galvani's theory.[19] In 1840 Carlo Matteucci had demonstrated the presence of constant currents between the surface of a muscular fibre and its cut extremity.[20] A few years later Emil du Bois-Reymond extended these observations to the peripheral nerves and identified the 'negative electrical oscillation', which represented the first report of what would later be known as the action potential. In 1850 Helmholtz was able to measure the velocity of transmission of an action potential in the sciatic nerve of the frog, showing that motility was not the immediate expression of voluntary activity but rather depended on a measurable biophysical phenomenon.[21] These discoveries, occurring in parallel with the development of the telegraph, suggested a comparison between the functions of the nervous centres and a network of telegraphic lines. Following completely different approaches, both anatomy and physiology were emphasizing the importance of the neural network over that of the individual nerve cells.

In fact, all the neuroanatomical models discussed above (above all the syncytial model of Gerlach, the most successful of them) represented a violation of the cell theory. On the other hand, the unique structure and function of the nervous system could well admit an infringement of the general rule. The physiological consequence of this approach was that brain processes would have to be considered the result of *unitary action* of a number of brain regions in direct anatomical and functional connection by means of anastomoses. The various reticular theories, but also Rindfleisch's hypothesis, were framed in a 'holistic' conception of the nervous system descending from the ancient Galenic hypothesis of a morphological–functional continuity in cerebral matter, and represented a cellular version of the fundamental continuity (*synécheia*) that Galen attributed to the nervous system.[22]

In the first half of the nineteenth century the major proponent of this 'holistic' conception of brain functions was Pierre Flourens. He was one of the first to carry out a series of 'mechanical' manipulations (particularly ablations, but also sectioning, slicing and cutting, very superficial pricking, puncturing, pinching, etc.) on portions of the central nervous system, especially of pigeons, in order to determine whether they were responsible for particular functions, as indicated by the loss or alteration of the function. With this method, he distinguished five fundamental parts of the nervous system, with each of which was associated its own particular 'class of functions'.[23] In the posterior tracts of the spinal cord he localized sensory functions; in the anterior roots and in the anterior half of the spinal cord, motoric functions; in the medulla oblongata, the 'principle of life' (Flourens was one of the first to identify the centres of respiration); in the cerebellum, the coordination of movements; and in the cerebral lobes, 'intelligence' (psychic activity). But his technique of ablating the cerebral lobes layer by layer led to the weakening and then disappearance of both intellectual and perceptual faculties simultaneously. On the basis of these results he concluded that the cortex functions in a unitary, global manner as an organ 'of intelligence', rejecting therefore any hypothesis of the localization of single psychosensory functions in particular cortical areas. In essence, the theory of Flourens recalled the dualistic hypotheses of Descartes (whom he took great pleasure in citing) of mind and body: *res extensa* and *res cogitans*, except that the cerebral cortex replaced the pineal gland as the site where sensory stimuli were transformed into ideas and then into movements.[24]

This conception was in complete opposition to the one propounded at the beginning of the nineteenth century by the phrenologists Franz Joseph Gall and Johann Caspar Spurzheim. According to phrenology, not just single psychic functions but also personality traits were localized in particular regions of the brain. The phrenologists' master plan was to draw a cerebral cartography of mental activities. They also believed that the development or regression of a cortical area would produce 'bumps' or depressions, respectively, in the overlying skull. From this came the idea that by palpating the skull one would be able to deduce the personality and the psychic characteristics of the person.

The idea that psychic faculties were localized was, however, antecedent to phrenology. In antiquity, for example, the cerebral ventricles had been assigned different psychic functions, and in the *Margarita Philosophica* of Gregor Reysch one finds a woodcut showing the ventricular localization of the faculties 'of the mind'. But in general the idea that the brain might be the seat of psychic functions encountered strong opposition, also because for a long time it was thought that the *res cogitans* might be localized in the heart. And even when it became clear that the brain was implicated in psychic functions the approach was to identify a zone that would serve as a unitary 'interface' between the brain and the *res cogitans* (as indeed the pineal gland was for Descartes), rather than distribute the single functions among various cerebral areas.

After the excesses of the phrenologists, a more rigorous version of cerebral 'localization-ism' was propounded and tested experimentally by Panizza, Paul Broca, Fritsch, Hitzig, and David Ferrier[25] and, in the twentieth century, by entire disciplines such as neuro-psychology and clinical and experimental neurophysiology.

It is clear that the reticular hypotheses of the first two-thirds of the nineteenth century were in perfect agreement with Flourens' holistic theory.[26] The atmosphere changed rapidly following the discovery by Paul Broca of the motor centre of language, a discovery that, although made public at the end of 1861, became influential only after 1870. Further impulse to the diffusion of cerebral localizationism was provided by the studies of Ferrier, Fritsch and Hitzig. When Golgi initiated his histological studies, however, the *Zeitgeist* was still favourable to a holistic conception of nervous system functions. In microanatomy, in particular, the prevailing models were all based on an almost dogmatic acceptance of the continuity among the ganglion cells and had not yet been reconciled with the cell theory. To change this situation it was necessary to clarify the fine structure of the nervous system.

Notes

1. Zanobio (1959).
2. *Ibid.* (1960; 1971).
3. Bracegirdle (1978); Shepherd (1991).
4. Golgi (1885, p. 20).
5. Deiters (1865).
6. Shepherd (1991, p. 47).
7. Schultze (1868; 1871).
8. Buchholz (1863).
9. Kölliker (1867).
10. Rindfleisch (1872).
11. Golgi (1875a).
12. Gerlach (1872). See also Golgi (1875a).
13. Stricker (1869–72). The Gerlach chapter was published in 1971 (Vol. II, pp. 665–93).
14. Shepherd (1991, p. 65).
15. Golgi (1875a).
16. Boll (1873).
17. Butzke (1872).

18. Shepherd (1991, pp. 30ff.).
19. Brazier (1958, p. 218); Gigli Berzolari (1993, p. 264); Pera (1986, p. 188).
20. Moruzzi (1973).
21. Cimino (1984, p. 52); Shepherd (1991, p. 31).
22. According to Galen, the peripheral nerves, the spinal cord, and the brain formed a morphological *continuum* that constituted an adequate substrate for perception and movement. These anatomo-functional concepts are discussed especially in *De Placitis Hippocratis et Platonis* (English edition: *On the doctrines of Hippocrates and Plato*, Book V and VII, P. De Lacy (ed.), Akademie-Verlag, Berlin, 1980; see especially pp. 445–59) and in *De usu partium corporis humani* (English edition: *On the usefulness of the parts of the body*, M. T. May (ed.), Cornell University Press, Ithaca, 1968, pp. 88–9, 392–423, 438–56, 682–708, *passim*). See also Lain Entralgo (1949, p. 135).
23. Cimino (1984, p. 171).
24. The holistic hypothesis of Flourens was taken up again in the second half of the nineteenth century by Friedrich Leopold Goltz, by Golgi, and in the twentieth century by Karl Lashley. The latter proposed the laws of 'mass action'and 'equipotentiality'on the basis of studies conducted in the rat. The first law held that the deficits caused by a cortical lesion depend only on the extent of the lesion. The law of equipotentiality states that the precise localization of the lesion bears no relationship to the behavioural performance (Lashley 1929; Beach *et al.* 1960). In reality, Lashley was much more reductionistic than might be apparent from these two laws. Incidentally, it should be remembered that, starting in 1970, a dualistic/interactionist version of the *mind—body problem* was developed by the neurophysiologist John Eccles. According to this conception, shared in part by the philosopher Karl Popper, the 'self-conscious mind' (an entity distinct from matter) interacts in a unitary manner with particular areas of the neocortex. Eccles' theory attempts to update the legacy of Cartesian dualism, rendering it compatible with the inescapable neurophysiological and neuropsychological reductionistic approach of modern neuroscience.
25. Among the works on the history of neurobiology that discuss the cerebral localizationism in the context of nineteenth-century science, those by Soury (1892; 1899) must be particularly mentioned.
26. Cimino (1984, p. 323).

8

Finding a way out of the labyrinth

Golgi remained at the Pie Case of Abbiategrasso until the end of 1875, a three-year period that was fundamental for his scientific growth. Armed with his new method, he now entered an immense new field of investigation, an enormous labyrinth to explore.

One of the more surprising aspects of his 1873 paper in the *Gazzetta Medica Italiana* is the cautious and vague description of the new method. There is no information about the duration of exposure to the two reagents, the optimal temperature, or how to prepare the tissues. However, Golgi had presented his study as a 'preliminary report'. The brevity of the methods section can be explained in part by the fact that in this early phase he was still unable to master satisfactorily the black reaction and therefore could not be precise about the optimal procedure. Two years later, in evaluating various techniques for the study of the nervous system, he wrote (italics added):

Because my method, among all others, is the one that has provided the best results (its use allowed me to stain in black the cells, or the nerve fibres, or the connective cells, or a combination of these elements, by making specific changes in the procedure), I want to mention very briefly in this note the procedures required to perform it, *with the premise, however, that I am still unable to provide with absolute precision the necessary procedures to obtain the best results. These are still partly determined by chance.*[1]

On the other hand, the importance of his first results mandated their preliminary publication.

As discussed in the previous chapter, the prevailing model of the nerve cell in the early 1870s was the one proposed by Deiters, in which the cylindraxis had no ramifications. Golgi discovered that, contrary to the opinion of Deiters, secondary ramifications branched off the cylindraxis, giving rise to a complex system of subdivisions distributed throughout the grey matter.

Beginning with O. Deiters, who, generalizing what he had observed in the spinal cord, was the first to affirm that, among the many processes of the nerve cells, one, called by him nerve process or *cylinder axis,* had unique characteristics and special functional relevance, because it continued directly into a nerve fibre; continuing with [Alexei Jakowlewitsch] Koschennikoff, who reportedly confirmed Deiters' conclusion; and down to Butzke and Boll, who most recently investigated this problem and who also claimed to have seen the direct continuation of the *cylinder axis* in a nerve fibre, all agreed that this process remains always undivided. Contrary to this unanimous opinion, I maintain that the process mentioned above, instead of remaining simple, gives rise to a great number of ramifications, which also branch out, producing a complex system of threads diffused throughout the grey matter of the brain.[2]

Before the discovery of the black reaction, neurohistologists had distinguished the nerve process from the protoplasmic processes due to the apparent absence of ramifications. On the basis of his new findings, Golgi concluded that this was no longer possible and, instead, he proposed a new criterion:

The presence of ramifications, far from abolishing the difference between the nerve process and protoplasmic processes, which are known to branch off in the most complex manner, provides a more definitive criterion for discriminating the two kinds of processes; that is, the manner in which the neural process branches off is so peculiar that it can be considered as one of its most distinctive characteristics; indeed, its secondary branches consistently depart at a right angle, and their appearance, their trajectory, and their manner of branching off are identical to that of the neural process; as for their direction, they run horizontally, sometimes for a short, sometimes for a long distance, then they turn upward reaching the periphery of the cortex, where they can be followed at a great distance from the cells from which they had originated. The branches of third and fourth order behave exactly in the same way. There is no better comparison for the manner of branching and for the general appearance of these filaments than the manner of distribution of the peripheral nerves, especially of the corneal nerves; it appears to me that this might have some relevance for the study of the physiological role of these filaments.[3]

Contrary to Deiters' opinion that the nerve process always continued into a nerve fibre in the white matter, Golgi discovered that in many instances the cylindraxis branched off in minute fibrils at a short distance from its origin. This discovery would be used later for the classification into Golgi Type I and Type II neurons (with long or short cylindraxis, according to Cajal[4]). The distinction between these two types of cells represented a great theoretical contribution by Golgi to the neurosciences because it made it possible to elaborate the concepts of local and long-distance circuitry. The different physiological role of these two types of neurons is indicated also by their different ontogenesis, since the Type II cells develop later at all levels of the nervous system.[5]

I believe that I can immediately challenge the prevailing opinion that it [the nerve process] always continues into the cylinder axis of myelinated nerve fibres, and at any rate this is not the general rule. The presence of its ramifications and progressive thinning is sufficient to invalidate the said opinion.[6]

In the second part of his study Golgi reported briefly on his earlier discoveries concerning the morphology of the protoplasmic processes, discoveries that were as original as those concerning the nerve process.

As we have seen in the previous chapter, the prevailing models of the structure of the nervous tissue were those proposed by Gerlach, who hypothesized the presence of anastomoses between protoplasmic processes, and by Rindfleisch, who thought that both the protoplasmic processes and the nerve processes ended in the interstitial granulo–fibrous substance. Golgi objected to both Gerlach's and Rindfleisch's model:

Another series of findings that I have been able to obtain thanks to my method concerns the characteristics of the so-called protoplasmic or ramified processes.

Among the various opinions concerning this topic, I mention here only those of Rindfleisch and Gerlach, which are very similar to each other. The former holds that the protoplasmic processes, after having branched in a series of extremely thin fibrils, would dissolve in the interstitial granular substance (diffuse nervous substance in the old conception of Wagner, Henle, etc.), and that also the *cylinder axis* of many myelinated fibres would end, after having likewise branched in a series of extremely thin fibrils, in the same substance. Gerlach, and recently also Butzke, Boll, and others, think instead that the protoplasmic processes, subdividing indefinitely in filaments, give rise to a neural reticulum *so fine that it could be demonstrated only with the strongest immersion methods*; bundles of filaments from this reticulum would originate the cylinder axes of the nerve fibres, and this would result in a continuous reticulum between the latter and the protoplasmic processes.

Also on this last point I must disagree with the above cited observers.

The protoplasmic processes, rather than subdividing indefinitely, either to end in the fundamental amorphous substance (Rindfleisch) or to give rise to a reticulum (Gerlach), end instead, when at the level of the third or more often the fourth order of ramification, on the cells of the interstitial tissue . . .[7]

Concerning the functional meaning of the cells on which the protoplasmic processes end, two other considerations can be made: either they serve to establish the anatomical continuity between nerve cells, or they are nutritional organs for these cells. It seems to me that it is not appropriate to relate here the arguments in favour of one or the other hypothesis; I would only note that I favour the second one, all the more so because it allows us to explain also the phenomena of functional connectivity, which, until recently, were thought to be explainable only by admitting the direct connection or anastomosis among protoplasmic processes. And indeed if, as in fact it is, the excitation, even psychic, of the brain nerve cells does result in an alteration of nutrition, that is, in acceleration of the processes of reduction and an increase in the absorption of nutrients, it appears likely that when a group of cells is excited there occur modifications in which other groups of cells participate, the roots of these latter cells taking nutrition from the same sources and probably being influenced by the same nutritive nervous filaments.[8]

Golgi not only denied that the protoplasmic processes could 'dissolve' in the interstitial granulo-fibrous substance, he also, most importantly, found no evidence for the anastomoses hypothesized by Gerlach. The relationship that these processes established with the cells of the interstitial tissue led him to think that they could play a role in the nutrition of the nerve cells.

The fact that Golgi was unable to observe the anastomosis between the protoplasmic processes had important implications for the development of his reticular theory. At the time it was thought that reflex actions required the 'fusion' of the processes of the nerve cells. Flourens' holistic neurophilosophy, of which Golgi was an advocate, was another powerful reason to think that the nerve cells were connected in a sort of syncytium. These theoretical assumptions led Golgi to locate these anastomoses at the level of the newly discovered ramifications of the nerve process. The complexity of the axonal ramifications of neighbouring cells in some preparations, especially from the cerebellum, made this speculation appear more as a 'positive fact' than a simple hypothesis. On the other hand, other prominent histologists had previously proposed the existence of anastomosis on the basis of even flimsier experimental evidence. In truth, the knowledge at the time was compatible with an explanation of reflex mechanisms on the basis of 'electric' transmission, an explanation that did not require anatomical continuity between nervous cells. Indeed, it would have been possible to hypothesize that electric current could 'jump' from a cell to a neighbouring, though unconnected, cell, discharging like a condenser once a threshold potential had been reached. A number of phenomena, including a century-old parlour game called the 'electric kiss', suggested this possibility. The pioneering work of Galvani first, and of Matteucci, du Bois-Reymond, and Helmholtz later, had demonstrated the importance of electricity in nerve physiology. However, until the end of the 1880s, the most obvious explanation for the transmission of electricity still required the anatomical continuity between nerve cells.

Following this line of reasoning, Golgi 'tried' to find a formulation that would account for his discoveries of the ramification of the axon and of the connections between dendrites and connective cells. This led to the doctrine of the *rete nervosa diffusa* (the diffuse neural net), as it would be called later. The dogma of the 'unity of action' in the central nervous system required (and, at the same time, was supported by) the physical continuity between nerve cells. This 'holistic option'[9] would influence all of Golgi's neurohistological work.

A hint of the diffuse nervous net theory can be seen as early as the first work with the black reaction:

. . . in addition, I could observe, albeit rarely, that the process in discussion behaved differently; in a few isolated cases I saw the process entering other filaments, identical to it, that ran obliquely downwards or horizontally.[6]

And few lines below, more explicitly:

I must also mention that I have found some evidence for the existence of anastomoses between the nervous filaments originating from the nerve process of the cylinder axis of several ganglion cells. If confirmed, this finding might have important implications for the physiology of the nervous system. And it is certain that in the cortex, and in the grey matter in general, one can observe a diffuse system of filaments reciprocally anastomized, which, because of their appearance, trajectory, manner of ramification, and connection with the granules, are identical to the filaments whose origin from the Deiters' process [that is, axon] of the ganglion cells can be easily ascertained.[10]

It appears, therefore, that Golgi was unconsciously conditioned by the scientific and cultural models with which he was imbued. The nervous cells 'must' be reciprocally anastomized, and if this was not the case for the protoplasmic processes, it had to be the case for the newly discovered ramifications of the nerve process.

Nevertheless, it is obvious in even the earliest of his papers that, contrary to the biased remarks by some of Cajal's biographers,[11] Golgi had immediately understood the importance of the black reaction:

right from his first paper, one can understand that he had immediately grasped the implications of the new method, and it is striking that such a modest man, who had always resorted to circumlocutions to refer to himself, used over and over: 'I found a method . . . with the method I have found'.

He must have been deeply satisfied by this new tool to emphasize that 'I' with such a delight and firmness.[12]

Golgi would stress again the relevance of his discovery from a historical perspective in an important review article published in 1875 in the *Rivista Italiana di Freniatria e Medicina Legale*, a journal founded by Carlo Livi, Augusto Tamburini, and Enrico Morselli, and of which Golgi, because of his growing reputation, had became an editor.

I think that an entirely new phase in the study of the fine neuroanatomy of the central nervous system has been opened by the findings that I have recently published. In the same way the phase initiated by Gerlach was characterized by Gerlach's development of the chloro-gold method, the present new phase could be said to have been ushered in by the silver nitrate method or black reaction (staining with silver nitrate of pieces hardened in dichromate) that I discovered.

It is interesting that the more the field advances the more the intimate relationship between chemistry and microscopic technique becomes clear. It could even be said that in our time histological discoveries are the result of the discovery of some new reactive or of the special effects of a reactive on the various elements and tissues.

I maintain that my method, based on the sequentially combined action of potassium dichromate and silver nitrate, is one of the most precious methods available in microscopy, and I believe that it is destined to play an important role in the solution of the problems that continuously emerge in the study of the central nervous system.

In the meantime, because of the results already obtained with this method, we must modify a number of assumptions that until now have been held as dogmas. In addition, we can say that by using this method we have rapidly and easily solved some of the problems that had so far defied the ingenuity of investigators.[13]

The period at Abbiategrasso was characterized also by other activities besides research. In addition to his duties as a physician, which did not take much time ('having the obligation of no more than one visit [to the wards] per day, a visit that usually lasts less than one hour'),[14] Golgi performed post-mortem examinations (averaging two autopsies a month, except during smallpox epidemics), which also provided some of the specimens for his research. In the spring of 1873, Golgi was a substitute for ten days for the municipal doctor of Morimondo, a neighbouring village, in exchange for a 'meagre reward'.[15] At the end of 1874 he was elected member of the Health Council for the Abbiategrasso district. By now 'he had acquired a good reputation' in the area around Abbiategrasso and he could have made money 'if he had not all too often refused to practise privately in order to keep from being distracted from his beloved histological studies', as Alessandro Golgi wrote to his brother-in-law.[16] Indeed, most of Golgi's time was spent at the microscope in his small home laboratory. Histology had became his mistress.

Golgi was also engaged in intense editorial activity. Between 1873 and 1875 he published in the *Rivista di Medicina, Chirurgia e Terapeutica* his reviews of the most important studies on the histology and histopathology of the nervous system published in Italian and in foreign journals,[17] including those of Gudden, Boll, Ranvier, Betz, Retzius, John Hughlings Jackson, and Jean Marie Charcot. He also published in the *Rivista* a summary of his work on the histology of gliomas and a summary *cum* commentary of his first paper using the black reaction, which appeared almost at the same time as the original paper (both in 1873). Golgi's commentary (in which he refers to himself in the third person) contains a statement that reveals the importance he attributed to his discovery, and indicates the ambitiousness of his research program (italics added):

How do nerve fibres originate? What are the laws that regulate the relationships between nerve cells and nerve fibres? Because of their importance from a physiological point of view, these two issues have received the greatest attention from investigators and yet they remain controversial . . . Although it is true that *his* findings are not yet a complete solution to these problems, *it is certain that they are of such importance as to lead us to believe that, by continuing on this path, he will be soon able to reach this goal.*[18]

In 1873 Golgi co-authored with Bizzozero a brief morphological study. This paper reported the results of experiments carried out on the rabbit, describing the alterations produced by the lesion of the sciatic nerve (atrophy and infiltration of adipose tissue in the muscles innervated by this nerve).[19] Synopses of this study were published in *Jahresberichte* in 1873 and in *Centralblatt* in 1874. Furthermore, Golgi's work was cited, together with a study by Mantegazza, in the prestigious six-volume *Handbuch der Physiologie* edited by Ludimar Hermann, Professor at the University of Zurich and a pioneer in electrophysiological research.[20]

Golgi was also taking advantage of the opportunities offered by the presence of the 'Incurables' in the Pie Case of Abbiategrasso. And incurables indeed these patients were. The Pie Case was the final destination for individuals who had received, unsuccessfully, all possible kinds of treatment in other hospitals. Among them were numerous neurological cases, which offered Golgi the chance to use his black reaction in a clinical context. A patient accepted into Tragella's ward in January of 1873 attracted Golgi's attention. This was a 42-year-old man affected by mental disturbances and involuntary, chorea-like movements, which were graphically described by Golgi:

no group of muscles is spared by the disease. His face is unceasingly tormented by the furrowing and unfurrowing of the forehead and of the eyebrows, the winking of the eyelids, the rotation of the eyeballs, the stretching in all directions of the lips and of the entire mouth rim. The trunk and the neck are restlessly bending forwards and backwards, leftwards and rightwards, in all possible postures. But above all, there are striking movements in the muscles of the upper limbs, which are thrown around in all directions, sometimes in a jerky manner, sometimes with countless contortions, in a continuous series of flexions, extensions, pronations, supinations, etc., etc., in the articulations of arms, hands, and fingers. The lower limbs are considerably less affected, although they too are unable to carry out voluntary movements in an appropriate manner, and the lack of harmony and proportion in the contraction of individual muscles is especially evident during walking, in such a way that the patient advances swinging, jolting from one side to the other, repeatedly stopping, as if to gather propulsive energy, and then advancing again in a precipitous and jerky manner, giving the impression that he is about to fall at any moment.[21]

Around the middle of October, the patient contracted pneumonia and died. Golgi carried out a thorough autopsy, reporting his findings in a study that deserves to be analysed from a historical perspective.

Almost two years earlier, on 15 February 1872, a recently graduated American physician, George Sumner Huntington summarized, before the members of the Meigs and Mason Academy of Medicine of Middleport, Ohio, a series of clinical cases concerning individuals with hereditary movement disorders, cases that had been gathered by his grandfather and father in East Hampton, Long Island, New York. Huntington emphasized the late onset of the disease, which made its appearance in middle age, and the presence of progressive intellectual deterioration with suicidal tendencies. In the East Hampton community the patients were known as those with 'that disease' and subsequent studies had demonstrated that they were all descendants of two brothers who had immigrated from England in 1630. During the seventeenth and early eighteenth centuries, some of these unfortunate individuals had been suspected of witchcraft and were persecuted because their movements appeared as a derisory pantomime of Jesus's suffering on the cross.[22] Huntington's study was published in 1872 in the *Medical and Surgical Reporter* and gained immediate international recognition, thanks to summaries in German made by Adolf Kussmaul and Hermann Nothnagel.[23]

Epidemics of a disorder similar to this had been already noticed in the Middle Ages. The bizarre, dance–like, movements were interpreted by the popular imagination as the influence of the devil or evil spirits. Against these superstitious beliefs, the Renaissance physician Paracelsus (Aureolus Theophrastus Bombastus von Hohenheim) proposed a classification of the disease, which he named chorea (from the Latin *chorea* = dance), in three types: imaginative (due to suggestion), lascivious (due to sexual desire), and compulsive (due to brain disease). In the seventeenth century Thomas Sydenham described a form of chorea occurring in young individuals (variously known as *chorea anglorum*, chorea minor, rheumatic chorea, or Sydenham's chorea), which is currently thought to be caused by an abnormal immune reaction to an acute streptococcal infection. Thus, Huntington had characterized another form of chorea (chronic degenerative chorea or Huntington's chorea), which was inheritable (through a single dominant gene, as we know now).

At the time of Golgi's study there was no precise information on the pathological anatomy of this disease, although some studies had reported a number of alterations, such as inflammatory processes in the meninges and in the spinal cord, and focal lesions of the brain. Golgi summarized the different opinions on the anatomical bases of chorea in the following way:

First, the great majority of pathologists think that gesticulatory chorea originates from alterations of nervous centres and more precisely of the brain, although it is generally believed that there is insufficient anatomical evidence for such an attribution.

Second, this belief about the lack of evidence should be attributed more to the putative discrepancy among positive findings than to actual presence of negative findings [that is, to the actual lack of alterations in the nervous system].[24]

Golgi emphasized that there 'were multiple centres for the coordination or control of muscles' the alteration of which could be responsible for chorea. Among these centres he examined in particular 'the corpora striata, which innervate all, or almost all, muscles'[25] and which, therefore, must be considered a 'centre responsible for the physiological coordination of almost all movements of the body, and, consequently, in the presence of certain alterations, for the choreic movements.' He then reviewed the work by Ferrier, Nothnagel, and Schiff, who had demonstrated that 'a severe lesion or the stimulation of one corpus striatum, can paralyse or excite most muscles on the opposite side of the body'.[26] Despite the importance of these findings, only two studies had so far hinted at a relationship between the corpora striata and the pathogenesis of chorea, and neither had included a thorough anatomical verification.

As early as the macroscopic examination, Golgi found 'both corpora striata greatly altered, particularly on the left'.[27] At the microscopic examination, which was conducted also with the black reaction, Golgi found in the fronto-parietal cortex an 'increase in the number and in the dimension' of the 'connective cells', that is, a reactive gliosis,[28] as well as a reduction in the number of nerve cells. The body of these nerve cells exhibited 'more or less pronounced thinning, protuberances, depressions'; the protoplasmic processes were mostly 'bumpy, tortuous, thin, and often filiform';[29] and the nerve process appeared to be thin and with a contorted course.

But 'even more severe and extensive' were the alterations found in the corpora striata. Here 'well preserved ganglion cells could be found in large number only in the deep portions of the grey matter; in the entire superior half, the alteration of the ganglion cells was almost complete'. Furthermore, 'there were numerous strips of grey matter in which the ganglion cells and their main processes are found in a state of complete calcareous degeneration' associated with an 'enormous amount of amyloid corpuscles'.[28] In addition, the connective tissue was greatly increased with an appearance that suggested a 'progressive interstitial growth of connective cells, with resulting atrophy of the nerve cells'.[30] Golgi also described minor alterations in the cerebellum (using the black reaction as well), where he found Purkinje cells in a state of calcareous degeneration, particularly in the fine peripheral branches of the protoplasmic processes. He would mention this finding in his acceptance speech for the Nobel prize as evidence of the putative trophic function of these fine branches.[31] Finally, he reported that the microscopic investigation of the spinal cord 'could not be carried out using my method with the silver nitrate because of the imprecise knowledge about the technique'.[32] It is likely that Golgi was still perfecting his technique while working on the spinal cord, and that he found optimal procedures only at the moment he began to study the cerebral cortex.

This study, published in 1874, is interesting for a number of reasons. The case he described may have been an instance of Huntington's chorea, although there was no evidence that it was inherited (his mother was indicated as an 'hysteric') and the reported 'rotation of the eyeballs' is atypical for this form of chorea (in which the eye muscles are usually spared). Golgi, however, cited Huntington's study, which he must have read in the abridged German version. In any case, the description of the alterations of the corpora striata, the fronto-parietal cortex, and the presence of 'gliosis' in both cortex and corpora striata, can be considered the first detailed report on the neuropathology of a case of chorea.

Shortly after the publication of this study, Golgi received a letter from Bizzozero (addressed jokingly to 'Dear Old Golgi,' although of the three Italian words for 'you,' the two friends were still using the formal *lei* and *voi* instead of the familiar *tu*) praising him in a jocular tone:

I have just finished reading the 'cap' on your chorea published in *Rivista Clinica*. Did I say cap? What cap am I talking about! This is a helmet with a crest, a crown, a papal triple crown!!—I have swallowed it in a gulp, a feat that I am not always able to perform with studies like this.[33]

Golgi's paper on chorea was immediately welcomed by Enrico Morselli as a 'stupendous work, which can be said to be the first Italian study that has tried to provide, instead of speculations, concrete, albeit difficult to investigate, neurohistopathological bases for the interpretation of mental disorders'.[34] Andrea Verga also reviewed Golgi's paper and although agreeing with the 'distinguished physician from Abbiategrasso' that his study represented one 'of the most eloquent in favour of the cerebral causation of chorea', he expressed the doubt that this specific case could be considered typical of this disease, which according to Verga was most commonly produced by a spinal affliction, hence the term 'spinal delirium'.

I beg forgiveness from my excellent friend Dr Golgi for insisting on this point. His name is already respected and pre-eminent, and if the form of 'gesticulatory chorea' he described were really typical, this would deal a deadly blow to the theory of a spinal localization of chorea, whereas the latter notion has been repeatedly ascertained by the research carried out in the last few years.[35]

Contrary to Verga's hypothesis, subsequent studies have demonstrated the validity of Golgi's conclusion. Golgi's paper received international recognition three years later when it was exhaustively summarized in an important work by Hugo Wilhelm von Ziemssen, who noted the use of the black reaction in the investigation of the corpora striata.[36] Although Golgi's contribution to the study of the neuroanatomical basis of chorea was acknowledged in the following years,[37] his name is now cited only infrequently in major historical reviews of chorea.

Between 1873 and 1875 Golgi carried out a number of studies using the black reaction. The first to be published was a study on the cerebellum,[38] followed by studies on the olfactory bulbs.[39] He then began to investigate the process of degeneration of nerve cells.[40] Finally, he extended the use of the black reaction to functional microanatomy: were there morphological differences between motor and sensory nerve cells?

His paper, 'On the fine anatomy of the human cerebellum', was published in 1874. From the first paragraph it is apparent that Golgi was now much more confident concerning the reliability of the black reaction. He discussed its differential staining properties as a function of the duration of the fixation in dichromate. By changing the procedure it was indeed possible to stain separately the nerve cells, glia, nerve fibres, or a combination of these elements at the same time. This study signalled, therefore, the passage from a 'histological' level of analysis, which characterized his first paper with the black reaction, to a 'neuroanatomical' one. Finally, and for the first time in the history of neurobiology, it was possible to visualize reliably the relationships among the different elements of the nervous tissue and to reconstruct its fine architecture. Furthermore, the black reaction was a powerful tool for distinguishing between nerve cells and glial cells.

The most important points in this study on the cerebellum are as follows:

1

The description of the fibres in the external layer of the cerebellar cortex, which 'run parallel to each other and, in most cases, are of considerable length, many of them running around an entire circumvolution'[41] (now known as parallel fibres). Golgi noted that 'they could be considered as originating from the granule layer'.[42]

2

The description of peculiar nerve cells which are very numerous in the molecular layer (the most external layer). They have assorted forms (irregularly polygonal, roundish, ovoid, fusiform, triangular, or conical) and 3–5, or more, protoplasmic processes and only one nerve process, which at a 'little distance from the point of origin (6, 10, 20 µ) . . . after thinning considerably, begins to emit ramifications, most of which are of extreme thinness and which, in turn, ramify further'.[43] It is noteworthy that only one year earlier Boll, in his ponderous monograph, had denied the existence of nerve cells in the molecular layer of the cerebellum.[44] The cells that Golgi describes are for the most part basket cells. They would later called 'small stellate cells' (*células estrelladas pequeñas*) by Cajal and 'terminal baskets' (*Endbäumchen*) by Kölliker. Golgi must have seen the baskets surrounding the Purkinje cells, because he reported that sometimes the nerve process 'descends vertically, almost to the level of the Purkinje cells, and then climbs upwards forming a loop of variable length and, throughout this long path, continuously gives off lateral filaments; sometimes taking bizarre shapes'.[43] The concept of an anastomotic net, however, was an obstacle to the identification of a characteristic spatial organization of the nerve fibres, which always had to give rise to 'a complex net'. The discovery of the baskets[45] was one of the most important successes of Cajal, who saw in them 'for the first time the real manner of termination of the nerve fibres in the grey matter'.[46] Later he demonstrated that in certain pathological conditions, such as 'general paralysis', or following section of the axon, the Purkinje cell degenerates while the surrounding basket remains intact, demonstrating the independence of the two.

3

Golgi offered a detailed description of the Purkinje cells as had never previously been possible. Their protoplasmic processes (dendrites) form

a system of ramifications originating from the entire contour of the protoplasmic processes, from the part close to the cell body to the most peripheral branches . . . ramifications that by subdividing, intertwining, and twisting in the most complex and bizarre manner, can, in fact, give rise to a uniform web, reticulum-like, which extends from the base to the periphery of the external cortical layer.[47]

No anastomotic net or nerve fibres originated from the terminations of these protoplasmic processes.

The cylindraxis of the Purkinje cell cuts across the entire granular layer (the third and deepest layer of the cerebellar cortex) and continues in a nerve fibre of the white matter.

Along this extremely long path, it does not remain undivided, as had been thought by researchers following Deiters' work, but it continuously emits ramifications, which in turn branch out in a complex manner . . . Concerning this system of filaments originating from the so called *cylinder axis* process of the Purkinje cells, two facts must be especially emphasized: first, the tendency of many of them to climb, turning upwards, towards the external cortical layer; second, their connection with the nuclei, a connection that occurs in a manner similar to that of the ramifications of the nerve fibres that originate from the medullary radiations.[48]

And about these nerve fibres: 'It can be seen . . . that the *fibres are interrupted along their path* . . . by nuclei surrounded by a layer of granular protoplasm with which the [protoplasmic] substance of the fibre appears to merge.' It appears that Golgi, in describing the course of the axon of the Purkinje cells, could see the recurrent collateral loop and it may be speculated that 'their connection with the nuclei' (which are described as small cells with little cytoplasm in which the fibre would 'merge') indicated a sort of connection with the stellate cells or (less likely) with the basket cells. Thus, as early as 1874 Golgi might have seen the neuroanatomical basis for the reverberating circuit originating from the Purkinje cells.

Between 1882 and 1885, Golgi published a series of articles in the *Rivista Sperimentale di Freniatria e di Medicina Legale* (republished in 1885 in a single volume) containing an impressive review of his findings on the structure of the central nervous system and in which he systematized and integrated all his earlier work. In discussing the cerebellum, he used almost the same words as in his 1874 paper (see above), but he did not mention the connection between nerve fibre and 'nuclei' (italics added):

Concerning this system of filaments emanating from the nerve process of the Purkinje cells, [one] must especially emphasize the tendency of many of them to climb, turning upwards toward the surface of the circumvolutions, into the molecular layer, *to participate in its complex system of local nerve fibres.*[49]

In this way the collaterals of the Purkinje cells, which in the 1874 paper appeared to establish somewhat of a connection with cell structures, ten years later would have no relationship with the 'nuclei' and would simply enter into the complex net of the molecular layer, becoming a component of the diffuse neural net.

If our interpretation is correct, we are presented with a prototypical example of the power of an 'epistemological filter', which not only acts as a guide in the interpretation of 'facts' but also selects, unbeknownst to the scientist, which observations are susceptible of becoming 'facts'. Indeed, the doctrine of the diffuse neural net, which was already hovering in the first paper using the black reaction, had become in the following ten years the theoretical beacon that guided Golgi in his investigation of the fine structure of the central nervous system. The diffuse neural net demanded the direct distribution of all branches of the nerve process in the net; the 'interruption' of the axons at the level of the 'nuclei' was incompatible with it.

4

Then Golgi described the cells of the granular layer; a layer that, in the subdivision of the cortical layers followed by Golgi, is located between the molecular layer, or external cortical layer, and the layer of white matter containing the myelinated fibres. Contrary to the opinion of the majority of the authors (including Boll) who had regarded them as connective cells (that is, glial cells), Golgi thought that 'the so-called granules must be generally considered as small nerve cells provided with three, four, five, and sometimes six processes, usually ramified' of which only one was a nerve process.[50] Although Golgi had observed that the nerve fibres running parallel to the external surface of the cortex originated in this layer, he had not identified the characteristic course of the axon of the granule cells, which ascends towards the most external region of the cortex and then bifurcates in the shape of a T, giving origin to the parallel fibres. This discovery would be made in 1888 by Cajal.[51]

In the granule cell layer Golgi identified two other cell types: fusiform cells with their larger diameter parallel to the surface of the circumvolutions, and cells with irregularly roundish or polygonal contour. These findings would be discussed again years later to conclude that:

(1) the fusiform cells present a nerve process that, branching off in tenuous fibrils, participates in the extremely complex system of nerve fibres of the granular layer';

(2) the globular cells (which are a little smaller than the Purkinje cells), found in the peripheral region of the granular layer, 'or even at the same level as the Purkinje cells', have a nerve process that after 20–30 μ branches out and sometimes gives rise to a complex net of fibrils, extending from the bottom to the periphery of the granular layer.'[52]

These two cell types are now collectively called Golgi cells.

5

Golgi was not able to provide a detailed description of the nerve fibres. Years later he would write on this topic:

In observing the area at the boundary between the granular layer and the external cortical layer, one can see a dense bush of isolated or bundled fibres, some of which are very thin whereas others are quite thick; these fibres cross the said area and enter the molecular layer, generally after having followed a tortuous course, often circling around the Purkinje cells, and branching out continuously along the way.[53]

This description suggests that Golgi had glimpsed bundles of the fibres that Cajal would later call 'climbing fibres' (*fibras trepadoras*),[54] but his obsession with the anastomotic net probably blinded him to the peculiarities of the different projection systems. Thus for Golgi there was a complex nervous plexus in both the granular and molecular layers. The latter originated from afferent fibres from the white matter, by the collateral fibres of the cylindraxes of Purkinje cells, and by the cylindraxes of the small cells of the molecular layer.

The work ended with some physiological inferences. If, as suggested by some authors, Purkinje cells are 'motor' cells and this function is mediated by their cylindraxis, then it is possible that the other nerve cells are 'sensitive' or 'psychic' cells. This concept was further elaborated in the section of *Sulla fine anatomia degli organi centrali del sistema nervoso* concerning the cerebellum.[55] In this monograph he subdivided the ganglion cells of the cerebellum into two types on the basis of their cylindraxis. In the first type, which included Purkinje cells, the cylindraxis (which, however, provided numerous collaterals that ended in the diffuse neural net) was well defined and continued in a medullated (myelinated) fibre. In the second type, the cylindraxis branched repeatedly in the granular layer, giving rise to the diffuse neural net.

On the basis of these findings, above all the striking differences in the relationship between nerve cells and the nerve fibres, I believe that it is justified to propose that the two types of cells and their respective fibres, described above, play fundamentally different functional roles. Indeed, I deem it obvious that the cells having nerve processes that give rise to a nerve fibre are organs that directly affect the periphery; therefore, it is conceivable that they are organs of motor activity.

In contrast, it appears likely that the other cells, for which we can safely exclude their direct connection with centripetal fibres, are organs of sensory activity, or, possibly, of automatic activity.[56]

Golgi insisted on this classification, although quite cautiously, in the following years. The reason for his hesitation was that, while there was abundant evidence in favour of the motor functions of nerve cells with long axons (in particular the fact that the nerve cells of the anterior horns of the spinal cord give rise to the nerve fibres for the muscles), there was very little evidence to support the putative sensory functions of the nerve cells with short axons.

In 1875, Golgi published a paper: 'On the fine structure of the olfactory bulbs'.[39] The study of the 'olfactory organ' at the University of Pavia dated back to Scarpa,[57] who had described the region of the palaeoencephalon connected to the olfactory structures of the periphery and had conducted extensive studies of comparative neuroanatomy on the olfactory systems of fish, reptiles, and birds. It is unlikely, however, that this was what motivated Golgi. Indeed, Golgi's interest in the olfactory bulbs appears to be an outgrowth of his study on the structure of the cerebellar cortex, as suggested by Morpurgo:

The hypothesis sketched out by Golgi in his study on the cerebellum led him to choose the olfactory bulb as a region of the brain certainly dedicated to the sensory functions and one in which he expected to find nerve cells having morphological features that matched such a function; but in his work on the olfactory bulb, Golgi did not state his intentions, as if he, although guided by a coherent and well thought-out research plan, was afraid of being conditioned by a thesis and wished to hide from himself the goal he was pursuing.[58]

Thus, Golgi may have chosen the olfactory bulbs to test his hypothesis on the functional dichotomy (motor versus sensory) between nerve cells with long versus short axons. This intent would be stated more explicitly in a 1882 paper on the olfactory lobe:

I considered such investigations most interesting because they concern a region of the central nervous system on the physiological function of which (perception of olfactory sensation) there is no disagreement, and, therefore, I thought that the knowledge of the fine [morphological] details of its structure could be generalized to make larger deductions on the meaning of similar [morphological] details that might be found in other [brain] regions whose physiological function is still unknown.[59]

Following a well honed routine, Golgi began his study with a synopsis of the work done on this topic by others, including Henle, Meynert, and Leydig, emphasizing the imprecision, nebulousness, and discrepancies of these earlier studies. In particular, he pointed out the terminological confusion produced by the abuse of such terms as 'granules' and 'nuclei', which most histologists had used to refer to the cells of the olfactory bulbs. He then divided the olfactory bulb into three layers. The first one included the peripheral nerve fibres arriving from the olfactory mucosa with the olfactory nerve. The second layer (grey layer) included the nerve cells and their processes. The third included the central nerve fibres of the *tractus olfactorius* (olfactory tract) and the nerve cells dispersed among them.

Finally he reported on the findings he had obtained using the black reaction on the olfactory bulbs of humans and other animals (dogs, cats, rabbits, hares, etc.), and described:

1. The convergence of the bundles of fibres that make up the olfactory nerve on the glomeruli located in the most external portion of the second layer.

2. The large and triangular cells (mitral cells) located in the second layer and their protoplasmic processes. These processes approach the glomeruli where 'they branch out repeatedly, generating a very intricate, fine, and elegant lace, which, being attached to the end of a very thick branch, assumes a quite bizarre appearance'. The cylindraxis of the mitral cells runs vertically toward the internal strata of the bulb and appears not to be ramified. Golgi speculated that the absence of ramifications could be due to an 'imperfect reaction'.[60]

3. Two other cell types in the intermediate layer:

   (a) small, ovoidal cells 'peculiarly clustered around the glomeruli [that is, periglomerular cells] ... one of the poles of which emits a extremely slender process having all the characteristics of a nerve process, whereas the other pole emits two or three protoplasmic processes. This latter pole, whatever the position of the cell body relative to the glomeruli, is always oriented towards these glomeruli, which are penetrated by the protoplasmic processes ... The slender nerve process, shortly after its origin, branches out in fine terminations, similar to the cerebral nerve fibrils. Some of these gracile filaments bend backwards to run in a direction opposite to that of the originating filament and penetrate, together with the bandlets of nerve arriving from the interior of the bulbs, into the olfactory glomeruli';[61]

   (b) 'Large cells irregularly disseminated'[62] with a protoplasmic process climbing towards the glomeruli and a branched nerve process descending towards the olfactory tract.

4. One type of cell in the internal layer of the nerve fibres of the olfactory tract, which have only protoplasmic processes (with associative functions like the amacrine cells of the retina), and a second cell type with both protoplasmic and nerve processes.

5. The penetration of the glomeruli by the nerve fibres arriving from the olfactory tract.

Golgi's detailed description of the architecture of the olfactory bulb was repeatedly confirmed, becoming the basis for all subsequent topographical models of the olfactory bulbs. The subsequent work of other neuroanatomists, including Cajal, on the topography of the olfactory bulb consisted in further subdividing the three-layer structure originally described by Golgi. On the basis of the relationships among nerve cells, nerve fibres, and glomeruli, Golgi sketched a physiological interpretation of the path travelled by olfactory stimuli to reach higher cortical structures after making relay in the olfactory bulbs.

Both the protoplasmic processes of the small and large cells of the grey layer and the nerve fibrils arriving from the olfactory region penetrate into the olfactory glomeruli and end in fine ramifications; thus, it might appear natural to reach the conclusion, previously embraced by Walter and Owsiannikow (although in the absence of the precise findings reported here), that the former [that is, the protoplasmic processes] continue into the latter [that is, the nerve fibrils] and vice versa.

Although such a conclusion appears to be inescapable, I do not feel any inclination to endorse it. It is sufficient to notice that the olfactory glomeruli represent a sort of meeting point for the various elements of the bulbs: blood vessels, connective cells, plasmatic cells, terminals of the protoplasmic processes, olfactory nerve fibres arriving from the periphery, and olfactory nerve fibres arriving from the [olfactory] *tractus*. All these components certainly establish very intimate relationships; however, the available evidence does not allow one to say whether in addition to a relationship of contiguity there is also a relationship of continuity, and, in case there is continuity, which of the elements are involved, besides the blood vessels and the plasmatic cells. Anyone who has pretended to draw more detailed conclusions, would simply be indulging, in my opinion, in the field of speculation. Nothing would be more speculative than to assert that the terminal branches of the protoplasmic processes of the small and large cells of the bulb continue into peripheral olfactory nerve fibres. Concerning this latter point, I want to offer here some considerations that will reinforce the doubts I indicated above.

One of the advantages of the method I have used is to stain in black separately, depending on specific modifications to the procedure for the preparation of the specimens, either the nerve cells and the extremely fine branching of their processes, or one of the different orders of nerve fibres [that is, each order of fibres could be stained separately from the others], or the interstitial connective cells, or a combination of these different elements, with various preponderances of one over the others. These different reaction products can be achieved also in the study of glomeruli. When the reaction is complete it happens that the interweaving within the glomeruli is so dense and complex as to make one believe that one set of filaments might simply continue into the other. When, as is often the case, the nerve fibrils are stained separately from the ramifications of the protoplasmic processes, or vice versa, it is immediately evident that the two systems of interweaving are quite different, and, above all, that the manner of ramification of the last branches of the protoplasmic processes is very different from that of the nerve fibrils. No matter how fine the filaments of the two systems might be, one can never observe a gradual continuation of one filament into the other.

On the other hand, the simple fact that the protoplasmic processes and the nerve fibrils are stained in black separately and at different points in time, is an argument that per se would be sufficient to lead to the conclusion that between the two systems of filaments there are substantial chemical differences; differences that would have no reason to exist if there were a continuity between the two systems. It must also be added that none of the above mentioned differences in appearance, manner of ramification and distribution, and chemical reactivity, are present when the peripheral nerve fibrils are compared . . . with the terminal ramifications of the single *nerve* process.

In contrast, we can accept a priori, on the basis of our knowledge of their functional relationship, the presence of an anatomical connection between the net of olfactory fibrils of the glomeruli and both the ganglion cells of the bulb and the nerve fibres of the *tractus*; a connection that we think can occur *indirectly* with the former [that is, the ganglion cells], through the numerous ramifications of the nerve process (indeed part of these ramifications penetrate into the glomeruli), and *directly* with the latter [that is, the nerve fibres of the *tractus*], through the bundles of fibres that, as we have described, cross the grey layer to penetrate the glomeruli.

Finally I want to emphasize that these considerations are presented here only to support my statement that we are still far from a solution to the problem of the manner of connection between the olfactory fibrils and the ganglion cells of the bulb.[63]

This latter point is extremely important. Golgi, after having demonstrated the discontinuity between olfactory fibres and the protoplasmic processes located in the glomeruli (proving incorrect the prediction from Gerlach's theory), could not accept *ipso facto* that olfactory pathways could pass from the former to the latter (to which he attributed a trophic function). Guided by his faith in a holistic model, he decided that the connection (which must exist a priori) between the two systems of nerve fibres (the afferents from the olfactory mucosa and the fibres of the olfactory tract) occurs through the axonal collaterals of the small periglomerular cells and the ascending fibres from the layer of the olfactory tract (third layer of the olfactory bulb; see above). Many years later two of his disciples, Monti and Pensa, reported that some collaterals of the axon of the mitral cells ascended among the fibres of the *tractus* to the glomeruli.[64] Obviously they considered these findings (which were rejected by a number of other histologists) as a confirmation of Golgi's hypothesis.

The presence of axon–axonal anastomoses in the glomeruli was later disproved, first by Cajal (who, on the contrary, found in the histological investigation of the olfactory bulbs the confirmation of his hypothesis of the contact between axons and dendrites), and then by Retzius, Michael von Lenhossék, Arthur van Gehuchten, and others.[65]

Of course, Golgi's 'holistic filter' not only altered what he saw at an anatomical level but also shaped his physiological model of the transmission of olfactory stimuli. He hypothesized that 'the functional connection between the bulb cells (centre of sensation) and those of the encephalon (centre of ideation) occurs as a whole through the fibres of the *tractus*; that is, there was not a series of isolated transmissions through single elements but only ensemble transmission'.[66] There remained to be discussed, however, the functional implications of the apparent lack of ramifications in the cylindraxis of certain nerve cells (mitral cells); a fact that might have suggested the possibility of 'isolated' transmission of the nerve impulse, as Golgi himself admitted:

However, I think that it is impossible to reject definitively the possibility that a set of cells of the bulb could function in a manner different from what has been proposed here, that is, that they could present isolated transmission. An example of this might be found in the large cells regularly aligned at the internal border of the grey layer, because I was not able to demonstrate the presence of ramifications in the nerve process of such cells; instead, I did find such ramifications in the nerve process of the ganglion cells of the cerebral and cerebellar cortices and of the posterior (sensory) horns of the spinal cord.[67]

Only few years later, however, we find no trace of these doubts in a paper on the 'olfactory lobes'.[68] In this later study (see Chapter 10) Golgi was most emphatic in stating the impossibility of 'isolated' transmission of nerve impulses. One possible explanation for this change of heart is that in the intervening years he had identified axon collaterals also in the mitral cells.[69]

As discussed above, the most likely, although not explicitly stated, initial aim of Golgi's work on the olfactory bulb was to find whether 'the cells of the putative olfactory centres,

present, in connection with a specific sensory function, also some morphological peculi-
arity, so that it would be possible to argue that also in the nervous centres the specificity of
the function is linked to a constitutional histo-morphological specificity'. In this respect,
both the 1875 and 1882 papers represented a disappointment because the presence of
various cell types and the complexity of their relationship prevented Golgi from reaching
any firm conclusion.

In the 1875 paper on the olfactory bulbs, Golgi used for the first time the *camera lucida*
invented by Oberhauser. He drew the nerve cells and the nerve fibres outlined with the
black reaction on a black and white plate (reproduced in colour in the *Opera Omnia*). In
addition, an appendix to the paper contained the first detailed description of the black
reaction, in which Golgi warned that the results were still partly determined by chance.

The exceptional importance of these first studies using the black reaction remained
undetected for many years. This is also surprising in light of the fact that these studies were
summarized in the most important journals. For example, a German summary of 'On the
structure of the grey matter of the brain' was published by Franz Boll on the *Centralblatt für
die medicinischen Wissenschaften*.[70] On this occasion Boll emphasized that Golgi's findings did
not support Gerlach's and Rindfleisch's theories. The studies on the cerebellum[38] and the
olfactory bulbs[39] were also summarized in German and English journals. In all cases it was
clearly reported that the nerve cells and their processes were stained in black. Golgi's work
with the black reaction had to wait until the second half of the 1880s to be recognized, and
even then only slowly. Clearly it was too much out of tune with the model prevailing at the
time, that is, the protoplasmic net of Gerlach.

Golgi's last experimental work in Abbiategrasso concerned the calcareous degeneration of
the nerve cells. The topic had been investigated previously by a number of German histo-
pathologists, including Virchow, who had linked the calcareous degeneration of nerve cells
to traumatic brain injury (concussion).

Golgi had already found calcareous degeneration of brain structures in his work on
chorea. During the period in Abbiategrasso he studied three other cases in which he found
deposits of calcium carbonate and calcium phosphate in different brain regions. Golgi's
excellent chemical background is indicated by the method he followed to distinguish
between carbonate and phosphate. He added sulfuric acid to the specimen: the disappearance of the deposits with a production of gas and crystals of calcium sulfate indicated the
presence of calcium carbonate; the absence of gas indicated instead the presence of calcium
phosphate. He found calcium phosphate in the nerve cells and calcium carbonate in the
connective membrane. In his conclusions, Golgi stated that the calcareous degeneration
was a non-specific consequence of tissue necrosis produced by a variety of conditions
(inflammation, nutritional deficits, and brain trauma).[40]

Golgi was now eager to leave his Abbiategrasso exile and return to academia. In October
1872 he had tried to obtain the professorship of Histology at the University of Pavia,[71]
but had been considered as not 'worthy of that position', as he bitterly complained to
Manfredi.[72]

At the end of the year he received a letter from Stanislao Cannizzaro, a world-renowned
chemist, who, inspired 'by the information received about you from reliable sources',

particularly Lombroso, promised to use his connections at the Ministry of Public Educa-tion to further Golgi's appointment to a professorship of Histology.[73] The most active on Golgi's behalf, however, was Boll, who had influential friends in Rome. One of them, the pathologist Corrado Tommasi-Crudeli, was a friend of Ruggiero Bonghi, who in 1874 became Minister of Public Education. Both Boll and Tommasi-Crudeli put pressure on Bonghi to 'do something for you, [it] being a great shame that you are not yet a professor'.[74] In November, in a 'long conversation' with Bonghi, Boll again defended Golgi's cause, emphasizing that his studies were 'among the most outstanding Italian works'. Finally, the Minister promised the professorship of Histology in Pavia to Golgi. He had not reckoned, however, with the hostility of the University of Pavia, which refused to approve the appointment. Bonghi bitterly complained to Boll that 'my hands are tied'. To console Golgi he promised: 'In the meanwhile I will make him [that is, Golgi] a Knight!!!!!!'[74] Indeed, on 12 January 1875 Golgi was made Cavaliere dell'Ordine della Corona d'Italia [Knight of the Order of the Crown of Italy]. 'This is the meagre result of my and Corrado Tommasi-Crudeli's efforts on your behalf' Boll wrote to Golgi few days later.[74]

However, Golgi's scientific reputation was on the rise and during the summer another attempt was made 'to get out of the swamp of Abbiategrasso'.[75] The professorship of Anatomy at the University of Siena was vacant and Golgi could compete for a non-tenured position. But he hesitated to accept such a precarious position, being also afraid of having to confront the hostility of the local academics, as had happened to Bizzozero in Turin. The latter, however, encouraged Golgi in a letter of 17 June, in which he wrote that anatomy, contrary to general pathology, would not expose him to accusations of being 'innovative' and that, therefore, Golgi did not risk attracting 'the wrath of the bigots'. At any rate, he suggested that Golgi keep his 'innovative ideas' to himself 'until tenureship will allow you to manifest them'. Once you have applied for the position, continued Bizzozero, 'pray to all the saints in paradise and all the archangels on earth, including Boll. I will do everything I can as you can easily imagine.' And wisely he added 'save money because, in case you are appointed in Siena, you will need it badly'.[76] Following Bizzozero's advice, on 24 July Golgi wrote to Boll to obtain his support. Boll immediately put pressure on Tommasi-Crudeli, who was an influential member of the High Council for Public Educa-tion and of the committee that decided the appointments to the professorships of Anatomy in Turin and Siena.[77]

What had appeared to be just a dream a few years earlier was now materializing. Like an underground river, Golgi's career re-emerged, after three years in the dark of Abbiate-grasso, into the light of the academic world.

He was about to leave for Siena when an unforeseen possibility opened up in Pavia. In mid-August, he was informed by the Rector, the chemist Tullio Brugnatelli, that he could be appointed *Professore Straordinario* of Histology.[78] We do not know whether the resistance of Pavia was overcome thanks to the pressure exerted by Cannizzaro on his colleague Brugnatelli, or by the pressure exerted by Bonghi on the Medical School. The Laboratory of Histology was temporarily housed in San Matteo Hospital[79] and later in a University building.

Toward the end of the year, Golgi asked 'to be released from the position' of Chief Physician,[80] but the regulations dictated that he could not 'abandon the position . . . until a replacement was in place'.[81] The replacement was eventually found[82] and Golgi was allowed to resign.[83] On 6 January 1876, Golgi formally resigned from the Pie Case degli Incurabili[84] and few days later left Abbiategrasso.[85]

Notes

1. Golgi (1875b; *OO*, pp. 127ff.).
2. Golgi (1873a; *OO*, p. 91).
3. *Ibid.* (*OO*, p. 92).
4. Cajal (1889).
5. Jacobson (1975).
6. Golgi (1873a; *OO*, p. 93).
7. *Ibid.* (*OO*, pp. 94ff.).
8. *Ibid.* (*OO*, pp. 97ff.).
9. Changeux (1983, pp. 10ff.); Cimino (1984, p. 287); Tanzi (1893, pp. 434ff.).
10. Golgi (1873a; *OO*, pp. 93ff.).
11. Cannon (1949, p. 134); Williams (1954, p. 108).
12. Perroncito (1926, p. 14).
13. Golgi (1875a, pp. 269ff.).
14. Alessandro Golgi's letter, 4 August 1872 (MSUP-II-7). Also in Riquier (1952, p. 58).
15. Certificate signed by the Mayor of Morimondo (MSUP-I-I-24).
16. Letter from Alessandro Golgi to Giulio Gioacchino Golgi, 23 March 1874 (MSUP-II-7).
17. Golgi (1873–75). Golgi reviewed also his own papers: 'Sulla struttura della sostanza grigia del cervello' (*Rivista di Medicina, Chirurgia e Terapeutica*, 1873, **2**, pp. 465–8) and 'Sui gliomi del cervello' (*Rivista di Medicina, Chirurgia e Terapeutica*, 1875, **1**, pp. 588–90). See also *Annuali Universali di Medicina e Chirurgia*, 1875, **232**, pp. 519–47.
18. *Rivista di Medicina, Chirurgia e Terapeutica* (1873, **2**, p. 465).
19. Bizzozero and Golgi (1873).
20. Mayer (1879, p. 206).
21. Golgi (1874; *OO*, pp. 885ff.).
22. DeJong (1953, p. 307).
23. Hayden (1981, p. 8).
24. Golgi (1874; *OO*, p. 874).
25. *Ibid.* (*OO*, p. 877).
26. *Ibid.* (*OO*, p. 878).
27. *Ibid.* (*OO*, p. 887).
28. *Ibid.* (*OO*, p. 891).
29. *Ibid.* (*OO*, p. 890).
30. *Ibid.* (*OO*, p. 892).
31. Golgi (1906; *OO*, p. 1279).
32. Golgi (1874; *OO*, p. 893).
33. Letter from Bizzozero to Golgi, 12 December 1874 (MSUP-VII-III-1).
34. Morselli (1875, p. 134).
35. Verga (1875, pp. 199ff.).
36. von Ziemssen (1877, p. 472).
37. Assagioli and Bonvecchiato (1878).

38. Golgi (1874a). Reviews–summaries of this work were published in *Rivista di Medicina, Chirurgia e Terapeutica* (1874, **1**, p. 100; by A. Lemoigne), in *Jahresberichte über die Fortschritte der Anatomie und Physiologie* (Leipzig: F. C. W. Vogel, 1875, for the literature of 1874, Vol. 3, pp. 190, 195, and 196). Summaries appeared also in *Centralblatt für die medicinischen Wissenschaften* (1874, p. 694) and in the *Quarterly Journal of Microscopical Science* (1875, **15**, pp. 192–3).

39. Golgi (1875b). The work was also summarized in *Jahresberichte über die Fortschritte der Anatomie und Physiologie* (Leipzig: F. C. W. Vogel, 1876, Vol. 4, pp. 222, 225–6). A list of Golgi's publications (*Rendiconti del Regio Istituto Lombardo di Scienze e Lettere*, 1926, **59**, pp. 776–81) includes: 'Piccole comunicazioni sulla fine anatomia del midollo spinale e del cervello' (*Rivista di Medicina, Chirurgia e Terapeutica*, 1874). The same reference is cited also by Golgi (1878–79; *OO*, pp. 143–8) but with a different date, 1875. However, I have been unable to find this paper in the *Rivista di Medicina, Chirurgia e Terapeutica*. It is possible that the above mentioned references does not refer to a full paper but to brief notes on the cylindraxis of the cells of the Rolando's substance (*Rivista di Medicina, Chirurgia e Terapeutica*, 1874, **1**, p. 511) and on the cells of the cerebral cortex (*Rivista di Medicina, Chirurgia e Terapeutica*, 1875, **2**, p. 310).

40. Golgi (1876). This work was reviewed the following year by Giuseppe Seppilli (1877). The date of publication is given incorrectly in a list of Golgi's publications published in *Rendiconti del Regio Istituto Lombardo di Scienze e Lettere* (1926, **59**, pp. 776–81).

41. Golgi (1874a; *OO*, p. 100).

42. *Ibid.* (*OO*, p. 101).

43. *Ibid.* (*OO*, p. 103).

44. Boll (1873).

45. Cajal (1888).

46. Cajal (1917, p. 74).

47. Golgi (1874a; *OO*, p. 104).

48. *Ibid.* (*OO*, p. 105).

49. Golgi (1885, p. 67).

50. *Ibid.* (1874a; *OO*, p. 106).

51. Cajal (1888a).

52. Golgi (1885, p. 74).

53. *Ibid.* (p. 77).

54. Cajal (1888a).

55. Golgi (1885).

56. *Ibid.* (p. 80).

57. Zanobio (1978).

58. Morpurgo (1926, pp. 37ff..).

59. Golgi (1882; *OO*, p. 251).

60. Golgi (1875b; *OO*, p. 117).

61. *Ibid.* (*OO*, p. 119).

62. *Ibid.* (*OO*, p. 118).

63. *Ibid.* (*OO*, p. 121).

64. Monti (1895, pp. 14ff.); Pensa (1961a, p. 447); Zanobio (1978, p. 11).

65. Cajal (1917, p. 107).

66. Golgi (1875b; *OO*, p. 126).

67. *Ibid.* (*OO*, p. 127).

68. Golgi (1882).

69. It was Cajal who first reported on the axon collaterals of the mitral cells (Cajal, 1890).

70. *Centralblatt für die medicinischen Wissenschaften* (1873, pp. 806–7).

71. Application sent to the Rector of the University of Pavia on 20 October 1872 (MSUP-I-I-23).

72. Letter from Golgi to Manfredi, 19 June 1873 (MSUP).

73. Letter from Cannizzaro to Golgi, 30 November 1873 (MSUP-VII-I-3).

74. Letter from Boll to Golgi, 23 January 1875 (MSUP-VII-III-22).

75. Letter from Golgi to Manfredi, 23 July 1873 (MSUP).

76. MSUP-VII-III-1.

77. Letters from Boll to Golgi, 9 August 1875, 23 August 1875, and 7 November 1875; and letter from Boll to Tommasi-Crudeli, 9 August 1875 (MSUP-VII-III-22). These letters are not included in Boll's correspondence edited by Belloni (1980).

78. Letter from Brugnatelli to Golgi, 14 August 1875 (MSUP-VII-I-2).

79. Letters from Brugnatelli to Golgi, 22 August 1875 and 12 October 1875 (MSUP-VII-I-2).

80. See the letter from the President of the Congregazione di Carità di Milano to the Director of the Pie Case degli Incurabili, 27 December 1875 (MGA) and Golgi's letter asking to be released from the position, 12 December 1875 (MSUP-I-I-27).

81. Article 6 of the *Istruzioni* (MGA).

82. During the session of the Congregazione di Carità di Milano, 24 December 1875, Golgi's request was acknowledged and, in a secret ballot, Ernesto Casazza was appointed to succeed him (Archivio Storico of the II.PP.A.B.). See also letter from the President of the Congregazione di Carità di Milano to the Director of the Pie Case degli Incurabili, 27 December 1875 (MGA). The appointment was communicated to Casazza on 29 December 1875 (MGA).

83. MSUP-I-I-28.

84. Golgi's letter of resignation (MGA).

85. See documents in MGA.

9

Professor at Pavia

On 5 February 1876 in the Anatomical Amphitheatre of our University, I initiated, with an opening lecture, the regular course of Histology that I then continued without interruption. I closed the opening lecture of that course affirming that I would be faithful to the flag carrying the motto 'Work, unrelenting work!'[1]

More than 40 years later, Golgi remembered with these words the beginning of his academic career at Pavia. In the same year Augusto Tamburini was appointed to the professorship left vacant by Lombroso, and Arrigo Tamassia took over the professorship of Legal Medicine.

Things had begun to move quickly for Golgi. In April of that year he had been appointed full Professor of Anatomy at the University of Siena, where he took up his duties on 1 May 1876.[2] Although the University of Siena Medical School was much less prestigious than the one at Pavia (which according to the Casati Law was considered 'First Class' along with Bologna, Turin, Rome, Naples, Padua, and Palermo), Golgi had promptly seized the opportunity to rise to the highest rank of an academic career. Indeed, the position of *Professore Straordinario* he would have had in Pavia, while tenure-track, would not necessarily lead to tenure. It was certainly worth the trouble of moving to a less important university in exchange for a tenured position. His friend Manfredi had done the same in 1874 when appointed Professor of Clinical Ophthalmology at the University of Modena. Furthermore, with an annual salary that had risen to 3000 lire, plus another 500 lire for directing the Laboratory of Anatomy, his economic situation had improved decidedly over the period at Abbiategrasso, even if costs rose in parallel.

Although Golgi remained at Siena for only six months, it appears that he enjoyed his brief stay in the Tuscan city, as we can deduce from a letter to him from his uncle Father Francesco Golgi, who wrote that he was 'pleased to hear that your students are industrious, that the people of Siena are pleasant, and that harmony reigns among the professors there'.[3] Preoccupied with his nephew's spiritual health, which he judged to be dangerously threatened by materialism, the priest advised him to make 'of science a means of serving God, and all the others that are made in His image'. But for Golgi science was a value in itself, actually the 'Supreme Value' to which he would dedicate his existence. All the rest were pious illusions.

Bizzozero invited him to Varese for the second half of August, hoping that 'you would keep me company for a while, and teach me the Tuscan accent, which could embellish my eloquence'.[4]

On 23 September 1876, Golgi was in Viareggio with the histologists Giuseppe Vincenzo Ciaccio and Salvatore Richiardi. Here they were joined by a party composed of Boll, Ranvier, and his factotum, E. Weber, 'a very courteous Alsatian, a polyglot who studied for his master all the histological literature written in a language different from French' as recalled by Boll in a letter to du Bois-Reymond.[5] Boll himself was not new to these scholarly sojourns in Viareggio where he was able to study the retina of marine animals and the electric organ of the torpedo ray. He had been Professor of Anatomy and Comparative Physiology at Rome for the previous three years and he was about to attain international fame with the discovery of the retinal pigment, which he called 'eritropsina' (currently known as rhodopsin). He was young and enthusiastic about scientific research and about Italy; he had a house in Rome overlooking the Coliseum and the Roman countryside with the Albani Hills, and he was well integrated into the scientific and political–diplomatic environments of the capitol. Unfortunately, his lungs were under-mined by tuberculosis which curtailed his stamina. We don't know if Boll had met Golgi before this;[6] certainly he considered Golgi to be one of the most outstanding Italian histologists and took it upon himself to make Golgi known in German circles. Boll also used his influence to find Golgi a university position. It appears that in Viareggio the five histologists tried to conduct some research together (Boll wrote to du Bois-Reymond that his Italian colleagues were 'extremely kind'), but there were too·many of them and they wound up hindering each other's efforts.

Meanwhile a new opportunity loomed in Golgi's future: a position as Professor of Anatomy at the prestigious Medical School of the University of Turin. Bizzozero had already been there for some years and Lombroso was about to arrive as Professor of Legal Medicine. By the end of the spring of 1876, thanks to the efforts of Bizzozero and Tommasi-Crudeli, the possibility of a professorship at Turin had became real. Bizzozero had decided to staff the Medical School with pre-eminent scientists of the positivistic school. To this end he had used all his influence to induce Lombroso and Golgi to come to Turin. On 6 June 1876 he announced to the latter that an agreement had been reached behind the scenes to have Golgi prevail over Carlo Giacomini and Vittorio Francesco Colomiatti. And he added that 'If things go as they should ... you will be Professor of anat. in Turin.—I hope that no one will ruin the party; however, we must remain vigilant.'[7]

Golgi, however, hesitated. There were rumours of 'hostility' towards him at the University of Turin, rumours that had been downplayed by Bizzozero who feared that Golgi could change his mind. Golgi was also aware of other rumours about his possible appoint-ment at Pavia, the city that by now he felt to be his own.

But Bizzozero was pressing hard from Turin. In a letter dated 18 June 1876,[8] he advised Golgi to abandon 'the microscope for a while' and to continue 'as you have already began to do, in the study of macroscopic anatomy'. Bizzozero added that with some skill in anatomical preparations and a grounding in 'a couple of areas of anatomy' Golgi would easily land a position in Turin 'annoying the chauvinists and the envious ones', and invited him to 'think about it'. He also suggested that he and Golgi should meet to talk things over and to overcome 'all your hesitations'.[8] The appointment at Turin, however, had to be approved by the Ministry of Education, and this was not forthcoming. Then Bizzozero asked Salvatore Tommasi for help[4] and in the end the last roadblocks were cleared.

For the University of Pavia this new transfer would have meant the definitive loss of another promising scientist and one, moreover, who was outside the various university cabals and therefore well accepted by the majority of the professors. Turin, unlike Siena, was considered one of the pinnacles of academia, and if Golgi went there, he was unlikely to leave. It was clear that this exodus of young and distinguished academics was seriously damaging the prestige of the University of Pavia. Already Bizzozero had 'gone to Turin because the Medical School of Pavia had not given him tenure'.[9] In order not to lose Golgi, too (whose apparently more malleable character promised not to be 'bothersome'), he was offered *ex professo* (that is, on the basis of his acknowledged professional competence) the professorship of Histology for the academic year 1876/77 and the complementary course of Microscopic Technique. The Consorzio Universitario Pavese (a consortium established in 1875 among City, Province, Hospital, and Collegio Ghislieri) offered to endow the professorship and to fund the Laboratory of Histology itself. Despite the pressure from Bizzozero and some opposition in Pavia, he 'opted for the university in which he had completed his studies'[10] and so, on 1 November 1876, he returned as a full Professor to his beloved Pavia.

Because of the new teaching duties, the transfer to Siena, and the return to Pavia, his research activity had virtually ground to a halt in 1876 and 1877. His first laboratory in Pavia was 'a huge undivided room, a kind of barn, in the Botanical Gardens'[11] and he was assigned Domenico Stefanini, former pupil of Bizzozero, as an assistant.[12] Students began to flock into Golgi's laboratory. The first was Giovanni Battista Grassi,[13] a student of the fifth year of medicine, already renowned in Pavia for his studies on intestinal parasites. Another was Giulio Rezzonico, who would later became known for his research on the structure of the myelin sheath.

These were also years of further recognition from the Italian scientific societies. In 1876 he was nominated Corresponding Member of the Accademia Medico-Chirurgica of Perugia and, in 1877, of the Accademia dei Fisiocritici of Siena.

Despite the distance and his refusal of the professorship in Turin, the contacts with Bizzozero did not slacken. On the contrary, Golgi's scientific stature and the fact that he lost no occasion to express his gratitude to Bizzozero, served to strengthen their friendship. As before, they sometimes spent their vacations together in Bizzozero's house in Varese and it is there that Golgi met Bizzozero's niece, Lina Aletti, 13 years his junior, with whom he fell in love. In the past his shyness had made it difficult for him to establish interpersonal relationships; but the recent improvement in his economic situation, and especially his newly attained academic prestige, worked miracles in building up his self-confidence. The social status and respect conferred by being a *Professore* at the University was a still palpable legacy of the Hapsburg era. Lina Aletti brought with her a suitable dowry and a heart-warming sense of security, exactly the kind of assets required for the wife of a young academic with great expectations.

So Golgi, after unburdening himself with his friend Manfredi and receiving his advice, decided to take the momentous step.

Having now secured a high social position and a certain economic security, victorious in the academic arena, like a knight of old after a tournament he went down on his knee before his lady, and offered his devotion and love to Lina Aletti.[14]

After some months of being engaged, he confided in a letter to Manfredi 'feelings never before experienced', a happiness 'I didn't believe was possible, when I think that she will be the companion of my life', his love for 'that good girl'.[15] The matrimony was finally celebrated in a civil ceremony at two in the afternoon of 28 October 1877 in the City Hall of Varese.[16] Witnesses were his brother Giuseppe for the groom and her uncle Giulio Bizzozero for the bride; also present were a few relatives and friends, including Manfredi.[17] The couple spent their honeymoon at Corteno[18] where Golgi introduced his wife to old friends and acquaintances. Lina Aletti was an affectionate companion who, by unanimous recollection of those who knew her, provided the ideal atmosphere for Camillo to continue his research undisturbed. She knew what kind of man she had married, and coming from a family that counted among its members a scientist of the worth of Giulio Bizzozero, she understood the importance of science for her husband. Lina took upon herself all domestic duties, seeking to relieve Golgi from daily nuisances and leaving him free in his scholarly activities and 'with the most delicate attentions, bringing . . . in days of sadness a soothing calm with the cheerful expansiveness of her soul'.[19] Occasionally she 'became involved in the stern rigour of scientific research', helping Golgi prepare his publications by drawing illustrations from histological preparations.

The Golgis lived for some years in a small apartment and then moved to a luxurious apartment building at No. 77 Corso Vittorio Emanuele (now Strada Nuova) close to the University.[20] They had no children, but a few years after their marriage they took into their home the beloved Carolina, daughter of Camillo's brother Giuseppe, who had died young.

This is how Carolina Golgi remembered her aunt and uncle in a letter sent to Giacomo Bianchi on 9 February 1972 (Lina Aletti is referred to as 'Aunt Luisa' perhaps because of an error of transcription):

My Aunt Luisa was for her husband the most worthy companion imaginable. Among the mementoes religiously kept by her, and just as much by me, there are, in a special case, all the cards, always accompanied by a flower, most often a fragrant acacia, that every year had been sent to her by Camillo, wherever he was, on 28 October, the day on which they were married and Aunt Luisa made her honeymoon trip to Corteno, the Corteno of more than one hundred years ago. I keep also the photo of Aunt Luisa's mother, thus not my grandmother yet much more than a true grandmother, because of the love and affection that she felt for me. She died in Pavia in 1913, while I was there to meet my husband, who was in the 90th artillery. She [that is, Lina's mother] was the widow of Giacomo Aletti and sister of Giulio Bizzozero, the celebrated professor of histology who held the professorship at Pavia and was mentor of Golgi. The Bizzozero family was from Varese and it is at Varese that Uncle Camillo got to know Aunt Luisa.[21]

And soon thereafter:

To find in the life of my uncle events or episodes outside his life as a scholar, is not easy. He lived with his thoughts, relieved of all the daily necessities of life by his companion, for whom he was like a divinity, and who followed, loved, and helped him in his work and social life, providing him with the most complete and intelligent support. My uncle was a person of few words, also with us children, but one glance of his was sufficient for us to understand and obey, yet without fear.[22]

Since Mantegazza's time, the professorships of Histology and General Pathology at the University of Pavia had been held by the same person. After Bizzozero's departure for Turin, the professorship of Histology remained vacant (until Golgi's appointment) while General Pathology was assigned to Achille De Giovanni,[23] an assistant of the clinician Francesco Orsi. De Giovanni was more interested in clinical medicine (even if from a biological perspective) than in general pathology. Indeed, he was also an instructor of *Practical Medicine* for the students of the Collegio Ghislieri. The return to Mantegazza's tradition became possible only when De Giovanni was appointed Professor of Clinical Medicine at the University of Padua in 1879, and Golgi could attach the adjunct professorship of General Pathology to the professorship of Histology. As a consequence, Golgi's laboratory was enlarged to include 'three rooms on the first floor of the same Botanical Garden' and few years later was moved again to 'four rooms on the ground floor, still at the Botanical Garden'.[24] The laboratory had no adequate equipment and its functioning depended largely on the enthusiasm and industriousness of the students and of the young graduates working with Golgi, and on their contribution to the lab expenses. Despite these difficulties, Golgi's laboratory was rapidly becoming the most important centre of biological research in Italy.

Finally, on 13 March 1881, Golgi was appointed Professor of General Pathology, and, at the same time, Adjunct Professor of Histology. The two-fold reason for this apparently bizarre carousel of professorships was that General Pathology was more prestigious than Histology and that keeping both professorships allowed Golgi, among other things, to have assistants in both disciplines.

Finally settled in his new laboratory in Pavia, Golgi took up research again with great fervour. Besides continuing his work on the structure of the central nervous system and striving to improve the black reaction, he began to investigate a topic very dear to contemporary physiology and psychophysics: the structure of the sensory nerve terminations in the tendons. The topic was of great interest because there was a gap between the model of tendon function suggested by the findings of clinical medicine and physiology, and the results of the few anatomical studies that had been carried out on the structure of the tendons. For some time it had been known that by tapping a tendon one could obtain a rapid contraction of the corresponding muscle. The involvement of cutaneous terminals had been excluded insofar as this phenomenon was not evoked by pinching the skin over the tendon but could be obtained by tapping the tendon after cutaneous anaesthetization. The participation of nerves in the joints had been also excluded because the contraction was not elicited by tapping in the direction of the joint or on the joint itself. There were some scientists who hypothesized a direct muscular contraction caused by mechanical stretching, but most physiologists thought that it more probable that the reflex action

free passage. That is, the cylinder axis appears to be sheathed by a series of conical funnels, each covering the successive one for about one-third or one-quarter of its length, with the smaller opening of the funnels circling the cylinder axis and the larger opening surrounding the external surface of the successive funnel. It is obvious that the largest diameter of the funnels corresponds to the transverse diameter of the nerve fibre, whereas their minor diameter barely exceeds that of the respective cylinder axis.[57]

At high magnifications, Rezzonico had the impression that they might be 'formed by a single very tenuous fibril, ribbon-like, wrapped into very tight coils which narrow progressively (hence the shape of the conical funnel)'.[58] Rezzonico concluded that these funnels had the function of holding 'in place the myelin and protecting the cylinder axis'[59] and that they should be considered 'analogous to the horny reticulum or horny sheets that are hidden in the medullary [that is, myelinated] nerve fibres of the peripheral nerves.'[60] He based his conclusions on previous research conducted mainly on the peripheral nervous system which had demonstrated the existence of a substance that could be digested by gastric juices and by tripsin (for example, the horny tissue), and which was called horny substance or neurokeratin.

In an appendix to Rezzonico's paper, there is a note by Golgi that pre-announced his discovery of a funnel-like structure also in the peripheral myelin.[61] Actually, Golgi's study was published a little earlier than that of Rezzonico. In it, Golgi completed the investigation that Rezzonico had begun, demonstrating the presence of funnels also in the myelin sheath of peripheral fibres, funnels that were more loosely bundled than those in the central nervous system.[62] Golgi then found a precise correspondence between the horny funnels and the striae of Schmidt−Lanterman (oblique clefts in the myelin sheath).

Today it is well known that when myelin, which is composed of alternating layers of lipids and protein (in the past called neurokeratin), is stained with silver nitrate, the silver is deposited on the protein layers, which appear as a system of filaments interposed between the lipids. The most likely interpretation is that the horny funnels of Rezzonico− Golgi, which had sometimes been thought to be artifacts,[63] correspond (in preparations using silver nitrate) to the striae of Schmidt−Lanterman, that is, to channels for nutritional exchanges.

The discovery of the funnel-like structure of myelin was promptly noted in Italy,[64] but it elicited mostly scepticism in the international scientific community. As early as 1881 Otto Pertik, when he was an assistant in the Anatomical Institute of Strasbourg, had criticized the work of Golgi and Rezzonico, maintaining that the horny funnels were optical illusions caused by the osmic acid, and accused Golgi of ignoring the fact that this reagent can produce artifacts.[65] The following year, a paper co-authored by L. Waldstein of New York and E. Weber, who had developed the anatomy course at the Collège de France, advanced their doubts of the existence of the funnel-like structures described by Golgi and Rezzonico.[66] Golgi was irritated by these criticisms and lamented that they had not 'given much credit to his [that is, Golgi's] observations'.[67] Golgi intervened at the Congress of the Italian Medical Association, to 'show the preparations confirming such peculiarities'. But the scepticism surrounding the results obtained by Golgi and Rezzonico persisted, especially in Germany, and in 1911 Grassi could still state that 'the best and most widely distributed German handbooks of histology appear to ignore, or at least do not report, the existence of the funnels of the nerve fibres discovered long ago by Golgi himself and his students.'[68]

However, an official and authoritative consecration came from Ranvier in his world-renowned treatise of histological technique.[69] All in all, this was not a bad outcome for work largely carried out by a student. These were the possibilities offered by the Laboratory of General Pathology in which there was, as Mantegazza said, 'every day a new discovery'.[70]

While still engaged in investigating the sensory terminals of the tendons, Golgi initiated a study on the histology and histopathology of voluntary muscles, which led to one of the earliest descriptions of the neuro-muscular spindle.[71] The initial part of this work painstakingly analysed the manner of connection between muscles and tendons, preceded by an exhaustive review of the scientific literature on the topic. On the basis of the results obtained with one of his methods of preparation, 'dissociation of the tendinous bands hardened in dichromate, showing the attachments of the muscular fibres',[72] Golgi reached the erroneous conclusion that there is 'a gradual passage of the muscular substance into the tendon tissue' and therefore that 'there is an uninterrupted continuation of the fibrils, which appear to constitute the primitive muscular fibre, into the [tendon] fibrils, the union of which gives rise to the tendon bandlets. This simple transformation happens by gradual disappearance of the specially distributed substance that constitutes the transverse striation of the muscular fibrils.'[72] On the contrary, as had already been suggested by some histologists cited by Golgi, at the border between the tendon and the fleshy part of the muscle there is continuity only between the muscle connective tissue (perimysium and endomysium) and that of the tendon.

Continuing his investigations, Golgi discovered a fact of primary importance.

In many muscles of humans and animals, regardless of age, there are numerous isolated bundles of muscle fibres, which can be discerned at a glance to be different from the common ones because of their young, in many cases embryonic, aspect.

These peculiar bundles could be easily seen in the transverse sections of the muscles, and are located, at times right in the middle of the muscle bundles of first order, more frequently in the strata of connective tissues (internal perimesial) that are between bundle and bundle ... These bundles consist of 5, 6 or at most 8 fibres, which can be easily distinguished from the others because: first, they are much thinner (although among them there are some of rather diverse dimensions; for example, some are very small and can reach a transverse diameter of 15–20 μ, whereas others have a diameter little inferior to normal); second, they consistently contain many more sarcolemmic nuclei (when there is a sarcolemma) than the normal fibres; third, they are consistently associated, throughout their entire length, with scattered nuclei situated in the muscle substance, many of which are encircled by a thin layer of protoplasmic granulation.

Furthermore, what contributes even more than the above mentioned characteristics to make these bundles noticeable and, one might say, unique is that they always appear to be surrounded by a special sheath, of remarkable thickness, consisting of compact connective tissue, of a homogenous aspect, slightly shiny like the tendon tissue, and provided with rather numerous nuclei. In some cases such a sheath presents a laminated structure, having some analogy with the shell of the corpuscles of Pacini.

Inside the sheath just described, near the bundle of muscle fibres, it is almost always possible to discern also a band of nerve fibres ... and one or two blood vessels of small or medium diameter.[73]

And then:

Therefore, when some portion of the above-mentioned bundles can be isolated in good condition (as a rule it is possible to isolate only short lengths) it appears as a tube with a well defined and isolatable wall, which consists of compact connective tissue of remarkable thickness, being, however, transparent enough to leave its content visible. This tube is not uniform in diameter at all, but presents gradual dilations, which occur repeatedly at not great distances ... The fibres contained in it, some of which are of very small and of medium diameter, and which, as has been said, are especially characterized by the richness in superficial and internal nuclei, are as a rule located in the centre of the tube; sometimes there is a considerable space between them and the sheath (in correspondence to the ampullar dilations), at other times the two are almost in contact.

These preparations also confirm that almost always within a tube there is a blood vessel of remarkable diameter, which provides branches, and 3 to 5, or even more nerve fibres, which are sometimes grouped together in a bundle or, more rarely, have an irregular distribution.[74]

It is clear that Golgi is sketching here the description of a neuro-muscular spindle, a description which, however, does not include a characterization of the nerve terminations. In truth, Golgi does hint at the similarities between the sheath of the structure described by him and that of the corpuscles of Pacini but he did not realize that he had identified a sensory corpuscle.

Golgi's description of the neuro-muscular spindle followed earlier hints contained in studies by Kölliker, August Weismann, and Wilhelm Kühne, but it was more precise. The work was accompanied by 14 figures[75] which had been drawn, directly from the preparations, by Lina.

With the discovery of the 'musculo-tendinous organ' (which would later carry his name), and of the corpuscles of Golgi–Mazzoni, and with the identification of the anatomical individuality of the neuro-muscular spindle, Golgi made a major contribution to the study of the anatomical bases of proprioceptive sensibility and therefore to the study of the sensory control of movement.

After this, Golgi turned his attention to the problem of muscular regeneration. He investigated this phenomenon by producing focal destruction of portions of muscle with injections of phenic acid and potash, or with ligation, and then sacrificing the animals at different times. He observed both the muscle regeneration and the formation of a connective scar, and saw that the magnitude of all these processes depended on the intensity of the inflammatory process caused by the toxic or mechanical insult. The greater the inflammatory process the greater the connective scar, and, correspondingly, the smaller the probability of muscular regeneration.

On the clinical side of the problem, Golgi studied the pathological anatomy of three cases of muscular disorders that had come to his attention. The first was the case of a 27-year-old patient affected by extreme stiffness of the inferior half of the muscle vastus and atrophy of the other muscles of the thigh and the trunk. In a small fragment of the muscle vastus externus obtained by biopsy, Golgi observed the co-existence of both atrophic and swollen fibres that had largely lost the transversal striation. Given the stiffness of the muscle, and especially the presence of fibres larger than normal but with degenerative characteristics, he labelled the affliction as 'pseudo-hypertrophy'. The pseudo-hypertrophic alteration of the muscles is common to a number of diseases (sarcoidosis, amyloidosis, congenital myopathies, etc.) but the description given by Golgi does not allow a precise nosographic classification of this case. His second case was an 18-year-old girl who had died of tetanus infection and who presented a 'minute fragmentation or breakage of muscle fibres'.[76] Finally, he investigated the muscular alterations in a case of 'locomotor ataxia'[77] in a 50-year-old woman who had died in the Hospital of Abbiate-grasso in 1874 after a very long paralytic illness. At the autopsy exam Golgi found 'an extensive sclerosis of the postero-lateral tracts of the spinal cord'[77] that was suggestive of spinal ataxia. Golgi had preserved several of her muscles in alcohol and their neuro-pathological examination showed many of the alterations already pointed out in the case of pseudo-hypertrophy (including the large differences in the diameters of the fibres, and the diffuse process of muscular segmentation), and this led him to conclude that muscular tissue can undergo, in particular conditions, a regression towards the less differentiated connective tissue. For this work Golgi again availed himself of the collaboration of his wife who drew the illustrations from the specimens.

The prodigious appetite of Golgi for apparently disparate research topics was also fed by his scientific collaboration with Bizzozero. The chance for a collaboration arrived in the autumn of 1879, probably when the two friends were vacationing together in Varese. Bizzozero had just invented the chromo-cytometer, an instrument that allowed the rapid and precise measurement of variations in haemoglobin and a few months earlier

Prof. [Emil Clemens] Ponfick of Breslau had reported that he had been able to transfuse blood in three patients via the peritoneal cavity . . . and with favourable success, since a low fever and slight abdominal pain occurred only for a brief time after the operation. Ponfick had been encouraged to make these attempts in humans by the results of a preliminary series of experiments in which he had injected pure defibrinated blood into the peritoneal cavity of dogs.[78]

Ponfick's method had therapeutic potential because it allowed the transfusion of considerable quantities of blood without the dangerous reactions that frequently occurred following intravenous transfusions prior to the discovery of blood groups. Ponfick had found that in the dog the blood was rapidly resorbed from the abdominal cavity and that there was no haemoglobinuria (haemoglobin in the urine), a clinical sign of massive destruction of red cells. He concluded, therefore, that the red blood cells transfused into the peritoneum passed directly into the bloodstream without being destroyed. A rigorous assessment of this interpretation required, however, a precise determination of the changes in the concentration of haemoglobin following blood infusion, which Ponfick had not been able to do.

The availability of the chromo-cytometer spurred Bizzozero and Golgi to test Ponfick's hypothesis. In experiments carried out in rabbits, they found that shortly after a intra-peritoneal infusion of blood haemoglobin began to increase (in an experiment it was detected after only 20 minutes), reached the maximum after about 31–48 hours, and, remarkably, was still elevated 'after 27 days, which is the longest period over which we have carried out continuous observations on the animals receiving the injection.'[79] Further-more, Golgi and Bizzozero found a certain degree of correlation between the amount of blood injected and the increase in circulating haemoglobin. The kinetics of the experiment indicated clearly that there was a passage of transfused blood into the circulatory system.[80]

On his return to Pavia, Golgi, energized by this success, was impatient to repeat the ex-periment in humans. The occasion to do so arrived in the form of a 38-year-old psychotic patient at the Psychiatric Clinic who was suffering from a severe form of anaemia. In collaboration with Antigono Raggi, Professor of Psychiatry and Director of the Mental Hospital of Voghera, Golgi attempted the transfusion of blood into the peritoneum of this patient. The results exceeded all expectations. An increase in haemoglobin was detected after only 18 hours and the level remained elevated through the 14th day when the cyto-metric determinations were suspended. In parallel, there was a marked improvement in the general conditions of the patient and in his psychiatric symptoms.[81] Golgi and Raggi repeated the transfusion in other patients, obtaining consistently positive results.[82] The interest for this type of transfusion technique was such that they were invited by the psychiatrist Augusto Tamburini to give a public demonstration before an audience of psychiatrists at the Third Freniatric Congress of Reggio Emilia, held in September 1880.[83] Two years later the technique had become an established procedure, and the work by Bizzozero and Golgi was rated very highly in a review 'On the transfusion of blood' published in the *Gazzetta degli Ospitali*,[84] a journal widely read by Italian physicians and students alike.[85]

By the end of the 1870s, Golgi had achieved national renown in the medical field. He was on the editorial and scientific boards of important journals, such as *Annali Universali di Medicina*, *Rivista Sperimentale di Freniatria e Medicina Legale*, *Archivio per le Scienze Mediche*, and was considered worthy of being listed in a biographical dictionary of 'contemporary writers' by Angelo De Gubernatis of 1879 (a kind of cultural 'Who's Who' of the time); this biography was later reprinted in the magazine *Il Patriota* of Pavia.[10] On 16 January 1879 he was nominated as Corresponding Member of the Reale Istituto Lombardo di Scienze e Lettere and soon after he was elected Member of the Italian Society of Hygiene.

On 19 December 1879 Franz Boll, Golgi's first international mentor, died in Rome. The discovery of retinal pigment, announced in 1876, had brought him fame among physio-logists and secured his election as Corresponding Member of the Accademia Reale dei Lincei and promotion to full Professor. His reviews in *Centralblatt* had brought to the atten-tion of German biologists some of the most important studies published in Italy, including the paper by Sertoli on the structure of the seminiferous tubule of the testicle.[86]

Boll might have been one of the first to try the black reaction,[87] but in the last years, undermined by consumption, he had restricted his interests mostly to theoretical studies on the mechanisms of vision. His life, like that of Deiters, had been abruptly interrupted at the dawn of a promising scientific future.

Notes

1. From a speech given on 29 June 1919 at the Fondazione Camillo Golgi-Pro Orfani di Medici. Reproduced in Mazzarello (1993, p. 341).
2. Royal Decree signed by Vittorio Emanuele II on 8 April 1876 (MSUP-I-I-32); 'Communication of the appointment to [the position of] Professor' at Siena, signed by the Rector of the University of Siena, 15 April 1876 (MSUP-I-I-33). The transfer to the University of Siena was not made without difficulty, owing the opposition of the Rector A. Corradi (see Linskens and Cresti, 1996, p. 47). References to Golgi's academic life before his departure for Siena can be found in letters from Bizzozero to Golgi dated 15 February (addressed to the 'Amiable Knight') and 4 April 1876. The letters of 18 June and 12 July are addressed to 'Prof. C. Golgi Via Nonna Agnese. 2. Siena'. In addition, there are other letters sent to Golgi at the Siena address between summer and autumn of 1876 (MSUP). Thus, there is no support for the notion that Golgi moved to the University of Siena in 1879, as reported by some (see for example Sala 1925, p. 42 and Pensa 1926, p. 11; 1961 p. 274).
3. Letter from Francesco Golgi to Camillo Golgi, 22 May 1876 (MSUP-VII-I-6).
4. Letter from Bizzozero to Golgi, 12 July 1876 (MSUP-VII-III-1).
5. Letter from Boll to du Bois-Reymond, 15 November 1876 (Belloni 1980, p. 398).
6. In the letter from Boll to Golgi dated 23 August 1875, the German scientist wrote that at the beginning of September he would be returning to Italy, passing via Milan, and he hoped that he would be able to 'get to know him personally' but we don't know if the meeting occurred (MSUP-VII-III-22). The letter is not included among the collection of letters of Boll published by Belloni (1980).
7. Letter from Bizzozero to Golgi, 6 June 1876 (MSUP-VII-III-1).
8. Letter from Bizzozero to Golgi, 18 June 1876 (MSUP-VII-III-1).
9. Grassi (1911, p. 64).
10. De Gubernatis (1879, p. 517); *Il Patriota*, 20 November 1879. For the passage of Golgi to Pavia, see also Royal Decree of 1 November 1876 (MSUP-I-I-34), the communication of the appointment signed from the Rector of the University of Siena of 5 November 1876 (MSUP-I-I-35) and the Ministerial Decree of 19 April 1877 (MSUP-I-I-36).
11. Perroncito (1926, p. 16).
12. The Laboratory of Histology was listed in the yearbook for the academic year 1877–78 and 1878–79. The direction was entrusted to Golgi. Domenico Stefanini is registered as an *assistant* even though in 1878 he published an article as an *associate* affiliated to the Institute of Histology. Some years later he became Instructor of Clinical Microscopy and Chief Physician at San Matteo Hospital.
13. That Grassi had been Golgi's first pupil (or one of the first) is reported by various biographers; see for example Belfanti (1926, p. 772); Perroncito (1926, p. 16); Rondoni (1943, p. 538; 1943a, p. 224); Pilleri (1984, p. 17). Grassi himself affirmed that he had been a pupil of Golgi (Grassi, 1911, p. 119). See also MSUP-VII-III-5.
14. Morpurgo (1926, p. 39).
15. Letter from Golgi to Manfredi, probably from the first half of 1877 (MSUP).
16. Golgi's wedding certificate is published in Goldaniga and Marchetti (1993, p. 63).
17. See Nicolò Manfredi's testimonial on the occasion of the celebration of Golgi's professional jubilee and 25th wedding anniversary (*Gazzetta Medica Lombarda*, 1902, p. 436).
18. See letter from Golgi's niece Carolina Golgi to Giacomo Bianchi (Bianchi 1973, p. 15).

19. See the report of the celebrations for the Golgis' professional jubilee and 25th wedding anniversary (*Gazzetta Medica Lombarda*, 1902, p. 435).
20. According to the Municipal Records, they took up official residence in Pavia only in 1880.
21. Bianchi (1973, pp. 15ff.).
22. *Ibid.* (p. 16).
23. Achille De Giovanni, former assistant at the Medical Clinic directed by Francesco Orsi, became Adjunct Professor of General Pathology in the academic year 1872–73 and *Professore Straordinario* of General Pathology in 1875–76.
24. Perroncito (1926, p. 16).
25. Golgi (1878; *OO*, p. 175).
26. Golgi (1878).
27. Golgi (1878a).
28. Golgi (1880).
29. Letter from Bizzozero to Golgi, 5 May 1878 (MSUP-VII-III-1).
30. Golgi (1878; 1880; *OO*, pp. 140 and 185).
31. Golgi (1878; 1880; *OO*, pp. 133 and 172).
32. Golgi (1880; *OO*, p. 180).
33. *Ibid.* (*OO*, pp. 180ff.).
34. *Ibid.* (*OO*, p. 182).
35. *Ibid.* (*OO*, p. 186).
36. Marchi (1880–81, p. 206).
37. Marchi (1880–81).
38. Marchi (1881).
39. Marchi (1882).
40. Golgi (1880; *OO*, p. 180).
41. *Ibid.* (*OO*, p. 184).
42. *Ibid.* (*OO*, pp. 184ff.).
43. *Ibid.* (*OO*, p. 186).
44. Lambertini (1990, p. 135).
45. Review by Löwe in *Centralblatt für die medicinischen Wissenschaften* (1879, pp. 725–6).
46. Thanhoffer (1882, p. 39).
47. Klein (1885, pp. 209ff.).
48. Perroncito (1926, p. 19).
49. Golgi (1878–79; *OO*, p. 144).
50. Golgi (1878–79). Summary by Löwe in *Centralblatt für die medicinischen Wissenschaften* (1879, p. 569).
51. Mondino (1885, p. 38).
52. *Ibid.* (pp. 39ff.).
53. Golgi (1885, p. 207).
54. Golgi (1891; *OO*, p. 608).
55. Stefanini (1877).
56. Rezzonico (1880, p. 79).
57. *Ibid.* (p. 82).
58. *Ibid.* (p. 83).
59. *Ibid.* (p. 87).
60. *Ibid.* (p. 88).

61. Annotations by Golgi regarding the peripheral nervous fibres (*Archivio per le Scienze Mediche*, 1880, **4**, No. 4, pp. 88–9).

62. Golgi (1879).

63. Jacobson (1993, p. 78).

64. Ceci (1881); Seppilli (1880).

65. Pertik (1881, pp. 54ff.).

66. Waldstein and Weber (1882, p. 3).

67. *Atti del Congresso della Associazione Medica Italiana* (Modena: G. T. Vincenzi and nipoti, 1883, p. 426). The congress was held in Modena; Golgi intervened in the fifth session which took place on 21 September 1882.

68. Grassi (1911, p. 6).

69. Ranvier (1875–86, p. 1058).

70. The phrase of Paolo Mantegazza is cited, among others, by Gravela (1989, p. 16) and by Medea (1966, p. 3).

71. Golgi (1881).

72. Golgi (1881; *OO*, p. 205).

73. *Ibid.* (p. 211).

74. *Ibid.* (pp. 212ff.).

75. Tables 8 and 9 in *OO*.

76. Golgi (1881; *OO*, p. 225).

77. *Ibid.* (*OO*, p. 227).

78. Bizzozero and Golgi (1880; *OO*, p. 923).

79. *Ibid.* (*OO*, p. 931).

80. The work was summarized in German (Bizzozero and Golgi 1879).

81. Golgi and Raggi (1880).

82. Golgi and Raggi (1880a; 1880b).

83. Seppilli (1881).

84. Sanquirico (1882).

85. An exhaustive account of the experiments by Golgi, Bizzozero, and Raggi ('Di alcuni trasfusioni di sangue nel peritoneo fatte in Italia') can be found in *Gazzetta Medica Italiana-Lombardia* (1880, Serie VIII, tome II, **40**, pp. 294–5).

86. *Centralblatt für die medicinischen Wissenschaften* (1872, pp. 263–4).

87. Letter from Boll (from Neubrandenburg) to Golgi, 4 September 1873 (Belloni 1980, p. 419), in which Boll expressed his intention to use the black reaction.

10

The structure of the central nervous system

From 1877 to 1880 Golgi's prodigious scientific activity achieved remarkable results in widely disparate areas. Nevertheless, as in Abbiategrasso, the central nervous system remained at the centre of his research interests.

During these years Golgi's work with the black reaction had acquired a certain recognition in Italy but his theory of the diffuse neural net was already encountering opposition. In February 1880, Giuseppe Bellonci presented a paper to the Accademia dei Lincei in which he criticized Golgi's theory and sided with the old protoplasmic net of Gerlach.[1] In his studies Bellonci used mostly osmic acid. He believed, in fact, that even though the black reaction allowed the demonstration of fine details, it was unreliable because it produced incomplete or illusory images. Less than one year later, Bellonci reported, again at a meeting of the Accademia dei Lincei, the presence of anastomoses between the protoplasmic processes of Purkinje cells. According to Bellonci, Golgi had been unable to demonstrate their presence because in the human brain they were too thin and complex to be detected.[2]

Golgi was not deterred by these criticisms. In recent years he had been patiently accumulating his findings instead of publishing them in brief notes. In September 1880 he was ready to answer his critics. He reported on his work at two scientific meetings in Genoa and Reggio Emilia.

At a medical congress in Genoa he 'caused a great sensation among the attending anatomists with the presentation of black reaction preparations'.[3] In his presentation ('On the central origin of nerves')[4] Golgi emphasized the following points:

1. Nerve cells have a single nerve process and therefore they should be considered functionally 'monopolar'; the nerve process at a 'more or less large distance from its origin emits a more or less large number of filaments, which are nerve fibrils'.[5]

2. The nerve process can either branch off completely, thus ending in the diffuse neural net (Type II cells), or maintain its anatomical individuality and, after having given rise to a few collateral branches ending in the diffuse neural net, continue into the cylinder-axis of a myelinated nerve fibre (Type I cells).

3. On the basis of their nerve processes, the nerve cells can be subdivided into cells with direct versus indirect connection with the nerve fibres; the former are motor or psychomotor cells; the second are sensory or psychosensory cells.

4. The diffuse neural net is distributed throughout 'all layers of grey matter of the central nervous organs'[6] and represents the system connecting sensory and motor cells.

5. 'The so-called protoplasmic process under no circumstances, either directly or indirectly, gives rise to nerve fibres and maintains independence from them; [the protoplasmic process] has, however, an intimate relationship with connective cells and blood vessels; thus, their functional role must be identified with the nutrition of the nervous tissue; that is, they represent the medium for the passage of nutritive plasma from the blood vessels and connective cells to the ganglion cells.'[7]

A few weeks later he attended the Third Meeting of the Italian Society of Freniatry, held in Reggio Emilia. In addition to demonstrating a peritoneal transfusion before the participants, and endorsing a pioneering atlas of histological microphotographs,[8] Golgi reported on his research on the spinal cord.[9] Again, he was eager to illustrate the physiological deductions that he had drawn from a wealth of anatomical 'facts':

1. Contrary to Kölliker's opinion, Rolando's gelatinous substance did not contain just glial cells but also numerous nerve cells.

2. In the grey matter of the spinal cord he was able to distinguish:

    (a) ganglion cells, the nerve process of which loses its anatomical individuality by giving rise to extremely thin fibrils that participate in their totality to the formation of a diffuse neural net;

    (b) ganglion cells, the nerve process of which, although sending off a few fibrils, keeps its individuality and forms the cylinder-axis of a nerve fibre.[10]

    And, as in his earlier studies on the cerebellar cortex, he attributed different physiological roles to these cell types:

    Since the first of these cell types is predominantly found in the areas of distribution of the posterior roots (posterior horns in general and more specifically Rolando's gelatinous substance), whereas the second type is predominantly found in the areas of distribution of the anterior roots (motor roots), it is natural to hypothesize that the cells of the first type have a sensory nature whereas the cells of the second type have a motor nature ... This speculation is greatly supported by the fact that in other regions of the central nervous system, such as in the more superficial layers of the *corpora bigemina*, which certainly receive sensory nerve fibres (fibres of the optical tract), one finds only, or predominantly, cells having nerve processes that subdivide repeatedly, losing their individuality;[10]

3. Also in the spinal cord there is a diffuse neural net, 'which, via the medulla oblongata, is connected to the fine neural net that also exists in all layers of the grey matter of the brain';[10]

4. The cylindraxes of the columns of the spinal cord (anterior, lateral, and posterior) have collaterals 'that enter obliquely and horizontally in the grey matter and there subdivide'.[11]

As we shall see in Chapter 14, in 1890 Cajal, who did not know about this work of Golgi, reported as a new finding his description of the collaterals of the axons of the columns of the spinal cord, angering Golgi and initiating a controversy that shortly thereafter would extend to their radically different views of the functional organization of the central nervous system.

5. The cylindraxis of the ganglion cells of the anterior horn project, as described by Deiters and Remak, to the anterior root 'sometimes quite directly, other times after a tortuous detour'.[12] Golgi also characterized a 'non-negligible number of cells'[12] of the anterior horns that send their processes in the white matter of the columns of the spinal cord to the opposite side via the white commissure (commissura alba or anterior white commissure).

6. The nerve process of some cells in the posterior horns of one side 'passing through the anterior commissure enter into contact with the nerve fibres of the anterior columns of the opposite side'.[12] Golgi also observed myelinated structures partly corresponding to the spinothalamic tract, which had not been described previously.

7. There are cells located in the area now called lamina VII, according to Rexed's topography, whose cylindraxis projects through the white commissure 'towards the lateral columns of the opposite side' and also to 'the lateral columns of the same side'.[12] Here Golgi was observing structures corresponding to those that will be later called spinothalamic tract, spinocerebellar tract, etc.

8. Sensory nerve impulses are transmitted to the motor fibres through the diffuse neural net; a fact that would also explain 'the so-called phenomena of diffusion, as well as the crossed and general reflex actions, which can occur in animals in which the brain, including the medulla oblongata, has been removed.'[13]

Three years later he would take up this argument again at the Fourth Meeting of the Italian Society of Freniatry held in Voghera, by emphasizing an important aspect of the histology of the spinal cord. Golgi had previously reported that many anterior horn cells send their nerve process to the anterior roots. But this time he added that 'when I could follow that [nerve] process for some distance within the anterior roots, it always appeared to be lacking secondary fibrils.'[14] This statement is surprising because in all his previous studies Golgi had suggested that the nerve process, even when maintaining its individuality, always emits collaterals connected with the diffuse neural net. But now Golgi admitted that the only nerve cell that could be considered beyond any doubt as a motor cell was quite different from other cells that were also considered as motor by him: that is, it appeared to have no collaterals.

Thus, the fact that the nerve process of the only cells that I could certainly consider as motor does not behave exactly as do the cells of the first type, which I have found in almost all regions of the central nervous system, invalidates the strongest argument that such cells of the first type are indeed motor cells.[14]

Thus, these new findings on the fine anatomy of the spinal cord were not compatible with the functional interpretation of the morphological dichotomy of nerve cells that Golgi had expounded since his 1874 work on the cerebellum.

Given this state of affairs, I must confess . . . I found a void that made me quite wary every time I felt it necessary to offer a physiological interpretation of such findings.[14]

To solve this dilemma Golgi decided to study the spinal cord in the newborn and in the fetus, anticipating thereby the methodological choice that Cajal later applied with great success. In the early phases of development, the 'different chemical conditions, especially the absence or the lesser development of the enveloping myelinated sheath, explain why, the younger the tissue is, the finer and more complete is the impregnation of the nerve cells.'[14] Under such conditions, even the nerve process of the motor nerve cell of the anterior horns 'emits, most of the time before, many times also after its entry in the anterior roots, some (usually only a few) faint fibrils, which turn toward the most internal portions of the grey matter and then branch off in a complicated and indistinct manner, dissolving in an extremely complex neural net.'[15] Having finally succeeded in demonstrating the presence of collaterals in the motor nerve cells of the anterior horns, Golgi had removed the main obstacle to his hypothesis (italics added for emphasis):

Indeed, it is clear that the demonstration that the cells of the anterior horns, which are certainly motor, are connected with the motor nerves *but not in an exclusive manner*, not only has an intrinsic relevance for the interpretation of many physiological phenomena concerning the spinal cord, but is also important for the interpretation of the findings I obtained in other regions of the central nervous system; only now do I feel authorized to suppress most, if not all, reservations to my interpretation of the physiological meaning of the two different types of cells.

. . . the motor nerve cells are in a direct but not exclusive relationship with the nerve fibres.

At this point it is not irrelevant to notice that the other cells, the nerve process of which subdivides in a complex manner, can now be considered, with greater reason, as sensory cells.[16]

In the early 1880s Golgi finally organized all the discoveries made with the black reaction and his theories on the organization of the nervous system in an imposing work of synthesis that would remain his most important systematic scientific work: *Studj sulla fina anatomia degli organi centrali del sistema nervoso* (Studies on the fine anatomy of the organs of the central nervous system). Golgi submitted it for the 1880 Fossati Prize, which was awarded by the Regio Istituto Lombardo di Scienze e Lettere to the best work concerning 'a finding in microscopic or macroscopic anatomy of human brain'. Three other works besides Golgi's were submitted. The committee, which included Serafino Biffi, Gaetano Strambio Jr, Carlo Zucchi, Andrea Verga, and Emilio Cornalia, while commending the works of Lorenzo Tenchini and those of the student Cesare Staurenghi (who received a 1000 lire prize), awarded the 2000 lire Fossati Prize to Golgi. *Sulla fina anatomia* was considered:

a grand and extremely meticulous work, illustrated by an atlas so rich, clear, and elegant that in itself would be worthy of the prize. The orderly, clear, and precise introduction immediately gains the readers' appreciation and sympathy, which grows further when they continue in the reading of the work. His excellence is demonstrated not only by the importance and complexity of the problems investigated, but also by the novel and masterful approach to them. With Germanic dedication and using methods of investigation superior to any other employed so far, the author offers here a general study of the central nerve cells, defining as such only the cells with a special, always single, nerve process; depending on whether this process is connected with the nerve fibre directly or indirectly, through a fine net in the grey matter, these cells can be considered, in agreement with the teaching of celebrated physiologists, either motor, psycho-motor, sensory, or psycho-sensory.[17]

The committee also commended the individual studies carried out by Golgi in the various regions of the central nervous system; cerebral convolutions, *pes hippocampi* ('he studied it both macroscopically and microscopically, in what almost amounted to a complete monograph'), *laminae albae cerebelli*, and striae Lancisi. On 15 November, Bizzozero jokingly congratulated Golgi and his robust wife ('*il Linone*', corresponding approximately to 'the big Lina') who had helped him with the drawings:

Many compliments to the Spouses for the prize received. Those bozos would have done a more deserving thing in awarding you also the other 1000 lire, which would have been more appropriate and deserved. In this way *il Linone* would have been able to afford an even longer train for her velvet dress.[18]

Golgi's prize-winning work was published in 1882 and 1883 in the *Rivista Sperimentale di Freniatria and Medicina Legale* (in five instalments with a slightly different title, *Sulla fina anatomia degli organi centrali del sistema nervoso*, and with modifications and bibliographic updates) and in 1884 in a single volume.[19] In 1885 two additional instalments (which were not included in the work submitted for the Fossati Prize) appeared in the *Rivista Sperimentale di Freniatria and Medicina Legale*, and in the same year the entire *Sulla fina anatomia degli organi centrali del sistema nervoso* as we know it now was published in a single volume[20] that also included a slightly modified version of the paper on the olfactory lobes.[21] Golgi dedicated the work to Bizzozero with sincere words of gratitude. Bizzozero, to whom Golgi had sent the text of the dedication prior to publication, wrote to his friend in Pavia:

Today I read once again the dedication you wrote and I cannot find anything wrong with the form. I have, however, some reservations about its substance, but you do not want to listen, and therefore I must shut my mouth before your benevolence.[22]

Sulla fina anatomia degli organi centrali del sistema nervoso (reprinted in 1886 by the publisher Hoepli of Milan)[23] was by far the most important work on the structure of the nervous system published up to that time. Using his revolutionary method, Golgi completely toppled the prevailing conceptions in neurohistology and neuroanatomy. Given the importance of this work, it is worth reviewing its content in detail.

The work comprises ten chapters, which can be subdivided into a histological–cytological, anatomical, and methodological parts.

Histology–cytology

The histological–cytological part includes: Chapter I, 'Preliminary notes on the structure, morphology, and reciprocal relationships of ganglion cells', in which he focused on his cytological findings and expounded his classification of Type I and Type II nerve cells;

Chapter II, 'The central origin of nerves', in which he expanded on his report to the Genoa congress (see above); Chapter VIII, 'Interstitial tissue of the central nervous organs', in which he reviewed his 1870–71 findings on glia and later works on glia carried out with the black reaction; Chapter X, 'The motor nerve cell', which contains the work communicated at the Fourth Meeting of the Italian Society of Freniatry.

Chapter I

This chapter deals with the cytology of the nervous system. In the nucleus of the nerve cells he observed granulations 'in continuous oscillatory (molecular) motion' (that is, Brownian motion), therefore arguing that 'this apparent vesicle is filled with fluid'.[24] However the main purpose of the first chapter was to review his previous descriptions and interpretations, building especially on the new morphological details discovered with his methods. Golgi expounded on the characteristics of nerve cells, the classification of the nerve cells in Type I (motor) and Type II (sensory), the trophic functions of the protoplasmic processes, and, above all, on his theory of the diffuse neural net.

Indeed, on the basis of his absolute certainty that all nerve cells establish a connection with the diffuse neural net, Golgi now boldly denies the very possibility of 'isolated transmission' of the nerve impulse, a possibility still considered viable in 1875 when he published the paper on olfactory bulbs:

Taking into account also the above described peculiarities of the connection between the nerve cells of the nervous centres and the nerve fibres, I believe that it is possible to state that it is too arbitrary to continue to entertain the notion of isolated transmission between peripheral points and putatively corresponding individual ganglion cells. On the contrary, I feel justified in stating that the law of isolated transmission, as far as the manner of functioning of ganglion cells and nerve fibres in the central [nervous] organs is concerned, is now completely without anatomical basis.

The histological evidence compels [us] to accept the existence not of isolated actions of individual cells but of the simultaneous actions of large groups [of cells], at least in most regions of the central nervous system.[25]

Chapter VIII

The portion dedicated to glia can almost be considered a separate monograph. Using the black reaction, Golgi investigated in great detail glial tissue of different areas of the central nervous system. He substantially confirmed the results he had obtained in 1870–72 using other methods, and sketched an ontogenetic study of glia using chicken embryos. Contrary to what has been suggested,[26] the advantages offered by the embryological approach to the study of the histogenesis of the nervous system had been appreciated early on by Golgi, although he made only a limited use of it.

Because I was convinced that the embryogenesis of central nervous organs provides the solution to a number of problems, which I have indicated here as being of particular physiological relevance, I thought it necessary to follow this approach as well, in conjunction with the use of methods that I have devised and that have been of great help in conducting purely histological research.[27]

Then Golgi considered Ranvier's criticisms of the similar descriptions of the glial cell given by Deiters and Boll. In examining Ranvier's findings, Golgi commented that 'the doubt immediately arises that Ranvier's description points not to the delusions of others but to his [that is, Ranvier's] erroneous interpretation'.[28]

Neuroanatomy

This portion of the book contains a thorough description of various brain areas studied with the black reaction and includes: Chapter III, 'Morphology and position of the nerve cells in the central anterior and occipital superior convolutions'; Chapter IV, 'On the fine anatomy of the cerebellar convolutions'; Chapter V, 'On the fine anatomy of the pes hippocampi'; Chapter VI, 'Notes about the superior surface of the corpus callosum'; and Chapter VII, 'Origin of the olfactory tract and structure of the olfactory lobes in humans and other mammals'.

The section dedicated to the cerebellum is an expansion of the research carried out in 1873–74 and has already been examined in Chapter 8.

Chapter III

Golgi's studies on the structures of the other brain regions are original, particularly his description of 'the anterior central [precentral] and superior occipital convolutions' to which he dedicated this entire chapter. Since his earliest studies with the black reaction, Golgi had tried to identify characteristic patterns that could be linked to the sensory and motor functions. This would have provided an anatomical basis for the many reports of localization of brain functions. His first unsuccessful attempt was reported in the 1875 paper on the olfactory bulbs. More promising were the results he obtained on the spinal cord,[29] where he found mostly Type I cells in the anterior horns and mostly Type II cells in the posterior horns.

Golgi's goal in focusing on the anterior central and superior occipital convolutions was to 'establish a comparison between convolutions that, according to the most recent research, should be attributed opposite physiological significance.' Indeed, 'following the now classical studies by Fritsch and Hitzig, almost all physiologists attribute motor functions to the anterior half of the brain (psycho-motor convolutions) and mostly sensory functions to the occipital convolutions.'[30] Betz, for example, had proposed that Rolando's fissure subdivided the brain into two domains, as was the case for the spinal cord: an anterior motor domain (analogous to the anterior horns) and a posterior sensory domain (analogous to the posterior horns). Thus, these two cortical areas 'can be thought of as having different histological constitutions', and thus 'as to their structure, they should be considered as opposite types.'[31] Meynert had in fact identified five layers in the precentral convolutions and eight in the superior occipital convolutions. Golgi rejected Meynert's cytoarchitectonics and proposed instead, for both convolutions, a classification of nerve cells into three main types and a three-layer organization.

The three cell types are:

1. Pyramidal cells of various dimensions ranging from very small to very large. They present six to ten processes, one of which is a nerve process.

2. Fusiform cells, located deep in the cortex, the nerve process of which, after emitting few collaterals, ends in the diffuse neural net.

3. Globular or polygonal cells with roundish edges, mostly located in the deep layers of the cortex.

The three layers are:

1. Superior or superficial layer, which includes the superior third of the cortex. It is rich in small pyramidal cells and to a lesser extent in 'globular or polygonal cells' (which might correspond to the granules and possibly to the small multipolar nerve cells later known as Martinotti's cells). In the current six-layer classification of the neocortex, Golgi's superior layer corresponds to the external granular layer (small pyramidal cell layer).

2. Intermediate layer, which includes the middle third of the cortex. It contains 'pyramidal cells that can be termed as medium and large. The latter are present near the inferior boundary of the layer [that is, internal pyramidal layer]'. The medium layer also contains other nerve cells that are 'pyramidal-shaped and that are the smallest [cells] of the cortex [probably the granules]'. In the current six-layer classification, Golgi's intermediate layer corresponds to the external pyramidal layer (medium and large pyramidal cells layer), the internal granular layer, and to the internal pyramidal layer (giant pyramidal cells layer).

3. Deep layer, which includes the inferior third of the cortex. It contains mostly fusiform cells, but there are also 'atypical globular or polygonal [cells]', and small and medium pyramidal cells. In the current six-layer classification, Golgi's deep layer corresponds to the fusiform cell layer. Golgi also described a submeningeal layer containing glial cells, which corresponds to the current plexiform or molecular layer.

In the end, Golgi was unable to find important cytoarchitectonic differences between the two brain regions. 'The only noticeable difference concerns the third or deep layer, and consists ... in the presence of numerous small nerve cells distributed in a small area in the deepest parts of the deep layer' of the superior occipital convolution.[32] It is puzzling that Golgi did not notice other obvious differences between the two regions, such as the presence of giant pyramidal cells (Betz cells) in the precentral gyrus. It is possible that the great level of detail produced by the black reaction paradoxically masked the presence of Betz cells, which are easily detectable with less sophisticated staining methods. Nevertheless, Golgi's cytoarchitectonics should be considered as the starting point for later studies of the cortex done by Cajal, Retzius, Kölliker, and Ludwig Edinger, using the black reaction.

Golgi thought that his study of the cerebral cortex, as well as that of the olfactory bulbs, fully confirmed his antilocalizationist position. He concluded Chapter III stating that:

The functional specialization of the various cerebral areas (convolutions, etc., etc.) is related not to the particular anatomical organization of these areas, but to the specialization of the peripheral organs connected to the nerve fibres originating from these brain areas.[33]

Chapter V

This chapter is dedicated to the 'fine anatomy of the *pes hippocampi*' and is presented by Golgi as containing 'the most detailed and precise assertions that can be made at this time on the general problem of the relationship between nerve fibres and cell groups'.[34]

Golgi considered the 'great *pes hippocampi*' as synonymous to 'Ammon's horn', but in fact he used the first expression to refer to all the structures of the ventral hippocampus (Ammon's horn, dentate gyrus, and fimbria). These structures are distinct from the para-hippocampal gyrus with which they are connected via the subiculum.

The chapter begins by highlighting major aspects of macroscopic neuroanatomy and by criticizing the most authoritative models of the anatomical structure of the ventral hippocampus, such as those proposed by Gustav Eduard Kupfer in 1859 and Theodor Meynert in 1867 and 1872. These authors had identified multiple layers in the cortex of Ammon's horn based on the relative density of nerve fibres and nerve cells. As was true of all neuroanatomical research carried out before the introduction of the black reaction, the scope of Kupfer's and Meynert's investigations was constrained by severe methodo-logical limitations. A self-confident Golgi, armed with the black reaction, disposed of Kupfer's *De Cornus Ammonis Textura* (On the structure of the Ammon's horn) stating that 'because of the imperfection of the methods and the scarcity of knowledge about the fine structure of the nervous centres, it is a typical product of the times.'[35] More severe was his criticism of Meynert, a celebrated and powerful neuroanatomist, and holder of a prestigious professorship at the University of Vienna. Meynert had discussed the anatomy of the hippocampus in his most important work *The structure of the cerebral cortex and its local variations, including a pathological-anatomical correlation*. Without hesitation Golgi wrote that 'Meynert's argument offers an abundance of evidence of this researcher's habit of adapting the anatomical data to his theoretical conceptions',[35] an opinion that would later be shared by others who referred to Meynert's neuropathological speculation on the aetiology of psychiatric diseases as a 'the mythology of the brain'.[36]

Golgi described the dentate gyrus as originating from medial longitudinal striae (Lancisi's nerves), contrary to the conclusions of Henle and Wilhelm Krause. He also criticized the prevailing notion that the ventral hippocampus 'simply results from the introflexion of a single convolution',[37] and proposed the alternative view that it was made up of two distinct convolutions: the 'convoluted grey lamina' (that is, Ammon's horn),[38] and the dentate gyrus. Golgi supported this position with geometric and structural arguments. He noticed, in fact, that between the two convolutions existed a space 'that is usually occupied by an extension of the pia mater or by a blood vessel',[37] and that the two convolutions were very different in the trajectories of their afferent fibres and in their cyto-architectonics. Although these observations were substantially correct, Golgi's conclusion was erroneous since the *pes hippocampi* is a phylogenetically ancient formation that had been pushed deep by the great development of the neocortex in mammals, undergoing a partial folding. During embryological development, the grey layers of the dentate gyrus and Ammon's horn, originally connected, undergo differential rotations and movements, and eventually separate. Even though the final result is the formation of two distinct anatomical structures, both originated from the introflexion of the same convolution.

Golgi then provided a detailed description of the microscopic neuroanatomy of the rabbit hippocampus.

1

In the alveus he observed the presence of numerous fibres that projected towards the underlying grey layer, continuing into the axons of local nerve cells (pyramidal cells). Golgi noticed that the axons of these cells emit, before entering the fimbria, collateral branches that 'assume a direction opposite' to that of the axon and 'return in the grey layer ... branching out in numerous filaments of great thinness' and contributing to the formation of 'the fine reticulum or net which extends throughout the grey layer'.[39] Thus, according to Golgi the pyramidal cells are connected with the fibres of the alveus either *directly* through their axons or *indirectly* through 'the diffuse net originating from the branches of the nerve processes'.[39]

Golgi also noticed that on the ventricular surface of the alveus is 'an epithelium' (that is, the ependima) 'identical to the one that lines the entire lateral ventricle' and immediately below he discovered 'a continuous layer of stellate connective cells' (that is, glial cells) the processes of which 'following a general rule for the connective elements ... in most cases make contact, through robust expansions, with the wall of the blood vessels. It appears that many basal protoplasmic processes of the nerve cells of the grey convoluted layer end on these [stellate connective] cells.'[40] These observations reinforced Golgi's conception of the physiological role of the glial cells and of their relationship with the protoplasmic processes of the nerve cells.

2

Deep below the alveus, Golgi analysed the convoluted grey layer (large ganglion cells layer) that corresponds to the actual *stratum oriens*, pyramidal layer, and part of the molecular layer. He described cells that 'appear as simple modifications of the pyramidal cells of the hippocampal convolution'[40] (parahippocampal convolution). They presented 'pyramidal, ovaloid, fusiform, atypical'[41] shapes and had a large dendrite that projects toward the cerebral surface and 'subdivides in 2 or 3 robust processes that continue to subdivide.' 'At the ventricular extremity, in contrast, the cells emit ... a true bush of fine processes, which after a series of dichotomous ramifications' reach 'the connective layer located immediately below the ventricular epithelium'.[41] Here it is clear that Golgi is describing pyramidal cells. Then Golgi noticed that among 'the numerous processes originating from the cell body, it is always possible to distinguish one of them which, because of its appearance, can be immediately identified as the nerve process.'[41] The nerve process 'emits a series of secondary filaments, which finely ramify in a complex manner, partly in the layer of the fibres and partly in the grey layer, remaining in it if they had originated from nerve processes projecting towards it, or returning to it if they had been emitted, as is almost always the case, from nerve processes that after their origin from the ganglion cells had [first] projected towards the ventricular white layer. Both participate in the formation of the diffuse neural net of the convoluted layer.'[42]

Also for this region of the nervous system, Golgi argued against Gerlach's description of anastomoses among dendrites; instead, he found, in agreement with his theory of glia function, that the terminal ramifications of the protoplasmic processes 'consistently make contact with connective cells and blood vessels'.[42]

3

The 'second or external layer of nerve fibres' (which Krause had called the *lamina medullaris circonvolta*, the actual external medullated layer), which is formed by fibres that occasionally 'penetrate obliquely into the near grey matter', subdivide 'in a very complicated manner and finally dissolve in the local diffuse neural net.'[43]

4

Concerning the dentate gyrus, Golgi disputed the prevailing subdivision into two layers (granule cell layer and molecular layer), remarking that 'the two zones are completely occupied by a single category of nerve cells'.[43] Subsequent cytoarchitectonic classifications would maintain the distinction between the granule and molecular cell layers and would add a third, the polymorphic cell layer.

The 'single category of nerve cells' described by Golgi consists of cells that were 'among the smallest of the central nervous system',[44] 'almost without exception globose or ovaloid',[43] and 'regularly aligned along a narrow zone, on a single, double, triple, or quadruple line.'[45] These cells are clearly the granule cells of the modern classification. Golgi found an analogy between granule cells and Purkinje cells in the manner in which their processes originated. He observed that 'the protoplasmic processes originate from one side whereas the nerve process emerges isolated from the other side.' The former project either to the free surface of the dentate gyrus or to 'the convoluted grey layer' (Ammon's horn) and make contact with the glia; the latter descend into 'that part of the convoluted grey layer that folds to occupy the space delimited by the dentate gyrus.'[45]

Golgi noticed that (emphasis added)

this nerve process penetrates with a straight or oblique trajectory into the marginal zone of the last expansion of the convoluted layer, and there, at a distance of no more than 25 or 30 μ from its origin, it begins to emit lateral fibrils (and continues to do so for a more or less long tract), which ramifying [repeatedly] so as to become extremely thin filaments, and by *intercrossing, and perhaps interconnecting* with those originating from other nerve processes, give rise to a complex nerve network that occupies an ill-defined zone, about 50–60 μ wide, starting near the strip containing the body of the small cells and extending along the concave surface of the dentate gyrus. The nerve process as such, despite the filaments that originate from it, can often be followed in its course for a long distance through the above-mentioned network and not infrequently one can observe its continuation with fibres coming from the fimbria or the alveus; sometimes, in contrast, it loses its individuality by ramifying into extremely thin filaments that disappear in the net, *giving the impression that it dissolves* to participate completely in forming this net.[46]

This passage indicates that Golgi was not entirely sure that the nerve process or its secondary branches always interconnected to form a diffuse neural net consisting of protoplasmic continuity. With great caution he suggested that the ramifications of the axons might sometimes intercross (without establishing connections). Thus it appears that

Golgi had considered this possibility many years before the formulation of the theory of the neuron.

Golgi did not explicitly describe the polymorphic cell layer, but in one of the plates accompanying his work[47] cell types different from the granules were drawn in the position occupied by the polymorphic cells. Golgi described rare instances in which the nerve processes of the cells of the dentate gyrus project to the fimbria and the alveus; these projections are characteristic of the axons of polymorphic cells.

The possibility of a simple intercrossing of nerve processes does not necessarily imply the 'isolated' transmission of nerve impulses (that is, the transmission of impulses without interactions between the ramifications of different nerve processes), but Golgi did admit the possibility of preferential transmission between single cells or groups of cells and distant regions.

Indeed (emphasis added):

If from purely morphological characteristics one is allowed to draw general conclusions about the manner of functioning of specific elements of the nervous system, it appears to me that on the basis of the details illustrated above, the isolated transmission from a single fibre to the corresponding cell is not admissible; instead it is evident here (probably because of the special connections in this layer) more than anywhere else that: (1) the nerve fibres probably establish, within the grey matter and before reaching the cells, reciprocal connections via a net of fibrils generated by the fine branching of their ramifications; (2) every nerve fibre that, coming from the white matter penetrates into the grey matter through its fibrillary ramifications, certainly establishes connections with numerous nerve cells, which can be even very distant from each other; (3) despite the numerous lateral fibrils *the main filament of the nerve process of many cells maintains its individuality even across the reticulum or the intercrossing formed by such secondary fibrils and even within the fibre layer; thus it cannot be excluded that there is also a preferential path of transmission, via individual fibres of groups of fibres, between single cells or groups of cells and corresponding peripheral areas.*[48]

Golgi ended this part of his study of the rabbit hippocampus with a physiological speculation based on the different behaviour of the fibres of the alveus and of the fimbria, which would be 'in direct (but not isolated) communication with the cells of the convoluted grey layer and of the dentate gyrus',[49] as opposed to those of the convoluted layer, which would be only indirectly connected (via the diffuse neural net) with those same cells.

Golgi was able to conclude, in agreement with his physiological conceptions (emphasis added):

In daring to make some general deductions about the physiological function of the areas investigated here, ... it appears to me that the following speculation naturally arises: the fibres of the convoluted lamina, which would take part in the formation *of the nervous intercrossing (or net)* that without identifiable limits can be seen throughout the entire convoluted grey layer etc., belong to *the sensory sphere*, whereas the fibres of the alveus and of the fimbria, which are in direct (not isolated with respect to the individual elements) connection with the nerve cells of the same convoluted grey layer and of the dentate gyrus, belong instead to the *motor and psychomotor sphere*.

It is not completely superfluous to state once again that these deductions, while reasonable, nevertheless belong to the realm of hypotheses, which require more solid support by further research.[50]

Then Golgi briefly discussed some minor differences between rabbit and human hippo-campus. He found that the cells of Ammon's horn in the human maintain a better defined pyramidal shape than those in the rabbit and he observed a greater number of cells 'irregu-larly distributed and with completely atypical shape (that is, with innumerable processes arrayed in all directions)'[51] in the part of Ammon's horn that is surrounded by the dentate gyrus. Apparently Golgi did not consider these images (which strongly suggest poly-morphic cells) to be particularly important.

Chapter VI

In this chapter, entitled 'Annotations about the superficial part of the corpus callosum', Golgi described the microscopic structure of the two *striae longitudinalis medialis* or striae of Lancisi. Contrary to the opinion of the few anatomists who had dealt with the topic and who considered them as 'nerve fibres running from front to back'[52] along the surface of the corpus callosum, Golgi thought that the striae of Lancisi contained 'grey matter . . . mixed with nerve fibres'.[53] He added that the 'relationship between these two components presents a number of differences and irregularities: a thin layer of fibres is constantly present, running longitudinally in the deep portion of the grey matter and therefore located between the latter and the transversal fibres of the corpus callosum.'[53] The nerve cells had a 'globular and fusiform or triangular shape; a well defined vesicular nucleus with nucleolus, and scarce cellular substance [that is, protoplasm]; thus they are small.'[54] Golgi could not precisely describe 'the course of their processes, of which there are many' because he had 'so far lacked the only reaction that can provide conclusive results', that is, the black reaction.[54] It is possible that even many years after its discovery the black reaction was still acting somewhat capriciously. Alternatively, the preparations on which Golgi based his description might have dated back to the mid-1870s at the time of his work on chorea, cerebellum, and olfactory bulbs, when his method was still being perfected.

Examining the sections in a progressively rostro-caudal direction, Golgi observed that, on the splenium of the corpus callosum the grey matter 'rapidly increases, to form soon a lamina of remarkable thickness, which . . . lies, assuming the name of dentate gyrus, in the groove of the *pes hippocampi*.'[55] In a footnote Golgi clearly indicated that the 'lamina of remarkable thickness' connecting the striae of Lancisi with the dentate gyrus, was the *gyrus fasciolaris* (or *fascia cinerea*). The continuity between striae of Lancisi and the dentate gyrus had been previously discovered by Luys, who, however, considered the former as contain-ing only nerve fibres. A description of the rostral continuation of the dentate gyrus would be published in 1882 by Carlo Giacomini, who described a small band surrounding the uncus of the hippocampus (band of Giacomini). The following year Giacomini would publish another study on the structure of the 'Dentate gyrus of the *pes hippocampi* in the human brain'.[56] Golgi and Giacomini were the two Italian anatomists who were providing, at the time, the most important contributions to the neuroanatomy of the hippocampus.

Also in this chapter Golgi condemned the habit of making assertions that were 'too often based on mere speculations'[57] the beneficiary of his contempt this time being Luys. Golgi, however, shared Luys' opinion that the fibres of the olfactory tract are connected to the *pes hippocampi*, an opinion that would be confirmed by subsequent neuroanatomical studies.

Golgi noticed that the striae of Lancisi presented 'remarkable individual differences'.[58] As a general rule they were more pronounced in younger individuals (particularly so in a female 26-year-old 'semi-idiot'. Differences in the morphology of the striae could also be found in other animals (monkey, horse, dog, and ox).

Golgi addressed the question of whether 'in the presence of facts that should lead one to admit that they [that is, striae of Lancisi] could be somehow considered as rudimentary convolutions, one might incidentally ask what their function could be, from a more general, anthropological point of view'. He continued (emphasis added):

for the moment I shall limit myself to express the opinion that the said striae must be classified with those structures of the body, which, while being remarkably developed in some classes of animals, are only rudimentary in humans, exhibiting a tendency toward progressive atrophy. Whether the so-called rudimentary structures must be considered as manifestations of *atavism* is a controversial issue, concerning which the greater or lesser development of the structure discussed here has for the moment only minor relevance. Perhaps even this detail may acquire greater relevance when the study is completed by further research.[59]

Golgi was referring here to the ongoing debate about the anthropological theory of 'atavism'. Lombroso had sketched out this theory in the early 1870s after having found a 'small median occipital fossa' in a 70-year-old brigand, a certain Villella, and had expounded on it in his 1876 book *L'uomo delinquente*.

Lombroso thought that this 'small median occipital depression' had been produced by an abnormal hypertrophy of the median portion of the cerebellum (*vermis cerebelli*). Since a similarly small fossa could be found also in some prosimians and rodents, Lombroso speculated that it might represent the remnant of an ancestral structure that re-emerged in criminals and, to a lesser extent, in psychotics and savages. With the theory of atavism, Lombroso interpreted criminality in an evolutionist perspective, considering it a form of regression, a step backwards in the human phylogenetic progression. The theory of atavism immediately elicited a spirited controversy. Andrea Verga claimed priority for the discovery of the occipital depression, denying that it had anything to do with the *vermis cerebelli*, and argued instead that it corresponded to the insertion of the *falx cerebelli*. Furthermore, Verga expressed strong doubts that this depression could be considered a 'stigma of criminality'.[60] To Lombroso's rescue came Bizzozero, who wrote an article, 'On the relationship of the cerebellum to the median occipital depression', in which he supported Lombroso's claim that this depression was related to an abnormal development of the medial cerebellar lobe.

Golgi, who had been a pupil of both Lombroso and Bizzozero, felt obliged to report findings that could have relevance to the controversy on atavism, but he was clearly not eager to elaborate on their possible implications.

Chapter VII

The section concerning the so-called olfactory lobes consists of his 1882 paper on the same topic, with minor modifications. In Golgi's terminology, the olfactory lobe refers to the superficial layer of the fibres of the *tractus olfactorius*, an underlying grey layer (now called the anterior olfactory nucleus), containing pyramidal, fusiform, globular, and irregular cells, and another layer of nerve fibres. Golgi thought that the grey layer of the olfactory lobe was analogous to the 'cortex of a convolution with some modifications'.[61] Other neuroanatomists shared this opinion and indeed the olfactory peduncles are sometimes called Retzius' gyrus.

Golgi classified the cells of the grey layer of the olfactory lobes as:

1. Ganglion cells whose nerve process subdivides almost immediately into extremely thin fibrils, thus losing its individuality and becoming part of a fine and intricate reticulum (or irregular net) distributed throughout the grey layer.

2. Ganglion cells whose nerve process emits a few extremely thin fibrils (which in turn subdivide repeatedly, participating in the formation of the aforementioned net) but which conserves its individuality and joins the nerve fibrils penetrating the grey layer; among such fibrils, of course, the nerve process can be considered as an individual nerve fibre.[62]

The nerve fibres of the olfactory lobes were also classified into two types. Some fibres were 'in direct connection with the nerve cells [of the olfactory peduncle] through nerve processes that maintain their individuality'[63] and project to the corona radiata (fibres originating from Golgi Type I cells), whereas other fibres have their origin in the diffuse neural net and are therefore only indirectly connected to the nerve cells of the olfactory lobes (Golgi Type II cells). Thus Golgi articulated the concept that nerve fibres can originate directly from the diffuse neural net. The relationship between the olfactory peduncle and the anterior commissure was later confirmed, even though Golgi's functional interpretation was clearly erroneous. The physiological corollary of the new neurohistological classification of the cell of the grey layer was in fact that:

From a physiological point of view, it appears to me that it is all too arbitrary to continue talking of isolated transmission between individual points in the periphery and corresponding individual ganglion cells. On the contrary, I believe that it is possible to state that there is no anatomical basis whatsoever for the so-called law of isolated transmission, *as far as its application to the manner of functioning of the ganglion cells and of the nerve fibres of central organs is concerned.*

At least as concerns most regions of the central nervous system, the histological evidence obliges us to conclude that there is a simultaneous action in large cell pools, rather than isolated transmission between individual cells.

The nerve fibre, as the organ for centrifugal and centripetal transmission, does not establish individual isolated connection with a corresponding ganglion cell but rather is connected with large cell pools; furthermore, each ganglion cell, of the [nervous] centres can be in relationship with numerous nerve fibres having different targets and, therefore, different functions.[64]

The description of the projection systems of the olfactory lobes was clearly distorted by Golgi's unconscious tendency to select findings consistent with the theory of the diffuse neural net. On the bases of this flawed evidence Golgi confidently elaborated a comprehensive interpretation of the functioning of the nervous system:

Even the concept of so-called localization of the cerebral functions, if one submits it to a rigorous examination, cannot be perfectly reconciled with the anatomical evidence; or, at least, the concept can be accepted only in a qualified and conventional manner. And indeed, it is difficult to understand how [cerebral] functions could be rigorously localized, considering that, for example, a nerve fibre is in relationship with large groups of ganglion cells and that the ganglion cells of a certain region, and of neighbouring regions, are connected by a diffuse neural net, to the formation of which all types of cells and nerve fibres of such regions contribute. At the most, it would be possible to grant that there are *predominant* or *elective* transmission pathways and that ill–defined regions, being *predominantly* or *electively* excited, *predominantly* respond to an actual excitation.[65]

The problem of the localization of cerebral functions, which at that time was a much discussed topic because of the clinical studies of Broca and Charcot and the neurophysiological research of Fritsch, Hitzig, and Ferrier, was discussed by Golgi on several occasions, including, as we shall see, in an 1882 paper entirely dedicated to this question.

Methodology

This is covered in Chapter IX. Golgi emphasized that 'the facts' discussed in the monograph 'represent progress in the knowledge of the fine anatomy of the central nervous system', a progress that was possible only because 'of the application of new methods'.[66] He then compared the different methods that he had used in this work.

Golgi described in detail the three methods of metallic impregnation that he had developed.

1. The first paragraph is dedicated to the black reaction (potassium dichromate, or ammonia dichromate, followed by silver nitrate), the basic method from which the others derive. He remarked that 'in the application of the method the most important variable . . . is the duration of the immersion of the pieces in potassium dichromate, before passing to the second phase, that is, to the reaction with silver nitrate.'[67] The optimal period varied according to the ambient temperature (one should not forget that at this time there were no temperature–controlled laboratories), the concentration of the potassium dichromate solution, the state of the specimens, etc. During the summer a successful reaction could be obtained after 15–20 days; during the winter longer periods were required (a month or more). Golgi suggested that in any case one should always 'repeat the reaction, that is, having a sufficient number of pieces available [in dichromate], transfer them at different times [that is, after different periods of immersion in dichromate] to the solution of silver salt, to verify whether the piece . . . is in the required state.'[68] Exposure to silver nitrate should last for at least 24–30 hours (even though the reaction sometimes occurs after only 2–3 hours); sometimes it may require a much longer duration. Golgi also discussed how best to preserve the preparations. The pieces were dehydrated and cut in very thick sections (100 μ or more) without previous embedding. The sections, cleared in turpentine, were layered directly on coverslips, covered with gum damar, and positioned over the aperture of a hollowed-out wooden slide.

2. In the second paragraph he discussed the methods based on 'osmium–dichromate mixtures and silver nitrate' (which had previously been used, in a slightly modified way, to demonstrate the horny funnel of myelin). This method allows the fastest staining of nerve cells in black. The silver nitrate reaction can be conducted after as few as 2–3 days of

immersion of the specimen in the osmium–dichloride solution. Its greatest inconvenience is that the silver reaction must be conducted within 10–12 days after the pieces have been immersed in the osmium–dichloride solution, although Golgi described a modification that extended this window to 25–30 days. The method was later used by Cajal and by the majority of *fin de siècle* anatomists.

3.   In the third paragraph he described the 'method in which the action of the potassium dichromate is followed by the that of mercury dichlorate'. He also discussed Mondino's modifications of the method.

Finally, Golgi described a new procedure for the fixation of the tissue by intravenous infusion of the dichromate.[69] This procedure allowed a 'homogenous hardening' of the piece, avoided 'cadaveric alterations', and shortened the period of immersion in dichromate.[70]

An objective appraisal of *Sulla fina anatomia* cannot hide its shortcomings. One of its most disappointing aspects is the author's inability to develop the concept of nervous pathway from a morphological point of view. Prisoner of the theory of the diffuse neural net, Golgi was unable to make coherent sense of the connections between nerve fibres and cell groups. Without the interpretative framework provided by the theory of the neuron and the law of 'dynamic polarization' any attempt to decode the organization of the central nervous system proved to be impossible.

Despite this, *Sulla fina anatomia* remains a book of exceptional value, full of new dis-coveries, original insights, and bold hypotheses. And above all it provided dramatic evidence of the powerful potential of the new methods discovered and developed by Golgi. The text includes 24 plates illustrating the morphological complexities of the nerve cells, each one of which would have been sufficient, when contrasted to the primitive and confusing images obtained with other methods, to convince an unprejudiced reader that Golgi had indeed achieved a breakthrough.

Golgi immediately sent copies of his work to Italian and foreign specialists, including Retzius. As we have seen, the work was initially reported in a series of articles published in the *Rivista Sperimentale di Freniatria*. Golgi was aware, however, that this journal was not an adequate international vehicle for its dissemination. In the second half of the nineteenth century, although Italian was still considered one of the four languages acceptable for publication in international journals (along with German, English, and French),[71] its status had deteriorated. During Golgi's lifetime, Italy had passed from being the third-ranking country in science to a distant sixth,[72] and Italian was now understood and spoken by fewer and fewer scientists outside Italy. It is not surprising, therefore, that Golgi decided to publish a French version of his work in a new journal, *Archives Italiennes de Biologie*, which had been founded in 1882 by Angelo Mosso, Professor of Physiology at the Univer-sity of Turin, and Carlo Emery, Professor of Zoology at the University of Bologna. It is emblematic that the only Italian biomedical journal with an international readership was published in French.

Between 1882 and 1886 Golgi published three papers in the *Archives Italiennes de Biologie*, which provided an exhaustive summary of his neurohistological work.[73] At the same time,

English translations of his works appeared in the journal *Alienist and Neurologist*[74] and summaries in German were published by Bizzozero and Grassi in *Jahresberichte für die Fortschritte der Anatomie und Physiologie*,[75] of which they were co-editors.

Despite Golgi's efforts, the prevailing attitude toward his neuroanatomical work was still one of scepticism and diffidence. Even if some of his papers had been quoted and summarized in foreign journals, he remained relatively unknown in the international arena, although he had consolidated his position in the Italian academic environment.[76] His election as an 'associate member' of the American Neurological Association in 1881 was a meagre compensation for the almost absolute neglect of his discovery in Europe. Giovanni Battista Grassi has left the following testimonial of the mix of diffidence and contempt with which the black reaction was met in Germany.

In 1880 I was in Heidelberg and I had with me a freshly published copy of one of those classical works by Golgi, which a quarter of a century later would contribute to his winning the Nobel prize. With a certain nationalistic pride I showed the paper to the celebrated Professor Kühne and gave it to him to read. The next day Kühne brought the paper back commenting that if Golgi had really succeeded, as in the figures, in staining the nerve process red and the protoplasmic processes black, he had certainly made a great discovery! The physiologist of Heidelberg had paid no attention at all to the substance of the paper.

Many years had to pass before Golgi's method of staining nerve cells would be recognized by learned Germany! And it might still be underestimated there if the renowned Kölliker had not imported it himself, after learning it personally in Pavia in 1887,[77] that is, many years after Golgi's discovery.[78]

One of the few foreign scientists who immediately understood the 'exceptional importance of the book by the Italian scientist'[79] was Cajal, who found in it the 'instrument of revelation',[80] the tool that would allow him to penetrate the mysteries of the nervous system and to achieve, within a few years, absolute pre-eminence in neuroscience.

Of course, Italian scientists who, like Grassi, had their national pride titillated, were quick to appreciate the importance of *Sulla fina anatomia*. The most unreservedly enthusiastic researchers were those who were already admirers of Golgi, like Bizzozero. In January or February of 1884 Bizzozero received the reprints of the instalments of *Sulla fina anatomia* published thus far and on 3 March 1884 he wrote to Golgi that he had intended

to write to you once I had finished reading your entire work. But, as usual, my many projects have so far allowed me to read only half of it; and on the other hand I do not want to delay further in thanking you for the magnificent work that you have completed (or rather, that you are about to complete). It reads very well (even though I now have trouble reading), because of the perfect consistency you have established between facts and deductions, structure and function. One comment only about all your discoveries: I would be delighted if you could make an expedition abroad to show and demonstrate them to that bunch of *barbaroni* [literally 'great barbarians', a facetious reference to North Europeans] who continue to strive without success by using methods that are so inferior to yours.[81]

We do not know whether or not Golgi followed Bizzozero's suggestion to travel abroad, but on 29 September 1884 the Prefect of Pavia issued a one-year passport to Golgi 'who would travel to the following countries: France, Belgium, Holland, Austria, and German Empire'.[82]

In the early 1880s Golgi made explicit his quite radical position on the controversial issue of the cerebral localization of psychic functions. Although the idea that some psychic functions were localized in specialized brain areas dates back to Ancient Greece, it was only with Gall's and Spurzheim's phrenology that it became the subject of a spirited debate in the scientific community and even in society at large. We have already seen how Flourens thoroughly exposed the unscientific basis of phrenology and became the major proponent of a holistic approach to brain function. Flourens' notion that the cerebral cortex is physiologically homogenous[83] and therefore lacks an anatomical substrate for specialized functions dominated neurophysiology during the first half of the nineteenth century. The first to demonstrate that certain brain functions were indeed localized was Golgi's mentor, Panizza.[84] Combining observations conducted in humans and animals, Panizza had demonstrated in 1855 that visual functions were localized to the occipital cortex (see also Chapter 3); he also reported a case of language impairment in an individual with a lesion in the left hemisphere. But Panizza was by now 70, and probably lacked the stamina to follow up on either of these discoveries. Unfortunately, during the second half of the nineteenth century, Panizza's name was only rarely mentioned in connection with the issue of localizationism (with few exceptions, such as the 1892 and 1899 books by J. Soury).

If Panizza's discovery went unnoticed, it was not so for Broca's 1861 report of a left hemisphere brain area responsible for language. At about the same time, using lesions and electrical stimulation, Hitzig (initially in collaboration with Fritsch) was able to identify the motor cortex and the visual area in the occipital cortex in the dog. In the following years a wave of anatomo-pathological and clinical studies, including those by Charcot, Jackson, and Ferrier, continued and extended this research, establishing the existence of precise connections between specific sensory and motor functions and various cortical regions.

These discoveries made it difficult to dismiss out of hand the claims of localizationists. However, a new divide immediately separated the most intransigent localizationists and more moderate scientists, such as Carl Wernicke, who adhered in principle to localizationism but were not willing to embrace it in a 'rigid' manner. A function was not 'located' in a specific region, but rather was produced by the special relationships that the specific region established with other areas.

An important bone of contention between these two positions was the phenomenon of 'recovery of function', that is, the spontaneous recovery of a previously impaired ability after a certain amount of time has elapsed since the brain lesion. Recovery of function was interpreted very differently by the 'hard' versus the 'soft' localizationists. Ferrier, a standard-bearer of hard localizationism, held that functional recovery was possible only for voluntary motor routines, which he thought were controlled by the *corpora striata* and which could be executed even in the presence of the cortical lesion. Thus, for Ferrier, recovery of function did not depend on the vicarious intervention of another previously uninvolved brain area, but simply followed from the automatic execution of motor programs that were already stored at the level of the *corpora striata*. Ferrier thought, in fact, that recovery of function was not possible in the case of unusual motor sequences.

In contrast, soft localizationists maintained that the cortical areas surrounding a lesion or the cortex of the opposite hemisphere could take over the function of the damaged cortex. Luigi Luciani and Augusto Tamburini, two Italian moderate advocates of localizationism, proposed that voluntary movements could be controlled not only by the cortex but also by subcortical structures, and they proposed that the latter were responsible for the recovery of voluntary motor functions after cortical lesions. They also suggested that the *corpora bigemina* and the thalamus allowed the persistence of visual perception after damage to the occipital cortex.[85] Actually, Luciani was the first to demonstrate that visual discrimination abilities can still be seen after bilateral lesions of Brodmann's area 17,[86] more than 80 years before similar findings with partial or extensive damage to area 17 were reported by researchers such as Nicholas Humphrey, Lawrence Weiskrantz, and others.[87]

There were, however, those who continued to reject localizationism altogether. After Flourens' death in 1867, the staunchest advocate of the holistic position was Goltz, who published a series of papers, beginning in 1876, criticizing the experimental procedures of the localizationists, especially Hitzig. Goltz thought that the immediate effect of a lesion or of stimulation was to produce a global alteration of cerebral activity. Other proponents of holistic and anti-localizationist positions were Alfred Vulpian and Edouard Brown-Séquard.

Both localizationist and holistic models were based on the findings of clinical neurology and pathological anatomy in humans and on the results of electrical stimulation and focal brain lesions in animals. Until the introduction of the black reaction, however, the primitive techniques available for studying the fine structure of the nervous system had been incapable of providing any evidence in favour of one or the other position—the only possible exception being the demonstration by Betz of giant cells in predominantly motor areas.

Golgi was acutely aware of the relevance of his neuroanatomical findings to the resolution of the controversy and he soon felt obliged to take a position in a study published in instalments in the *Gazzetta degli Ospitali*,[88] which was published also in French in the *Archives Italiennes de Biologie*.[89]

In this study Golgi first outlined 'the histo–morphological criteria that can be considered necessary a priori to state that anatomy, with its own findings, is in support of the doctrine of localization'. That is:

1. Structural peculiarities of the cerebral cortex that correspond to functional specialization of its various areas.

2. Segregated projection of the nerve fibres from the [sensory] organs . . . to the respective cortical areas.

3. A more or less precise physical delimitation, or line of demarcation, of the different regions responsible for the voluntary activation of specific groups of muscles, or for the perception of the different sensory stimuli received from the periphery.[90]

Golgi dealt with the first point by noting that between 'the central anterior convolution and the superior occipital convolution there are no relevant differences in the form of the ganglion cells scattered throughout the two cortices.'[91] Furthermore, he underscored the lack of 'differences in the diameter of cell bodies'[92] and the presence of cells similar to the giant Betz cells also in the sensory cortex. Finally, he denied the existence of differences in the cytoarchitectonics of these two cortical areas, emphasizing that Type I cells (which he considered motor) and Type II cells (which he considered sensory) are equally represented in the two cortices and that therefore both areas were implicated in both motor and sensory functions. On the basis of these arguments he concluded that the first criterion had not been met.

Then Golgi disposed of the second point on the basis of the existence of the diffuse neural net, which makes it impossible for nerve fibres to establish exclusive connections with 'precisely delimited central areas of projection'; the most one could concede was that there are 'areas of prevalent or more direct distribution; areas, therefore, with which the nerve fibres coming from the periphery, or projecting toward it, would have a closer and more direct connection than with neighbouring or even distant areas, which are also in connection with the same fibres but in a less direct and less close manner.' From a functional point of view, this led to the conclusion that there are 'prevalent or elective transmission pathways and areas, with completely undetermined boundaries, which, to the extent that they are prevalently or electively excited, will prevalently respond in the appropriate manner to the succeeding excitations.'[93]

Moving from these premises, Golgi had no difficulty explaining the phenomenon of functional 'compensation' or 'substitution'.

I think, therefore, that the compensation of the functional alterations, which follows the destruction of different cortical areas, depends on the functional development and augmentation of other areas; this is related to the pathways of the nerve fibres and their connections with the different areas of the [nervous] centres. And indeed, taking into consideration the histological data on the course and behaviour of the nerve fibres that I have discussed, it is completely obvious to suppose that once an area of prevalent or more direct central distribution of a nerve fibre is suppressed, this must increase the activity of a neighbouring or distant area with which the same fibre is also connected, albeit in a less direct way, and that while the functional activity of this area increases, the respective secondary transmission pathways become stronger.[94]

Concerning the third point, Golgi noticed that 'not only is there no evidence of physical delimitation of cortical areas, there is a continuity of structure, or better, a deep reciprocal connection between the different areas of the cortex, including those that are supposed to be responsible for completely different functions.'[95]

Golgi concluded that the available evidence did not support the three criteria required by the 'doctrine of localizations'. Thus, 'the functional specialization of the various cerebral areas would be determined by specialization of the organ to which the nerve fibres project peripherally and not by the specialization of the anatomical organization of those areas.'[92]

At the end of the paper Golgi commented on the hypothesis that specific cognitive functions could be localized in specific cortical areas. Hitzig, for example, had localized 'abstract thought' in the frontal lobes. Despite his resolve not to discuss issues that were beyond experimental investigation, Golgi was unable to hide his disagreement with this idea. For him there was no doubt 'that the meaning we usually associate with the word psyche refers to the overall activity of the different parts of the central nervous system, activity that is certainly the more complex (psychic) the more complicated or developed are the parts interacting.'[96] Five years later, in a letter to Lombroso who had requested an opinion on an article in which G. Pouchet claimed that intelligence was located in unique formations called 'Myelocites', Golgi dismissed Pouchet's theory as an 'anatomo–pathological fantasy' and argued that true 'anatomical reasoning' should lead one to the conclusion that 'intellectual functions represent the sum of the coordinated activity of all nervous elements (without exclusion of any category).'[97]

In the end, Golgi's position on the problem of localization was a direct consequence of his personal neurohistological conceptions. His belief in the diffuse neural net and in the presence of sensory and motor cells equally distributed throughout the cortex led Golgi inescapably to take a radical anti–localizationist position, just at the moment when the nascent neurosciences were moving in the opposite direction.[98] At a time when Flourens' theory was beginning to be regarded as obsolete, Golgi, confident that he had proven beyond doubt the existence of cortical isomorphism and cortical equipotentiality, concluded that

we have come closer to Flourens and Goltz, who, as we know, accept the functional homogeneity of grey matter; or at least, to the extent that we have distanced ourselves from Hitzig, we approach Flourens and Goltz.[95]

Notes

1. Bellonci (1880, p. 176).
2. Bellonci (1881, p. 47).
3. Morpurgo (1926, p. 41).
4. Golgi (1880–81).
5. Golgi (1880–81; *OO*, p. 247).
6. *Ibid.* (*OO*, p. 248).
7. *Ibid.* (*OO*, p. 246).
8. Golgi (1881a).
9. Golgi (1880–81a).
10. Golgi (1880–81a; *OO*, p. 237).
11. *Ibid.* (*OO*, p. 238).
12. *Ibid.* (*OO*, p. 240).
13. *Ibid.* (*OO*, p. 241).
14. Golgi (1883–84; *OO*, p. 540).
15. *Ibid.* (*OO*, p. 540ff.).
16. *Ibid.* (*OO*, p. 542).
17. *Rendiconti del Regio Istituto Lombardo di Scienze e Lettere* (1880, series II, **13**, pp. 636–9).
18. Letter from Bizzozero to Golgi, 15 November 1880 (MSUP-VII-III-1).
19. The work was published in five instalments in 1882–83 in the *Rivista Sperimentale di Freniatria e Medicina Legale* and summarized by A. A. Torre in *Archivio per le Scienze Mediche* (1884, **8**, pp. 91–7). The entire memoir was published as a single volume the following year (Golgi 1884b). In 1885 Golgi added two further papers on neuroglia and methods of investigation, which appeared in the *Rivista Sperimentale di Freniatria e Medicina Legale* as a continuation of the five instalments published in 1882–83 (Golgi 1882–85).

20. Golgi (1885).
21. Golgi (1882).
22. Letter from Bizzozero to Golgi, 11 November 1883 (MSUP-VII-III-1).
23. Golgi (1886).
24. Golgi (1885, p. 10).
25. *Ibid.* (p. 43).
26. Williams (1954).
27. Golgi (1885, pp. 178ff.).
28. *Ibid.* (p. 157).
29. Golgi (1880–81a; 1883–84).
30. Golgi (1885, pp. 50ff.).
31. *Ibid.* (p. 51).
32. *Ibid.* (p. 63).
33. *Ibid.* (pp. 63ff.). Recent studies seem to support Golgi's hypothesis, at least in part. The functional specialization of cortical areas that are similar in cytoarchitectonics and neural circuitry appears to depend on the specialization of the afferents (see Mountcastle 1995, p. 293).
34. Golgi (1885, p. 81).
35. *Ibid.* (p. 88).
36. Papez (1953, p. 66).
37. Golgi (1885, p. 86).
38. *Ibid.* (p. 87).
39. *Ibid.* (p. 97).
40. *Ibid.* (p. 98).
41. *Ibid.* (p. 100).
42. *Ibid.* (p. 101).
43. *Ibid.* (p. 103).
44. *Ibid.* (p. 105).
45. *Ibid.* (p. 104).
46. *Ibid.* (pp. 105ff.).
47. Golgi (1885 and 1886, Tav. XX; OO, Tav. 29).
48. Golgi (1885, pp. 107ff.).
49. *Ibid.* (p. 109).
50. *Ibid.* (p. 110).
51. *Ibid.* (p. 111).
52. *Ibid.* (p. 112).
53. *Ibid.* (p. 114).
54. *Ibid.* (p. 115).
55. *Ibid.* (p. 116).
56. Fusari (1898).
57. Golgi (1885, p. 117).
58. *Ibid.* (p. 113).
59. *Ibid.* (p. 118).
60. Raggi (1898, p. 83).
61. Golgi (1885, p. 124).
62. Golgi (1882; OO, p. 252).
63. Golgi (1885, p. 126).

64. Golgi (1882; *OO*, pp. 258ff.).
65. *Ibid.* (*OO*, p. 259).
66. Golgi (1885, p. 182).
67. *Ibid.* (p. 185).
68. *Ibid.* (p. 186).
69. Jacobson (1993, p. 192).
70. Golgi (1885, p. 197).
71. Grassi (1911, p. 6).
72. de Candolle (1873, pp. 176ff.).
73. Golgi (1882a; 1883; 1886a).
74. Golgi (1883a; 1885a; 1886g).
75. *Jahresberichte über die Fortschritte der Anatomie und Physiologie. I. Abtheilung: Anatomie und Entwickelungsgeschichte* (Leipzig: F. C. W. Vogel, 1880, Vol. 8, p. 12; 1881, Vol. 9, pp. 59 and 65–6; 1883, Vol. 11, pp. 177–8; 1884, Vol. 12, pp. 199–206; 1885, Vol. 13, pp. 90–1; 1886, Vol. 14, pp. 119–21; each volume reviews the literature for the previous year). Bizzozero edited the summaries up to Vol. 13. Grassi, who became co-editor of *Jahresberichte* in 1886, edited the summaries in Vol. 14. See also Belloni (1975, pp. 164ff.).
76. In 1878 the publisher Vallardi began the publication of the *Enciclopedia Medica Italiana* with contributions from the best Italian specialists. Golgi was asked to write the entries for 'Nervous System' and 'Neuroglia' (Golgi, 1882d; 1882e).
77. The first documented visit of Kölliker to Golgi took place on April 1889 (Belloni 1975, p. 145).
78. Grassi (1911, pp. 5ff.).
79. Cajal (1917, p. 55).
80. *Ibid.* (p. 54).
81. Letter from Bizzozero to Golgi, 3 March 1884 (MSUP-VII-III-1).
82. MSUP-I-I-5.
83. Cimino (1984, pp. 160ff.). Finger (1994, pp. 34ff.).
84. Mazzarello and Della Sala (1993). Finger (1994, p. 85).
85. Luciani and Tamburini (1878–79). See Cimino (1984, pp. 127ff.).
86. Luciani (1884).
87. See Weiskrantz (1997).
88. Golgi (1882b).
89. Golgi (1882c).
90. Golgi (1882b, p. 498).
91. *Ibid.* (p. 529).
92. *Ibid.* (p. 530).
93. *Ibid.* (p. 546).
94. *Ibid.* (p. 554).
95. *Ibid.* (p. 569).
96. Golgi (1882b, p. 553).
97. Letter from Golgi to Lombroso, 15 March 1887, reproduced in *Archivio di psichiatria, scienze penali ed antropologia criminale*, (1887, **88**, pp. 206–8). See also Cimino (1984, pp. 339ff.).
98. Cimino (1984, p. 341).

11

Controversies and various studies

In the early 1880s, after many years of intense investigation of the nervous system, Golgi was eager to broaden the scope of his research. He was beginning to have both material and human resources to accomplish this ambition.

As we have seen in chapter 9, his position in the University had been strengthened in 1881 by the double appointment to the professorships of General Pathology and Histology. In the same year he had become Chief Physician *ad honorem* of a small clinical unit consisting of Wards 'O' and 'P' (and later a ward called 'Ward B Women') of the San Matteo Hospital.

His scientific prestige was also on the rise. On 30 January 1881 he was elected, along with Ernst Haeckel, Corresponding Member of the Royal Academy of Sciences of Turin. In the same year he was made Chair of the committee of the Istituto Lombardo di Scienze e Lettere that awarded the Cagnola Foundation Prize, the theme of which, for 1881, was 'On the nature of pollution and contamination'. On 9 December Golgi read 'during a special session of the society' the decision of the committee (which he had probably written), severely criticizing the only work presented to the competition, considering it unworthy 'of a prize, or of any other honourable mention as a form of encouragement' and deploring 'that there has been someone who, lacking preparations of any kind, had ventured to discuss a subject that requires deep knowledge, erudition and practical experience of research methods'.[1]

Meanwhile, the few rooms of the Laboratory of Histology had begun to swarm with pupils. The person in charge of the premises and responsible for supervising the undergraduates and, to some extent, the graduate students, was the laboratory technician Domenico Germanò. Having come to Pavia from his native Calabria to perform his military service, Germanò was hired by Golgi 'in the early days after his appointment to the professorship of Histology. The laboratory [of General Pathology] had no secrets for Germanò, who also knew perfectly well the habits and needs of the Chief (which actually were few and simple) and those (faulty and reproachable, according to him) of the assistants; he was also very cunning in exploiting situations in the most imaginative way to turn things to his advantage and to fulfil his duties satisfactorily (there was no doubt about this) with minimum effort'.[2] As a collaborator, he was 'invaluable in assisting and helping with the experiments on animals, but one could not expect more than this from him'.[3] A handsome man of quick intelligence, 'ladies' man and sensual, prone to sexual intemperance and disorder', he apparently led an 'abnormal family life, managing to keep a legitimate wife and a concubine, with offspring from both'. The students endeavoured to ingratiate themselves to Germanò 'with flatteries and above all with silver coins. When broke or deficient in laudatory initiative, one could be certain of Germanò's wrath.'[2]

One of the brightest student in Golgi's laboratory during the early 1880s was Romeo Fusari who later pursued a brilliant academic career.[4] Golgi became acquainted with him through his brother-in-law Siro Campagnoli.[5] In 1873 Fusari had been obliged to interrupt his studies after the first two years of grammar school because his father, an impecunious elementary school teacher, could no longer support him. Fusari, however, continued to study on his own and managed to take the courses required to enrol in the School of Pharmacy at the University of Pavia. To pay for his studies in Pavia, Fusari found employment as a clerk in Siro Campagnoli's pharmacy. Golgi took an interest in this tenacious youth, as he was always ready to encourage anyone who demonstrated a willingness and desire to learn, advising Fusari to prepare for the grammar school certificate while continuing to take pharmacy courses at the University. In 1881, Fusari graduated from grammar school and was awarded a full scholarship at the Collegio Ghislieri. With the credits he had obtained in his pharmacy courses, he was able to enrol directly in the third year of Medical School, and was immediately accepted in Golgi's laboratory, where he became assistant in 1884, one year before graduation.

Another of Golgi's pupils in this period was Livio Vincenzi, Assistant in Histology in 1882–83, who worked under Golgi's supervision on a dissertation on the origin of some of the cranial nerves. Vincenzi's findings were judged by Golgi to be worthy of publication.[6] Vincenzi remained in the Laboratory of Histology for a few months after his graduation and then in 1885 moved to the University of Modena as an Assistant of Pathological Anatomy. Also among Golgi's pupils in that period were Eugenio Brugnatelli (Assistant in 1883–84), and A. Saccozzi (Assistant in 1884–86), who studied the regeneration of peptic and intestinal glands.

The entrusting of a small clinical unit to the direction of Golgi continued a tradition that could be traced back to Mantegazza. Its rationale was to give the students of general pathology an opportunity to complement their experimental studies with the direct observation of patients. Golgi was 'an excellent physician, even if he never considered private practice'.[7] As recorded by Pensa, in his account of the early 1890s, Golgi's clinical unit was directed 'with modern and scientific criteria and with great dedication' and there the patients received 'diagnoses and cures that bordered on the miraculous'.[8] Every morning the Chief Physician visited the patients, followed by the Assistants and some students. After the visit they set off together for the Laboratory. Along the way there was room only for 'very serious conversation, which sometimes was as intimidating as an exam. If, as sometimes happened, the master had some preoccupation, the journey would be made in silence; any attempt to begin a conversation of any kind immediately faded away.'[9]

One of the main consequences of Golgi's daily contact with the patients of his clinical unit was the rekindling of his passion for the study of infectious diseases. The emergence of this research interest is clearly indicated by a critical review on lung infections that Golgi published in two instalments in January 1882. Here he discussed the nosographic, epidemiological, clinical, and anatomo–pathological aspects of infectious diseases in the light of the various microbiological theories proposed in the wake of Robert Koch's and Pasteur's discoveries.[10] As we shall see in the following chapter, Golgi's new interest in microbiology brought his laboratory to the forefront in the fight against malaria and rabies.

It is easy to imagine why Golgi's double professorships caused some resentment within the University. But even more unbearable was the fact that Golgi, a general pathologist, had been put in charge of a clinical unit. This situation in particular was unacceptable to 'the misoneists to be found especially in [the Institute of] Clinical Medicine' directed by Francesco Orsi and 'to the physicians who adhered most strenuously to the position of this master. From this quarter came criticisms, cutting remarks, and backbiting based on distorted or invented facts.'[8] Golgi's worst enemy, however, was the pathologist Sangalli who, as we have seen, was a bitter opponent of the doctrine of cellular pathology. As Pensa recalled, Sangalli

exercised his malice in two ways: either by seeking to discredit the activity of the physicians of [Golgi's] unit, and particularly of the Chief Physician himself, on the basis of factitious interpretations of the autopsy reports concerning individuals who had died on that unit; or by obstructing the execution of autopsies by the personnel of the unit, claiming the exclusive right [to carry out autopsies] for himself. Occasionally this led to situations that were macabre and comical at the same time, such as clandestine autopsies or autopsies interrupted by injunctions and altercations, and resumed after ridiculous compromises.

The battleground of these skirmishes was the morgue and two filthy and poorly ventilated rooms, which were in a kind of no man's land contested by the pathologist [Sangalli] and the San Matteo Hospital.[8]

Sangalli had a combative and aggressive character and nobody could 'endure for more that a year or two being his assistant, putting up with his arbitrariness and bad temper.'[11] The only one who remained at his side for many years 'with the admirable submissiveness of a faithful dog' was his laboratory assistant Giuseppe Rizzi, 'a tall, thin, haggard and bearded man, dirty and impregnated with all sorts of smells and foul odours coming from the autopsies and the macerations for the preparation of the skeletons.'[12] Sangalli's vendettas on students were carried out during the final exams and in the dissertation committees. Being cyclothymic, it took next to nothing to make him lose his temper and on the frequent occasions when this happened he usually accompanied his altered mood with the phrase, 'Here ends the comedy and begins the tragedy'.[13] The students who were known to be Golgi's pupils, and those who were so daring as to mention cellular pathology, were his preferred targets. There were those who feared Sangalli's wrath so much that they transferred to other universities to defend their doctoral dissertation. Emilio Veratti, one of Golgi's pupils, graduated from Bologna for exactly this reason.

The feud between Golgi and Sangalli was not limited to the jurisdiction over autopsies. They frequently argued during faculty meetings and now and then engaged in scientific arguments. The most sensational of these quarrels occurred at a meeting of the Istituto Lombardo, of which Golgi had been a regular member since April 1882. These meetings were often the scene of heated discussions and Sangalli had already been involved in contentious squabbles. In 1872, he and Luigi Porta had scornfully attacked the poor Lombroso, who was exhibiting two chickens that he thought had contracted pellagra after being administered oil extracted from 'spoilt maize'. The debate between Golgi and Sangalli began on 20 July 1882, when Golgi presented a communication 'On the immunity against anthrax'[14] written by Luigi Griffini, Professor at Messina and one of Bizzozero's former pupils. Griffini, who had come for a brief period of study in Golgi's laboratory, was investigating the possibility of placental transmissibility of the *Bacillus anthracis*, the agent responsible for anthrax. The bacillus had been discovered in 1850 by the French physician Casimir Joseph Davaine who had described, in the blood of a goat suffering from anthrax, small rod-like corpuscles to which, at first, he had not attributed a precise biological significance. In the early 1860s, when the idea that microbes could provoke diseases began to emerge in the wake of Pasteur's studies on fermentation, Davaine proposed that the rod-like corpuscles were the cause of anthrax, an hypothesis later confirmed by the work of Koch and Pasteur.

Davaine had noted that the blood of a fetus from a mother suffering from anthrax did not contain the bacilli, and suggested that the placenta was acting like a filter. In agreement with Davaine, Griffini found that the 'blood of guinea pig fetuses of various stages of development, whose mothers had been infected and killed by anthrax, did not contain the *Bacillus anthracis*', but it did contain '*durable spores of the same bacillus*, which, if the blood samples were sealed under paraffin, quickly developed into bacilli, and, when placed with blood in culture chambers, produced the flora characteristic of *Bacillus anthracis*.'[15]

A few weeks later Sangalli presented findings on the same subject at the Istituto Lombardo: 'Bacteria of anthrax in the fetus of a heifer killed by this disease'.[16] Although Sangalli was exceedingly scornful of discoveries of bacteriology, he used microbiology when it suited his urge to castigate his enemies. In a fetus of a 'heifer that died during pregnancy' he found bacilli, but 'only in the liver and in the spleen'.[17] On the basis of these observations, Sangalli claimed that he had proved that Davaine's research was incorrect, insofar as he had demonstrated the transmission of anthrax to the fetus, not only by means of spores as maintained by Griffini and his patron Golgi, but also by a direct route. Sangalli added that at the beginning of July, his collaborator, Innocente Nosotti, inspector of the public slaughterhouse of Pavia, had talked about this finding to Griffini to whom he had provided 'blood of heifers vaccinated with the preservative liquid of Pasteur',[17] blood which Griffini used in his experiments on guinea pigs carried out in Golgi's laboratory. Sangalli concluded that 'the preliminary report of Prof. Griffini, which was based on results of experiments on the guinea pig, had been anticipated by our earlier direct observations on the heifer',[18] and accused Griffini of not having mentioned this fact in his communication. Golgi immediately took the floor to contest these criticisms and subsequently wrote a searing and aggressive critique of Sangalli's work.[19] Golgi stated that it was 'unfortunate that, in his exposition, Prof. Sangalli had suggested that Prof. Griffini, in his report to this Institute, had exploited private information concerning the observations of the same Prof. Sangalli',[20] while 'the facts communicated here by Griffini were observed by him in his laboratory in Messina a considerable time before coming to Pavia. In my laboratory in Pavia he only completed his study with other experiments that had the value of confirming these earlier observations.' He then criticized the thesis of Sangalli, 'whose observations do not serve at all to demonstrate what they are purported to demonstrate', and noted that Sangalli had not tried to cultivate the bacilli or to inoculate animals with the bacilli to ascertain whether they were indeed the agent responsible for anthrax. Golgi proposed two possible explanations for Sangalli's findings: (1) Sangalli had in reality observed in the fetus bacteria developed from durable spores that had passed through the placental barrier as had been demonstrated to be possible by Griffini; and (2) 'the bacilli seen by Prof. Sangalli were not anthrax bacilli but rather bacilli of septicaemia'.[21] And to corroborate this second hypothesis Golgi pointed out that 'owing to the kindness of the veterinarian Signor Ghisio' he too had received 'at the same time as Sangalli pieces of spleen and other organs belonging to the above heifer', which, in a test of inoculation of dogs rapidly caused their death. And he added that so quick a death certainly cannot be 'attributed to an anthrax infection, but rather to septicaemia'. However, 'together with the bacilli of septicaemia, there were in the heifer the bacilli of anthrax' as demonstrated by the 'flora characteristic of *Bacillus anthracis*'[22] obtained in culture.

Thus, Golgi concluded, the bacilli observed by Sangalli in the fetus, if they were indeed anthrax bacilli, must have entered in the form of spores as Griffini asserted; but if they were not *Bacillus anthracis*, then he must have been dealing with the germs of 'septicaemia'.

Naturally, such a harsh attack was resented by Sangalli, who in his 'Counter-observations',[16] was determined to 'answer with composed words, suitable to the dignity of our Institute, also to the comments that Prof. Golgi has made in the subsequent discussion'.[23] His reply to Golgi's criticism that he had not carried out experiments to identify the anthrax microorganism was that he did not believe it was 'necessary to indicate . . . if and which experiments had been made to ascertain . . . the nature of the bacteria' because 'he knew he was talking to cultured persons, who, by their nature, are inclined to trust the studies of others'.[24] And he cited some experiments of Nosotti on the rabbit and of his assistant Emilio Parona 'carried out in the full light of day' in the presence of witnesses 'so nobody would dare contest their truth'. He then accused Griffini of impropriety for having 'kept his observations hidden' from Nosotti, who had given materials to Griffini to continue his observations and who had 'candidly' acquainted him 'with their similar findings'.[25] Sangalli responded then to Golgi's hypothesis that the bacteria observed may not have been anthrax but rather 'septicaemia', accusing him of having changed the cards on the table:

In his rebuttal before the members of the Institute he had already manifested the suspicion that the bacteria seen by me in the fetus . . . could be those of putrefaction; now he changes the charge and maintains that they could have been those of septicaemia. But does Prof. Golgi believe that the microbes responsible for the former and the latter are the same?[25]

Citing the noted parasitologist Edoardo Perroncito, Golgi's brother-in-law, he reminded Golgi 'that he [Perroncito] wrote: *the cause of the septicaemia is not a bacillus but a micrococcus. This micrococcus is exactly the one that Klebs calls* septicum.' And to show that despite his scepticism for microbiological research he was up to date with the most recent literature on the topic, he added polemically: 'Golgi can see that I am acquainted even with Klebs' work!'[26]

He then contested Golgi's assertion that 'the anatomical characteristics alone, absolutely cannot suffice to establish the differential diagnosis between the anthrax bacillum and other bacterial forms'[27] and that 'distinctions like this cannot be made without cultures or grafts',[28] that is, without a biological proof. Nevertheless he emphasized that he had also confirmed the results of his experiments with this last procedure. At this point Sangalli commented on Golgi's reticence in taking a position on the problem of the pathogenesis of malaria. As we shall see in the next chapter, in 1879 Albrecht Edwin Klebs and Tommasi-Crudeli had proposed that a bacillus, called *Bacillus malariae*, was the causal agent of this disease. Sangalli had learned that Golgi was conducting experiments on the *Bacillus malariae* and although Golgi had refused to divulge his results, Sangalli suspected that he had been unable to confirm Klebs and Tommasi-Crudeli's hypothesis. He now relished the idea that such a champion of the microbiological theory of infectious diseases could be responsible for the demise of the bacterial hypothesis of malaria. In mock admiration of Golgi's reserve, Sangalli added sarcastically that it was

to be deplored that Prof. Golgi, so well-versed in the culture of spores and bacilli, did not want to put his expertise to the test on that theory, vented some time ago in the Ticinian University [that is, the University of Pavia] of the presence of malarial bacilli in the blood of those affected by intermittent fever; and in so doing he has not come to the aid of the new doctrine, demonstrating that such objects, found perhaps more frequently in the blood of healthy individuals, could truly be the much sought-after parasites.[28]

And he concluded his 'counter-observations' by confirming that he had demonstrated '*the passage of both of spores and bacteria from the carbuncular heifer to its fetus* notwithstanding all sorts of contrary observations from Prof. Golgi.'[29]

On 9 November 1882 Golgi presented at the Istituto Lombardo a study on the compensatory hypertrophy of the kidneys,[30] which was published also in French.[31] Although it was a well established fact that the congenital lack of a kidney, or its 'acquired loss', would result in 'a perfect compensation through the doubling of the work carried out by the remaining, or the only active, kidney', little was known about the microscopic modifications in the remaining kidney. Utilizing as an index of cellular duplication the presence of typical modifications of the nucleus (karyokinesis), Golgi was able to demonstrate that in the 'urinary ducts' of the residual kidney 'because of the nephrectomy, the nucleus of many epithelial cells undergoes the various metamorphoses that on the whole are characteristic karyokinesis.'[32] At the end of the presentation Golgi and Sangalli had an 'exchange of observations',[33] we do not know to what extent polemical.

Golgi's interest in renal physiopathology did not end with this work. In 1827 the English physician Richard Bright had been the first to demonstrate that in many cases of generalized oedema with loss of proteins in the urine (albuminuria) the illness is caused by an alteration of the kidneys. For many years the symptomatic triad of oedema, albuminuria and kidney alterations, came to be used synonymously with Bright's disease. Successive studies showed that this syndrome picture could not refer to a single renal disease but must be the end-point of many different conditions. With time, the meaning of the eponym came to be narrowed and modified according to the anatomo-pathological descriptions and to the various pathogenic interpretations of renal diseases.

Some studies had suggested that the renal epithelium had the potential for regenerating in the course of various renal diseases, but this hypothesis was supported only by indirect data. Two fatal cases of Bright's disease that had came to Golgi's attention allowed him to contribute to the solution of this problem.

On 15 February 1883 a certain Boffi was hospitalized in Golgi's ward. This patient was affected by a 'classical form of parenchymal nephritis' characterized by a 'great diminution of urine (only 200–300 cc in 24 hours), by abundant albuminuria . . . and by great quantities of epithelial cells, granulous and hyaline casts, and blood in the sediment'. While the disease was improving, the patient was stricken by a fulminating pneumonia, which quickly led to death. On the following 19 December Golgi treated a boy of 15, from the town of Chignolo Po, who was also afflicted by 'parenchymal nephritis', which evolved acutely over a few days, leading to uremic coma and death.

Golgi realized that these two patients would allow him to investigate two different phases of Bright's disease (in its original meaning): the initial stage (second patient) and the phase of improvement (the first patient having died from pneumonia while the renal pathology was regressing). In the kidneys of the first patient Golgi observed a process of cellular duplication widely distributed 'in the more superficial tubules of the cortical substance', and similar to that described 'in the experimental study of the compensatory hypertrophy of the kidney'.[34] On the contrary, he observed no karyokinetic images in the kidneys of the second patient. Golgi's physiopathological interpretation was that the proliferation of cells was not a 'primary phenomenon' (otherwise it should have been present also in the initial phase of the illness) but only the expression of a reactive regenerative process to compensate for the cells 'which are lost through degeneration and disintegration'.[35]

These two case studies have largely been forgotten, but they are very important because they rigorously demonstrated, for the first time, the regenerative and reparative potential of the renal parenchyma by studying the presence of karyokinetic images. This is a typical example of Golgi's masterful ability to interpret apparently disparate findings coming from both clinical and experimental observation within a unified coherent model.

In 1883 Achille Monti, a pupil of Collegio Ghislieri, joined the Institute of General Pathology for an internship. The previous year he had participated in the student Irredentist demonstrations that erupted after the hanging of the patriot Guglielmo Oberdan by the Austrians. Small, strong-willed and ambitious, he immediately met the favour of Golgi. Soon after he started attending the laboratory, he had the opportunity to initiate an experimental study under the direct guidance of the master. On 20 November and 15 December of that year two terminally ill patients were hospitalized in the clinical ward of the Institute. In both patients the examination of the faeces showed the presence of parasitic larvae. At the autopsy Golgi and Monti observed 'intestinal anguillule' in the duodenum and jejunum, and in the lumen of the gland of Lieberkühn; the presence of eggs in the same segments of intestine; and the presence of larvae from the anus up to the beginning of the duodenum.

At the time that Golgi and Monti were making these observations, a controversy was in progress among parasitologists on the identity of this worm, a parasite of the human gastrointestinal tract. In particular, it was debated whether *Anguillula intestinalis* and *Anguillula stercoralis* were two distinct nematodes or different forms in the biological cycle of the same organism. The first hypothesis was supported among others by Edoardo Perroncito, Professor at the Veterinary School of Turin; the second had been advanced the year before by Grassi, based on studies he had been carrying out since 1878 in collaboration with Ernesto Parona, Assistant at the Institute of Clinical Medicine. Until that moment nobody had been able to observe *Anguillula stercoralis* in the intestine, although it was visible in cultures of faecal material, or verify its 'simultaneous presence in the intestinal contents and in the culture'.[36]

Golgi and Monti, having identified the parasite in the intestine, decided to culture the larvae 'directly from the small intestine as soon as it was cut, placing them in fresh faeces, which a detailed microscopic examination had proven to be free of any species of worm'.[37] After three days of culturing, they observed the *Anguillula stercoralis*, thus confirming Grassi's suggestion that this was the free form of *Anguillula intestinalis*. The preliminary results of this study were communicated at the Istituto Lombardo[38] and were then presented by Giulio Bizzozero at the 15 November session of the Academy of Sciences of Turin.[39] A full report was published one year later.[40]

Nowadays this worm is called *Strongyloides stercoralis* and the illness it causes is called strongyloidiasis. The larvae are excreted with the faeces and evolve in the ground into filariform larvae, which can enter the human body through the skin. The larvae are then transported by the blood to the lungs, from whence they ascend in the respiratory tree to the pharynx, and are swallowed. In the small intestine they mature, nesting in the mucosa of the jejunum. Monti had proven that he was an outstanding researcher, dedicated and prepared. Soon he was appointed Assistant in Golgi's clinical unit,[41] where he was mostly involved in carrying out autopsies under the guidance of Domenico Stefanini, the post-mortem pathologist at the San Matteo Hospital.

In 1884 Golgi found another assistant in Vittorio Marchi. As a medical student in Manfredi's laboratory, Marchi had demonstrated that the neurotendinous organ was present also in eye muscles (see chapter 9) and had proposed that these structures be named after Golgi, something that certainly must have delighted Golgi. After obtaining his medical degree in 1882 he was hired as a post-mortem pathologist at the San Lazzaro Psychiatric Hospital of Reggio Emilia. But Marchi's interests lay in the study of the central nervous system. Using the black reaction he conducted a study on the anatomical structure of the corpus striatum, finding support for the theory of the diffuse neural net and for the classification of nerve cells into Types I and II.[42] We don't know exactly when Golgi became acquainted with Marchi, but certainly the two met at the Congress of the Italian Society of Freniatry, held in Voghera in 1883. Marchi showed Golgi his preparations 'on the pathological histology of progressive paralysis', which he then confidently presented to the Congress audience, specifying that they had been 'checked by Prof. Golgi'[43] (another indication of the degree of authority achieved by Golgi in this area of research).

In that same year Marchi joined Golgi's Laboratory thanks to a government fellowship. When he arrived he was already an expert on histological technique and immediately began neuroanatomical research. Using the black reaction he studied the structure of the normal brain, particularly the thalamus, but he was also interested in neuropathology. He found, probably by modifying Golgi's methods, that the myelin sheath of degenerating axons could be selectively stained by osmic acid after fixation in dichromate. Marchi understood immediately that this would allow him to identify the course of myelinated fibres, from their origin until almost their termination, opening enormous possibilities for the study of nerve pathways. In 1884 he was appointed Assistant, the beginning of what appeared to be regular career progressions. But the following year, with an inexplicable decision (perhaps he had financial difficulties), he left Golgi's Institute and returned to the San Lazzaro Psychiatric Hospital.[44] There he developed, in collaboration with Giovanni Algeri, a method for staining myelin (Marchi's stain), which he applied to the study of the descending degeneration produced by lesions of the cerebral cortex. The method, probably glimpsed at Pavia and clearly derived from Golgi's methods, was presented during a medical congress held in Perugia in September of 1885, and was soon thereafter published with the affiliation of the San Lazzaro.[45] Marchi's stain produced, 'by the action of the osmic acid, an intense black staining of the droplets of myelin within individual nerve fibres undergoing the degenerative process'. In this way it was possible to 'detect the nerve fibres in degeneration, even when they are sparse and therefore completely undetectable with the usual carmine staining'.[46]

Marchi's method had a remarkable influence on the development of neuroanatomy. It provided a certain marker of neuroanatomical degeneration, thus stimulating a great deal of experimental work on the alterations of the nerve pathways following selective lesions of the nervous system. It was adopted, among others, by Vladimir Mikhailovich Bechterew and Constantin von Monakow, who used it to demonstrate the projections of the ascending pathways to the thalamus, initiating a new area of neuropathology concerned with the alteration of sensory functions following cerebral lesions.

The year 1885 was particularly happy for neuroanatomical studies also because of the development of the aniline staining method by Franz Nissl, which ushered in a new era in morphological studies of nervous structures.

The collaboration between Golgi and Manfredi had not been interrupted by their separation. The two friends continued to write and exchange advice, and Manfredi continued to hope that one day he would finally be able to return to Pavia. In 1884, he was appointed Professor of Clinical Ophthalmology at the University of Pisa and his return to Pavia seemed imminent. In the Italian university system the hurdle was, in fact, obtaining a professorship; afterwards, an academic could obtain a transfer to another university carrying the position along. When in 1881 Quaglino left the University of Pavia (temporarily replaced by Roberto Rampoldi), 'Certainly it must have seemed natural that the most illustrious disciple of that school [that is, Manfredi] should succeed Quaglino in that prestigious professorship.'[47] In 1886, however, because of an 'indecent cabal against him, and despite his being the most illustrious pupil and the most worthy successor, [Manfredi] was prevented ... from succeeding Quaglino on the Pavian Chair'.[48] Evidently, 'malevolent' rumours had instilled in 'the elderly Quaglino ... diffidence towards Manfredi'.[49] The best names in Italian medicine (among others Bizzozero, Lombroso, Golgi, and Giacomini) revolted against this gross injustice and drafted a letter of solidarity with Manfredi, in which they expressed their disappointment 'in seeing your aspirations unjustly deluded, and in seeing that you have been ranked below others in a competition that we thought had been conducted only in homage to the greatest formality, but that in your case should have been deemed superfluous by a Medical School that should have felt honoured by your arrival'.[50] So were dashed Golgi and Manfredi's hopes of becoming colleagues in the University where they had begun their scientific careers.

On 5 November 1883 Golgi inaugurated the academic year with a Rectorial lecture on 'Experimentalism in Medicine', an important essay in which he described the epistemological guidelines of his research for the first time. In a brief historical *excursus* he discussed how the emancipation of medicine and biology from the old prejudices had had to wait for physics and chemistry to attain 'such a grade of perfection as to provide a secure base and the required experimental methods'.[51] Among these advances he listed the microscope 'thanks to which ... the new science, histology, which was destined to become a common ground for all branches of medicine, had been able to develop'.[52] Golgi listed also the main achievements of anatomy and physiology from the fifteenth century onwards: the discovery of the circulation of blood, the description of capillary vessels by Marcello Malpighi, the anatomo-pathological work of Morgagni, the doctrine of tissues of François Xavier Bichat, the cell theory, and cellular pathology. In accord with the positivistic programme he advocated a reductionist approach: 'in order to understand the complex vital activity one must turn to the [study of] individual cellular activity'. And therefore life has lost 'much of the wholeness so favoured by the ancient spiritualistic ideas'.[53] For Golgi, medicine must refute these ideas in the name of the experimental method, but it must also refute materialism as an a priori interpretative system, which he considered 'irreconcilable with the experimental method ... because it too somehow presupposes as already explained what science is currently unable to explain'. Materialism 'would therefore be a dogma that attempts to replace another [dogma]', something that must be refuted 'in the name of experimentalism'.[54]

   For Golgi anything that can be said about the phenomenon of life derives necessarily from the application of the laws of physics and chemistry; 'but medical science doesn't try to hide the fact that between the extreme reach of a physical–chemical reading of living phenomena and the true understanding of the most elevated examples of them. [e.g. consciousness], there is an abyss that science currently does not know how to cross.' Still, 'before this abyss, [science] does not retreat disheartened, nor does it endorse certain aphorisms with which some standard-bearers of science pretend to demarcate the confines of human knowledge.'[55] The reference here is to the physiologist Emil du Bois-Reymond who, in a famous conference in Leipzig on 14 August 1872, had posited insurmountable limits *in principle* to the scientific investigation of human consciousness and of concepts such as matter and force.[56] This agnostic choice, which established boundaries to human knowledge, had been expanded upon in another conference 'The seven enigmas of the world', with the addition of five other unsolvable problems (in part reducible to the first two): the nature of motion, the origin of life, the teleology of nature, the problem of free will, and the nature of thought. Such enigmas, according to du Bois-Reymond, could not be attacked by the only form of scientific knowledge available to humans: *mechanistic knowledge*, that is, the phenomenalistic investigation in terms of classic mechanics. Their transcendent nature renders them not only unknowable now (*ignoramus*) with the limited means at the disposal of science, but unknowable forever (*ignorabimus*). But for Golgi it was not appropriate to place limits or boundaries on knowledge, despite the enormous problems that science faces; on the contrary, from the

surprising progress that biology has made in the course of a few decades, [science] receives fresh energies to continue in the battle; a battle not of grandiose ideas but of facts accumulated with the pertinacity of patient and tireless work, knowing that the progress achieved in this way, no matter how small, will be imperishable, opening the way to new conquests.[57]

The only acceptable faith for a scientist 'is the faith in the facts that can be documented with experiments.'[58] But the experimental data have no absolute value; building on the contribution from other disciplines, medicine must 'verify and re-examine everything that is already known, ever ready to find imperfect and erroneous tomorrow what today seems complete and certain.'[59]

Golgi's adherence to positivism was not uncritical and fideistic. Distancing himself from the extremist positions of radical materialism and dogmatic scientism, Golgi retreated within the pragmatic approach 'of small daily steps', which, using a felicitous phrase, can be characterized as 'positivism without myths'.[60]

Golgi made exactly the same points over 30 years later in a conference on 'The modern evolution of the doctrine and of knowledge of life' in 1914,[61] and in the autobiographical speech that he read in 1919 on the occasion of the celebrations for his retirement. The fact that this 'positivism without myths' had already been precisely delineated in 1883 shows that, contrary to what some have asserted, it was not an expression of caution linked to the emergence of idealistic and anti-positivist tendencies during the twentieth century, but rather represented one of the fundamental traits of Golgi's personality and intellectual coherence dating back to the early phases of his scientific development.

The speech on experimentalism in medicine also contained a reference to the 'veiled threats' against the University of Pavia. There were rumours of an attempt to transfer to Milan some of the Schools of the University of Pavia, first and foremost the Medical School, or even, much more ominously, to create a university in Milan. And this 'threat' was fed by the many problems of the University of Pavia, from those of space and logistics to those of management. There were many who complained that at Pavia 'science was restricted within narrow confines' and who therefore were pressing for a Milanese solution. Thus Golgi warned of the necessity for a rapid approval of provisions for the renovation of University facilities, 'then ... no one will challenge Pavia's glory'.[62]

The speech was received favourably by the academic body of the University. Bizzozero wrote Golgi of having 'heard with pleasure the news of the success of your speech' of which he did not 'doubt a priori' knowing 'for some time that you have a head that thinks, ponders, and produces stuff of the highest quality'. He asked for a copy of the speech 'as soon as it is printed, because I have a burning desire to gulp it down.'[63] And he did so soon as he received it:

I have read also in one gulp, as soon as I received it, your Inaugural Lecture. You have dealt with the argument most appropriately; and certainly it deserved to have a great impact, if we weren't in Italy, where the gossip of the politicians, the lotteries, and the Carnivals is infinitely more interesting than the questions concerning education, progress and the true welfare of the country.[64]

In 1883 Golgi was elected Corresponding Member of the Royal Academy of Medicine of Turin. He was also asked to serve on various committees awarding scientific prizes; in 1883 and 1884 he was Committee Chair for the Fossati Prize[65] and the following year he was on the committee for the Brambilla Prize[66] of the Istituto Lombardo.

One of the best indicators of the growth of science during the nineteenth century was the creation of numerous scientific societies linked to the most important European universities. These societies were places for interdisciplinary exchanges and they often published the proceedings of their meetings. Such a need was felt also at Pavia, where 20 years earlier Bizzozero had sought to organize a multidisciplinary group of scientists around a scientific journal. Even though this initiative had failed, the need from which it had arisen did not die out but actually became even more urgent, especially because the biomedical field was undergoing a tumultuous expansion after the recent breakthroughs in microbiology. And so, in October–November 1885, Arturo Guzzoni Degli Ancarani, Assistant at the Obstetrical and Gynaecological Clinic, began to promote among the physicians of the province of Pavia an initiative to establish a medical–surgical society. The project quickly gained momentum, and on the following 8 December the first meeting of a new scientific society, consisting of 41 Pavian physicians, was held on the premises of the San Matteo Hospital.[67] A committee of five members, including Golgi, was charged with drafting a founding constitution, which after some discussion and modification was approved in the course of the second meeting six days later. The first Article established that the new Società Medico-Chirurgica (Medical–Surgical Society) was founded 'for the purpose of promoting and encouraging the study and the progress of medicine, surgery, and allied sciences'.

The third meeting, held on 18 December with 39 members present and presided over by Giovanni Zoja, was dedicated to the election of the officers. Golgi was elected President,[68] and Guzzoni Degli Ancarani Secretary. The 61 founding members included representatives from the academic and medical community of the province: 13 professors, headed by Camillo Golgi, 13 assistants, headed by Guzzoni Degli Ancarani, 5 chief physicians of San Matteo Hospital, and other physicians with various titles.[67] At the meeting of 11 January 1886, Golgi initiated his presidential duties by thanking 'with noble and affectionate words [the colleagues] who wanted me to be President' and warning them, modestly, that 'he did not have the necessary endowment to cover such an honourable position, but that he will dedicate himself to it with all his energies.' Then Golgi presented the bylaws, which were approved, and it was established that the sessions would be held in the afternoon of the first and third Saturdays of each month. On the following Saturday Golgi presided over the first scientific meeting of the new society with 36 members attending. During the meeting Fusari presented a report on 'The blood platelets in various diseases'. It is possible that, with the presentation of his assistant, Golgi intended to honour Bizzozero who on 9 December 1881 had made a thorough description of blood platelets (establishing their role in coagulation) in a communication to the Academy of Medicine of Turin, of which *The Lancet* carried a full page report on 21 January 1882.

The Società Medico-Chirurgica of Pavia quickly became internationally renowned and its bulletin (*Bollettino della Società Medico-Chirurgica di Pavia*) was read in hospitals and laboratories throughout Europe. Important discoveries, such as that of the Golgi apparatus, Negri's bodies, and the cycle of the malarial parasite in humans, were announced at its meetings. Naturally, an association dominated by Golgi (who published some 33 articles in the *Bollettino*) was snubbed by Sangalli and Orsi, neither of whom ever presented any scientific reports there.

The Laboratory of General Pathology had now become a magnet for Italian researchers interested in the structure of the nervous system. In 1884 there arrived Casimiro Mondino who had been a student with Giacomini and Bizzozero at the University of Turin, and who immediately after graduation had been appointed Director of the Laboratory of Pathological Anatomy of the Mental Hospital of Turin. Here he had conducted histological studies on the circulatory system of the liver and perfected the mercury dichloride method first devised by Golgi. He was surrounded by an aura of mystery because it was rumoured that he was an illegitimate son of a high member of the royal family (according to some, the King himself).

Mondino was particularly interested in neuroanatomical studies. Soon after his arrival in Pavia he set about studying the structure of peripheral nerve fibres and published a work in which he was harshly critical of Pertik and Waldstein for their superficial criticisms of the works of Golgi and Rezzonico on the horny funnels.[69] He also conducted macroscopic and microscopic studies on the neuroanatomy of the claustrum and the amygdala.[70] The following year he published a monograph titled *Macro and microscopic research on nervous centres*, which he submitted for the 1886 Fossati Prize. The committee was chaired by Golgi and included Verga and Biffi. The Prize was awarded to Mondino, whose work was ranked ahead of four other papers, which nevertheless were judged worthy of publication.[71] Under Golgi's sponsorship, Mondino was appointed Professor of Histology at the University of Palermo in 1886.

Meanwhile, the translation of Golgi's work on the nervous system into English and French began to bear fruit in the international arena. One of the first foreign researchers to become interested was the Swiss psychiatrist August-Henri Forel, director of the Burghölzli Psychiatric Hospital. Fascinated by Golgi's extraordinary descriptions of nerve cells, he asked his collaborator Eugen Bleuler to test the method of metallic impregnation. The results were some preparations of the cerebral cortex of the rabbit, which were shown at the meeting of 5 December 1885 of the *Gesellschaft der Aerzte* of Zurich,[72] attended also by von Monakow. The images of the nerve cells obtained with this method represented a revelation for Forel.[73] By a trick of fate it was thanks to the images produced by the black reaction that he developed the concept of the individuality of the nerve cells.

Independently of Forel, Wilhelm His Sr also developed similar ideas in the same period. The 'theory of the neuron' was taking its first steps.

At the end of the nineteenth century, American science was still poorly developed and enterprising American researchers travelled to Europe, especially Germany and Austria, to visit the most celebrated research centres in the world. Upon returning to America, they worked with great determination to elevate American medical research to the standards of the 'Old World'. Americans were particularly interested in new developments in micro-biology and therefore one of their primary destinations was the laboratory of Koch, which was visited by, among others, Henry William Welch, the pathologist from Johns Hopkins University. Another American from Johns Hopkins, Henry Herbert Donaldson toured the great neurological centres of Europe, including visits to Forel in Zurich, Gudden in Munich, and Meynert in Vienna. In their laboratories he became aware of the growing importance of Golgi's work and so decided to make a brief stop in Pavia at the beginning of 1887.[74] During a two-day visit in the poorly equipped Laboratory of General Pathology of the Botanical Gardens he was able to observe perfectly outlined nerve cells demon-strated by the very discoverer of the black reaction.[75]

Donaldson was not the first non-Italian scientist to visit Golgi's laboratory. Just before him the laboratory had hosted the Norwegian Fritjof Nansen.[76] Born near Christiania (Oslo), the handsome Nansen had since youth demonstrated a remarkable passion for the natural sciences, hunting, fishing, and adventurous travelling. When 21 he participated in an exploration of the polar ocean, in the course of which he made zoological observations of marine biology; on his return he was appointed curator of the Zoological Museum of Bergen. In 1885 he published his first scientific work on the microscopic anatomy of worms.[77] Very soon he became interested in the nervous system of invertebrates. When he discovered the black reaction and realized its potential for his work, he determined to learn it, and after some unfruitful attempts in Bergen decided to visit Pavia to acquire the method from Golgi himself. He spent a week of the spring of 1886 in Pavia working (as his daughter remembered) with Golgi and Fusari, familiarizing himself with the black reaction. Immediately after Pavia he visited Venice, Florence, and Rome, and arrived 'a mia bella Napoli [in my beautiful Naples]'.[78] He remained in Naples from April to June to experiment with Golgi's method on the amphioxus (with scant results) and to collect bibliographic materials for his thesis. Back in Bergen, he wrote a warm letter of thanks to Golgi 'for the splendid days spent at Pavia' and 'for what I have learned' during my 'too brief' visit; of this 'I shall be grateful, to you, dear professor, for the rest of my life'.[78] Nansen added that he had taken up again 'with great zeal' the studies of the nervous system and that 'your outstanding method works very well here and I have already found many interesting things', although he regretted that he was unable to stain the nervous processes well and that 'the preparations are not permanent and I am far from having achieved ideal conditions'. Nansen promised that as soon as he was able to obtain entirely satisfactory results, he would send some preparations to Golgi 'so that you can decide whether you can be proud of your pupil'. He sent his greetings to Fusari and Monti, and promised again to send a photograph of himself to Golgi and his wife, whom he thanked 'for all her kindness'. In the following months Nansen worked hard to complete his doctoral thesis, which was published in 1887.[79] As promised, he sent Golgi, as a memento of the visit, a photograph of his handsome Scandinavian face dated Bergen 9 March 1887.[80]

Between 1893 and 1896 Nansen became known throughout the world for his polar expedition with the ship *Fram*. In 1902 he again wrote to Golgi that he would never forget the time passed in the Laboratory of General Pathology and the kindness with which 'the young and unknown Norwegian student' had been welcomed, and that he 'always remembered with gratitude all that you taught me' and professed that the dream of his late life had been to return to the studies of the nervous system 'which I began with you', although he feared that this dream would never be realized.[81] And in fact for the rest of his life his many political and diplomatic activities absorbed him totally, keeping him far from his youthful love of biology. Nansen had an important role in the events that led to the independence of Norway in 1905 and was later Ambassador to England. Because of his work as High Commissar for the refugees of the First World War and for the humanitarian spirit that animated his activity he received the Nobel Prize for Peace in 1922.

Notes

1. Report of the Committee for the Premio Straordinario di Fondazione Cagnola (*Rendiconti del Regio Istituto Lombardo di Scienze e Lettere*, 1881, Serie II, **14**, pp. 732–3).
2. Pensa (1991, p. 69).
3. Medea (1966, p. 3 *bis*).
4. Bruni (1919).
5. Siro Campagnoli was born in Pavia on 17 August 1841; in 1865 he took over the Cazzani Pharmacy on Corso Cavour (Arch. communale IV.4.1.B); his second marriage was to the sister of Golgi, Maria Teresa, with whom he had five children.
6. Vincenzi (1883).
7. Rondoni (1943, p. 542).
8. Pensa (1991, p. 97).
9. *Ibid.* (p. 98).
10. Golgi (1882f).
11. Pensa (1991, p. 105).
12. *Ibid.* (pp. 105ff.).
13. See note by Prof. Bruno Zanobio in Pensa (1991, p. 106).
14. Griffini (1882).
15. *Ibid.* (p. 546).
16. Sangalli (1882).
17. *Ibid.* (p. 671).
18. *Ibid.* (p. 672).
19. Golgi (1882g).
20. *Ibid.* (p. 672).
21. *Ibid.* (p. 673).
22. *Ibid.* (p. 674).
23. Sangalli (1882, p. 675).
24. *Ibid.* (p. 676).
25. *Ibid.* (p. 677).

26. *Ibid.* (p. 678).
27. Golgi (1882g, p. 673).
28. Sangalli (1882, p. 679).
29. *Ibid.* (p. 680). Perroncito was in Pavia for a few days during the Carnival holidays in 1881. During his stay he was also able to talk with Nosotti about his observations on the placental transmissibility of anthrax. As soon as he returned to Turin he began to investigate the problem and on 15 December 1882 he reported preliminary results of his studies to the Academy of Medicine of Turin. On 4 February 1883 he presented to the Accademia dei Lincei a more extensive report in which he concluded that 'we have to admit the passage of the anthrax virus from mother to fetus, although this occurs only sometimes . . . Furthermore, the virus can be found in the fetus in the form of bacteria and not of spores, as the experiments demonstrate in a clear-cut manner.' (Perroncito 1883 p. 210.)
30. Golgi (1882h). The work was cited also by Podwyssozki (1886, p. 279).
31. Golgi (1882i). The work was cited also by Podwyssozki (1886 p. 279).
32. Golgi (1882h; *OO*, p. 954).
33. *Rendiconti del Regio Istituto Lombardo di Scienze e Lettere* (1881, Serie II, **15**, p. 590).
34. Golgi (1884a; *OO*, p. 964). The work was taken up again by Podwyssozki (1886, p. 279).
35. Golgi (1884a; *OO*, p. 967).
36. Golgi and Monti (1886; *OO*, p. 976).
37. *Ibid.* (*OO*, p. 979).
38. Golgi and Monti (1884).
39. Golgi and Monti (1885–86). Bizzozero was very interested in Golgi's studies on the 'anguillule'. In a letter sent on 3 March 1884 he asked Golgi to send him 'as soon as possible' the 'eggs and larvae, and adult anguillule' and in a following letter dated 21 March 1884 (with the salutation '*Caro Golgione*'—'Dear Big Golgi', a typical Italian way of expressing affection), he wrote: 'I await with impatience your work. I would also be very happy to receive some of your material, or some of your preparations; especially the ovules and the larvae from fresh faeces, and everything that can serve a diagnostic purpose.' From a letter Bizzozero wrote to Golgi on 3 December 1885 we know that Bizzozero received the study on the anguillulae only 'a quarter of an hour before' he left for the meeting of Academy of Sciences where he reported Golgi's findings (MSUP-VII-III-1).
40. Golgi and Monti (1886).
41. Monti (1935, p. 3).
42. Marchi (1883).
43. Marchi (1883a, p. 221).
44. According to biographical notes on Marchi (Belloni 1974; Rizzoli 1990; Roizin 1953), he was Assistant for one year (1885) in the Institute of Physiology of Florence, directed by Luigi Luciani, who had been a pupil of Karl Ludwig. However, the works published by Marchi in 1885 bear the affiliation of the Mental Hospital of Reggio Emilia. Therefore it is possible that, having left Golgi's laboratory, he returned for a brief period to the San Lazzaro Hospital before moving to Florence. But even in Florence Marchi did not remain long: after barely a year he returned to Reggio Emilia as a post-mortem pathologist. An exhaustive list of Marchi's bibliography is found in Belloni (1974).
45. Marchi and Algeri (1885).
46. *Ibid.* (pp. 493ff.).
47. Alfieri (1916, p. 407).
48. Gualino (1936, p. 14).

49. Alfieri (1916, p. 405).

50. The letter is kept in the private archives of the Manfredi family at Bosco Marengo and is dated 'Rome 28 September 1886'. It has been published in Gualino (1936, pp. 15ff.) with the incorrect year (1868). The competition at Pavia was won by Roberto Rampoldi, but Golgi managed to have it invalidated (making an enemy of Rampoldi) by the High Council of Public Education, of which he had become a member in 1886, on the basis of a technicality. The notice of the annulment, which appeared to leave some hope for Manfredi, was received with great satisfaction by Bizzozero: 'I thank you [Golgi] for the promptness with which you have telegraphed me the magnificent news; the annulment of the competition … demonstrates that you have made a brilliant entry into the high Conclave!' (letter from Bizzozero to Golgi on 26 October 1886; MSUP-VII-III-1). But Manfredi was not appointed to the professorship; it was only finally assigned in 1888, to Francesco Falchi.

51. Golgi (1884, p. 20).

52. *Ibid.* (p. 29).

53. *Ibid.* (p. 34).

54. *Ibid.* (pp. 37ff.).

55. *Ibid.* (p. 36).

56. du Bois–Reymond (1891).

57. Golgi (1884, pp. 36ff.).

58. *Ibid.* (p. 38).

59. *Ibid.* (p. 37).

60. Cimino (1984, p. 265).

61. Golgi (1914).

62. Golgi (1884, p. 66).

63. Letter from Bizzozero to Golgi, 11 November 1883 (MSUP-VII-III-1).

64. Letter from Bizzozero to Golgi, 3 March 1884 (MSUP-VII-III-1).

65. *Rendiconti del Regio Istituto Lombardo di Scienze e Lettere* (1883, Serie II, **16**, pp. 1027–8; 1884, Serie II, **17**, p. 766).

66. *Rendiconti del Regio Istituto Lombardo di Scienze e Lettere* (1885, Serie II, **18**, p. 616). See also *Rendiconti del Regio Istituto Lombardo di Scienze e Lettere* (1886, Serie II, **19**, pp. 36–8).

67. *Bollettino della Società Medico-Chirurgica di Pavia* (1886, Anno 1, pp. 3–7). See also Zanobio (1986).

68. Golgi remained President until 9 December 1888 when the Professor of Hygiene, Giuseppe Sormani, was elected.

69. Mondino (1884, pp. 54ff.).

70. Mondino (1885a).

71. Prizes of encouragement were proposed for three participants: Vittorio Marchi, Livio Vincenzi, and Lorenzo Tenchini. *Rendiconti del Regio Istituto Lombardo di Scienze e Lettere* (1887, Serie II, **20**, pp. 48–58).

72. *Correspondenz-Blatt für Schweizer Aerzte* (1886, **16**, p. 155). See also Belloni (1975 p. 143).

73. Akert (1993, p. 427).

74. Postcard of Forel to Golgi, 23 January 1887 (MSUP-VII-II-F); and letters from Donaldson to Golgi (MSUP-VII-II-D). See also Conklin (1939, p. 230), Pilleri (1984), and Saffron (1980, pp. 160ff.)

75. Donaldson remained in Europe for 18 months from February 1886 to autumn 1887; after his return to America he pursued an outstanding career, first as a Professor of Neurology at the University of Chicago and then as Director of the Wistar Institute of Anatomy and Biology

of Philadelphia, where he selected the famous Wistar strain of albino rats still used throughout the world. Saffron (1980, pp. 160ff.).

76. Aarli (1989, p. 73); Shepherd (1991, pp. 117 ff.).

77. Nansen sent to Golgi a copy of his first scientific work *Bidrag til Myzostomernes Anatomi
og Histologi*, published by the Museum of Bergen, with the dedication: 'Professor M. C.
Golgi—with the compliments of Fridtiof Nansen' (kept in the Institute of General Pathology of the University of Pavia).

78. Letter from Nansen to Golgi, 12 October 1886 (MSUP-VII-III-12).

79. Nansen (1887).

80. The original photograph is at the MSUP, and is reproduced in Pensa (1961b, p. 21; 1991,
p. 262).

81. Letter from Nansen to Golgi, 12 December 1902 (MSUP-VII-III-12).

12

The secret of the intermittent fevers

Golgi's experimental work on intestinal parasites and the transmission of anthrax in the early 1880s was not a momentary fancy after many years of almost exclusive focus on the nervous system. Indeed, Golgi's long-lasting interest in the study of infectious diseases had been overshadowed only by his passion for neurohistology. The electrifying discoveries made in microbiology at the beginning of the 1880s, however, would be instrumental in transforming what had been only a latent interest into the main focus of his research activity.

The notion that living organisms, invisible to the naked eye, could produce severe diseases had been advanced since the first century BC by Marcus Terentius Varro,[1] but it was only with the discoveries of Pasteur and Koch in the 1870s that the study of microbiology reached maturity. After the discoveries of the *Mycobacterium tuberculosis* (1882) and the *Vibrio cholerae* (1884—although in fact this comma-like micro-organism had already been observed by Pacini in 1854) by Koch, and of the *Corynebacterium diphtheriae* by Klebs, medical laboratories around the world began a feverish search for the microbes responsible for infectious diseases. The guidelines for this search had been established by Koch (Koch's postulates) in 1882–83. A micro-organism could be specifically linked to a disease only if it is present in all patients with that disease, it can be cultivated outside the patient, and its inoculation in healthy animals produces the disease.

The Laboratory of General Pathology was ready to participate in the 'hunt for the microbe'. The University of Pavia Medical School already prided itself on a glorious tradition in microbiology. In the last decades of the eighteenth century Spallanzani had successfully refuted the theory of spontaneous generation of micro-organisms (the 'little animals of the infusions') and envisaged their possible pathogenic actions, and half a century later Bassi conclusively demonstrated that micro-organisms were responsible for the infection of the silkworm. Bassi also demonstrated in the 1830s that physical and chemical agents (sunlight, milk of calcium, and sulfurous anhydride) could block that infection. And in 1863 Enrico Bottini, who later became Professor at the University of Pavia, used phenol for the first time in treating surgical infections at the Hospital of Novara. Bottini published his findings in 1866, one year before the publication of similar results by Lister.

It is not difficult to understand why, among the many infectious diseases afflicting mankind at the turn of the century, Golgi decided to focus on malaria. Malaria was a world-wide scourge, striking millions of individuals, especially in tropical regions, and since antiquity had been endemic in large areas of Italy, including the Po Valley, the Italian North-East, Tuscany, Sicily, Sardinia, and the countryside around Rome. In the first century AD Aulus Cornelius Celsus identified three forms of the disease on the basis of the duration of the intervals between febrile bouts: one day in quotidian malaria; two days in tertian malaria (because the fever occurred on the first and third days of the cycle), which could be benign or malignant; and three days in quartan malaria (because the fever occurred on the first and fourth days of the cycle).[2] The name of the disease (*mala aria* being 'bad air' in Italian) reflected the old theory of the miasmic origin of the disease. Indeed, the occurrence of malaria in regions with marshes, swamps, or lagoons (whence: marsh, paludal, or swamp fever) was taken as evidence that the disease was produced by the noxious, putrid vapours emitted by stagnant water.

In the early 1880s the controversy surrounding the aetiopathogenesis of malaria had reached a high point. During a meeting of German naturalists held at Kassel in 1878 Tommasi-Crudeli and Klebs planned to conduct a field study on the aetiology of malaria. The Roman countryside was probably chosen because it was one of the most dramatically affected regions in Europe. In the winter of 1878–79, Tommasi-Crudeli began a preliminary investigation of the spread of the disease and its relationship to the distribution of water reservoirs, especially those underground.[3] In the following spring Tommasi-Crudeli and Klebs began to work in a laboratory that Stanislao Cannizzaro had made available to them in the Institute of Chemistry in Rome.[4] On 1 June 1879 the two scientists made a sensational report to the Accademia dei Lincei in which they claimed to have identified a rod-like micro-organism, the *Bacillus malariae*, in the ground of malarial regions.[5] They hypothesized that the *Bacillus malariae* ascended from the ground to pollute the lower layer of the atmosphere and to infect humans. Tommasi-Crudeli and Klebs claimed also to have experimentally infected rabbits, which exhibited a febrile disease similar to human malaria. As was the case for the just identified *Bacillus anthracis*, the *Bacillus malariae* also generated spores. The study was immediately published in German,[6] creating quite a stir, and the findings were soon corroborated by others. Ettore Marchiafava, a former student of Tommasi-Crudeli and Assistant of Pathological Anatomy at the University of Rome, found bacilli similar to the *Bacillus malariae* in the blood of three individuals who had died of pernicious malaria, as well as a black pigment (similar to that found by Tommasi-Crudeli and Klebs in the rabbit) in their spleen and bone marrow. Furthermore, a collaborator of Marchiafava, Giuseppe Cuboni, found similar bacilli in the water and mud in Ostia (a small seaside town near Rome) during an epidemic of malaria. And there was more. Cuboni found the bacilli also in his own sweat and in that of an accompanying person, suggesting that the *Bacillus malariae* could indeed spread from the ground to the lower layers of the atmosphere.[7]

At the end of 1880, while the excitement for what promised to be one of the greatest discoveries in bacteriology was mounting around Tommasi-Crudeli, Alphonse Laveran, a French Army physician at the Military Hospital of Constantine in Algeria, found peculiar formations in the blood of an individual with malaria, which suggested the presence of a parasite quite different from the *Bacillus malariae*.[8] Laveran's discovery was met by indifference and scepticism everywhere, including France. Indeed, similar alterations in the blood of malarial patients had been described by Virchow, Marchiafava, Friederich Theodor Frerichs, and others, but none had suggested that they could be related to a new micro-organism. These researchers, and Tommasi-Crudeli, considered the formations to be the result of haemoglobin degradation ('necrobiosis') produced by the malarial fever. Undeterred, Laveran continued to propound that the oscillating filaments outside the red cells of malarial patients were a new parasite, *Oscillaria malariae*, and in 1884 he reiterated this hypothesis in his *Traité des fièvres palustres* (Treatise of paludal fevers).[9] One of the few who took him seriously was another Army physician, Eugène Richard of the Military Hospital of Philippeville (currently Skikda) near Constantine. Laveran entrusted him with verifying the presence of *Oscillaria malariae* in the blood of malarial patients. Very soon Richard concluded that Laveran was substantially right, although his own findings were slightly different (initially he could find the micro-organisms only inside the red cells).[10]

The greatest threat to the *Bacillus malariae*, however, was brewing in Italy. Francesco Orsi, after making several attempts to verify the results of Tommasi-Crudeli and Klebs, began to nurture 'very strong doubts, and in order to dispel them, I thought it well to appeal, at beginning of this year [that is, 1881], to Prof. Golgi'.[11] Despite the strained relationship with Golgi, Orsi must have thought that only a virtuoso of the microscope could provide a definitive answer to his doubts. Golgi and Orsi decided to carry out some haematological observations during the Carnival holidays (the week before Lent), taking advantage of the presence of the noted parasitologist Edoardo Perroncito, who had planned to spend a few days in Pavia.[12] On 26 February they chose the patients and the controls to be included in the study. The blood tests were carried out on 3 March in the ward of Clinical Medicine by Bassini, Domenico Stefanini, and Pietro Grocco under Orsi's supervision; and again, two days later, in Golgi's laboratory. As in Tommasi-Crudeli and Marchiafava's study, the blood was examined not immediately after withdrawal, but several hours later, thus allowing the samples to be easily contaminated by micro-organisms. Orsi (who was the only one to know the origin of each blood sample) concluded that 'the most numerous micro-organisms and those which most resemble those thought to be the unique biological cause of the paludal infection, were found in completely healthy subjects ... and in those who never suffered from intermittent fever'.[11]

Tommasi-Crudeli was extremely upset by these conclusions and complained that 'two serious scholars' such as Golgi and Perroncito had 'let themselves be drawn' by Orsi into an asinine scientific error. And, in a letter to Golgi, he pointed out that Marchiafava had already shown that 'in malarial regions those bacillary forms could be found in the blood of individuals who were either healthy or affected by other diseases'. Tommasi-Crudeli thought that 'this parasite [that is, *Bacillus malariae*] nests in the spleen and in the bone marrow' where it can 'live for a long period of time' and then pour into the blood in a 'number of individuals [parasites] sufficient to produce fever'.[13] Marchiafava also complained to Golgi that the Roman scientists had clearly stated that the bacillus could be found in 'apparently healthy' subjects, even though it was present 'invariably and always in the greatest number in the blood of febrile individuals, and precisely during the chill'. Marchiafava added that the problem should be dealt with in a 'more serious and less hurried manner than that adopted by Mr Prof. Orsi'.[14]

Meanwhile Orsi was preparing another attack. He had asked some physicians with whom he was in contact to send him blood samples from individuals who had never lived in malarial areas. Orsi found again the controversial micro-organisms and, half annoyed and half contemptuous, wrote a brief note in which he attributed the presence of the bacilli to the 'decomposition' of the blood.[15] At this point the controversy touched on operetta, with Tommasi-Crudeli writing to Golgi that Orsi 'seems to me ready for the Lunatic Asylum', that 'it is a case of waiting until he acquires better titles of competence before discussing such complex matters with him',[16] and that Orsi was a typical example 'of the difficulty in explaining . . . a scientific problem' to someone who has received only 'a medical education'.[17]

Golgi tried to maintain a neutral position in the squabble but must have begun to suspect that the results of the Roman scientists were at least problematic.

Although in 1880 Marchiafava had provided independent support for Tommasi-Crudeli and Klebs' pathogenic theory of malaria, it is possible that by 1882 he had already began to nurture some reservations about the *Bacillus malariae*. In that year he met Laveran, who was conducting research on malaria in the Medicine ward of the Santo Spirito Hospital in Rome, directed by Guido Baccelli.[18] Baccelli, who was also Professor of Clinical Medicine at the University of Rome and, from 1881, Minister of Public Education, had been proposing for some years that malaria was a disease of the blood, in particular of the red cells, and was therefore quite interested in the work of the French physician. When Laveran visited Marchiafava's laboratory and saw the slides with the *Bacillus malariae* his suspicion was confirmed that the micro-organisms isolated by Tommasi-Crudeli and Klebs bore little relevance to malaria. Then Laveran showed Marchiafava the parasites that he had found not only in the blood of the Algerian patients but also in the blood of patients at the Santo Spirito. Laveran's visit made quite an impression on Marchiafava, who, however, could not afford to show much support for the point of view of the French Army physician. At that time Marchiafava was hoping to succeed Tommasi-Crudeli in the professorship of Pathological Anatomy at the University of Rome and did not want to lose the support of his powerful mentor.

Once the professorship was in his pocket, however, things changed. Marchiafava began collaborating with Angelo Celli, who had just returned from a period of study in the Munich laboratory of Max Joseph Pettenkofer (one of the founders of experimental hygiene) and was now an Assistant at the newly built Laboratory of Hygiene of the University of Rome, directed by Tommasi-Crudeli. The two scientists spent most of the summer and the first half of the autumn of 1883 studying the 'black pigmentations' in the blood of malarial patients from Santo Spirito. At first they concluded that these pigmentations were 'of regressive nature' and were produced by the 'necrobiosis of the red cell, in which haemoglobin is transformed into melanin',[19] as suggested by Tommasi-Crudeli. The latter was delighted by these findings and presented some of Celli and Marchiafava's preparations at an international medical congress held in Copenhagen in 1884.

Very soon, however, Marchiafava and Celli were able to identify 'roundish corpuscles' in the blood cells of malarial patients, and made some veiled references to the putative parasitic nature of such formations. At the same time they advised two physicians of Santo Spirito, Ugo Mariotti and Gaetano Ciarrocchi, to conduct experiments on the transmissibility of malaria through inoculation of blood. They injected blood of malarial patients subcutaneously into patients with chronic mental disorders who had been certified as free from malaria. Such experiments had been successfully conducted previously but Mariotti and Ciarrocchi demonstrated that the periodicity of the malarial fever in the recipient was identical to that of the donor.[20] The use of individuals with mental disorders as guinea pigs for medical experimentation, although offensive to modern sensibility, was a common practice during the nineteenth and early twentieth centuries.

Between 1884 and 1885 Marchiafava and Celli became convinced that the 'roundish corpuscles' were indeed the parasites responsible for malaria and that once the malaria parasite has 'penetrated the human organism it produces in the blood, and precisely in the red cells, dramatic and characteristic alterations'.[21] In a paper published in 1885[22] and immediately translated into German,[23] they described a variety of pigmented formations inside and outside the red cells, confirming Laveran's findings, and adding an imposing number of new morphological details about the malarial parasite. Although Laveran had been the first to establish a connection between the haematological alterations of malaria and the presence of a specific parasite, it was only with the detailed study by Marchiafava and Celli that the *Plasmodium malariae* came into the spotlight.

The pair also continued the experiments initiated by them in 'some patients affected by chronic nervous diseases who were happy [sic] to participate in our experiments'.[24] The inoculation of infected blood in these unhappy individuals (whatever Marchiafava and Celli thought) not only produced the expected intermittent fever but also resulted in the presence of the pigmented formation in their blood.

In the summer of 1885 Marchiafava and Celli made a concerted effort to rescue their master's aetiopathogenic hypothesis but the bacteriological analysis of the 'bad air' of the Paludi Pontine gave consistently negative findings. It was now clear that the *Bacillus malariae* was simply a blunder of Tommasi-Crudeli and Klebs.

The collaboration between Marchiafava and Celli was not limited to malaria but extended also in other directions. In 1883 they studied an epidemic of cholera in chickens and the following year they identified the presence of a micro-organism similar to the gonococcus (*Neisseria gonorrhoeae*, agent of gonorrhoea) in two cases of meningitis. Three years later Anton Weichselbaum established that this meningococcus (*Neisseria meningitidis*) was the causal agent of the epidemic cerebrospinal meningitis.

Marchiafava's laboratory suddenly acquired world-wide renown. In the middle of November 1885, George M. Sternberg, who had unsuccessfully attempted to replicate Klebs and Tommasi-Crudeli's findings in New Orleans, visited the Institute of Pathological Anatomy and left with the absolute conviction that malaria was caused by the micro-organism discovered by Laveran. Other American specialists followed suit. And in September 1885 Marchiafava and Celli were visited by Golgi, who stayed in Rome for ten days. The latter had followed the unfolding of the controversy on the aetiology of malaria with great interest, and the sensational findings from Rome had convinced him that a personal visit was necessary. Golgi was fascinated by what he saw.

Between August and October of 1885 Marchiafava and Celli studied 120 malarial patients from Rome and from the Paludi Pontine, where 'the endemia was the most severe of the last five years.'[25]

Golgi was able to verify personally the accuracy of Marchiafava and Celli's conclusions:

1. 'In the red cells of individuals stricken by recent malarial infection one can notice the presence of parasitic organisms made of a block of homogeneous protoplasm, characterized by extreme amoeboid motility and distinctly stainable. Because of these characteristics and because they can be found only in malarial infection they might be called malarial plasmodia and haemoplasmodia.

2. 'Within the haemoplasmodia can often be found a reddish or brownish pigment, which is not an integral part of them [that is, haemoplasmodia], but arises because of the transformation of haemoglobin, which is taken from the invaded red cells, into melanin. The presence of the pigment within the haemoplasmodia is not constant and might be absent even in cases of extremely severe fever (pernicious fever). According to whether there is production of the pigment or not, the malarial infection may or may not be accompanied by melanaemia.

3. 'A process of scission transforms the haemoplasmodia into masses of corpuscles . . . This scission occurs both in plasmodia that are pigmented and in those that are not . . . and it is probable that this is how they multiply within the human body.

4. 'The malarial infection is transmissible to humans through intravenous injection of malarial blood . . .'[26]

5. 'With the progression of the infection [the plasmodia] progressively increase in the blood of the inoculated [individual], whereas they rapidly decrease, became immobile, and then disappear with specific therapy and the end of the disease.'[27]

During his sojourn in Rome, Golgi became convinced that further inroads into the nature of malaria could come only by correlating the different stages in the development of the parasite with the clinical picture. Back in Pavia he immediately tried to 'recruit' malarial patients but without great success. 'He did not have abundant clinical material, but only a few patients, sometimes found at their private residence or encountered by chance' and 'in these researches, as on the other hand in all the others, he did not receive any substantial collaboration.'[28] To increase his case load Golgi was obliged to study the malarial patients of other clinical units. His collaboration with Orsi had not healed the bad relations between the two academics and this meant that the many cases of malaria in the wards of the Institute of Clinical Medicine were off-limits for him. Fortunately, Pietro Grocco, a former pupil of Orsi and now Professor of Propaedeutic Clinical Medicine, was more cooperative and allowed Golgi to take blood samples from some of his patients. Also cooperative was Alessandro Cuzzi, Director of the Obstetrics and Gynaecology Clinic. Between October and December 1885 Golgi managed to study 40 malarial patients, mostly cases of quartan. Twenty-two of these patients were studied for 2–5 bouts of fever; the remaining 18 (probably patients of other wards and therefore difficult to monitor), underwent only blood sampling which demonstrated haematological alterations in 16 of them.[29]

We have seen that Marchiafava and Celli had observed 'images of scission' in the pigmented bodies and had hinted at the hypothesis that the 'corpuscles' produced by the scission represented a newly formed generation of parasites. Golgi was soon able to determine the entire cycle of the parasite's development, and by November was certain that he had cracked the mystery of the 'intermittence' of the malarial fevers, establishing a correlation between 'figures of scission' and febrile bouts. The importance of these findings mandated their immediate publication. On 20 November[30] Bizzozero reported Golgi's discovery at the Academy of Medicine of Turin ('Golgi's law'): the febrile bouts coincided with the 'scission of the parasite'.[31] On 20 December Golgi finished writing his paper 'On the malarial infection', which was published a few months later,[32] and on 3 April 1886 he presented a report on malaria (the first of a long series) to the newly founded Società Medico-Chirurgica of Pavia.[33]

'Thanks to his patience and his spirit of observation, perhaps also assisted by his exceptional memory for local history, [Golgi] was able to find the right points of reference and to recognize the regularity of a cycle in a congeries of [clinical] forms that seemed to be unrelated and to alternate in a random, disorderly manner.'[34] In this he was helped by the fact that his patients were almost exclusively affected by quartan. Indeed, quartan (popularly known as 'long fever') was the most common form of malaria during autumn in the region around Pavia. This also had a long-lasting effect on the terminology used for the malarial parasites. Golgi had adopted the term introduced by Marchiafava and Celli to indicate the parasite responsible for malaria, *Plasmodium malariae*. When it became clear that the different forms of malaria were produced by different parasites, the name *Plasmodium malariae* continued to be used but exclusively for the aetiological agent of quartan malaria.

Golgi maintained the morphological distinction between plasmodia (non-pigmented amoeboid parasites) and pigmented bodies, although he realized that the latter were only 'a modification of the former'.[35] In his description the plasmodia were small elementary forms of the parasite, whereas the pigment bodies corresponded to the trophozoites which, during the three days before the febrile bout, progressively enlarged to reach the dimensions of the schizont (or mature trophozoite) which would then segment into numerous merozoites.

The main point of Golgi's paper was that

In quartan malaria the pigmented bodies complete their development in the period between two bouts; the maturation and the incipient or actual segmentation of the same bodies occurs just before a new bout; therefore, in the same way that the presence of mature forms and segmentation predict the imminent onset of a febrile bout, other, different phases of development can predict whether the bout will occur within one day or two days.[36]

The identification of a cycle of 72 hours allowed Golgi to interpret the nature of more complex clinical pictures, such as the double quartan (characterized by two days of fever and one day of remission) and some forms of quotidian malaria (characterized by daily paroxysms), which he attributed to infection by two (double quartan) or three (quotidian) distinct groups of *Plasmodium malariae*, segmenting 24 hours out of phase from each other. Golgi realized, however, that no combination could account for the tertian and predicted that in this case 'the parasite responsible for the malarial infection must have a different reproductive cycle'.[37] At the time, however, Golgi was not necessarily thinking of a different species of *Plasmodium*. For example, the different forms of malaria could be attributed to the effect of certain environmental and seasonal conditions on the life cycle of the particular parasite.

Golgi noted also that the 'white cells containing lumps of pigment are found almost exclusively in the periods of high fever and those of defervescence'; indeed 'the process of segmentation releases the small pigmented masses which are encysted by the white cells.'[38] Finally, he described and drew the different phases of the process of maturation of the trophozoite[39] and the 'daisy-like' formation that preceded its segmentation into merozoites.

During the winter of 1886 the incidence of malaria had decreased but in the spring a new epidemic made its appearance around Pavia, and Golgi had the opportunity to study the new patients who arrived in Wards 'O' and 'P' of his unit, and some patients in other wards.[40] This time it was the turn of the tertian! Golgi could thus verify his hypothesis on the pathogenesis of this form of malaria.

Golgi demonstrated that the biological cycle of the parasites in the red cells of these patients 'takes place between two bouts, that is, in two days, whereas the pigmented bodies of the quartan complete their cycle in three days.'[41] He also demonstrated that some forms of quotidian could be explained by two independent cycles caused by two different strains of *Plasmodium* that were out of phase by one day. He realized that the biological cycles of the tertian and of the quartan (Golgi's cycle) were morphologically different, allowing a differential diagnosis for the two forms (both in the first phases of development and during the process of segmentation). He also hinted at the idea that the two forms of malaria might be caused by two different micro-organisms. Finally, he confirmed the 'presence of pigmented bodies within the white cells' and proposed that the process of phagocytosis could play a role in the spontaneous termination of the infection.

In the early 1800s, Giovanni Rasori had hypothesized that malarial fevers 'are caused by parasites that produce the [febrile] bout at the moment of their reproduction which happened more or less frequently according to the different species. Thus arise the intermittent quotidian, tertian, and quartan fevers.'[42] This oracular hypothesis was fully confirmed by Golgi's findings.[43] On 5 June 1886 Golgi reported to the Società Medico-Chirurgica the results of his new studies on tertian malaria,[44] which were later published in full in *Gazzeta degli Ospitali*.[45] Since he had made reference to phagocytosis in his work, Golgi thought that it was appropriate to send a reprint to the pre-eminent scholar of this phenomenon, Metschnikoff, who directed a bacteriological institute in Odessa. A few months later, Metschnikoff was invited to write a summary of his theory in the first issue of *Annales de l'Institute Pasteur*. In this essay he proposed that phagocytosis was an adaptive mechanism against biological insults, and emphasized the importance of Golgi's work and his hypothesis that the process of phagocytosis could lead to the spontaneous extinction of the infection.[46]

The work of Marchiafava, Celli, and Golgi on *Plasmodium malariae* had exasperated the poor Tommasi-Crudeli who continued to believe in the existence of the *Bacillus malariae*, but who was rapidly losing his eyesight and so not in a condition to carry out new experiments. Therefore, one can imagine his delight when he received 'as a gift' ten microscopic preparations with bacterial cultures from malarial regions, which were very similar to those he had obtained seven years earlier in collaboration with Klebs. These preparations came from Bernardo Schiavuzzi, a physician from Pola in Istria, who had analysed the 'bad air' of that region in the hope of identifying a micro-organism that could be responsible for the intermittent fevers. Tommasi-Crudeli saw in these results the possibility of vindicating his theory, and decided to communicate Schiavuzzi's findings to the Accademia dei Lincei. In this brief note, after emphasizing the resemblance between the micro-organism isolated by Schiavuzzi and his own *Bacillus malariae*, Tommasi-Crudeli advised Schiavuzzi to carry out a biological test of transmission by inoculating the bacterial culture in 'male rabbits to avoid any possibility that the results of the experiment could be complicated by the consequences of pregnancies, child births, or post-partum period.'[47] However, he still had to counter the interpretation proposed by Marchiafava, Celli, and Golgi. The occasion arose in the subsequent session of the Accademia dei Lincei on 2 May. Tommasi-Crudeli presented a paper in which he restated his hypothesis that the alteration of red cells during malaria was of a 'regressive' nature, contrary to the opinion of Marchiafava, Celli, and Golgi. In particular he contested Golgi's notion that the images of 'segmentation' represented the moment of reproduction of a micro-organism, considering them instead to be a regressive phenomenon comparable to that observed in a red cell undergoing the action of various agents.[48]

Meanwhile, Schiavuzzi was continuing his research. By 'passing air through a vial containing five cubic centimetres of sterile gelatin' and utilizing portable air aspirators (including Koch's apparatus for the analysis of large volumes of air), he found a 'constant presence of this bacterium in the environment in all malarial areas' but not in the environment of healthy areas. When cultivated on gelatin, the bacterium formed 'quite viscous white plaques'.[49] Schiavuzzi also tried the biological proof suggested by Tommasi-Crudeli. And indeed, the inoculation of bacterial cultures in rabbits appeared to produce intermittent fevers 'of tertian and quartan type' as indicated by the temperature curves in the inoculated animals. Furthermore, 'in the red blood cells, especially in one of the infected rabbits, some primary alterations were identified ... which were considered as pathognomonic signs of malarial infection.'[50] Galvanized by these results, Tommasi-Crudeli returned to the fray at the Accademia dei Lincei during the session of 5 December 1886 with a note in which he presented the most recent findings by Schiavuzzi.[51] Among those who read this note was Ferdinand Julius Cohn, Professor of Botany at the University of Breslau, who had been one of the first to give credence to Koch's research on anthrax[52] when the latter was a simple municipal doctor. True to his vocation as a talent scout, and possibly finding an analogy between Schiavuzzi and the young Koch, Cohn decided to go 'to Pola for the purpose of assessing first-hand Schiavuzzi's research'.[53] Fully convinced by what he saw,[54] Cohn went so far as to declare Schiavuzzi's findings 'decisive' for the solution of the aetiological problem of malaria and to present them at a meeting of the Schlesische Gesellschaft für vaterländische Cultur, announcing that he would publish a full report by Schiavuzzi in the prestigious *Beiträge zur Biologie der Pflanzen*.

Engulfed in the controversy, Golgi had not remained idle. Despite the difficulties in gathering patients, his case load continued to increase, thanks also to field studies in the Tuscan Maremma and in malarial areas of Sardinia.[55]

In the spring of 1887 Tommasi-Crudeli found another unlikely ally in Angelo Mosso, a pre-eminent physiologist from the University of Turin and personal friend of Golgi. On 3 and 17 April, Mosso reported the results of experiments on the degeneration of red cells to the Accademia dei Lincei. Two or three days after injecting dog blood into the abdominal cavity of hens or pigeons, he sacrificed the bird to observe the modifications of the dog's red cell in the abdominal cavity and compared them not 'to the blood of malarial patients but the figures and descriptions provided by Laveran, Richard, Marchiafava, Celli, and Golgi'.[56] He concluded that:

in the blood of dog left for three days in the abdominal cavity of a hen can be found alterations of corpuscles [that is, red cells] and hyaline and pigmented formations similar to those that Laveran, Richard, Marchiafava, Celli, and Golgi have described in their studies on the malarial infection; this resemblance applies not only to the morphology but also to the movements.

 . . . [the facts] emerge with such evidence that far from being something audacious, it is a logical necessity to think that what so far has been considered as the consequence of processes of development or growth should be rather regarded as the consequence of a process of degeneration.[57]

While professing the greatest esteem and admiration for the work of Marchiafava, Celli, and Golgi, Mosso openly took sides with Tommasi-Crudeli. Now Golgi had also to confront a scientist of the stature of Mosso, who, adding injury to insult, pretended to solve the problem of the haematological alteration of malaria with the bizarre experiment of inoculating dog blood into the abdominal cavity of birds. Being present during Mosso's report, Golgi expressed all his dissent, and commented on 'the enormous gravity of the things asserted by you [Mosso]'.[58] The person most satisfied by Mosso's report was obviously Tommasi-Crudeli. On 1 May 1887, he summarized the state of knowledge on malaria, and in particular the findings by Schiavuzzi and Mosso, in a report to the Accademia dei Lincei. Tommasi-Crudeli restated forcefully that the haematological alterations of malaria 'occur following various kinds of physical or chemical insults, and the segmentation of the *Plasmodium* described by Golgi was simply a fragmentation of the degenerated red cell followed by its complete destruction'.[59] He complained, feeling victimized, that 'in 1885 I was left alone preaching to the deaf'[60] and that nobody had 'listened, because in that period there was in Italy and abroad a true infatuation for this hypothetical *Plasmodium malariae*'. But finally the matter had been 'solved, brilliantly solved' by Mosso.[61] He then concluded that thanks to the work of Mosso and Schiavuzzi it was clear 'that the cause of malaria is a bacterial schizomicete, quite common on the entire surface of the earth, capable of maintaining its potential life for long periods of time deep in the soil and of vegetating in the ground of the most different geological composition—sometimes swampy, more often non-swampy—provided that the ground in which it is contained be moderately humid during the hot season and in direct contact with the air.'[61] He also predicted that, although at the moment his point of view was shared by no more than two dozen scientists in all of Europe, 'it was destined to become the opinion of everyone in the next generation of scientists'.[62] Tommasi-Crudeli had staked his scientific reputation on the *Bacillus malariae*, entrusting to the existence of this micro-organism his hope of entering the Hall of Science as the discoverer of the aetiological agent of one of the most important infectious diseases.

Enraged by Mosso's conclusions, Golgi had already taken countermeasures by instruct-
ing his assistants Cattaneo and Monti to check his results. And Marchiafava and Celli were
doing the same. Cattaneo and Monti easily demonstrated that the formations described by
Mosso had nothing to do with what Golgi had observed. On 7 May 1887 they presented
some preliminary findings to the Società Medico-Chirurgica.[63] At the end of Cattaneo's
presentation, Golgi could not hide his irritation with Mosso:

[Golgi] wishes to state how there is not the least correspondence between the alteration of red
blood cells injected into the abdomen of a chicken and those of malaria. He finds it bizarre that
Professor Mosso could have stated such a thing. This surprises him greatly, but he believes that
everything derives from the fact that Mosso had not [directly] examined the blood of malaria
patients.[64]

Ten days later, a sad event drew Golgi's attention away from this bitter controversy. His
mother Carolina died. For a few days all the family members gathered around the elderly
Alessandro. Golgi received a touching note from Bizzozero:

I am truly desolated by the drama that has stricken you, right at a time when many preoccupations,
one more serious than the other, demand your attention. This is one of those wounds, I know
from having gone through it myself, that not even time can heal.

Saddened, his friend and mentor added: 'Every time we take a look at the past, whenever
we go back to the memories of our youth, a painful stab reminds us that it [youth] exists no
more', and concluded 'have courage; working will give you relief'.[65]
And so it did. Mosso, disconcerted at having stirred up such a hornet's nest with his
report, declared that he wanted to submit his findings for review by a panel of authoritative
scientists, including Golgi himself. The latter replied on 27 May thanking him for his trust
and assuring that 'I cannot even fathom the possibility feared by you that for such a
controversy our friendship could be in any way shaken.'[58] But then he added, completely
confident in Cattaneo and Monti's findings:

I do not hesitate in expressing my opinion in the most firm manner; the differences between the
two categories of formation are so great that I believe that anyone who had compared them could
not confuse them.

And he continued, expressing 'the absolute certainty that this is what will happen as
soon as you will verify my observations at the microscope in the same way I have verified
yours.'
On 29 May Mosso's results were contested by Marchiafava and Celli in a communication to the Academy of Medicine of Rome. Even his friend Bizzozero tried to avoid
Mosso as much as possible because at the moment it was impossible 'to influence his ideas'
or even 'discuss' the matter without 'causing bad blood needlessly'.[66] But Mosso himself
was beginning to fear that the blood gone bad in the bird's abdomen could also cause bad
blood between him and Golgi and Bizzozero. Minimizing the importance of his experiment, which had instead been magnified by Tommasi-Crudeli, Mosso told Marchiafava
that he had found himself trapped in this squabble only by chance, and that he was not
particularly interested in dealing with this matter. To Golgi he wrote that 'To say that the

two formations are similar does not imply that they are identical; in the same way in which we cannot say that two people who resemble each other are brothers or sisters.'[67] Even Mosso was distancing himself from Tommasi-Crudeli.

A few weeks later, however, a clinician from Genoa, Edoardo Maragliano, came to the rescue of the supporters of the 'degenerative' hypothesis. In a report on 27 June 1887 to the Academy of Medicine of Genoa, he claimed that he had reproduced the alteration of red cells described by the supporters of the *Plasmodium* simply by treating normal blood with a solution of soda and methyl-violet and sealing it in paraffin.

Once again Golgi charged Cattaneo and Monti with checking the validity of the challenge. And sure enough the two assistants were able to demonstrate that the alterations of the red cell described by Maragliano had nothing to do with the malarial infection[68] and a French version of their paper was published in *Archives Italiennes de Biologie*, of which Mosso was Editor-in-Chief.[69]

In 1887 Golgi was elected President of the local organizing committee for the Twelfth Congress of the Italian Medical Association, to be held in Pavia from 19–25 September, and in which 800 Italian physicians would participate, including the most important exponents of Italian medicine, such as Cantani, De Giovanni, Lombroso, Morselli, Tamburini, and Tamassia. In his opening address, Golgi emphasized the importance of a meeting of 'general medicine' because only by maintaining a connection with this 'common mother' could one find 'a remedy against the exaggerated tendency toward specialization'.[70] Cattaneo and Monti presented the results of the experiments in which they compared the degeneration of red blood cells with the haematological signs of malaria. During the meeting, however, the degenerative hypothesis of Mosso and Maragliano found another ally in Grassi. He presented a report in which he stated his opposition to the idea, proposed mostly by French and Italian scientists working on *Plasmodium*, that protozoa could cause an infectious disease. Grassi thought that there was no evidence that *Plasmodium malariae* was a protozoan, a position similar to that held by Tommasi-Crudeli.[71] Grassi's presentation wounded Golgi, already under strain because of the superficiality of the objections against the findings from his laboratory.

The aetiopathogenesis of malaria was not the only controversial issue concerning this disease. The timing for the treatment with quinine was also hotly debated. On the strength of his pathogenetic theory, however, Golgi thought that he had the solution of the problem at hand. The right moment to administer the drug was during the process of segmentation of the *Plasmodium*. After several clinical trials, he concluded that the optimal moment was a few hours before the onset of fever, and that it was advisable to repeat the treatment two or three times. He reported this finding to the Società Medico-Chirurgica on 17 March 1888.[72]

He also continued to study the phenomenon of phagocytosis. Golgi established that 'phagocytosis is a process that occurs periodically as a regular function of white cells, a function that is carried out with precise modalities on the occasion of certain phases of the life cycle of malarial parasites and in certain periods of each febrile bout.'[73] He also established that the phagocytosis begins with the bout, increases during the following 3–4 hours, and stops a few hours after the end of the bout, for a total of about 8–12 hours or slightly more. If in the initial phases of phagocytosis there are white cells containing entire forms of segmentation, in the following phases the white cells will contain pigment, whole *Plasmodia*, and debris. Golgi carried out splenic biopsies and discovered that phago-cytosis occurs in the spleen to a greater extent than in the blood, and hypothesized that the same should occur in the liver (although a liver biopsy was uninformative) and in the bone marrow. At that time most scientists thought that phagocytosis played an exclu-sively 'waste removal' role by eliminating dead micro-organisms and debris from dead cells. In contrast Golgi, in agreement with Metschnikoff's theory, concluded that phagocytosis could also involve live *Plasmodia*, as an active response of the organism to limit the infection. On 19 May 1888 he delivered his findings to the Società Medico-Chirurgica.[74]

So far Golgi had maintained the most unwavering confidence in his pathogenetic theory, which was based 'not on dogmatic conclusions or superficial experiments but on hundreds of observations scrupulously collected and repeatedly checked'.[75] He had looked upon the overblown statements of Tommasi-Crudeli with 'a feeling of sadness because of the manner with which they had been made'.[76] He was not worried by Cohn's paper either, because he regarded Cohn as a competent botanist but not an expert on animal research. However, Tommasi-Crudeli's repeated claims that the publication of Schiavuzzi's findings would finally bring the controversy to an end continued to command Golgi's attention. 'And since the kernel of the problem was represented by Schiavuzzi's findings with the bacillus that he had isolated from the air around Pola' Golgi decided to ask 'Dr Schiavuzzi himself to provide an authentic culture of the bacillus in question.'[77] Schiavuzzi, who was in the process of moving to Parenzo as a municipal doctor, sent Golgi an agar culture of the bacillus. Golgi immediately began to experiment with inoculations of the putative *Bacillus malariae* in rabbits. But then he decided to suspend this work, waiting for the publication of Schiavuzzi's paper with a precise description of the experimental protocol.

Finally, the long awaited paper by Schiavuzzi appeared in April 1888.[78] Armed with it Tommasi-Crudeli marched triumphantly into a session of the Accademia dei Lincei thundering that 'this putative parasite, called by some *Plasmodium malariae* . . . does not exist.'[79] Golgi had to wait (undoubtedly with a certain degree of anxiety) until mid-May before being able to read Schiavuzzi's paper. His 'disappointment with the content of this work'[80] was as great as the expectation with which it had been awaited. Indeed, all that Schiavuzzi had done was to carry out two inoculations of pure culture of his bacillus into rabbits at an interval of about one month, measuring the temperature curves in four different experiments. But the most important flaw in Schiavuzzi's study was the lack of reliable controls. Amazingly, he interpreted as bouts of fever the normal circadian variation of a few tenths of a degree in the body temperature of the rabbits. The experiment was flawed also by the fact that abscesses had formed at the site of the injections, which could also produce increases in body temperature. In addition, Schiavuzzi claimed that he had cultured the *Bacillus malariae* from blood, spleen, and abdominal lymphatic glands, but his procedure could not rule out contamination from other bacteria. Finally, the haemato-logical alteration so trumpeted by Tommasi-Crudeli had nothing to do with those described by the supporters of the *Plasmodium* theory. Schiavuzzi had found, in addition to normal red cells, deformed red cells that appeared to have lost part of their contents, and others with a small and shiny central densification. A simple comparison with the haematological alterations of a malarial patient would have revealed the colossal differences between the two conditions.

Nonplussed by the superficiality of his opponents, Golgi decided to put to rest once and for all the story of the bacillus. He was now in a position to attack the problem in the most appropriate manner. He knew the experimental protocol of Schiavuzzi and was in possession of the putative *Bacillus malariae*. First, he found that the temperature curves of healthy rabbits used as controls completely overlapped those of the rabbits that Schiavuzzi had thought affected by malaria. Second, in rabbits injected with culture of *Bacillus malariae*, or with innocuous micro-organisms present in the air, he sometimes observed slight and transitory increase in temperature, but never above the maximum observed in the healthy untreated controls. He concluded, therefore, that this was an increase in temperature due to local inflammation and not to a specific pathogenic action. Third, he compared the haematological findings in these rabbits with those obtained in malarial patients, and found that they were completely different, the former consisting simply in deformations of the red cells. Finally, he demonstrated that the *Bacillus malariae* did not produce any of the anatomo-pathological alterations typical of malaria, and that once inoculated they were rapidly destroyed by leucocytic phagocytosis.

Golgi presented his findings in a paper in which he ridiculed Schiavuzzi's work and accused Tommasi-Crudeli of having given credit to flawed experimental data only because of self-serving purposes.[81] Golgi was not surprised that Cohn too had given credit to Schiavuzzi's temperature curves: 'If they were considered pathological by physicians [that is, Schiavuzzi and Tommasi-Crudeli], why wouldn't they be considered the same by a botanist?', from whom, however, 'one would have expected greater soundness of judgement in things that were not in his area of strict competence.'[82] To give the greatest resonance to this devastating dismissal of the *Bacillus malariae*, he published a German version of his paper in the prestigious *Beiträge zur pathologischen Anatomie und zur allgemeinen Pathologie*.[83] Despite the efforts of Mosso, Maragliano, Schiavuzzi, Tommasi-Crudeli, and Cohn, the plasmodial hypothesis for malaria was gaining international recognition, thanks not only the work of Golgi's laboratory but also to the studies of Sternberg, William Thomas Councilman, William Osler, and Metschnikoff.

Since his early studies on malaria, Golgi had acknowledged the important differences between the life cycle of tertian and quartan. After studying a few cases of tertian, he had begun to suspect that the micro-organisms responsible for the two forms of the disease were two different species. After collecting hundreds of cases of malaria from Lombardy, Piedmont, Sardinia, and Tuscany, his suspicion became a virtual certainty. He reviewed the biological differences between the *Plasmodium* of tertian and that of quartan[84] and the principles of differential diagnosis for the two forms of malaria in a special paper, in which he pointed out that 'the peculiar course of tertian fever is due to the development of a micro-organism different both biologically and morphologically from the one that produces a similar but not identical fever, quartan fever.'[85] He presented this work to the Società Medico-Chirurgica on 2 February 1889.[86]

Besides intermittent fevers with cycles of three and four days, Golgi had repeatedly observed forms of malaria that could not be reduced to combinations of tertian and quartan. Since antiquity, fevers with longer periodicity had been reported in the medical literature. Galen, for example, had reported cases of quintan; Tissot and Morgagni of septan; others had also reported more irregular periods. For many researchers, however, these alternative forms either did not exist or were determined by the suppression of some bouts by quinine.

Golgi was convinced that there were indeed other forms of malaria, different from tertian and quartan, and the frequent occurrence of 'crescents' in these forms provided him with haematological criteria for differentiating them. The crescents had been demonstrated already by Laveran and others, and were due to the fact that the parasite assumes a sickle-shaped form having a major axis about twice that of the red cell, which therefore stretches and then breaks, releasing the protozoan. Golgi had already observed and drawn sickle-shaped structures in his first 1886 paper, and now he found the same images in the forms of malaria with long intervals. A patient in his clinical unit was prototypical. He was a 12-year-old boy from Breme, near Pavia, who was hospitalized on 3 January 1889. Since August 1888 he had been affected by an irregular fever and presented a complex haematological picture (crescents, pigmented intracellular bodies, flagellated forms). After a few days without fever, the haematological picture became simplified, with the exclusive presence of crescents. The febrile bouts occurred at intervals that ranged from 5–12 days, and were accompanied by the presence in the blood of small non-pigmented parasites. Taking into account similar cases, and what he found in the literature, Golgi concluded that the crescents were undergoing a process of maturation of variable duration, and that the young forms derived from them would undergo a process of maturation and segmentation giving rise to the febrile bout. The irregularity in the occurrence of the febrile bouts depended, according to Golgi, on the irregularity of the maturational process of the crescents.

We now know that the crescents are characteristic of the malaria produced by *Plasmodium falciparum*, and represent the sexual form, whose further development depends on the passage into the anopheles. This kind of *Plasmodium* can indeed produce not only the malignant tertian, but also irregular forms of malaria. Golgi had the intuition to correlate the latter with the crescents, although the physiopathological interpretation of the febrile bout as the moment of maturation of the crescent would prove to be wrong. He reported these findings in April 1889 at a meeting the Società Medico-Chirurgica[87] and in September at the congress of the Italian Medical Association in Padua.

Between 1889 and 1890 Golgi obtained good microphotographs of the malarial parasite (that he now classified as in the genus *Amoeba*), which he sent to Carl Flügge, professor of Hygiene at the University of Breslau.[88] The use of photography in microbiology had been introduced ten years earlier by Koch, but until 1890 the figures that Golgi had used in his scientific publications had all been drawn from microscopic observation, usually by him and sometimes by his wife, especially at the beginning of his career, or by his Assistants Fusari and Monti. On 8 February he presented the photographic documentation of the biological cycle of the parasites of quartan,[89] and on 17 July of the parasites of tertian,[90] to the Società Medico-Chirurgica, emphasizing the differences between them. This photographic material appeared so convincing to him that he made it the theme of his report to the Tenth International Congress of Medicine held on 8 August 1890 in Berlin.[91] But Golgi returned from the Congress with the feeling that he had not been able to dissipate 'the manifest scepticism' still surrounding his hypothesis on the pathogenesis of the disease. He then decided to write to the editors of *Zeitschrift für Hygiene* (Flügge and Koch) asking them to publish his photographs in their journal in order to assure their maximal international diffusion.[92] Both editors answered positively, asking only for a reduction in the number of photographs.[93] The work was published in 1891 and in it Golgi proposed that malarial parasites should be considered as a sub-species and gave the quartan form the name *Amoeba malariae febris quartanae*.[94]

At the end of 1889 Grassi changed his mind about the pathogenesis of malaria and proposed that the disease was caused by an amoeba-like micro-organism, of which he and his collaborator Raimondo Feletti thought they had identified two species, the *Haemoamoeba malariae* (which included the parasite of tertian and quartan previously identified by Golgi), and the *Laverania malariae* (which included the parasite of the irregular fevers). Although this position had some points in common with the plasmodial hypothesis, its main effect was to reshuffle the cards in an area where some sort of order had already been achieved. Golgi could not but be resentful about this and found a powerful ally in Bizzozero, who entered the arena with all his scientific ascendancy and polemical witticisms. He wrote a biting critique of Grassi's hypothesis, accusing him of having simply added the names of two micro-organisms to the controversy on the pathogenesis of malaria, and of having criticized Golgi's solid work with meaningless scientific arguments.

Grassi was devastated by this criticism and on 8 March 1890 he wrote from Catania, where he was then teaching, to his former teacher:

The note by Bizzozero . . . had such a painful effect that my nerves are again shaken and I can no longer sleep or eat or work seriously. This painful impression is not due to the fact that B. wounded my pride, but to the fact that I can see that I have done, *completely against my will*, a thing that can displease you who have always shown affection toward me.[95]

However, Grassi disagreed with the essence of the criticism, and cited Bizzozero's own 1888 treatise of pathology, which did not classify the *Plasmodium* among blood parasites. And then he added:

Thus, Mr Esq. Professor and Maestro, as much esteemed as loved by me, in the name of that little of affection which you have always exhibited to me, I beg you to convince me that I am wrong and I will be extremely happy to send to the *Centralblatt f. Parasit.* a retraction; it would be a retraction that will bring dishonour to my scientific reputation but it will be the action of a gentleman, which I believe I am . . .

I conclude by offering my apologies even though I am not convinced that I am wrong.

The next day Grassi and Feletti wrote a paper in which they refuted all of Bizzozero's accusations point by point.[96]

But Grassi was rapidly 'convinced', whether he wanted to be or not, by Golgi's answer, which must have hit with devastating effects. Indeed, on 20 March a contrite letter, betraying a deep psychological crisis and almost physical suffering, was sent to Pavia.[97] Grassi wrote that he had begun to consider the idea 'of abandoning scholarship' in the conviction, 'which I am beginning to entertain, of not being able to carry out any serious work'. And he disclosed that:

Whatever the matter is, I no longer have those grand aspirations that I once had; I see that many and much younger [individuals] than I are superior to me and I esteem and admire them sincerely; and I am happy only about two things: that of belonging to an insignificant university, and that therefore I can keep my position without feeling bad, and that of having some time ago started a family, which compensates for the mediocre results I have achieved with so much study and work.

Recalling his youth he added:

Ah, dear Professor, many years have passed since I was in Pavia. Then I was young and full of illusions but now I am old and full of disillusions, and you do not recognize me any more.

And, in an attempt to assuage the situation, he announced

that I, publishing a note on the parasites of malaria in birds, will find a way to demonstrate the depth of my admiration for everything you have done on malaria, cutting short any qualms you may have. I shall state that you were right to believe that the plasmodia were the parasites [of malaria], and that I was mistaken in good faith, and that I did not intend to formally contradict your opinion. And then Feletti and I shall include in the full report on malaria [subsequent to the note on the malaria in birds] a dedication to you which will publicly confirm that I never had the least intention of diminishing the very great merits of your work on malaria. If I can do more, tell me and I shall do it. After this explanation I hope you will not shrink from shaking my hand, with profound respect,

Catania 20 March, 1890 Devotedly Prof. B. Grassi.[97]

The tone is that of a person covering his head with ashes. Considering that Grassi had a difficult and unaccommodating character, we have a measure of the awe that Golgi now inspired at the height of his world-wide fame.

In his letter Grassi also told Golgi that he wanted his work on malaria 'to go ahead as far as I can go, if only for the determination of demonstrating that even I can achieve something.'

Unfortunately, he made another scientific *faux pas*. On the basis of the data obtained working with Feletti he hypothesized that the encysted malarial parasite could freely diffuse in the air and then penetrate humans and birds. In support of their hypothesis the two researchers described encysted malarial parasites in the dew and in the nasal cavities of birds of malarial areas.

But Golgi later demonstrated that these encysted formations were no more frequent in malarial than non-malarial areas. In a series of experiments he also showed that the encysted micro-organisms could not be the same as those that produce malaria in humans (for example, they did not cause febrile episodes), notwithstanding the biological similarities between the two species.[98]

It is a testament to Grassi's stubbornness and scientific skills that after these inauspicious beginnings he was still able to make outstanding contributions to the study of malaria. In 1898 he demonstrated that the *Anopheles* mosquito is the vector of malaria, and described the sporogonous cycle of the *Plasmodium* in this intermediate host.

Of course, malaria was not the only research activity in Golgi's laboratory. The importance of the black reaction was gaining recognition outside Italy, a fact that certainly had not escaped Golgi's notice, who kept himself up to date with the neuroanatomical literature, also because of his work as a reviewer.[99] Neurohistological research with the black reaction was conducted by Romeo Fusari and Grocco, who collaborated in a study on polyneuritis. During Nansen's visit in the spring of 1886, Fusari was assigned by Golgi to teach the Scandinavian the best procedures for the black reaction. The work on the Golgi's organ was continued by Alfonso Cattaneo, Assistant of General Pathology, who in 1886 completed a study on the alteration of the neurotendinous organ following section of the nerves.[100]

Golgi's interest in neuroanatomy was also kept alive by his crucial friendship with Kölliker, one of the most influential European neuroanatomists of the era. At some point during the first months of 1887 Golgi sent some of his black reaction preparations to the Swiss scientist (we do not know if it was at the request of the latter) who, notwithstanding his 70 years, was still extremely lucid and active. Kölliker immediately realized the great importance of the black reaction and began a correspondence with Golgi that would later flower into a deep personal and professional relationship.[101]

In 1889 Golgi revised the chapter on the nerve cells for Monti's Italian translation of the celebrated treatise of human histology by Samuel Leopold Schenk; as would be expected, the chapter was integrated with the discoveries made with the black reaction.[102]

During the second half of 1880s Golgi also studied other infectious diseases besides malaria, particularly rabies. Pasteur's vaccination in July 1885, of an Alsation child who had been bitten by a rabid dog, had created the need for a diagnostic method that could rapidly demonstrate the presence of the disease in the animal so that it could be decided whether the bitten person should undergo vaccination or not. At the end of 1886 Golgi received from Perroncito a rabbit infected with rabies, to be used in the research on histological alterations specific to this disease. On histopathological examination, Golgi found only a non-specific 'active enlargement of the nuclei of different types of cell of the nervous tissue in various regions of the brain and spinal cord, due to karyokinesis',[103] and on 29 January 1887 he presented a brief report to this effect to the Società Medico-Chirurgica. This first unsuccessful attempt did not discourage Golgi who, as we shall see, returned to the work on rabies in the following years.

Another line of research on infectious diseases was initiated in 1885–86 by a most remarkable student, who had arrived in the Laboratory of General Pathology to conduct research on the aetiology of puerperal fever (post-partum septicaemia) for her doctoral dissertation. Anna Kuliscioff[104] was born near Simferopol in Crimea, daughter of the Jewish Russian merchant Moisey Rosenstein. Blond, blue-eyed, and very beautiful, she had escaped, like many Russian intellectuals of the time, from her fatherland, which was choking under the Czarist regime, and taken refuge in Switzerland where she gave up her paternal family name. In Switzerland, she initiated contacts with socialist and anarchist exiles, mostly Russian. She became the companion, in life and in political battle, of the anarchist (later socialist) Andrea Costa, and acquired a certain notoriety, which extended well beyond the environment of the Italian radical left.[105] Starting in April 1882, she began to attend classes at the University of Bern Medical School, and enrolled as a regular student in 1883.[106] The following year, thanks to the support of Costa and Giovanni Bovio, and the sponsorship of Arnaldo Cantani, Professor of Clinical Medicine, she managed to enrol provisionally in the fifth year of Medical School of the University of Naples, where she began to work on her doctoral dissertation.[107] Consistent with her feminist convictions, she chose to study the aetiology of puerperal fever, an extremely controversial topic following the discovery of its infectious nature by the Hungarian physician and former pupil of Skoda, Ignaz Philipp Semmelweis, who died insane without receiving appropriate recognition for his achievements.[108] But the encounter in April 1885 with the emerging leader of Italian Socialism, Filippo Turati, changed the destiny of Anna Kuliscioff, who meanwhile had received a confirmation from the High Council for Education that she would be allowed to abbreviate her curriculum, which had already been granted by the Medical School. In love with Turati, Kuliscioff decided to follow him to Milan, and petitioned to be transferred to the University of Pavia Medical School. Confident that her petition would be accepted, she asked the Rector to allow her to 'attend clinical courses and to prepare an experimental dissertation, while waiting for the regular exam session'.[109] In order not to lose time, she began working as an internal student in the Laboratory of General Pathology where Golgi had just discovered the temporal correlation between the segmentation of the *Plasmodium* and the bouts of malarial fever. In line with microbiological research done in the laboratory, she resumed her studies on the aetiology of puerperal fever. Not being prejudiced against women, and possibly even being a sympathizer of the left at that time,[110] Golgi immediately accepted her in his lab. Six years earlier, Pasteur had been able to grow streptococci in cultures of blood and other organic materials from women affected by puerperal fever. But the methods for the isolation of micro-organisms had greatly improved thanks to the efforts of Koch. Applying some of Koch's methods to the secretions of the uterine mucosa in the post-partum period, Kuliscioff was able to isolate some bacterial species that were present under normal conditions. Only large amounts of these micro-organisms injected subcutaneously or intraperitoneally would infect experimental animals. Kuliscioff could thus conclude that

although it is not possible to draw definitive conclusions about the pathogenic potential of the described species . . . three types of micro-organisms of putrefaction might play an important role during pathological post-partum processes when they are allowed to reproduce abundantly because of the retention of residual portions of the placenta, or blood clots, or following deep lacerations, producing forms of sapraemia, septicaemia, and piaemia.[111]

These results were quite different from those obtained by Pasteur.

On 6 April 1886, Kuliscioff had the unpleasant surprise of seeing her request for transfer denied by the Pavian Medical School because her scholastic standing had not been adequately documented, and some clarifications from the Ministry of Public Education were required.[112] This completely unexpected response obliged her to return to Naples where there were fewer bureaucratic obstacles. In the academic year 1886–87 she became the first woman to graduate as a physician from the University of Naples Medical School, and she was later nicknamed *la dottora* (female doctor in Milanese vernacular) in the socialist working class environment in Milan.

But Kuliscioff had the satisfaction of seeing her work appreciated by Golgi, who on 30 June 1886 presented to the Società Medico-Chirurgica of Pavia the report ' "On the micro-organism of the normal secretions of the uterine mucosa during the post-partum period", research conducted by Mrs Anna Kuliscioff in the Laboratory of General Pathology'.[113]

Shortly after Kuliscioff's departure, new research on the puerperal fever was carried out by Innocente Clivio, Assistant of Histology, and by Achille Monti, Assistant of General Pathology, who took up Pasteur's idea of the pathogenic actions of streptococcus, publishing some papers on this topic in 1887 and 1888.

Golgi's scientific eclecticism during the second half of the 1880s is indicated also by his work on the functional anatomy of the kidney, which can be considered a continuation of his 1883 research on the histopathology of renal failure. In December 1887, while the controversy on malaria was raging, he decided to characterize the course of the renal tubule from its origin in Bowman's capsule to its opening in the collecting tubule. The usual preparations, however, were only partly demonstrative because these were thin layers of kidney tissue, which did not allow a good discrimination of the different portions of the renal tubule. Golgi tried to develop a method that would allow the isolation of a few nephrons at a time. He found that by immersing pieces of kidney cortex for 4–10 days in 'a 1% solution of arsenic acid to which an amount of alcohol equal to a fourth of its volume had been added' it was possible to obtain 'an extensive detachment of the renal canaliculi [tubulus]' with 'conservation of the epithelial elements', allowing one 'to obtain the isolation of entire systems of canaliculi from their origin to their outlet in the collecting canaliculi recti'.[114] Using this method he discovered that immediately after its origin the renal tubule runs for a length in the cortex where it forms the tubulus contortus. Most important, however, was the observation that 'the ascending limb of the loop of Henle, climbing in the cortical substance, invariably returns towards its [Bowman's] capsule of origin, against which it adheres (by a small amount of connective tissue) in correspondence with a point opposite that of emergence [of the renal tubule], and precisely where the afferent vessel enters and the efferent vessel exits'.[115] Thus, it was Golgi who first established the unique anatomical relationship between the distal tubule and the vascular pole of the Malpighian glomerulus, which, as would be discovered many years later, plays an important and delicate role in a number of physiological functions including the regulation of blood pressure. Preliminary results of this study were reported on 21 January 1888 to the Società Medico-Chirurgica.[116]

The method he had used to isolate the nephrons could also be applied to the study of their histogenesis. According to some authors, the tubulus contortus had a different origin from that of the tubulus rectus. It was also thought that Bowman's capsule pre-existed the vascular glomerulus and that they came into contact by encapsulation of the latter by the former. Golgi demonstrated that 'the canaliculus contortus originates from the canaliculus rectus, owing to continuous proliferation of the epithelium of the latter'. Furthermore, he established that 'the vascular glomerulus originates at the same time as its capsule of epithelial origin, within which it remains enclosed because of the parallel development of epithelial cells and vascular loops'.[117] Even in his minor contributions, Golgi demonstrated great originality and an uncanny flair for developing new methods to solve histological problems.

The studies on malaria had further contributed to establish Golgi's scientific and academic prestige in Italy and abroad. Royal Decrees appointed him to serve on the High Council of Public Education in 1886 (he would be reappointed to the same office until 1901) and on the High Council of Public Health in 1887. In August 1887 Golgi was elected Corresponding Member of the Section of Pathology of the Accademia dei Lincei (at the same time his former first student, Grassi, was elected in the Section of Morphology and Zoology). He was also elected Corresponding Member of the Academy of Medicine of Rome in 1887; of the Societas Medicorum Svecana of Stockholm and of the Accademia Medico-Fisica of Florence in 1888; of the Società Medico-Chirurgica of Bologna in 1889; and honorary member of the Italian Society of Freniatry. And despite the election of Sangalli as Dean of the Medical School in 1888, Golgi's power in the University remained intact or even increased.

In December 1889 Golgi was sent by the Minister of Internal Affairs to Paris to collect information on an epidemic of influenza that was wreaking havoc in France, and on the prophylactic measures and therapies that the French physicians were adopting. The Italian authorities were evidently eager to prepare appropriate countermeasures to prevent the spread of the disease to Italy and turned to the member of the High Council of Public Health who was an expert infectologist. On the evening of 15 December Golgi was in Paris, where he visited the Val de Gràce Hospital directed by Laveran, and then other hospitals in the city. On his return he reported his observations to the *Società Medico-Chirurgica*.[118] Surprisingly, the infectious nature of the disease was accepted only by a minority of the physicians interviewed and Golgi maintained that its contagiousness had not been definitely proven or disproven, despite his having contracted the influenza himself.

Despite his personal ascent Golgi continued to lead a simple life, divided between home, laboratory, and lecture hall. During the summer months, when the heat and humidity became insufferable in Pavia, he spent his vacation in a house in a residential area of Varese near the market square and next door to Bizzozero. So the two friends often spent their vacation together, opening their homes to 'famous Italians such as Lombroso, Mosso (who vacationed on the nearby Lago Maggiore), and Bozzolo (who owned a beautiful eighteenth-century villa in Val Cuvia), and foreign personalities such as Van Gehucten [sic], Retzius, etc.'[119] They frequently organized group trips around Varese, as a young relative of Bizzozero, Eugenio Medea, recollected:

A beautiful trip to Campo dei Fiori above Varese is still fixed in my mind, taken on a wonderful day in early autumn (I believe in 1888 or 1889 because I was in grammar school at the time).

The trip to Campo dei Fiori was not easy in those times: on the road to the Chapels of Sacro Monte, Bizzozero—who was very fond of the region of Varese—owned a villa in the form of a chalet (which, remodelled and enlarged, still exists between the twelfth and thirteenth Chapels) where he used to spend some weeks in the middle of the summer.

There were no automobiles or cable cars; one went by carriage up to the first Chapel, and from then on by foot. We arrived by dinnertime at Villa Bizzozero; we slept for a few hours and then we left very early in the morning for Campo dei Fiori and as soon as we reached the summit we ate a huge *panettone*, which had been carried up there in triumph (we were a jolly group, among whom

I remember dear Prof. Fusari, anatomical disciple of Golgi and poor hiker, which made him an object of mockery for us kids). I shall always remember the good humour, the simplicity of the two great Masters, whom I would a few years later see in the lecture hall and in the laboratory! The wives of the two professors with their exquisite grace made the trip particularly pleasant and worthy of being remembered.[120]

Notes

1. Marcus Terentius Varro (*Script. Rei Rust.*, Lib. I, Ch. xii).
2. Aulus Cornelius Celsus (*De Medicina*, Lib. III, Sect. 3).
3. Tommasi-Crudeli (1879).
4. Tommasi-Crudeli was the driving force behind the foundation of the Laboratories of the Institute of Hygiene of the University of Rome, of which he became the first Director and which were under construction at the time of his collaboration with Klebs.
5. Klebs and Tommasi-Crudeli (1879).
6. Klebs and Tommasi-Crudeli (1879a).
7. Cuboni and Marchiafava (1881).
8. Laveran (1880; 1880a). See also Fantini (1992, pp. 50ff.).
9. Laveran (1884).
10. Richard (1882). See also Fantini (1992, pp. 56ff.).
11. Orsi (1881, p. 91).
12. Golgi and Edoardo Perroncito married two sisters, Lina and Erminia Aletti, respectively, who were nieces of Giulio Bizzozero. The following family tree is modification from Trautmann (1988, p. 28, bibliography) and Pensa (1991, p. 41).

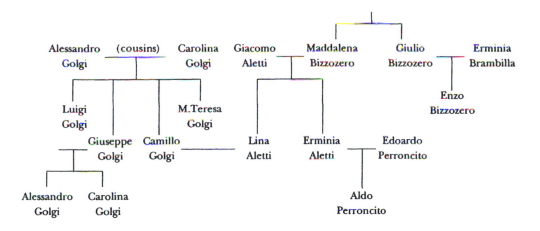

13. Letter from Tommasi-Crudeli to Golgi, 23 March 1881 (MSUP-VII-I-14).
14. Letter from Marchiafava to Golgi, end of March or beginning of April 1881 (MSUP-VII-III-9).
15. Orsi (1881a).
16. Letter from Tommasi-Crudeli to Golgi, spring 1881 (MSUP-VII-I-14).
17. Letter from Tommasi-Crudeli to Golgi, probably at the end of March or beginning of April 1881 (MSUP-VII-I-14).

18. Laveran (1884, p. 51; 1887, p. 273).
19. Marchiafava and Celli (1884, p. 394).
20. Mariotti and Ciarrocchi (1884).
21. Marchiafava and Celli (1885, p. 311). See also Fantini (1992, pp. 65ff.).
22. Marchiafava and Celli (1885). The paper described: (a) corpuscles with a 'central vacuole, with the coloured protoplasm of the red cell showing through it', which appears as 'light rings of various size' sometimes exhibiting 'clear-cut amoeboid movements' (p. 313); (b) 'pigmented masses', also mobile, within which the pigment assumes the aspect of 'granules or rods'. Sometimes they noticed granules of pigment detaching from the pigmented masses, granules that 'either remain in the protoplasm of the red cell, or are extruded almost with violence into the plasma, where they continue to move with the same speed, and then vigorously disappear among the red cells' (p. 315); (c) 'pigmented semilunar bodies' (pp. 315ff.) previously described by Laveran; (d) 'roundish formations, provided with processes' corresponding, according to Laveran, to the complete parasite; (e) 'roundish pigmented bodies, in which there is a hint of scission, others in which [the scission] is complete, so the entire body appears as a mass of corpuscles . . . The volume of these masses of corpuscles is progressively reduced by the detachment of such corpuscles; free corpuscles can be observed . . . although their aspect is identical to those contained in the red cells . . .'(p. 322).'. . . what is the meaning of the bodies undergoing scission? We have seen that the resulting corpuscles have the same aspect as those in the red cells during the initial phases of the scission. Might they represent the new generations of parasitic elements? Also on this point, for the moment, we cannot answer with precision' (pp. 327ff.). Thus, Marchiafava and Celli had described, unknowingly, many of the intermediate forms assumed by the four malarial parasites, *Plasmodium vivax* and *Plasmodium ovale* (causal agents of the benign tertian), *Plasmodium falciparum* (causal agent of malignant tertian), and *Plasmodium malariae* (causal agent of quartan) during the hematic phase. But since their patients were a non homogenous clinical group, with different febrile curves and different chronologies for the clinical symptoms, it was impossible for them to interpret the different morphological forms as sequential stages of development of different parasites. Worth noting is their description of the scission of what we currently call schizont (mature trophozoite) into merozoites, new parasites that can infect other red cells.
23. Marchiafava and Celli (1885a).
24. Marchiafava and Celli (1885, p. 328).
25. Marchiafava and Celli (1886, p. 186).
26. *Ibid.* (p. 210).
27. *Ibid.* (p. 211). The results of these studies immediately became known outside Italy because the publication was translated into German (Marchiafava and Celli, 1885b).
28. Veratti (1942–43, pp. 101f.). But see Achille Monti, who wrote 'I collaborated with him [that is, Golgi] in all the studies on malaria done in Pavia, in Rome, and elsewhere.' (Monti 1935, p. 3.)
29. With reference to the two negative cases, Golgi wrote: 'If in two of the very first cases I found negative results, I can now state with confidence that those two cases were either not malarial or, more likely, that the observations were not frequent enough. In all subsequent cases, examined with greater diligence and repeatedly, there were no negative findings. When in some cases, presented to me as malarial, I could find no parasite, the further course of symptoms demonstrated that those cases were due to other types of infection.' (Golgi 1889; *OO*, p. 1063.)
30. In the full report Golgi (Golgi 1886b, p. 109) wrote that he presented a summary of his data on 15 November 1885, whereas in the *Opera Omnia* (p. 989) the date is 5 November 1885.

According to the *Giornale della Regia Accademia di Medicina di Torino* (1885, **33**, pp. 734) Bizzo-zero reported on Golgi's research in the meeting of 20 November 1885.

31. *Giornale della Regia Accademia di Medicina di Torino* (1885, **33**, pp. 734–5). 'The member Bizzo-zero, on behalf of Corresponding Member Professor Golgi, reports on research done by the latter on malarial blood. According to Golgi's observations, concerning especially quartan fevers, the pigmented bodies in the red cells, which are quite small in the first day of apyrexia, grow progressively until they fill the entire red cell in the period that precedes the bout; and finally, in the hours immediately before the bout and during the bout, they exhibit two characteristics: the lumping of the pigment in the centre of the corpuscle and the segmenta-tion of the peripheral substance of the corpuscle, resulting in a series of small corpuscles which surround the pigment as a crown. This segmentation, therefore, coincides with the appearance of the febrile bout and can possibly be considered as the source of a new genera-tion of parasitic elements.' See also Belloni (1978b, p. 36).

32. This paper achieved immediate international recognition because a summary of it was published in German by Carl Günther (*Fortschritte der Medizin*, 1886, **6**, pp. 575–8) and the following year it was translated into French (Golgi 1887).

33. Golgi (1886c).

34. Veratti (1942–43, p. 102).

35. Golgi (1886b; *OO*, p. 991).

36. *Ibid.* (*OO*, p. 993).

37. *Ibid.* (*OO*, p. 1007).

38. *Ibid.* (*OO*, p. 1001).

39. Golgi noticed that immediately following the febrile bout the red cells contain extremely small parasites exhibiting amoeboid movements. These parasites enlarge in the two days without fever, wearing out the red cells and transforming haemoglobin into a 'melanaemic' pigment. On the day of the febrile bout the parasites almost completely fill the red cells and appear as white−transparent bodies containing sparse dark pigments. Before the chill the pigments migrate towards the centre of the parasite and radial sulci began to form, sub-dividing the parasite into roundish sections in which a nucleus can be seen. The final product is a body containing a central 'melanaemic' mass and many corpuscles disposed like petals in the corolla of a daisy. Then the petals detach (segmentation) releasing the mass of pigment. The new generation of parasites will infect new red cells giving rise to a new cycle. The pigment released by the destruction of the red cell will be phagocytized by the white cells.

40. Golgi (1886e; *OO*, p. 1015).

41. *Ibid.* (*OO*, p. 1016).

42. Quoted in Belloni (1951, p. 17).

43. Belloni (1978b, p. 37).

44. Golgi (1886f).

45. Golgi (1886e). A summary of the publication in German was published by Carl Günther (*Fortschritte der Medizin*, 1886, **6**, pp. 692–3).

46. Metschnikoff (1887, p. 328).

47. Tommasi-Crudeli (1886, p. 225). Being unable to participate in the 4 April 1886 session, Tommasi-Crudeli asked the anatomist Francesco Todaro to present Schiavuzzi's findings on his behalf.

48. Tommasi-Crudeli (1886a).

49. Tommasi-Crudeli (1886b, p. 329).

50. *Ibid.* (p. 330).

51. Tommasi-Crudeli (1886b).
52. Garrison (1929, p. 578).
53. Tommasi-Crudeli (1888, p. 306).
54. *Botanisches Centralblatt* (1887, **31**, p. 288).
55. Golgi (1889a; *OO*, p. 1037).
56. *Ibid.* (p. 335).
57. Mosso (1887, p. 337).
58. Rough draft of a letter to Mosso, 27 May 1887 (MSUP-XXVIII-II-2).
59. Tommasi-Crudeli (1887, p. 357).
60. *Ibid.* (p. 361).
61. *Ibid.* (pp. 355ff.).
62. *Ibid.* (p. 360).
63. Cattaneo and Monti (1887).
64. Transcripts of the session (*Bollettino della Società Medico-Chirurgica di Pavia*, 1887, Anno II, p. 40).
65. Letter from Bizzozero to Golgi, 19 May 1887 (MSUP-VII-III-1).
66. Letter from Bizzozero to Golgi, 6 June 1887 (MSUP-VII-III-1).
67. Letter from Mosso to Golgi, 2 June 1887 (MSUP-VII-I-8).
68. Cattaneo and Monti (1888).
69. Cattaneo and Monti (1888a).
70. Golgi (1888, p. 8).
71. Grassi (1888).
72. Golgi (1888b). A few years later, Golgi published a more exhaustive report of his research (Golgi 1892) which was published also in French (Golgi 1892a) and German (Golgi 1892b). In this full report he extended the research he had done four years earlier (Golgi 1888b) on the optimal period for the treatment with quinine, and thoroughly discussed the action of quinine on malarial parasites, also reviewing the literature on the clinical and pharmaco-kinetic aspects of the treatment.
73. Golgi (1888c; *OO*, pp. 1027ff.).
74. Golgi (1888c). The article was published in French (Golgi 1889c).
75. Golgi (1889a; *OO*, p. 1037).
76. *Ibid.* (*OO*, p. 1036).
77. Golgi (1889a; *OO*, p. 1038).
78. Schiavuzzi (1888).
79. Tommasi-Crudeli (1888, p. 307).
80. Golgi (1889a; *OO*, p. 1039).
81. Golgi (1889a).
82. *Ibid.* (*OO*, p. 1037).
83. Golgi (1889d).
84. As far as the biological characteristics are concerned, Golgi pointed out the following differences: (1) a cycle of 2 days for the tertian and 3 days for the quartan; (2) more vigorous amoeboid movements in the tertian; (3) rapid decolouration of the protoplasm of the red cell during the early phases of the parasite cycle in the tertian, whereas in the quartan the red cell maintains a characteristic yellowish–greenish colour until the last phases of its destruction; (4) red cells that tend to shrink in the quartan and to swell in the tertian.

    Among the morphological differences, Golgi listed: (1) the lighter and more delicate aspect of the tertian parasite; (2) in the quartan the pigments of the parasites look like granules or thick rods, whereas in tertian they have the appearance of thin rods; (3) the process of segmentation has constant characteristics in the quartan, but not in the tertian. The new plasmodia (merozoites), originating from the process of segmentation, are smaller and number 15–20 elements in the tertian (here Golgi is referring to the *Plasmodium vivax* whereas the *Plasmodium ovale*, which also causes tertian, segment into 8–10 merozoites) whereas they number 6–12 elements in the quartan. It must be noticed that in these descriptions Golgi was not studying a single *Plasmodium* but rather a mix of *vivax* and *ovale*, which had not yet been differentiated.

85. Golgi (1889; *OO*, p. 1078).
86. Golgi (1889e). On the differential diagnosis between tertian and quartan fever, Golgi published extensive papers in Italian (Golgi 1889), French (Golgi 1891a), and German (Golgi 1889f).
87. Golgi (1889g). Full reports were published in Italian (Golgi 1890), French (Golgi 1891b), and German (Golgi 1890a).
88. Flügge thanked Golgi in a letter dated 8 January 1890 (MSUP). See also Belloni (1978b, p. 41).
89. Golgi (1890c).
90. Golgi (1890d).
91. Golgi (1891c).
92. Letter sent to one of the two directors, 14 September 1890 (in Belloni, 1978b, pp. 42ff.).
93. See letters of Flügge to Golgi, 17 October and 10 November 1890 (MSUP). See also Belloni (1978b, pp. 43ff.).
94. Golgi (1891d).
95. MSUP-VII-III-5.
96. The note by Feletti and Grassi, *Risposta alla critica fatta dal prof. Bizzozero alla nostra nota preliminare sulla malaria* (Answer to the criticism by Prof. Bizzozero of our preliminary note on malaria) was printed in Catania in 1890 (a copy of it can be found in the Institute of Comparative Anatomy of the University of Rome 'La Sapienza').
97. MSUP-VII-I-6. An excerpt of the letter was published in *Rendiconti dell'Accademia Nazionale dei Lincei* (1954, **16**, pp. 574–6), and it appears in full in *Symposia Genetica* (1956, **4**, 169–71).
98. Golgi reported on his work on the malaria of birds in a note in the *Trattato di Medicina*, ed. J. M. Charcot, C. J. Bouchard, and E. Brissaud. (Turin: Utet, Vol. I, 2nd part, p. 368).
99. Golgi (1886d).
100. Cattaneo (1886).
101. Belloni (1975).
102. See note to the chapter 'Cellule gangliari' (Ganglion cells) in *Elementi di istologia normale* (Elements of normal histology), ed. S. L. Schenk. (Milano: Vallardi, 1889, pp. 92–7).
103. *Bollettino della Società Medico-Chirurgica di Pavia* (1887, Anno II, p. 25). A full report was published in both Italian (Golgi 1887a) and French (Golgi 1887b).
104. Sometimes the spelling is Koulisciof.
105. Addis Saba (1993).
106. Belloni (1978, p. 112).
107. Belloni (1978a, p. 342).
108. Céline (1952).
109. In Belloni (1978, p. 113).
110. In the 1890s Golgi would openly take sides with the moderates but from hints contained in an article in *La Provincia Pavese* (28 June 1899) it appears that at an earlier time he had leftist sympathies.

111. Kouliscioff (1886, p. 613).
112. Belloni (1978a, p. 344).
113. Kouliscioff (1886).
114. Golgi (1889b; *OO*, p. 543).
115. *Ibid.* (*OO*, p. 544).
116. Golgi (1888a).
117. Golgi (1889b; *OO*, p. 551). The results of the histogenetic research on the kidney were communicated to the Società Medico-Chirurgica of Pavia on 7 July 1888 (Golgi 1888d).
118. Golgi (1890b).
119. Medea (1966, p. 2). According to Rossi, 'Between 1877 and 1913, Golgi used to spend his vacation in Varese, surrounded by the affection of his family, and in serene harmony with Giulio Bizzozero; and here, as in Abbiategrasso, he set up a laboratory in which interesting research was carried out' (1927, pp. 16ff.). Notable among these research projects was the one on peritoneal transfusions. Reference to Golgi's sojourns in Varese can be found also in Pensa (1991, pp. 116ff.).
120. Medea (1966, p. 3). See also Sacerdotti (1947, p. 4).

13

The prophets of the neuron

By the mid-1880s the black reaction, although discovered more than ten years earlier, was still known to only a small number of researchers. Only a few years later, in the early 1890s, the most important neurobiologists were hailing it as a breakthrough. It was an irony of fate that a crucial role in this dramatic change was played by a young Spanish scientist who would later become Golgi's most formidable scientific opponent.

In fairness, it must be noted that, even before beginning his work on malaria, Golgi had already attained a certain international renown. His studies had been repeatedly cited, his work on glia had played an important role in the international debate on the nature of this tissue, and the newly discovered neurotendinous organ now bore his name. But the true value of the black reaction, his greatest achievement, had been slow to be appreciated.

Although his first paper with the black reaction had been immediately reviewed in Italy and abroad, for several years Golgi had been the only one to use the method. At the beginning of the 1880s Giuseppe Bellonci, while recognizing its superior ability to define fine morphological details, criticized it because he thought that it could produce partial impregnation and artifactual images.[1] In Italy, the first scientists to use it outside the Pavian group were Giuseppe Magini in Rome, beginning in 1882, Giacomini in Turin, who studied the brain of three microcephalic patients and published his findings in 1885 in *Archivio di Psichiatria e Scienze Penali*, and Ferruccio Tartuferi, who applied it to the study of the retina. At the 12th Congress of the Italian Medical Association held in Pavia in 1887, the use of the black reaction was discussed by Ciro Bernardini, who between 1886 and 1887 applied the method to investigate various pathologies (progressive paralysis, epilepsy, idiocy), and in a major way by Giuseppe Magini,[2] who studied the fetal nervous system (particularly the cortex) of various mammals, including humans, and provided a precise description of radial glia and the periventricular proliferative zone. He also observed roundish cells, which probably represented migrating immature neurons. Those, like Lombroso, who had followed the progress of Golgi's work recognized his greatness to the point of defining him in 1887 as 'greatest perfecter' of the 'fine histology of the nerve centres'.[3]

Around the middle of the 1880s Golgi's neurobiological work was known only to a small group of European researchers. His studies had been summarized in the *Jahresberichte* for anatomy and physiology and in the *Quarterly Journal of Microscopic Science*; in 1873 Franz

Boll had published a critical review of his work 'On the structure of the grey substance of the brain' in the important *Centralblatt für medicinischen Wissenschaften* soon after its publication in the *Gazzetta Medica Italiana*.

In 1881 Gustav Schwalbe, in his classical manual of neurology, emphasized Golgi's findings, especially those on the anatomy of the olfactory bulbs, and gave the impression that he shared some of Golgi's functional conjectures.[4] Edinger[5] and Obersteiner[6] also appeared to have taken notice of the new method. Kühne, who in 1880 had mortified Grassi by his cavalier attitude towards Golgi's findings, four years later, while visiting Bizzozero's laboratory in Turin, marvelled over brain preparations stained with the mercury dichloride method. He then began to use the technique but with less than satisfactory results.[7] More successful were the attempts made by Forel and Bleuler, and by van Gudden.[8]

The visits by foreign scientists such as Donaldson and Nansen, as well as his appointment (under the auspices of Bizzozero) to the Editorial Board of the prestigious *Internationale Monatsschrift für Anatomie und Histologie,* are good indicators of Golgi's international reputation toward the middle of the 1880s.

Despite this, the prevailing opinion about the black reaction is well represented by Ranvier's criticisms in his *Traité Technique d'Histologie*. For the French histologist (to whom Golgi might have shown some preparations during their meeting in Viareggio and who probably tried the reaction), the black reaction, while sometimes providing the most beautiful images of the nerve cells, in most cases produced an irregular deposit of silver granules.[9] It should be noted that Ranvier, on the basis of Golgi's discovery that the axons are ramified, elaborated an ingenious theory to explain 'referred' sensation and pain. Sometimes, the sensation of pain produced by stimulating a skin region is localized (referred) to another region located at a distance on the body surface. Ranvier thought that the nerve fibres originating from the irritated region and those originating from the region to which the sensation is referred converge on the same nerve cell, causing the spatial dislocation of the sensation. And he emphasized how the old concept of Deiters of the non-ramified axon could not explain this phenomenon.[10] Ranvier's elegant physiological model of referred pain represents a good example of the powerful implications of Golgi's discovery. In 1885 the black reaction was adopted also by Kölliker, Retzius and others, but again with results that were less than satisfactory.[11]

After the publication of *Sulla fina anatomia degli centrali del sistema nervoso*, and the French and English translations of his works, the enormous potential of the new method finally began to be appreciated. On 6 March 1886, Wilhelm Biedermann, of the Institute of Physiology of the University of Prague, wrote to Golgi that he was very interested in his neurohistological research and in their physiological implications, and asked the Italian to lend him some preparations.[12] The Russian Wladimir Podwyssozki, on 29 March 1887, asked Golgi to send him 'the latest of your very important publications on the nervous system, so I can report on them in the Russian Literature'.[13]

When Kölliker and Golgi began their correspondence in 1887[14] the latter sent his Swiss colleague some of his preparations on the nervous system. On 3 May 1887, Kölliker thanked Golgi for having shown him the most beautiful nerve cells that he had ever seen,

congratulating him for having developed a method that allowed their processes to be outlined in such great detail.[15] Kölliker, who had some pieces of human cerebellum and horse
brain hardened in dichromate, immediately tested the method, obtaining positive results.
The evening of the following 21 May, during a session of the Physikalish-Medicinische
Gesellschaft of Würzburg, Kölliker showed the preparations obtained both by Golgi
(human brain and cerebellum; spinal cord of kitten) and by himself. In his report,[16] and
in a subsequent paper,[17] he expressed his great appreciation for Golgi's method and for
some of his conclusions (such as the notion that the protoplasmic processes end with free
terminations), but criticized Golgi's physiological interpretations. In particular, he rejected
the idea that the dendrites had no *nervous* function (for Golgi, they mostly had a role in
cellular trophism) and advanced doubts about the existence of the diffuse neural network.

On the following day, Kölliker wrote to Golgi to inform him of the communication of
his data to the Physikalish-Medicinsche Gesellschaft and enthusiastically pronounced that
Golgi's method 'heralded a new era' in the micro-anatomy of the central nervous system.
He then added, 'you would not be offended if, although embracing your discoveries, I do
not agree with all your conclusions . . . Your achievements in this area are so great that a
little bit of disagreement would only give them greater prominence.'[18] We do not know
if Kölliker and Golgi met or exchanged letters in the next two years, but Kölliker was
certainly a guest of Golgi in 1889, probably on 22 and 23 April,[19] and presumably they
spent the little time available examining slides and discussing the nervous system. Kölliker,
in his memoirs, proudly took credit for having introduced the black reaction in
Germany.[20]

Retzius, who was in correspondence with Kölliker, was also quick to appreciate Golgi's
'wonderful method' and the 'epoch-making' importance of *Sulla fina anatomia degli organi
del sistema nervoso* (of which he had received a complimentary copy).[21] Nevertheless his
attempts to apply the black reaction were disappointing and on 10 January 1888 he asked
his Italian colleague for some of his preparations to show at a session of the Swedish
Medical Society.

In 1887 Golgi's method was applied by P. Kronthal in the study of progressive paralysis.
In the medial frontal, anterior, and central convolutions, and in the insula on the right, he
found that the gangliary cells were reduced in number, smaller, and with fewer processes.
On the contrary, he observed an increase in the number and dimensions of glial cells, that
is, reactive gliosis.[22] These results were contested by L. Greppin, who obtained beautiful
preparations with the black reaction,[23] but did not observe the specific alterations
described by Kronthal. Greppin was one of the first to understand the importance of the
black reaction and suggested some technical modifications to enhance the preservation of
the sections.[24]

The black reaction was also making inroads in France. The Lyonnais anatomist Renaut,
who was appreciative of Golgi's studies on glia, began to experiment with the new method
after reading *Sulla fina anatomia degli organi del sistema nervoso*. On 14 February 1888 he wrote
to Golgi that he 'had already studied some preparations obtained with your method of the
black reaction, and I am preparing others with the same technique to be included in my
histological treatise, now in press, because the results you obtained appear remarkable to
me, and worthy of being diffused in France.'[25]

In 1888 Golgi became a member of the Editorial Board of the prestigious journal *Beiträge zur pathologischen Anatomie und zur allgemeinen Pathologie* while the black reaction received an official consecration in the important treatise of histology by Karl Toldt, who gave great emphasis to Golgi's description of nerve cells.[26] And, in the same year, Obersteiner reviewed the technical advantages of the black reaction and discussed the theory of the diffuse neural net.[27] In 1889 Golgi's method was also employed by Edinger, who discussed it in his monograph on the structure of the nervous system,[28] and again by Sehrwald, who published a study on the technical aspects of the method, in which he suggested how to treat the histological sections in order to avoid the formation of artifacts due to the deposition of silver granules.[29]

A radical criticism of the black reaction was published in 1888 by M. J. Rossbach and E. Sehrwald, who, while paying homage to the originality of the method, suggested that it did not stain nerve cells but rather the lymphatic vessels of the brain, particularly those of the cortex.[30] At that time a debate was raging on the very existence of lymphatic pathways in the nervous system. His Sr and Obersteiner, among others, advocated the existence of perivascular or pericellular spaces, while others, including Golgi, contested this hypothesis. The controversy was still alive in the 1880s; in 1884 His Sr had reiterated the existence of the perivascular spaces, and Obersteiner, in 1888, that of pericellular spaces. Rossbach and Sehrwald maintained that Golgi's method was without equal for the demonstration of these spaces; according to them the black precipitate formed a sleeve around the cells, vessels and their ramifications. They provided a number of reasons for this peculiar interpretation. The ganglion cells appeared to be larger, stockier, and roundish when stained with Golgi's method;[31] in some preparations there were interruptions in the black stain of the nerve process and thus it was possible to see a length of unstained cylindraxis connecting two thicker stained portions; often it was possible to see, in partially stained cells, a black ring of encrustation surrounding a smaller unstained cell body. Another argument used by Rossbach and Sehrwald to support their theory was the presence of drop-like or leaflet-like small processes emanating from the large dendritic processes of the Purkinje cells, images that they interpreted as varicose expansions of the lymphatic spaces. What they actually described were dendritic spines, which in the same year had also been glimpsed by Cajal, who drew them as small irregularities on the outline of the Purkinje cells.[32] These formations had been described in 1864 by Philip Owsjannikov, but his report had been forgotten.[33] According to Rossbach and Sehrwald, the long processes of glial cells were also none other than lymphatic canaliculi that contained a cell process for only a short length. They found, as indirect evidence for their conclusion, that the application of Golgi's method in plants resulted in the black staining of the lymphatic canaliculi and lacunae.

Rossbach and Sehrwald's conclusions were immediately endorsed by Kronthal,[34] but rejected by Ernesto Belmondo, an Assistant at the Psychiatric Clinic of Modena, who tested their hypothesis in studies conducted in the Laboratory of Histology of the Mental Hospital of Reggio Emilia. Belmondo thought that if the theory of the vascular spaces were correct, perpendicular sections of the pyramidal cells, obtained by cuts parallel to the cerebral surface, should demonstrate a 'black ring (pericellular space in which the silver chromate crystals should have been deposited), containing an unstained cell body' whereas 'we never saw such a ring, and the cell section appeared to be homogeneously stained black or filled with brown'.[35]

Although more and more neurohistologists were acknowledging the importance of the black reaction, Golgi's ideas on the non-neural function of dendrites, the different functional significance of Type I and II cells, the modality of connections of the axons, and on the neurophysiology originating from these structural bases, triggered no small perplexity. Golgi's name began also to be associated with that of Gerlach, as the champion of a reticular model, without much attention being given to the substantial differences between the two theories.[36] Both Golgi and Gerlach, however, were destined to face a formidable new theory that was then gaining ground among neuroscientists.

In fact, in 1886 a scientific event of the greatest importance had occurred. In October Wilhelm His Sr, who was then at the University of Leipzig, published an article in which he advanced the hypothesis that the cell body and its processes constitute an independent unit.[37] Disciple of such great biologists as Johannes Müller, Robert Remak, and Claude Bernard, His Sr was an undisputed authority in embryology. His established that the processes of the nerve cells originate from the soma by a process of growth in which the axon develops before the dendrites. Discussing how the axons freely end in the motor plate and the sensory fibres in the peripheral receptors such as the Pacinian corpuscle, His hypothesized that this might also be true for the terminals of the nerve processes in the central nervous system. Golgi (who was cited by His), on the other hand, had already shown free terminations of dendrites, demolishing the reticular hypothesis of Gerlach. His' hypothesis of free terminations of axons, combined with Golgi's discovery of axon ramifications, made it possible to envision a neuroanatomical basis for the enormous number of connections among nerve cells predicted by physiological models.

At the same time that His was formulating these hypotheses, another Swiss scientist, Forel, was arriving at similar conclusions from a different direction. He had learned the degeneration method in Gudden's laboratory in Munich, and had become renowned for having identified the subthalamic structures that are now known as the fields of Forel. In 1879 he became director of the Burghölzli Psychiatric Hospital and professor of Psychiatry at the University of Zurich. Studying some preparations stained with the black reaction by Bleuler, he was able to confirm the presence of ramifications in the nerve process and free terminations in the protoplasmic process, but he could not visualize Golgi's diffuse neural net. Thus he wondered whether the nervous tissue, contrary to Golgi's theory, was instead discontinuous; all the more so as the experiments of his teacher Gudden had demonstrated that, after selective lesions of groups of nerve cells, only their respective nerve processes degenerated but not the nerve cells with which they were connected, indicating that this connection was purely functional. While vacationing at Fisibach, he developed the idea further and discussed it in an article published in the influential *Archiv für Psychiatrie und Nervenkrankheiten*.[38] Unfortunately for Forel, the article appeared only in 1887,[39] thus depriving him of priority in what a few years later would be called the *theory of the neuron*. However, Forel's insight immediately found a place in the treatise that Obersteiner completed in October 1887 and published the next year. Obersteiner declared that Forel's model made it unnecessary to accept a priori a protoplasmic continuity between nerve cells, as was also evident by examining the best histological preparations obtained with the black reaction.[40]

Another important contribution to the emergence of the theory of the neuron was the publication of Nansen's dissertation in 1887.[41] Heavily influenced by Golgi's neurohistological theory, Nansen embraced Golgi's classification of nerve cells (Type I and Type II) and his idea that dendrites have a primarily trophic function (he saw them ending near blood vessels), and rejected Gerlach's reticular theory. But Nansen explicitly declared that there were no anastomoses either between the axons or between their finer ramifications. He considered the dotted substance of Leydig to be nothing more that an interlacing formed by the finer subdivisions of the cylindraxes, without protoplasmic continuity.[42] In fact, an outline of this idea had already been sketched by Golgi himself,[43] and it is probable that Nansen expanded on it because of his association with Golgi's laboratory. Thus from an anatomical point of view, the concept of nerve cells as independent units was formulated at about the same time by Nansen, His, and Forel. Physiologically, however, Nansen's interweaving in the 'dotted' substance (currently, the neuropil) carried out the same function as Golgi's diffuse neural net as the actual locus of nervous activity; the nerve message would pass from the ramification of one axon to another (evidently jumping the protoplasmic gap), whereas the cell body had only a simple trophic function. From this he concluded that the development of intellectual functions was proportional to the degree of complexity of the 'dotted' substance. Although it is clear that Nansen's model of the nervous system was derived from that of Golgi, his explicit rejection of anastomoses places him among the pioneers of the theory of the neuron.[44]

In 1887, the Spanish psychiatrist Luis Simarro Lacabra, who had studied with Charcot and Ranvier in Paris, returned to Madrid, bringing the latest innovations in histological techniques, including some preparations with the black reaction. Indeed, although Ranvier had given only a brief and partially positive description of the black reaction in his treatise, by 1887 most French neurohistologists must have been acquainted with Golgi's method.

In his house at No. 41 calle Arco de Santa Maria, Simarro received a visit from a young professor from the University of Valencia, Santiago Ramón y Cajal, who was eager to hear about the latest developments in science. Cajal was born in 1852 in a small Spanish village on the Pyrenees, near the French border. His father, who came from a line of poor farmers, had made heroic sacrifices, first to attend the School of Surgery at the University of Barcelona and then, when already married and the father of four children, to realize his dream of graduating as a doctor of medicine from the University of Zaragoza. After a rebellious adolescence in which his artistic aspirations were frustrated by his strict father, Santiago followed in his father's footsteps and graduated in medicine from the University of Zaragoza in 1873. Immediately after graduation he was drafted into the military and in 1874 was sent to Cuba to fight in the Spanish–American War. In Cuba Cajal contracted malaria and was discharged. Back in Spain he fell victim to tuberculosis and almost died of a pulmonary haemorrhage. However, he recovered completely from these misfortunes and progressed to become the Director of the Anatomical Museum of Zaragoza and, at the age of 31, Professor of Anatomy at the University of Valencia. Around the mid-1880s

Cajal became attracted to a new theory by Jean Baptiste Carnoy and others, who posited the existence of a reticular structure (made of anastomosed filaments) in the cytoplasm of a variety of cell types, particularly those endowed with motility. Indeed, this reticulum was thought to be responsible for all phenomena of cell motility, from the propulsive movement of the amoeba to the contraction of skeletal muscle fibres. And there were those, such as the British scientist B. Melland, who held that the peculiar striations of the muscles were simply an artifact without functional relevance to muscle contraction. This theory is a typical example of what Sir Andrew Huxley called the 'principle of uniformity of nature'.[45] One of the staunchest supporters of this idea was van Gehuchten, a pupil of Carnoy, who propounded it in two massive papers in *La Cellule*.[46] Cajal, who had begun corresponding with van Gehuchten, became another advocate of the role of cytoplasmic reticulum in muscle contraction.[47] In the end, however, Cajal abandoned this theory, which had been subjected to devastating criticism by Kölliker (who vigorously maintained that muscular contractions depend on a mechanism originating from the muscle striations), and it is possible that as a consequence of this he developed a permanent aversion to reticular concepts.

By 1887 Cajal had published some scientific papers in Spanish journals and, thanks to Krause's endorsement, also an article in a German journal. When he visited Simarro, he was in the process of publishing a manual of histology in instalments, and wished to bring himself up to date with the latest innovations in microscopic technique. In the home laboratory of Simarro, Cajal admired some excellent preparations made with the Weigert–Pal method, but he was literally dumbfounded when Simarro showed him a slide stained with Golgi's method. 'Cajal's surprise and emotion were enormous when he saw in the microscope the nerve cells with all their processes',[48] realizing 'with his own eyes the marvellous revelatory power of the silver chromate reaction.'[49] He was unable to pull his eyes away from the microscope. The sight of a perfectly stained neuron was a revelation and that night he was unable to sleep in anticipation of returning to look at Simarro's extraordinary nerve cells again.[50] He quickly decided to dedicate his scientific career to the study of the nervous system using this powerful tool discovered by Golgi. It was true that Golgi had already written an entire book on the findings obtained by using this method or its variants, but an enormous amount of work still had to be done. Back in Valencia, he set to work applying the black reaction 'on a grand scale' and with all the tenacity and perseverance of which he was capable. He used Golgi's book, which he had borrowed from Simarro, 'like a Bible'. His first attempts fully confirmed Golgi's descriptions of the free terminals of dendrites but also suggested that there remained an entire continent to explore. Meanwhile, Cajal was given the choice of a professorship at Zaragoza or at Barcelona. He decided in favour of the latter because 'For a man devoted to an idea and who has decided to dedicate himself completely to it, big cities are preferable to small ones.'[51] At the beginning of 1888, 'my pinnacle year, my lucky year',[52] the quantity of new findings that he was obtaining and his impatience for their quick publication was such that he decided to establish a journal, *Revista trimestral de Histología normal y patológica*, the first issues of which were dedicated entirely to his research. Initially only 60 copies of each issue were printed and sent to the principal histologists of the world (presumably gratis).

The first issue appeared in May of 1888 with an opening article on the structure of the cerebellum in birds.[53] Compared to Golgi's studies, it contained some novelties, such as the characterization of basket cells, dendritic spines (described previously by Owsjannikov and studied also by Rossbach and Sehrwald at the same time as Cajal), and mossy fibres. Cajal was surprised that Golgi had not described the basket cells and thought that this might be due to the fact that they were much less visible in mammals than in birds. Most important, in one paragraph Cajal discussed the connections of the cerebellar nerve cells and concluded that there were no anastomoses, thus rejecting the theory of the diffuse neural net. In the second article of this first issue he examined the structure of the retina, which had already been studied by Ferruccio Tartuferi who had reported the presence of anastomoses. Cajal sketched a model of connections between the bipolar and gangliary cells in which the dendrites of the latter come 'in contact' with the descending ramifications of the bipolar cells without interposition of the diffuse neural net. In another article, which appeared in the August issue, Cajal reported the discovery of peculiar nerve fibres (*fibras trepadoras* = climbing fibres) that arise from the white matter and climb on the body and dendrites of the Purkinje cell, but maintain their anatomical autonomy.[54] The existence of climbing fibres and basket cells represented for Cajal the critical evidence for 'the transmission of nervous impulses by contact'.[55] From that moment on, the notion of the nerve cell as an anatomical unit would remain the cornerstone of Cajal's theoretical model of the nervous system. With this idea solidly in his head and convinced that 'scientific conquests are the creation of the will',[56] Cajal threw himself body and soul into the decoding of the nervous puzzle using Golgi's method. He realized, however, that he would have to improve the method to make it less capricious. First of all, he decided to use a more intense stain. While this might sometimes obscure the image, it had the advantage of permitting the visualization of finer details.[57] But the most critical decision was that of using tissues from embryos or young animals, whose structures are simpler and whose nerve fibres are largely unmyelinated (allowing the penetration of silver into the fibre). This approach had already been developed by Giuseppe Magini with his work on the fetal cerebral cortex (which Cajal knew very well). It was one thing to study a small stand of trees and something else entirely to take into consideration an inextricable forest.[58] As we have seen, Golgi had at one time adopted this approach too, but had not pursued it. One possible reason was that the very complexity of the nerve structure in the fully developed animal was more consistent with Golgi's theory of the diffuse neural net. Of course, the contrary was true for Cajal.

With the self-assurance of one who has discovered a new truth, Cajal became 'categorical, vehement in his affirmation'.[59] In February of 1889 he published in *Anatomischer Anzeiger* a French version of his study on the retina. In a paragraph dedicated to 'retinal connections', he denied the existence of anastomoses and proposed that 'nervous activity ... is transmitted by contiguity [between nerve cells] or by a kind of induction'.[60] In a review paper, published on the following 2 October, he wrote that Golgi, despite having demonstrated the individuality of nerve cells, had resorted to the idea of anastomoses probably because he was 'still influenced by the doctrine [of the reticulum]'.[61] In the same paper he proposed that nervous impulses were transmitted through a specialized cell apparatus (which Sherrington would call the synapse in 1897), and suggested as an example that the nerve impulse was transmitted from the stellate cell to the Purkinje cell through the baskets. In this paper, he hinted at the idea of the directionality of the nerve impulse, which would be fully developed a little later by Cajal and van Gehuchten into the 'law of dynamic polarization'.

It is already evident in these first studies that Cajal had a tendency to take clear-cut and argumentative positions. Of course, the accusation of being 'influenced' by reticularism (an accusation that Cajal would repeat in the following years), incensed Golgi who saw himself as a devotee of rigorous and unbiased research. Reading Cajal's memoirs (*Recuerdos de mi vida*), one can understand how, at the end of the 1880s, he conceived the reticular hypothesis as a 'formidable enemy',[62] which must be engaged in an all-out battle to impose the '*new truth,* laboriously obtained'.[52] In a feverish crescendo of discoveries and publications (between 1888 and the beginning of 1892 he published 48 papers in Spanish and foreign journals), Cajal was by this time the major champion of the theory of the neuron. One of the factors that magnified the impact of his papers was his natural talent for graphic art, which allowed him to illustrate his findings so effectively.

Between the second half of 1888 and the first half of 1889 he sent all his publications in Spanish to the most pre-eminent neuroanatomists, including Golgi,[63] even though he was sure that 'my ideas will upset the reticularists, and particularly those of the Golgi school'.[64] However, he suffered from a twofold disadvantage. First, the fact that he was from a country completely lacking in scientific traditions exposed him to the risk of being ignored, or worse, being treated with contempt. Second, most scientists to whom he had sent his work were unable to read Spanish. In fact, most neuroanatomical publications of 1889 either did not cite his works or referred to them only in passing. The publication of French versions of his works on the cerebellum and the retina in 1889 did little to obviate this problem. Cajal was indeed devoured by a 'fever of publicity',[65] and wanted an immediate response ('all authors aspire to the approval, and if possible the applause, of their public').[64] Incapable of contenting himself with national fame, he decided to attempt 'the direct and personal conquest of the great German anatomists, knowing full well that with it would come the recognition of the international scientific world.'[66]

The appropriate occasion came on 10–12 October 1889 at the Third Meeting of the Anatomische Gesellschaft, attended not only by German, Austrian, and Hungarian anatomists, but also representatives from many other nations, such as the Scandinavians. The Congress was held in Berlin and Cajal decided to present his findings, planning also to visit some of the principal foreign scientific laboratories. On 27 August he wrote to Golgi, announcing his intention to visit Pavia on the return trip from Berlin.[67] In the same letter he informed Golgi that he was studying 'the structure of the olfactory bulb, a subject that I consider extremely important for establishing the mode of connection between the sensory fibres and the central nerve cells', and asked him for a copy of his 1875 work on the olfactory bulbs. After thanking him for reprints of papers on malaria that Golgi had sent to him, he continued:

My discoveries on the embryonic medulla which you have seen in my *Revista* are so unique that I must show my preparations before making a French translation of my work. Fortunately, my preparations are so clear, so analytical, that all doubts concerning certain facts are absurd.

Golgi certainly understood what those 'certain facts' were and one can imagine his irritation at the effrontery of the unknown Cajal.

Cajal packed all his preparations and his beloved Zeiss microscope and set off on his travels, pausing at Lyons, Geneva, and Frankfurt. It was the first time that he had left Spain, apart from the period of military service in Cuba. In the course of the trip he was able to meet Weigert, Edinger, and Paul Ehrlich, the inventor of the methylene blue staining method. At the Congress, he could not participate actively because he didn't understand German. But eventually his moment came. In the room reserved for demonstrations he set up his Zeiss and requested another two or three microscopes. He arranged his preparations of cerebellum, retina, and spinal cord, engaging the curious onlookers who approached in his broken French. Initially, the reactions were incredulity and scepticism. But when such authorities as His Sr, Waldeyer, Schwalbe, Karl Bardeleben, and particularly Retzius and Kölliker saw the beauty of Cajal's preparations, he won the day. Suddenly, he became an authority; the coveted fame was finally attained.

Golgi's method had finally triumphed at the international level, not at the hands of its author but at those of Cajal. The latter garnered the fruit of Golgi's hard work over many years.

Cajal's presentation had an immediate impact on all who were interested in the structure of the nervous system. Retzius remembered the event, during his Croonian Lecture at the Royal Society of London in 1908:

Cajal's first studies had an electrifying effect upon those who were working in the same field. For my part I shall never forget the overwhelming impression that the demonstration by Cajal, at the Berlin Anatomical Congress of 1889, of a large series of his preparations produced upon those of us who were specially interested in the subject. Albert von Kölliker and I were enchanted by the sight of the preparations which Cajal placed before us. Both he and I were converted and we started home to begin working afresh with Golgi's method, which was not in great repute among other anatomists of that day. Kölliker, as well as von Lenhossék, working then in Kölliker's laboratory as his prosector, succeeded in applying Golgi's method, and published several excellent new researches. At the same time I, in Stockholm, and Van Gehuchten, in Louvain, were applying the same method, while Cajal himself went on with one investigation after another, and Golgi and a couple of his pupils continued pursuing their various researches.[68]

Actually, as we have seen, Kölliker was already familiar with Golgi's method and was well aware of its revolutionary potential. Even if Cajal's preparations were more demonstrative than Golgi's, it cannot account for Kölliker's interest in a method that he already knew. It must have been the power of Cajal's ideas, even if expressed in broken French, that had conquered Kölliker. Certainly it must have been extraordinary to hear about streams of electrical current flowing from one nerve cell to the next in a preferential direction, after so many decades of theories positing that nervous energy was dispersed throughout an inscrutable reticulum. If Cajal was right, there now existed the possibility of reducing the nervous structure into many circuits similar to those of the nascent electrical technology.

After the Congress, inebriated with success, Cajal visited Krause in Göttingen, and then he went to Lucerne and Turin, where he meet Bizzozero and Mosso. It is not known what he and Bizzozero talked about but certainly whatever he said would have been quickly related to Golgi. It is, however, reasonable to hypothesize that in the euphoria of the moment he had delved into his discoveries and his neuronistic ideas. He probably reported the interest that his preparations had elicited in Kölliker and the other neuroanatomists and perhaps he talked about Golgi's diffuse neural net, one can imagine in what terms. Then he arrived in Pavia, ready to pay his respects to the man who had provided the basis for his success. But the discoverer of the black reaction was not there and unfortunately no record exists of Cajal's visit to Pavia. It is not known how he was welcomed in the laboratory, or by whom. In the end, Cajal regretted not having been able to meet Golgi, to show him his preparations and to express his admiration, because this might have avoided the later controversies. In his *Recuerdos* Cajal wrote that Golgi was in Rome busy fulfilling his duties as Senator. But this is not possible because Golgi was made a Senator for life more than ten years later. Perhaps Golgi avoided Cajal intentionally; he must have been irritated by Cajal's bold statement that he had never seen an anastomosis and by the accusation that Golgi was the unwitting victim of a reticularist prejudice.

After Pavia, Cajal made a short visit to the University of Genoa, where he was cordially welcomed at the Institute of Anatomy, and finally, passing through Marseilles, he returned to Barcelona.

Golgi's impatience with the new anti-reticularist attacks in the second half of 1889 is demonstrated also by the change in his relationship with Kölliker. Although always very tactful, Kölliker had never hidden from Golgi his disagreement with the theory of the diffuse neural net, and, though with much circumspection, tended to take sides with Forel, His Sr and, after the Berlin Congress, Cajal. After the stay in Golgi's house, where he was hosted in a 'more than amicable'[69] manner, Kölliker sent to Golgi the first volume of the sixth edition of his handbook of histology, fresh from the printer. On the next 7 July he received from Golgi a letter of thanks, then nothing for several months, not even in response to Kölliker's wishes for a Happy New Year. Perhaps Bizzozero had told Golgi of his meeting with Cajal, and his irritation been increased by the fact that Cajal's theory had been so welcomed by Kölliker and the other neuroanatomists in Berlin. In any case, in the second half of 1889 Golgi interrupted, without explanation, his correspondence with Kölliker. The research from his laboratory gave the impression of hostility towards the Swiss histologist,[70] and on 13 March 1890 Kölliker wrote a letter to Golgi[71] in an attempt to smooth over the disagreements and re-establish a climate of friendship. Concerned by Golgi's silence he appealed to Bizzozero for help. On 23 March he wrote a letter to the pathologist in Turin,[72] stating that he was preoccupied that Golgi had 'taken offence at the fact that I cannot accept all his conclusions'.[69] And he concluded writing:

If I have wounded Golgi in whatever manner, I have done it quite involuntarily and I am ready to say it to anyone who wants to listen to it, and at the same time I am at pains to do everything possible to overcome the bad opinion that Golgi might have of me.[69]

It is worth noting that Kölliker, a world authority, was much older than Golgi, and had always behaved correctly with him. The letter indicates how good-natured he was (a fact also attested to by others such as Cajal), how ready he was to understand and to make amends where possible in order not to lose the friendship and esteem of his Pavian colleague, whom he considered to be one of the most important biologists of the world. In addition, Kölliker deeply loved Italy and the Italians. The friendship with Golgi was only the last in a series of personal ties with Italian scientists. He had been a great friend of Filippo De Filippi, who died in Hong Kong from an hepatic abscess, and to whose memory he had dedicated the fifth edition of his *Handbuch der Gewebelehre*. One of his most brilliant pupils had been Alfonso Corti, with whom he had studied the retina and the optic nerve. Kölliker used to spend his spring vacation on the Italian Riviera. Thus, for many personal motives, affective and scientific, he wanted to remain Golgi's friend.

Bizzozero immediately intervened on Kölliker's behalf, and wrote Golgi:

> You are a great lazy one. Read this letter from Kölliker . . . I wrote to him immediately that it was impossible that you could have the feelings towards him that your obstinate silence has made him suppose, but I added also that you would be writing him yourself. And this is what I hope you will do, so that excellent man is spared the nightmare of your anger.
>
> Sometimes I reprove myself for my laziness in writing; but I see that I am a pigmy compared to you![73]

But certainly it was not only a matter of laziness. Eventually, both Golgi and his wife wrote cordially to Kölliker and on the following 12 April Kölliker responded to both of them declaring himself happy that their friendship was intact.[74]

In the aftermath of the Berlin Congress many European laboratories began to adopt Golgi's method. But the theoretical framework within which the findings were interpreted was that provided by Cajal. As Cajal's observations were endorsed by the likes of Retzius, van Gehuchten, Kölliker and Lenhossék, so also was his theory. Golgi's joy at receiving, with much delay, the appropriate recognition of his achievement was poisoned by the fact that at the same time this obscure professor from a university placed at the periphery of the scientific world was displacing him from the spotlight.

The moment had come to mount a defence of reticularism.

Notes

1. Bellonci (1880).
2. Bernardini (1888), Magini (1888, 1888a). See also Bentivoglio *et al.* (1997); Bentivoglio and Mazzarello (1999), and *Rivista Sperimentale di Freniatria e di Medicine Legale* (1887, **13**, pp. 129 and 207–8).
3. Lombroso (1887, p. 6).
4. Schwalbe (1881, pp. 743ff.).
5. Edinger (1889, p. 4).
6. Obersteiner (1883, pp. 467ff.).
7. Letter from Kühne to Golgi, 15 April and 18 May 1884 (MSUP-VII-II-K).
8. Papez (1953a, p. 47).
9. Ranvier (1875–86, p. 1062).
10. *Ibid.* (p. 1099).
11. Retzius (1908, p. 417).
12. Letter from Biedermann to Golgi, 6 March 1886 (MSUP-VII-II-B).
13. Letter from Podwyssozki to Golgi, 29 March 1887 (MSUP-VII-II-P).

14. The Kölliker–Golgi correspondence is kept at the MSUP and has been published by Belloni (1975). It includes 53 letters (No. 7 and No. 31 are postcards) from Kölliker to Golgi, 4 letters from Kölliker to Golgi's relatives, and the hand-written drafts of 4 letters from Golgi to Kölliker. In the present book the letters are cited as 'No. X' following the progressive numbering established by Belloni.

15. Letter No. 1 (Belloni 1975, p. 157). The envelope has the word 'Koelliker!' in Golgi's hand-writing, indicating the satisfaction of having awakened the interest of such a great world authority of histology. In 1899 Kölliker affirmed that he had gone to Pavia in 1887 to meet Golgi and to observe the application of his method (Kölliker 1899, pp. 169 and 233); whereas in a speech given on 20 April 1900 in Pavia he referred instead to having gone in 1888 (Kölliker 1900, p. 5). From the letters it is clear that their first contacts were of an epistolary nature and that Kölliker became aware of the importance of the black reaction after having seen the preparations that Golgi had sent to him. The Kölliker–Golgi correspondence indicates that the first visit took place in April 1889. See also Belloni (1975, pp. 145 and 159).

16. Kölliker (1887).

17. Kölliker (1887a).

18. Letter No. 2 (Belloni 1975, pp. 157ff.).

19. See letter No. 3 sent by Kölliker to Golgi from Nervi on 14 April 1889 (Belloni 1975, p. 159) and letter No. 3 *bis* that he sent on 23 March 1890 to Bizzozero (Belloni 1975, p. 160).

20. Kölliker (1899, pp. 169 and 233).

21. Letter from Retzius to Golgi, 10 January 1888 (MSUP-VII-III-15).

22. Kronthal (1887).

23. Greppin (1889).

24. Greppin (1888).

25. MSUP-VII-II-R.

26. Toldt (1888, pp. 172ff.).

27. Obersteiner (1888, pp. 124ff.).

28. Edinger (1889).

29. Sehrwald (1889).

30. Rossbach and Sehrwald (1888).

31. It is now known that Golgi's method tends to overestimate the size of the body and the nerve processes because of the silver precipitate on the surface of the cell.

32. Cajal (1888).

33. Jacobson (1993, p. 58).

34. Kronthal published a critical review of Greppin's work in which he aligned himself with Rossbach and Sehrwald and contested the reservation that Greppin had expressed toward his own work, *Neurologisches Centralblatt* (1888, No. 21, p. 602).

35. Belmondo (1888, p. 356). The thesis of Rossbach and Sehrwald was contested also by Falza-cappa (1889), Cajal (1890), and Monti (1890).

36. Edinger (1887, p. 149).

37. His (1886).

38. See Shepherd (1991, p. 115). The source is Forel (1937). Interesting information can also be found in Forel's correspondence (1968).

39. Forel (1887).

40. Obersteiner (1888, pp. 124ff.).

41. Nansen (1887).

42. Nansen (1887a, p. 5).

43. Golgi (1885, p. 105).
44. Aarli (1989, p. 75); Shepherd (1991, pp. 122ff.).
45. Huxley (1977). See also Shepherd (1991. p. 134).
46. Shepherd (1991, p. 200).
47. Cajal (1917, p. 52).
48. De Castro (1952, p. 36).
49. Cajal (1917, p. 56).
50. Sherrington (1935, p. 430).
51. Cajal (1917, p. 63).
52. *Ibid.* (p. 67).
53. Cajal (1888).
54. Cajal (1888a).
55. Cajal (1917, p. 75).
56. *Ibid.* (p. 70).
57. Shepherd (1991, p. 139).
58. Cajal (1917 p. 69).
59. Riquier (1952, p. 68).
60. Cajal (1889a, p. 120).
61. Cajal (1889, p. 341).
62. Cajal (1917, p. 76).
63. At the MSUP is a postcard dated 22 May (1889) that Cajal sent from Barcelona, accompany-
    ing or after sending his *Revista trimestral de Histología*, and some reprints of his work contain-
    ing some 'discoveries that your admirable method has permitted us to achieve (MSUP-VII-
    III-14). Other copies of the issue were sent to Fusari, Angelo Petrone and Giuseppe Magini.
    See also Pensa (1991, p. 262) and Belloni (1975, p. 147).
64. Cajal (1917, p. 89).
65. *Ibid.* (p. 70).
66. Belloni (1975, p. 147).
67. The letter arrived in Pavia on 29 August as indicated by the postmark but was not received by
    Golgi, who was in Varese. It was then forwarded to this city, through Milan on 30 August,
    and was received by Golgi on the same day (MSUP-VII-III-14).
68. Retzius (1908, pp. 420ff.).
69. Letter No. 3 *bis* (Belloni 1975, p. 160).
70. Martinotti (1890).
71. The reference to this letter, which is not found in the collection of letters kept at the MSUP, is
    in letter No. 3 *bis* (Belloni 1975, p. 160).
72. Letter No. 3 *bis* (Belloni 1975, pp. 159–60). Bizzozero is the only plausible recipient of this
    letter.
73. Letter from Bizzozero to Golgi dated 25 March 1890 (MSUP-VII-III-1).
74. Letter No 4 and 4 *bis* (Belloni 1975, pp. 161ff.).

14

Seemingly a matter of priority

At the beginning of 1890 Golgi certainly had became aware of the triumphal success of his black reaction at the Congress of Berlin. At the same time, however, he must also have realized the threat that Cajal now represented for his theory of the diffuse neural net. All the more so because Cajal's heresy found favourable conditions in a scientific ground already prepared by the work of His Sr and Forel, and by the perplexities of Kölliker.

Golgi conceived of histology as a 'science of organization'. For him, however, the rigorous description of living forms was not an end in itself, but a necessary precondition of a physiological interpretation of life phenomena, following the motto 'the structure unveils the function'. Thus, he could not content himself with the resounding international recognition of his discovery of 'facts' (which, on the other hand, he worshipped in the most classical Pavian tradition). He wanted to be acknowledged as the one who had pointed the way to a new 'global physiology' of the nervous system. The 'facts' he had discovered went hand in hand with his 'theoretical' interpretation of them. It is not surprising that he was greatly irritated by work, such as that of Rossbach and Sehrwald, that exploited his method to challenge his theory. Even in Italy he had been criticized. For example, in 1889 Ernesto Falzacappa, of the Laboratory of Comparative Anatomy of the University of Rome, reported to the Accademia dei Lincei the findings he had obtained on the spinal cord using Golgi's method. On the basis of his findings Falzacappa rejected Golgi's classification of nerve processes as 'long' and 'short', depending on whether the cells were motor or sensitive.[1] Furthermore, Falzacappa completely ignored Golgi's study on the spinal cord[2] and vaguely embraced Gerlach's theory.

The appearance of Cajal on the international scene, however, accelerated events so dramatically that Golgi was left utterly bewildered. His recent research activity had focused almost exclusively on malaria, a task that was not yet completed. He was also busy with his research on rabies. On 15 March 1890 he communicated to the Società Medico-Chirurgica the results of studies carried out on animals experimentally infected with rabies. In the nerve cells (especially Purkinje cells) of these animals, he found alterations that he 'designated with the terms *rarefication*, *vacuolization*, and *vesicular transformation*', which he considered 'as progressively more severe phases of the same process'. 'Rarefication' was also accompanied by cell swelling that caused the cytoplasm to be 'here and there more

In fact, in the first works on the central nervous system carried out with the same methods and with the same approach as in my own work, which came to be published subsequently by numerous scholars, there was no mention of my results, which were, in fact, not even cited; and these same works, which in addition contained *only a fraction of the findings that I published a long time ago,* were presented as if entirely new!

Even if this neglect might be attributed in part to the limited diffusion of the Italian language, and to the unsatisfactory conditions of scientific publishing in our country (putting aside for the moment the diffidence that until recently met my results, so novel were they compared to those that were until now considered classics), still I cannot believe that such a neglect is completely justifiable, nor that I should continue to bear it, primarily because the most authoritative foreign journals, including the German ones, had mentioned and summarized my published studies at the time.[17]

The paper mentioned the studies on the cells of Type I and Type II, motor and sensory, respectively, and their different distributions in the anterior and posterior horns of the spinal cord, and then reminded the readers that he had demonstrated 'that the nervous fibres forming the different (anterior, lateral, and posterior) tracts of white matter, in their course along these tracts, continuously emit fibrils, which penetrate the grey substance and take part in the formation of the diffuse neural net.'[18] And he emphasized that he had thoroughly described these findings, had remarked on their importance, and had also unambiguously reviewed them in his article on cerebral localization,[19] of which he had published a version in French in the *Archives Italiennes di Biologie.*[20] And now the same findings were not only described as new but also interpreted from a functional (physiological) point of view.

While the dispute with Cajal was in the making, Golgi participated in the International Congress in Berlin. As many as 144 Italians gathered in the German city, including the most important names from all Italian universities: Baccelli, Bottini, Foà, Mosso, Maragliano, Cantani, Celli, Bozzolo. Before the scientific proceedings began, Virchow, President of the Congress, turned the podium over to Baccelli, whose polished Latin had earned him the appellation, 'Cicero of Medicine' (a title previously reserved for Celsus, one of the creators of medical Latin). The official languages were German, French and English, but Baccelli maintained that in learned Germany all would be able to understand it and gave his speech in Latin to an appreciative audience. After this address, at the suggestion of Virchow, the Italian was made Honorary President of the Congress. Baccelli, taking the podium again, suggested Rome as the site of the next international congress planned for 1894, and this proposal was accepted unanimously.

Many of the Italians attending the meeting in Berlin had had substantial experience outside the country, spoke German or French well, and were able to move comfortably in the cosmopolitan environment of the meeting, crowded as it was by several hundred doctors and biologists from around the world. For Golgi, on the contrary, it was the first time he had actively participated in an international congress. By this time, however, he was a celebrity and the studies that had made him famous were at the centre of two fundamental areas of scientific research. The most celebrated scientists were now approaching him as a colleague of equal rank. He was included in the scientific secretariat of the

Congress in the Anatomy Section. Many participants (among them His Sr and von Len-hossék), cited him in their presentations, but more often than not his name was associated with that of Cajal, who, in little more than two years of work, thanks in part to his direct and aggressive style, had also acquired a position of pre-eminence. And, naturally, Golgi was nonplussed at the thought of his many years of obscure work and the slow recognition of his merits compared to the immediate fame garnered by the Spanish histologist, who had essentially done no more than apply his method (or so Golgi thought).

The Italian histologist and his wife spent a great deal of time in the company of Kölliker, who introduced them to other important anatomists. It is likely, however, that Golgi's excessively reserved character did not help him in establishing international connections. Golgi's personality was the opposite of Cajal's: the latter was warm and extroverted, the former shy and reserved. Golgi was 'almost insufferably' embarrassed when His Sr 'during the official banquet unexpectedly raised his glass to extol Golgi's studies on the nervous system'.[21] As soon as he was back in Italy, and restored 'to the quiet of this autumnal sojourn' (he was probably vacationing in Varese), Golgi wrote Kölliker to express his gratitude:

To my great surprise, in Berlin I was surrounded by manifestations of esteem and respect; I am all too aware, however, that such honours were substantially due to you; I feel that in a certain way I took advantage of the glorious aura surrounding your name.[22]

As we know, at the meeting Golgi presented a series of photomicrographs illustrating the various stages of the life cycle of the protozoan *Plasmodium malariae*. Baccelli's and Celli's presentations were also concerned with malaria. The attention of the participants was, however, dominated by Koch's communication of a new treatment against tuberculosis. In truth, the German bacteriologist had presented his finding without great fanfare, and, on the grounds that his experiments were still in progress, had provided no technical information about the weapon he had devised to fight the terrible scourge. But an announcement of such importance, made in the presence of hundreds of scientists, was bound to spread rapidly around the world. Golgi was so impressed by Koch's experiments that he attempted to replicate them a few months later in Pavia.

By the time the meeting was over, there were hardly any neuroanatomists who had not read Golgi's article in the *Anatomischer Anzeiger*. It is not difficult to imagine how irritating the 'not very amicable' tone of that paper must have been for Cajal. His answer was ready by 20 August and was delivered in an article sent to the same journal.[23] After conceding to the Italian the priority in the discovery of the collateral fibres, he remarked how strange it was that such an important observation had been published in a journal unfamiliar to most anatomists, and, in addition, in an 'obscure' paragraph barely five lines long that had never been cited by those who had worked on the spinal cord in those years. Golgi himself, Cajal noted, had underplayed the relevance of his own findings to the point of making only indirect mention of them in his treatise on neuroanatomy. This was not completely true, because, although Golgi had not explicitly mentioned the discovery in his book, he had written about it in the *Archivio Italiano per le Malattie Nervose* and in the *Rivista Sperimentale di Freniatria*,[24] and had further discussed it in an article about cerebral localization published both in the *Gazzetta degli Ospitali* and, most importantly, in the *Archives Italiennes de Biologie*. Cajal complained also that Golgi, upon receiving his article in Spanish, had reciprocated by sending a collection of papers that did not include the study at the centre of the controversy, and that no issue of priority had been raised by the Italian scientist at the time. Finally, Cajal accused Golgi of having failed to fully describe the experimental conditions necessary to observe the collateral fibres, and claimed that these could be successfully stained only with 'my [that is, Cajal's] modification of the rapid [Golgi] method' (immersion in osmium–dichromate solution for 12–36 hours followed by immersion in potassium dichromate). Having defended his good faith, Cajal continued his review of the most important findings on the neuroanatomy of the spinal cord illustrated in his, but not in Golgi's, study, and then wrote:

I admire the work of Golgi and profess the greatest respect and utmost consideration for his scientific persona. We are indebted to him and to his seminal and path-breaking experiments for the precious method that allows us to discern the innermost structure of the nervous system with the clarity of a diagram; his great merits and the well-deserved renown that surround the persona of the pioneer, however, do not excuse him from acknowledging the modest merits of those who, while confirming the merits of the master, are honoured to call themselves his disciples and followers.[25]

Immediately after these flattering words, however, Cajal began a severe analysis of the 'theoretical speculations' of the master. 'Golgi's work presents two aspects: the facts and the hypotheses. Most facts are proven', but 'as far as the hypotheses are concerned it is a completely different affair.' Then, with great ability he proceeded to develop a tight and compelling critique of the three main neurohistological hypotheses proposed by Golgi:

(1) the existence of a diffuse neural net;

(2) the presence of two types of nerve cells corresponding to sensory and motor neurons;

(3) the exclusively nutritive function of the protoplasmic processes (dendrites).

Concerning the first point, Cajal noticed that, despite having examined about 20 000 sections (6000 of which were successfully stained) in four years, he had been unable to identify with confidence a single anastomosis. He then wrote that, despite Golgi's efforts, there was no certain criterion for the distinction between motor or sensory nerve cells (both could be found in sensory and motor areas), and finally, recalling also the perplexity already expressed by Kölliker, he expounded many reasons why the protoplasmic processes should be considered as playing a role in nervous transmission.

The quarrel between Golgi and Cajal on the specific issue of the collateral fibres in the medullary tracts came to an end a few months later with the publication of a paper in which Golgi gave a systematic exposition of the functional meaning of the diffuse neural net.[26] In a footnote, Golgi replied point by point to Cajal's criticisms. To the accusation of having buried his discovery of the collateral fibres in a journal unknown to most anatomists, he replied by quoting in full the passage on the collaterals from the paper on cerebral localization published in French in the *Archives Italiennes de Biologie*, the Italian scientific journal with the largest international readership. Concerning the impregnation method used by Cajal to visualize the collaterals, Golgi objected that except for insignificant modifications it was substantially identical to the one he had described in *Sulla fina anatomia degli organi centrali del sistema nervoso*, and furthermore he found it 'peculiar' that the Spaniard could have referred to it as 'my modification of the rapid method'. Golgi then remarked that the collateral fibres could be visualized on 'a large scale and with even greater resolution and abundance of detail, using other methods', such as, for example, impregnation with mercury dichloride. As for the accusation of brevity, Golgi argued that he was unable 'to add other words ... since I deemed unbecoming to a serious student of anatomy the practice of diluting the facts with prolix descriptions.'[27] Having disposed of Cajal's criticisms, Golgi added:

Having made these rectifications, I would like to declare, for the sake of exactitude and in all fairness, that the phrase contained in my article in *Anatomischer Anzeiger*, the phrase that gave Prof. Ramón y Cajal reason to write a note addressed to me, insofar as it concerned this same colleague Ramón y Cajal, was not deservedly applied. I hold this young scientist in the greatest consideration and I not only admire his productivity and creativity but also appreciate the importance of his original findings. The few differences between his conclusions and mine do not have, nor could they have, any consequence for my feelings, being, on the contrary, deeply convinced that such divergences, by spurring research, are always beneficial to science.[28]

Re-examining the facts at a distance of a century, we can safely say that the existence of axon collaterals in the medullary tracts had been concisely but unambiguously described in Golgi's papers and that the discovery had also been reported in an international journal, the *Archives Italiennes de Biologie*. It is clear, however, that for Golgi the apparent bone of contention was only a pretext to attack Cajal. Indeed, the squabble exploded only when the Spanish anatomist began to emerge as a protagonist in the faction opposed to Golgi's reticular theory. The rudeness of Golgi's reaction reflected the state of mind of one who feels unfairly relegated to a second-rank position and who demands that the primacy of his studies be acknowledged. Cajal, on the other hand, was certainly acting in good faith. He was familiar with the neuroanatomical treatise by Golgi and with some of the papers that the latter had sent to him (but probably not with the study on cerebral localization in which Golgi had discussed the existence of collateral fibres) and was right in lamenting that Golgi had not raised the issue of priority at the time. As Guido Cimino wrote, 'The fact is that, if the pen of Golgi were guided by the anger of one who feels unfairly overlooked and superseded, the pen of Cajal was guided by the youthful boldness of one who finds approval and applause around him.'[29]

At this point, the gulf between Golgi and Cajal became unbridgeable, with the two scientists looking at each other from opposite shores. As happened with Galvani and Volta, the scientific debate evolved into personal animosity.[30]

In the following years Golgi would continue to defend his reticular theory and every now and again (often through his disciples) he would attack the rival theory. Meanwhile, Cajal would further develop and refine the neuron theory, soon to be known as the 'neuron doctrine', of which he would become the undisputed *maîtres à penser*. These are all the ingredients for the final drama, which would be consummated more than a decade later during the award ceremony for the Nobel Prize.

But this was still the early 1890s. Like a machine, Cajal continued to grind out paper after paper, finding more and more proselytes along the way. Even the great Retzius in Stockholm now asserted the independence of neurons and the existence of free axon terminals in the crustacean ganglia.[31] Kölliker himself, in a review on the spinal cord (in which he mentioned Golgi's contribution), did not hide his sympathy for the anti-reticularist field and for the notion that the dendrites participated in the transmission of the nerve impulses.[32] Finally, on 11 October 1890, Cajal published a paper titled 'Origin and termination of the olfactory nerve fibres', in which, after confirming all Golgi's findings, he completely rejected Golgi's interpretations. Specifically, he maintained that the olfactory fibres transmitted the nerve impulse directly to the dendrites of mitral cells at the level of the glomeruli. Following his custom, Cajal send copies of the paper to the experts in the field, including Kölliker. At the end of December the latter wrote to Golgi, asking for a reprint of his 1882 paper on the olfactory bulbs and for an opinion on Cajal's hypothesis.[33] Although we do not know the contents of Golgi's reply, we know that he immediately sent Kölliker reprints of his papers on the olfactory tract (1882), the olfactory bulbs (1875), and the horse retina (1872). At any rate, it is somewhat shocking to realize that while Cajal was flooding the desks of all important neuroanatomists with reprints of all his papers, Golgi, who had been corresponding with Kölliker for the last three years, had not yet send him copies of such important papers. In his reply, Kölliker thanked Golgi and noted that 'you should stop publishing your works in journals that are little circulated and known'.[34]

All the scientists working on the nervous system were now using the black reaction and methodological papers suggesting modifications and special applications were being published.[35] Golgi's satisfaction was, however, poisoned by the emerging rejection of his reticular theory. It was time for a comprehensive theoretical work that would formulate, in an organized way, the ideas that had been scattered here and there in a number of little-known papers.

Notes

1. Falzacappa (1889).
2. Golgi (1880–81a).
3. Golgi (1890e, p. 42). Session of 15 March 1890.
4. Cajal (1890).
5. Golgi (1880–81a; *OO*, p. 238).
6. See Cajal (1890a, p. 580).
7. Cajal (1890 p. 88).
8. Letter No. 4 from Kölliker to Golgi, 12 April 1890 (Belloni 1975, p. 161).
9. Letter from Bizzozero to Golgi, 20 May 1890 (MSUP-VII-III-1).
10. Kölliker (1890).
11. Letter No. 5 from Kölliker to Golgi, 26 May 1890 (Belloni 1975, pp. 163ff.).
12. Letter No. 6 from Kölliker to Golgi , 27 May, 1890 (Belloni 1975, p. 165).
13. Session of 17 May 1890. The communication (*Sulla fina anatomia del midollo spinale*) is cited but not published in the Bulletin (*Bollettino della Società Medico-Chirurgica di Pavia*, 1890, Anno V, p. 59).

14. Golgi (1890f).
15. Letter No. 7 from Kölliker to Golgi, 24 June 1890 (Belloni 1975, p. 166). In the letter, Kölliker informed Golgi that he had reserved, from 2 August, a room with two beds at the Central-hotel of Berlin for his Italian colleague and his wife.
16. Golgi (1890g).
17. Golgi (1890f; *OO*, p. 556).
18. *Ibid.* (*OO*, p. 558).
19. Golgi (1882b, p. 546).
20. Golgi (1882c).
21. Perroncito (1926, p. 43).
22. Rough draft of a letter from Golgi to Kölliker. Undated, but probably written soon after the Berlin Congress. (Belloni 1975, p. 167).
23. Cajal (1890a).
24. Golgi (1880–81a).
25. Cajal (1890a, p. 583).
26. Golgi (1891e).
27. *Ibid.* (*OO*, p. 597).
28. *Ibid.* (*OO*, p. 598).
29. Cimino (1984, p. 359).
30. Notwithstanding their argument, Cajal continued to send his works to Golgi. A copy of Cajal's study 'On the structure of the cerebral cortex of some mammals' (*La Cellule*, 1891, **7**, pp. 125–76) dedicated 'To the anatomical savant C. Golgi, as a demonstration of consideration and esteem by the author' is kept in the Institute of General Pathology of Pavia (see Piccolino *et al.* 1988, p. 20). The publications of Cajal between 1890 and 1912 are kept in the 'Collezione Golgi' of the Institute of General Pathology of Pavia (Nos. 229-1 to 229-6, 10-3, 10-4, 10-6, 10-7, 10-8, and 10-10 to 10-14).
31. Retzius (1890). The Swedish histologist sent the work to Golgi with the dedication, 'Al Illustrissimo Professore Cam. Golgió—Ommagio [sic] del Autore' ['To the most illustrious Professor Cam. Golgió—With the respects of the author']. The reprint (with the successive series) is kept in the Institute of General Pathology of the University of Pavia.
32. Kölliker (1890a).
33. Letter No. 8 from Kölliker to Golgi, 22 December 1890 (Belloni 1975, p. 168).
34. Letter No. 9 from Kölliker to Golgi, 2 January 1891 (Belloni 1975, p. 169).
35. Obregia (1890).

15

Protoplasmic pantheism

At the beginning of the 1890s, support for Golgi's diffuse neural net was confined to the circle of his direct or indirect pupils. Gerlach's version of the reticular theory continued to be much more popular in Italy and elsewhere. There were also other reticular theories, sometimes touching on the bizarre. The Lithuanian, Alexander Stanislavovich Dogiel, for example, wishing to mix oil and water, maintained that in the retina there existed a double intercellular reticulum; one was inter-cylindraxial (similar to that of Golgi); the other inter-dendritical (similar to that of Gerlach). And then there was even a suggestion that there might be three reticula, with the third consisting of a connection between dendrites and axons.[1] The most important scientists, however, were embracing the theory of the neuron with more and more conviction.

For Golgi, the support of reticularism was not an end in itself, nor was it a matter of siding with one group or the other, although Cajal's arrival on the scene might have been instrumental in pushing him to rigidify his position. Golgi was convinced that the diffuse neural net was the model that best accounted for the wealth of new findings on the physiology of the nervous system published in the 1860s and 1870s, and the only one to offer the beginning of a solution for important neurophysiological problems.

As we have seen, the concept of the diffuse neural net had arisen early in Golgi's scientific development, immediately after the discovery of the black reaction. At that time his thinking was heavily influenced by the reticularist *Zeitgeist*, which to some extent pervaded all contemporary theories on the organization of the brain. Golgi was probably so astonished by the discovery of axonal ramifications and by the absence of dendritic anastomoses that he automatically thought of a reticulum formed by the union of various collateral branches of the cylindraxes. And the illusory superimposition of these ramifications would certainly have reinforced this idea. It is evident, however, that even before seeing the images created by the black reaction, Golgi, in common with the others who were studying the structure of the nervous system at the time, was conditioned by a conceptual framework requiring direct communication between nerve cells. This initial choice affected all his subsequent research on the central nervous system, becoming a *heuristic model* with which he explained and interpreted all the observed data.

Golgi admired Flourens and his holistic conception of cortical activity, but he disagreed with the French scientist's 'metaphysical' ideas, such as the notion that psychic phenomena might be the expression of a unitary 'soul' (a *res cogitans*) ontologically distinct from matter,

The Plates

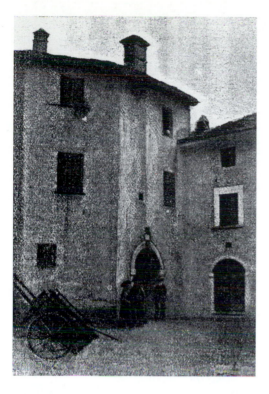

Plate 1   Top left: La casa di Corteno, birthplace of Camillo Golgi; top right: the announcement for the position of Chief Physician at the *Pie Case degli Incurabili* of Abbiategrasso. Courtesy of the Institute Camillo Golgi of Abbiategrasso. Bottom: Golgi's degree diploma in Medicine and Surgery. Courtesy of the Museum for the History of the University of Pavia.

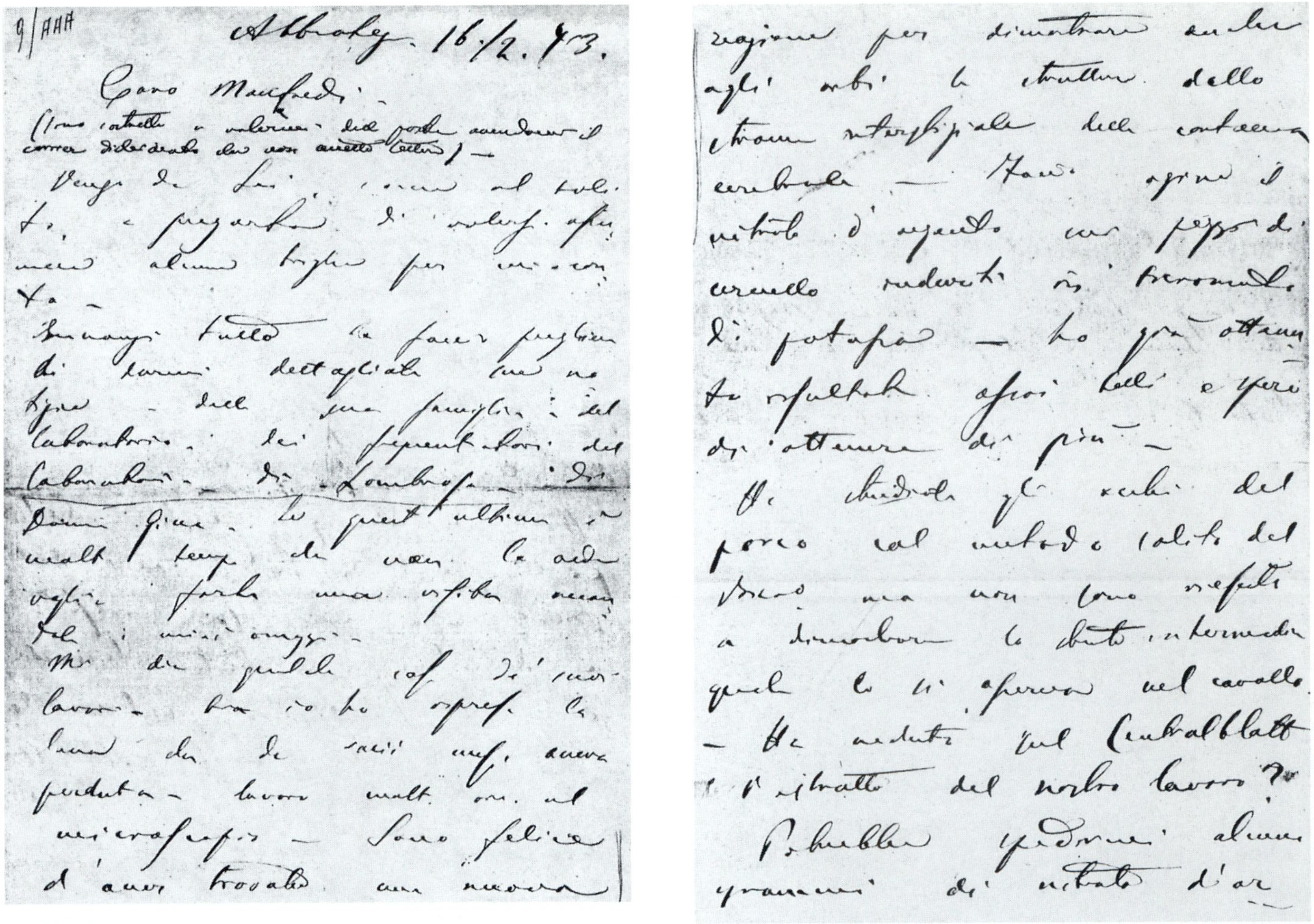

Plate 2 Letter from Golgi to Manfredi, 16 February 1873, with the first announcement of the black reaction. Courtesy of Museum for the History of the University of Pavia.

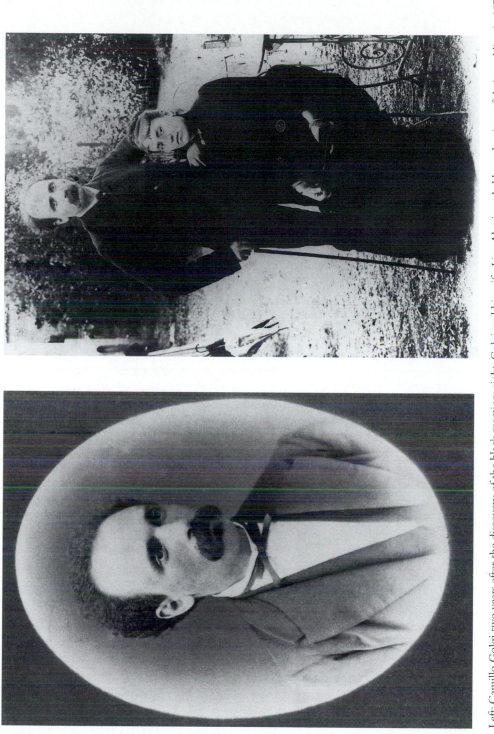

Plate 3 Left: Camillo Golgi two years after the discovery of the black reaction; right: Golgi and his wife, Lina Aletti, probably at the time of their wedding in 1877. Courtesy of the Institute of General Pathology of the University of Pavia.

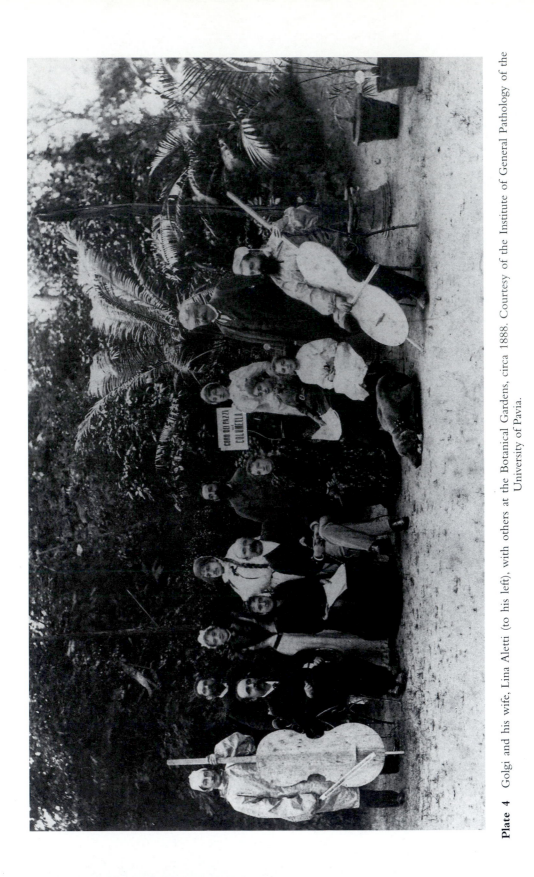

Plate 4 Golgi and his wife, Lina Aletti (to his left), with others at the Botanical Gardens, circa 1888. Courtesy of the Institute of General Pathology of the University of Pavia.

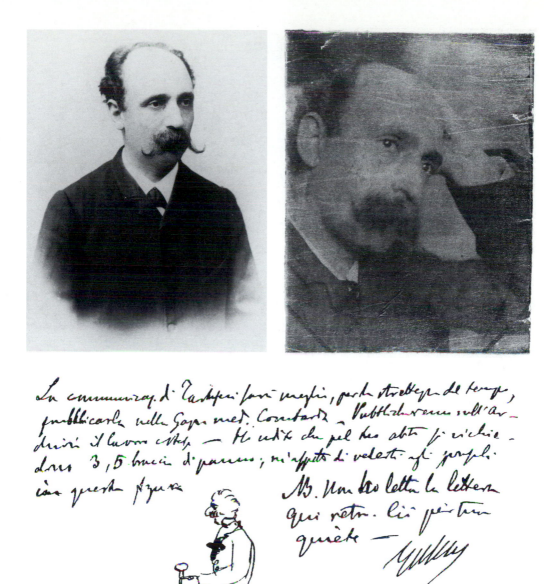

5. Golgi visto da Bizzozero attorno al 1888

Plate 5   Top left: Golgi at the time of his studies on malaria; top right: a contemplative Golgi. Courtesy of the Institute of General Pathology of the University of Pavia. Bottom: Golgi seen by Bizzozero, circa 1888. Courtesy of the Museum for the History of the University of Pavia.

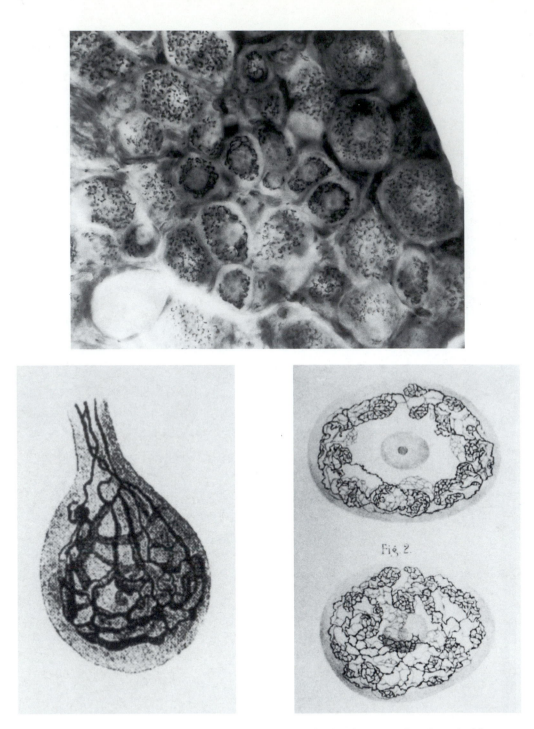

Plate 6 Top: microphotograph of an original preparation of a dorsal root ganglion from the laboratory of Camillo Golgi. The impregnation of the structure defined by Golgi as internal reticular apparatus, and now known as Golgi apparatus, is clearly evident, stained in black. Note the detachment from the cell membrane and the perinuclear location, which Golgi emphasized in his reports. Bottom left: Golgi's first drawing of the internal reticular apparatus in the body of a Purkinje cell of the cerebellum in 1898; bottom right: drawings by Camillo Golgi of a partial or total impregnation of the internal reticular apparatus in spinal ganglion cells. Reproduced from Golgi (1898; 1899).

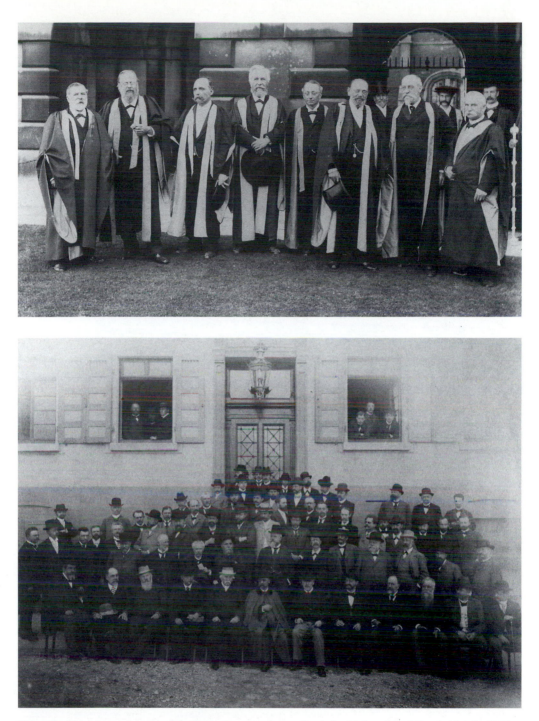

Plate 7 Top: the recipients of the honoris causa degree from the University of Cambridge in 1898, a few months after the discovery of the Golgi apparatus. From the left: Etienne-Jules Marey, Anton Dohrn, Camillo Golgi, Ernst Haeckel, Ambrosius Arnold Willem Hubrecht, Wilhelm Kühne, Henry Bowditch, and Hugh K. Kroneker. Courtesy of the Institute of General Pathology of the University of Pavia, bottom: Tübingen 1899, meeting of the Anatomische Gesellschaft when it was officially decided that it would be held in Pavia the congress of the following year. Courtesy of the Institute of General Pathology of the University of Pavia.

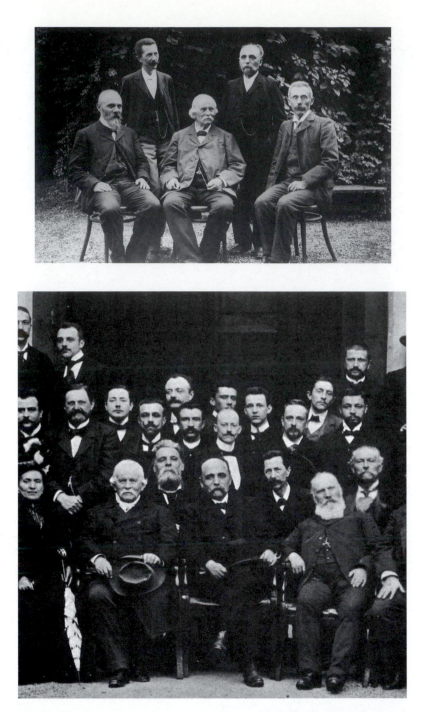

Plate 8   Top: from the right, first row: Romeo Fusari, Albert Kölliker, and Edoardo Perroncito; second row: Camillo Gogli and Glulio Bizzozero, 1900. Courtesy of the Institute of General Pathology of the University of Pavia; bottom: some of the participants of the Anatomical Congress of Pavia, 1900. Sitting from the right: Wilhelm Waldeyer, Camillo Golgi, Albert Kölliker, and Lina Golgi. Second row from the right: Enrico Bottini, Giulio Bizzozero, and Guglielmo Romiti. Near the left door-post: Guido Sala. Near the right door-post: Carlo Martinotti, on his right is Edoardo Gemelli. A very young Aldo Perrocito is to the right of Gemelli. Behind Golgi and Romiti is Giovanni Marenghi. Courtesy of the Institute of General Pathology of the University of Pavia.

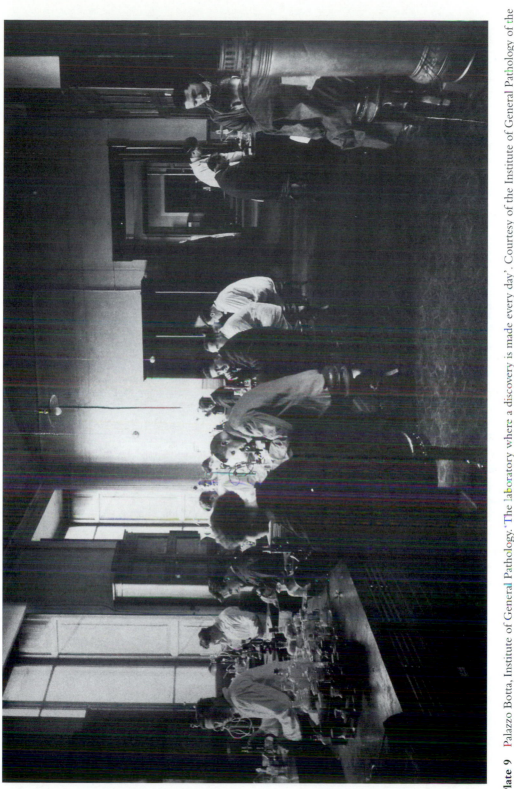

Plate 9 Palazzo Botta, Institute of General Pathology. 'The laboratory where a discovery is made every day'. Courtesy of the Institute of General Pathology of the University of Pavia.

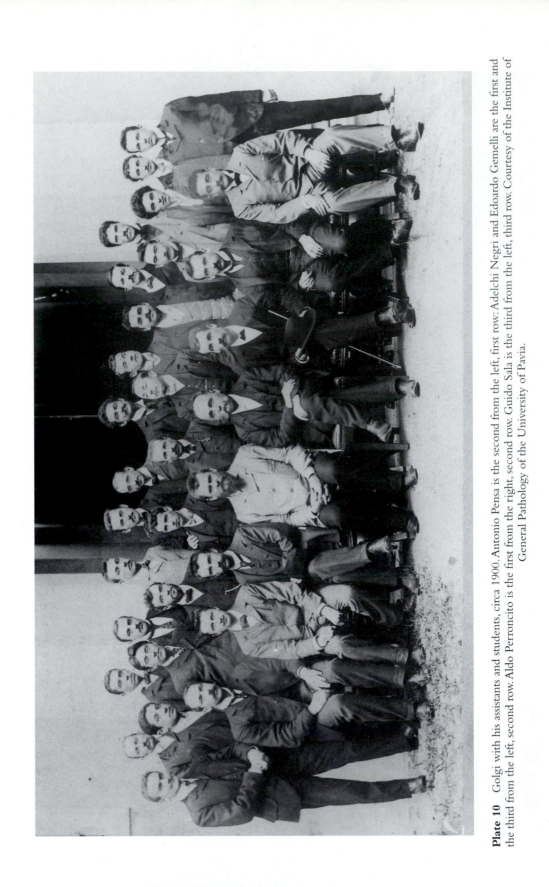

Plate 10 Golgi with his assistants and students, circa 1900. Antonio Pensa is the second from the left, first row; Adelchi Negri and Edoardo Gemelli are the first and the third from the right, second row. Guido Sala is the third from the left, third row. Courtesy of the Institute of General Pathology of the University of Pavia.

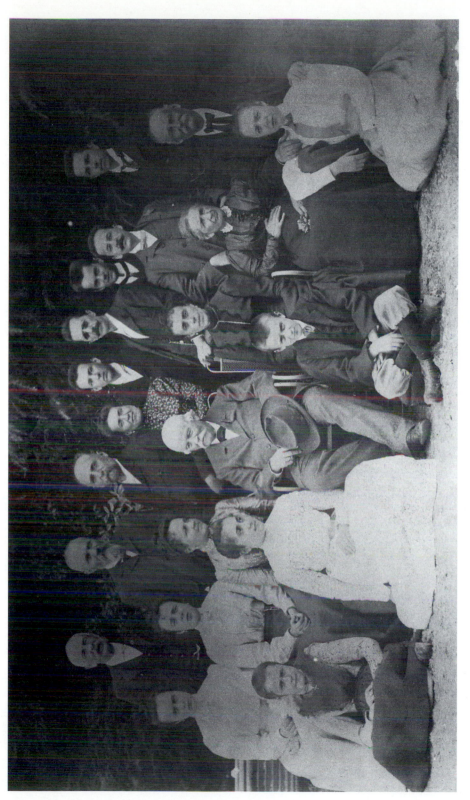

Plate 11 The Golgi, Bizzozero, and Perroncito families gathered around Albert Kölliker. Carolina, the adopted daughter of Golgi, is the second (sitting) from the left, first row. Courtesy of the Institute of General Pathology of the University of Pavia.

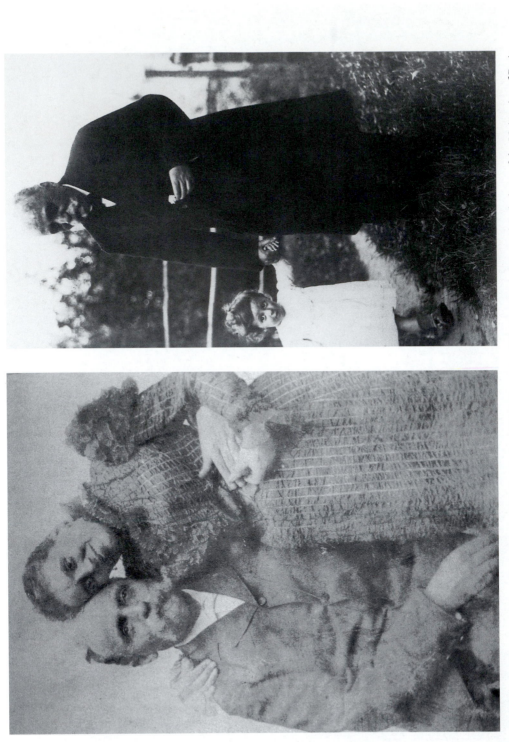

Plate 12 Left: Golgi and his wife; right: a tender Golgi, circa 1915. Courtesy of the Institute of General Pathology of the University of Pavia.

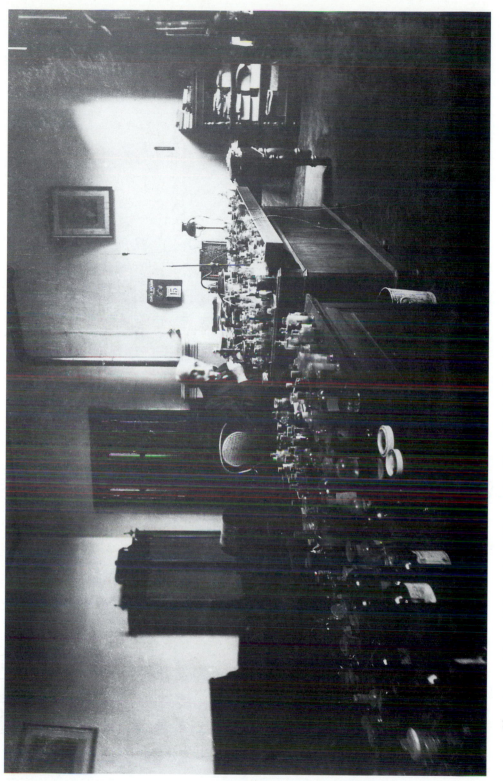

Plate 13 Golgi at work in his laboratory at the age of 77, 1920. Courtesy of the Institute of General Pathology of the University of Pavia.

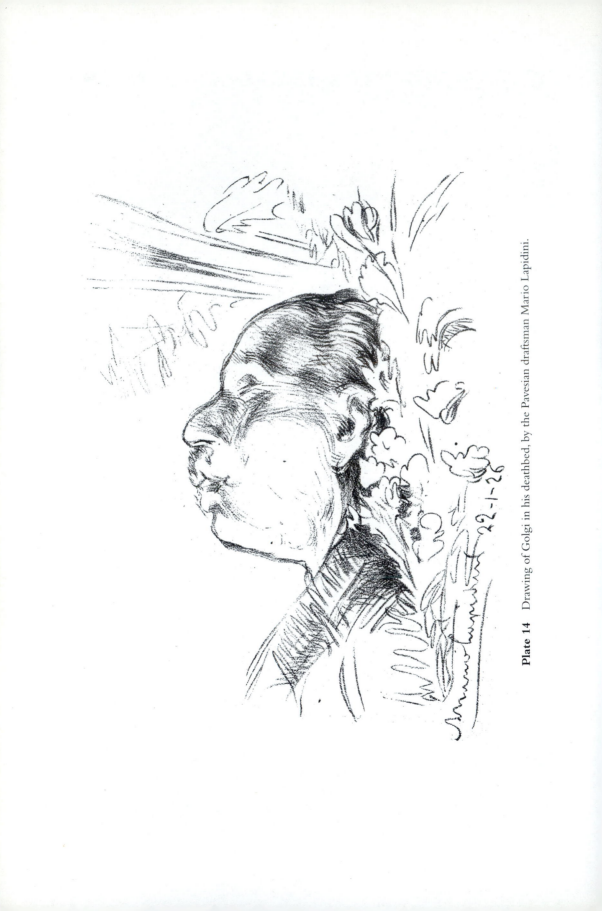

Plate 14 Drawing of Golgi in his deathbed, by the Pavesian draftsman Mario Lapidini.

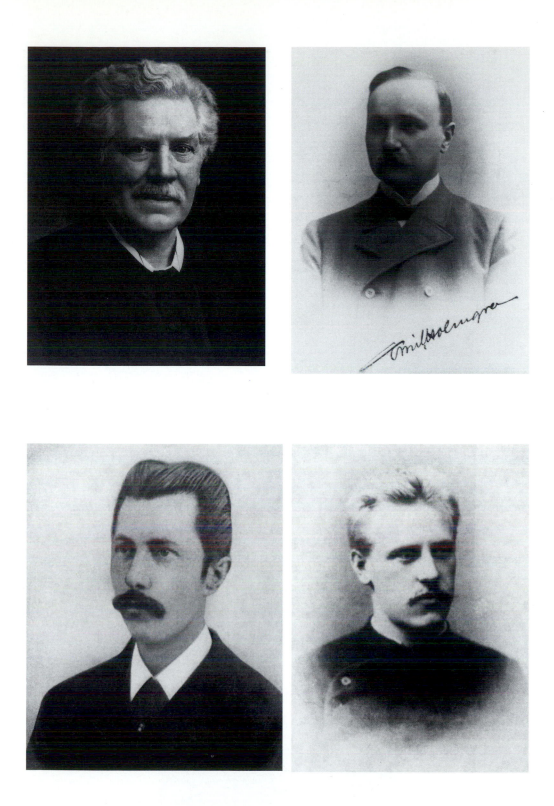

Plate 15 Top left: Gustaf Retzius; top right: Emil Holmgren; bottom left: a very young Giulio Bizzozero; bottom right: Fridtjof Nansen.

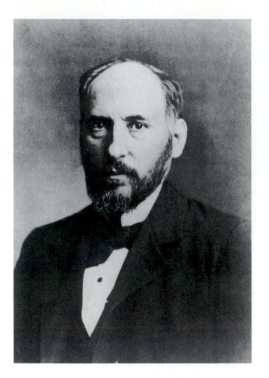

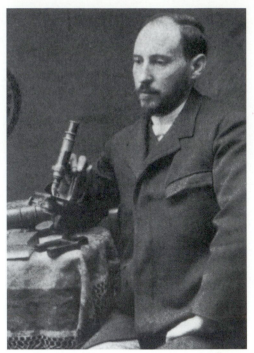

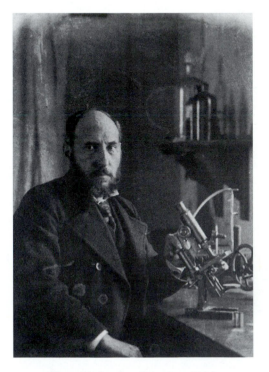

Plate 16 Santiago Ramón y Cajal.

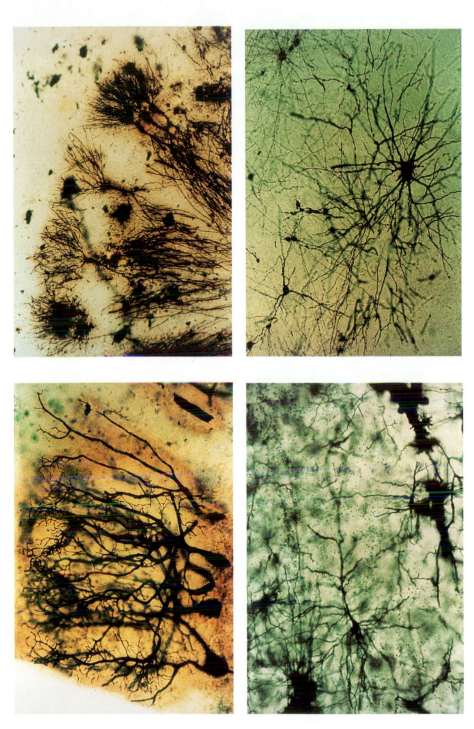

Plate 17 Top left: microphotograph from an original preparation of the cerebellum from Golgi's lab impregnated by the black reaction; top right: microphotograph from an original preparation of *pes hippocampi* from Golgi's lab, impregnated by the black reaction; bottom left and right: nerve cells stained by the black reaction. Original preparations from Golgi's lab. Courtesy of the Institute of Pathology of the University of Pavia.

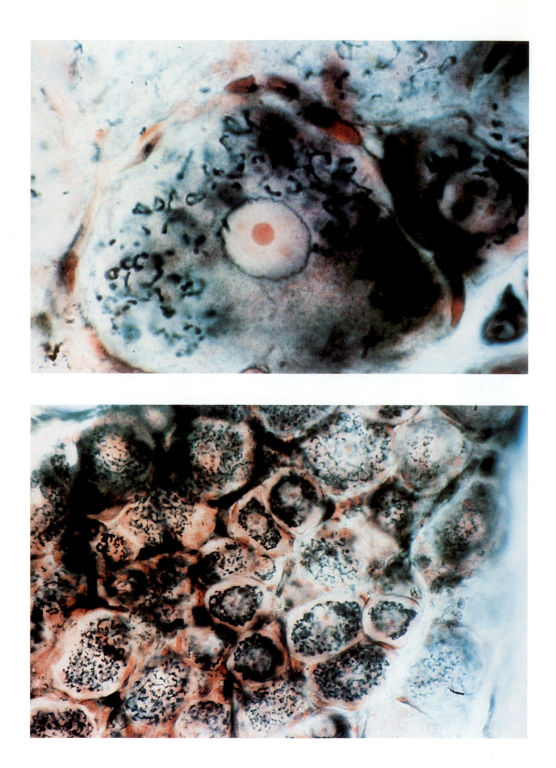

Plate 18 Top: photomicrograph of a dorsal–root ganglion neuron stained by the Golgi reaction, from an original preparation from Golgi's lab. Golgi apparatus is stained in black; bottom: photomicrograph of the Golgi apparatus stained in black in the dorsal–root ganglion neurons. Original preparation from Golgi's lab. Courtesy of the Institute of General Pathology of the University of Pavia.

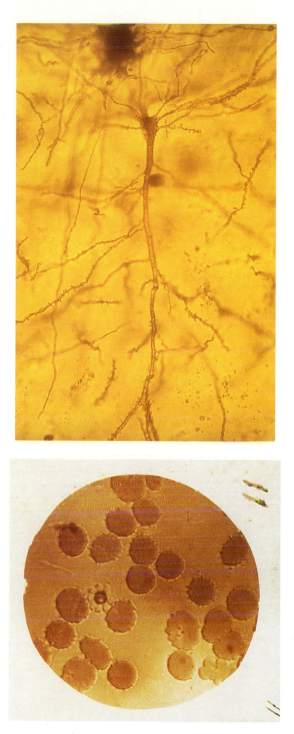

Plate 19 Top: photomicrograph of a pyramidal neuron from an original preparation of Casimiro Mondino, showing numerous dendritic spines, the axon hillock, and the beginning of the axon. Golgi method with potassium bichromate and mercuric chloride. Courtesy of the Institute of General Pathology of the University of Pavia. Bottom: original photomicrograph of Golgi from a blood preparation, showing a 'daisy-like' formation from a malarian patient. Courtesy of the Museum for the History of the University of Pavia.

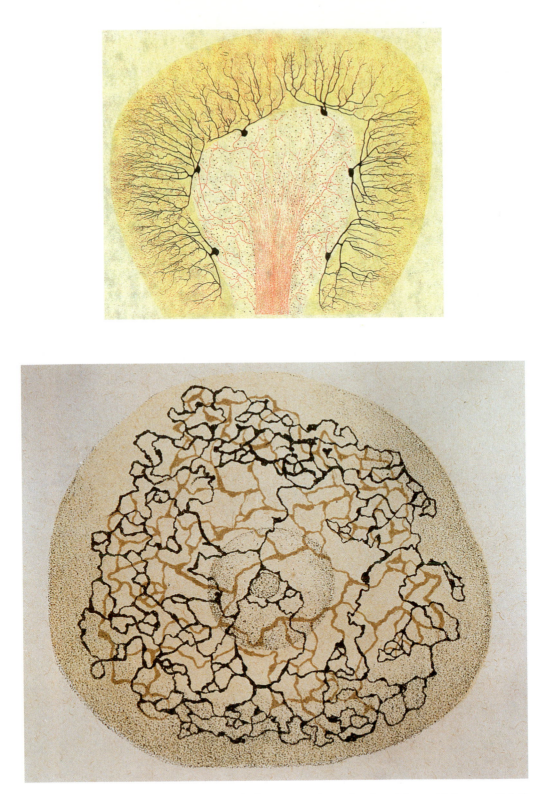

Plate 20 Top: Golgi's drawing of the cerebellum. From *Opera Omnia*, vol. I, tav. 16; bottom: Golgi's drawing of the internal recticular apparatus. From *Opera Omnia*, vol. II tav. 38.

with which it interacted in the cerebral hemispheres. The notion of a diffuse neural net allowed him to distance himself, as a good positivist, from the philosophical presuppositions of the French scientist, thus rescuing a neurophysiological 'holistic' theory that he considered to be particularly appealing. We do not know if Golgi as a young man had read Flourens,[2] and thus there is no way of knowing how much Flourens influenced Golgi's initial holistic choices, but Golgi cited him in 1882 in his essay on cerebral localization, and continued to cite him and declare his admiration for him again and again in the following years.

The theory of the diffuse neural net incorporated, in a logical and coherent way, new neurocytological discoveries into the 'holistic' framework. It was a mature conception considering the times in which it was formulated. It emphasized, for the first time, the role that axons have in connecting nerve cells, a role that had been unthinkable prior to the discovery of their ramifications. And Golgi deserves credit for the notion that the axon is the fundamental element in these connections, a notion that completely overturned all the preceding morphological/functional perspectives.

The cultural climate of neurology and psychiatry began to change radically in the 1880s, just as Golgi was shifting his research interests to other topics. But it is unlikely that Golgi would have changed his position even if he had continued to focus primarily on neuro-histological studies because by this time he had invested too much of his scientific reputation in the theory of the diffuse neural net. Of course, there was nothing wrong with changing one's opinion. Preeminent scientists like Kölliker, Waldeyer, and Retzius, who had been reticularists, did defect to the other camp. But for Golgi to change his opinion would have been to admit to himself and to all the scientific world that he had made inaccurate observations with the black reaction, that he had misinterpreted the evidence, in sum, that he had made mistakes. As Blaise Pascal wrote, 'We are more easily convinced, usually, by reasons we have found by ourselves than by those which have occurred to others.'[3] Golgi undoubtedly had difficulty reconciling the astonishing flexibility of the brain with the idea of many small watertight compartments (that is, neurons) that were rigidly separated and independent. How, for example, would they be able to explain 'the more or less rapid disappearance or compensation of paralytic phenomena or sensory disorders after the destruction of various cortical zones; ... [or] the process of recovery in severe cases of paralysis (hemiplegia), which from a clinical and, sometimes, from an anatomo-pathological point of view appear to be caused by a true disorganization of the nerve bundles.'[4] On the contrary, with his anatomical results, he was convinced that he had found 'an obvious explanation' for phenomena of this type, which otherwise would have remained 'inexplicable'.

On his return from the Berlin Congress, Golgi felt the need to gather ideas, to better define his hypothesis, and especially, to defend it in the face of attacks from others. He decided, therefore, to expound his reticularist credo in a systematic work, putting together various thoughts that up to then had been scattered in many different publications. The results were reported at a meeting of the Istituto Lombardo,[5] and then in a summary form to the Società Medico-Chirurgica.[6] These were followed by a substantial work in French in the *Archives Italiennes de Biologie*,[7] which was a translation of the text presented at the Istituto.

To his contemporaries, the diffuse neural net looked like an almost isotropic system of 'communicating vessels'. The tremendous theoretical obstacles presented by such a system were repeatedly thrown in Golgi's face by his rivals. How could the nervous energy be channelled through preferential pathways in 'discrete' fluxes without decaying and dispersing to reach a state of equilibrium and massive entropy? Claiming that everything communicates with everything and therefore that nervous energy tends to distribute itself isotropically and bidirectionally through the nervous processes led to a sort of *protoplasmic pantheism* that was paramount to 'declaring the absolute unknowability of the organ of the soul'.[16]

As we have seen, Golgi was convinced that nerve cells were interconnected *per continuitatem* by means of axonal anastomoses (as he often stated explicitly). Yet Golgi did not rule out the theoretical possibility that axons could cross each other without forming an anastomosis, that is, forming an intercrossing similar to the vines in the jungle (to use one of Cajal's images). This hypothesis was not new; in fact, Golgi had alluded to it indirectly some years before[17] and Nansen had propounded a version of it when he had described the 'dotted substance' as a very fine matrix caused by axonal subdivisions.

The hypothesis that axons could overlap without actually forming anastomoses, was explicitly restated by Golgi in 1891, and came to be interpreted by some as a conversion to anti-reticularism. Kölliker himself, participating in the fifth meeting of the Anatomische Gesellschaft held in Munich on 18–20 May 1891, reported that Golgi had never, in conversations or letters, stated with absolute certainty the existence of anastomoses. Naturally, Kölliker, who was Golgi's friend but did not share his reticularism, was more than willing to emphasize this aspect of Golgi's position. The news caused a certain stir at the Munich Congress, because everyone looked to Golgi as a champion of the continuity between nerve cells and they were naturally curious about this apparent shift to the opposing camp. Even Waldeyer in his famous 1891 review (in which he introduced the term *neuron*)[18] made reference to Golgi's putative repudiation of reticularism.

In fact, Golgi had not modified his position; even in the past he had admitted that the net could be an optical illusion, but this did not prevent him from forcefully arguing for the existence of intercellular continuity. Furthermore, even in the absence of anastomoses, Golgi's idea of a neural net could still survive. 'From the moment that the studies on electricity demonstrated that electric currents could act without direct continuity on the part of the conductors, and that it was not even necessary that they be in contact, why couldn't the same be true for the nervous system?'[19] Even without protoplasmic continuity, it was still possible to have an organ in which transmission occurs through electric conduction, with properties that are physiologically equivalent to that of an anastomotic net. In conclusion, it was the modality of interaxonal transmission of the nervous stimuli that characterized Golgi's net, not its exact anatomic architecture.

The theory of the diffuse neural net was immediately attacked by the supporters of the neuronal theory, including van Gehuchten and Michael von Lenhossék. The former had been in touch with Cajal for several years and both of them had fallen into the trap of the reticular theory of muscular contractions. In 1888, when this theory was already falling into disgrace, van Gehuchten received a letter from Cajal in which the Spaniard communicated his fresh interest in the study of the nervous system using Golgi's method. Following a route parallel to that of Cajal, van Gehuchten also came to repudiate the reticular protoplasmic theory, and joined the neuronists. He quickly obtained good preparations using the black reaction. In October 1889 he was among those who witnessed Cajal in action at the Berlin Congress and, of course, like the others, was impressed. Convinced, as Cajal was, of having found a good trail to follow, van Gehuchten started to work indefatigably on the structure of the nervous system using Golgi's method and soon began to publish evidence in support of the theory of the neuron.

Michael von Lenhossék was the son of the anatomist Joseph; he also was converted to the black reaction by Cajal in Berlin and very soon was able to report findings favourable to Cajal's interpretations.

Unfortunately for Golgi, in the very year in which he was most strenuously propounding his theory of the diffuse neural net, the mounting tide of the neuronists became unstoppable. And at the end of 1891 even the high priest of anatomy, Wilhelm Waldeyer, gave his official blessing to the theory of the neuron. In a six-instalment review on the latest developments in neuroanatomy and neurohistology, Waldeyer reached the conclusion that the nervous system is formed by many elementary units, anatomically, physiologically, and genetically independent, which he called *neurons*.[18] Incidentally, it is worth noting that periods of tumultuous development of biology always pose new problems for medical nomenclature and Waldeyer demonstrated an extremely well tuned ear for their solution (he also introduced the term *chromosome*).

In Italy, Golgi's theory was subjected to a searing criticism by the psychiatrist Eugenio Tanzi, who perceived some of its inconsistencies. In particular, discussing Golgi's interpretation of the images of 'intercrossings' as a reticulum with anastomoses, Tanzi stated (emphasis added):

In one of his communications to the Istituto Lombardo and in another in the *Anatomischer Anzeiger* he [Golgi] expressed a doubt whether one is dealing with a true net rather than simple intercrossings and admitted explicitly the theoretical possibility of transmission by contiguity. But in substance and despite this doubt, his earlier ideas remain unchanged, and correspond perfectly to the reading of them by Ramón [y Cajal], Kölliker, Waldeyer and Lenhossék. If the interstitial fibrils are, as Golgi states, diffuse and continuous; if moreover, as is his conviction, they have no individual trajectory and can establish connections with an unlimited number of central [nerve] cells, and with the most diverse and distant parts of the nervous centres; if finally (using his words) the entire nervous network is ramified so as to favour the greatest possible level of complexity, extension and closeness of relationship between fibres and cells, it is difficult to understand what is the difference between such a net and the interpretation of the reticulum that the interpreters and the critics of the Pavian school have put forward. This is so true that as a conclusion to his paper Golgi had no hesitation in rejecting again the possibility of isolated conduction.

In my opinion, by rejecting [the possibility of isolated conduction], Golgi completely ruined not only the theory of rigorously delimited localization, but also the theory of relative localization, which he was willing to accept. In other words, Golgi accepted Luciani's notion of functional centres with unlimited and overlapping boundaries. In agreement with this notion that today is contested by none, one should accept that the distribution of nerve fibres in the cortex can vary in some regions where they can establish more direct and close contact than elsewhere: that is, there are elective pathways. Now, this electivity is nothing but an equivalent of individual conduction and can hardly be reconciled with the diffuse and continuous net which according to Golgi connects every nerve fibre with an unlimited number of cells. It appears that if one accepts Golgi's net or intercrossings up to its ultimate consequences, one is required to abandon the theory of functional localization, even in Luciani's weak version. Any other continuous reticulum between fibrils that conduct nerve waves encounters the same incompatibility. And indeed, if [one accepts the notion that] a sensation of the external world—penetrating as a neural event into a sensory fibre—*instead of being channelled into a more or less isolated anatomical system in which it cannot deviate, were to find itself within an unlimited net in which it will necessarily disperse*, not only one does not understand the theory of localization and is compelled to reject it, but one must also give up the simplest and most likely explanation of an undeniable fact, that is, that thought has laws and rules of temporal sequence from which it cannot escape.[20]

Tanzi continued with great acuity (emphasis added):

Golgi's hypothesis, which one should nevertheless accept if the evidence supports it, has caused embarrassment and pause to physiological psychology. Once the belief in isolated conduction, and thus in a *division of labour* between different brain compartments, is removed, psychology is left with no other way to conceptualize objectively psychic functions than to accept that in each thought there is *participation of the entire encephalon*. To explain the various occurrences of thought, one must suppose in this unitary and homogenous (?) organ the disposition to as many different dynamics as the number of possible different thoughts. In the absence of an answer from histology, psychology must in the end put all its hopes in an extremely complicated and perhaps chimerical physio-mechanics of which at any rate we do not even know the alphabet.[21]

Then Tanzi pointed out that

minimal interruptions between neighbouring and functionally connected neurons would also explain in a sufficiently satisfying manner the well-known fact, originally brought to light by Helmholtz, that nervous processes, crossing the grey substance, suffer a reduction of velocity. The cause of this delay would reside in the difficulty in crossing the open space [between neurons].[22]

In a paper written at about the same time, van Gehuchten pointed out that the reduction in the speed of conduction through a reflex arc in the spinal cord could be accounted for by the presence of an anatomical interruption between sensory and motor fibres.[23] Thus the idea that nerve cells were independent units was beginning to find support in the electro-physiological data. And, as predicted by Tanzi, it provided the basis for a new physiological psychology. Indeed, Tanzi made the first remarkable attempt to create a theory of learning and memory based on synaptic modifications induced by external stimuli.[24] According to this theory, an activated neuron, 'is not different from a muscle that has been used', and would become hypertrophic, thus reducing the distance between the terminal expansion of its axon and the soma, or dendrite, of the nerve cell with which it makes connection. This modification could be temporary in the case of a single stimulation, or permanent as a consequence of repeated stimulation. Depending on the circumstances, the 'nerve wave' could travel from one cell to another with more or less facility. The reduction of the interneuronal distance would thus provide the physical basis for learning. Thus Tanzi anticipated by half a century a similar theory by Hebb.[25]

Another attempt to elaborate a biomechanical psychological theory based on the inter-actions of neurons separated by a 'contact barrier' (a concept strikingly similar to that of the synapse) was developed in 1895 by Freud, who since the early 1880s had begun to think vaguely of nerve cells as independent 'units'. In the next few years, despite the fact that his interests had shifted toward clinical neurology and psychiatry, he continued to keep himself abreast of the latest structural studies carried out with the black reaction. In 1893, in a work on the differential diagnosis of organic motor paralysis versus hysteria, Freud referred to the 'new histology of the nervous system … based on the work of Golgi, Ramón y Cajal, Kölliker and others'.[26] Naturally, he was ready to accommodate Waldeyer's concept of the neuron and the idea that neurons could be functionally polarized. Freud thought that this new histology could provide the basis for a physiological psychology in which affective and mental dynamism could be described on the basis of the principle of the conservation of energy, just as physics had done in the fields of hydrodynamics, thermodynamics, and 'electrology'. The result was the unfinished work *Project for a scientific psychology*, written in 1895 but published posthumously. If neurons are separated by 'contact barriers' one might speculate that in this discontinuity resides the possibility of compartmentalizing nervous energy. For Freud, neurons differed on the basis of their ability to transfer this energy to the level of the 'contact barrier' in permeable or 'phi' (ϕ) neurons (those receiving sensory stimuli from the environment without registering them) and impermeable or 'psi' neurons (Ψ). The latter were endowed with the ability to aug-ment slightly their permeability to the 'excitatory flux' across the 'contact barrier'. The trace of this event would constitute the neurobiological basis of the memory process. Thus, Freud was one of the first, along with Tanzi and then Cajal, to hypothesize that memory depended on synaptic modification. But he also tried to establish a connection between this hypothetical neuronal physiology and the new psychoanalytical categories he was characterizing. The Ego (which did not yet have the full significance that it acquired in psychoanalytic theory) derived from a particular neuronal organization; consciousness arose from processes of excitation of particular nerve cells called 'omega' (ω) neurons; and the experience of pain and psychological gratification corresponded to discharges of energy. However, his attempts were too far ahead of their time; they led, together with some brilliant intuitions, to a purely speculative neuronal physio-mechanics without experimental basis. Eventually, Freud, dissatisfied with the limitation of his theory, decided to put it aside.

Although a number of important Italian neurologists and psychiatrists, including Tanzi and his collaborator Ernesto Lugaro, readily embraced the theory of the neuron, Golgi's diffuse neural net continued to exert a persistent influence in Italy, especially after the 1890s when Golgi's pupils became professors of Histology, Anatomy, and General Pathol-ogy in the most important Italian universities.[27] In general, all those who had received their scientific training in the Istituto di Patologia Generale of Pavia remained staunch followers of the theory, also because this had become for Golgi the critical measure of their loyalty and respect. He interpreted as a personal affront any compromising with the theory of the neuron. During a conference, Eugenio Medea, who was very close to him, dealt with the theory of the neuron:

Whatever might have been my personal opinion with respect to the debated question, I was always very careful, out of respect for the Maestro, not to assume an attitude favourable to that doctrine, which I knew was not only not shared but tenaciously opposed . . . Some people (there always existed 'obliging' troublemakers) reported my words maliciously to the Maestro, and I know that he was hurt. I always regretted that I unintentionally caused him a small displeasure. Later all was explained and I continued to have a very good relationship with him.[28]

Golgi remained steadfastly faithful to his theory, which he expounded repeatedly in the following years, in particular in his Nobel Prize lecture[29] and in two important works of a 'philosophical' nature.[30]

Notes

1. Tanzi (1893, p. 432).
2. The BUP holds various theoretical and experimental works by Flourens, some of which were presumably in place in the decade 1860–70, including *Researches expérimentales sur les propriétés et les fonctions du systéme nerveux, dans les animaux vertébrés* [Experimental researches on the properties of the nervous system, in the vertebrate animals] dedicated to Scarpa: 'to Mr Scarpa. Homage of respect and of admiration. The author. Flourens'. (I thank Prof. Giovanni Berlucchi for bringing this to my attention.)
3. *Pensées*, English translation, by H. Levi, *Pensées and other writings*. Oxford University Press (1995), from fragment 617, p. 135.
4. Golgi (1910, p. 41).
5. Golgi (1891e).
6. Golgi (1891f). Meeting of 18 April 1891.
7. Golgi (1891g).
8. Golgi (1891e; *OO*, p. 580).
9. *Ibid.* (*OO*, p. 583).
10. *Ibid.* (*OO*, p. 586).
11. *Ibid.* (*OO*, p. 587).
12. *Ibid.* (*OO*, p. 589).
13. *Ibid.* (*OO*, p. 592).
14. *Ibid.* (*OO*, p. 600).
15. Golgi (1885, p. 44).
16. Cajal (1917, p. 78).
17. Golgi (1885, p. 105).
18. Waldeyer (1891).
19. Golgi (1891e, p. 593).
20. Tanzi (1893, p. 433ff.).
21. *Ibid.* (p. 435).
22. *Ibid.* (p. 439).
23. van Gehuchten (1891).
24. Tanzi (1893, p. 468); see also Buchtel and Berlucchi (1977, p. 287).
25. Hebb (1949).
26. Freud (1893, p. 29). James Strachey (editor of the English translation of Freud's works) maintains that the first part of this work, which is more neurological in nature, came out in 1888 or

earlier. The reference to Cajal (who was still relatively unknown in 1888) and to Kölliker, who had only recently learned of Golgi's method, would seem to contradict this dating, unless the references to these authors were added later.

27. It is sufficient to remember that the great neurophysiologist Giuseppe Moruzzi, working under the guidance of Antonio Pensa, one of Golgi's pupils, began his research activity at the end of the 1920s with a work titled *La rete nervosa diffusa (Golgi) dello strato dei granuli del cervelletto* [The diffuse neural net (Golgi) of the granular layer of the cerebellum].

28. Medea (1966, p. 5 *bis*).

29. Golgi (1906).

30. Golgi (1910; 1914).

16

Golgi versus Cajal: holism versus reductionism at the dawn of the neurosciences

In 1891, while Golgi was making a last attempt to convince his critics of the reality of the diffuse neural net, Cajal and van Gehuchten developed a physiological model in which dendrites, cell body, and axon played well-defined roles in the mechanism of nervous transmission. In contrast to the static model propounded by His Sr and Forel, Cajal was in fact propounding a more dynamic vision of the nerve cell, and van Gehuchten moved in the same direction, albeit with some small differences. We have seen that Cajal began to hint at the idea of directional flow of nerve currents in 1889 while investigating the relationship between the basket cells and Purkinje cells. Two years later, this vague intuition became the 'law of dynamic polarization', according to which the dendrites (and the cell body as well) receive nerve impulses, which are then transmitted to the cylindraxis (the conduction apparatus), which in turn distributes them to the terminal varicose arborization (emission apparatus).[1] If the cells of the exocrine glands were functionally polarized in terms of their secretory activity, the same could be true of neurons in their role of transmitting nerve impulses.

The law of dynamic polarization was immediately successful because of its simplicity and elegance. From that moment on, the task of identifying 'the exit' from the labyrinth of the nervous system became much easier. What had appeared until then as meaningless ideograms suddenly acquired meaning. The nerve currents were not getting lost in an uncharted ocean but rather were following clear-cut 'directions'. The direction of the nerve currents could be established by identifying the somato-dendritic complex, the axon, and the master plan of neuronal connections. If Golgi's method was the Rosetta Stone of neuroanatomy, the law of dynamic polarization was its 'Ariadne's thread', a sort of elementary grammar that allowed the extraction of pieces of information from the nervous mosaic. But all grammatical rules have exceptions, and modern neurophysiology has shown that this law is not valid in all cases. Nevertheless, it was of fundamental importance in guiding neurosciences at the turn of the century. In contrast to the chaotic structure of the diffuse neural net, in which the complication of the net guaranteed the greatest possible number of intercellular connections, Cajal's model simplified things; it pointed to well-defined structures and worked as a filter that allowed spatial configurations to emerge from the chaos. While Golgi allowed the tree to grow unchecked, Cajal pruned it to identify the trunk and main branches. In this way Cajal was not obliged to consider all possible connections but could focus on the most promising types of configuration. He possessed a 'morphological algorithm' that allowed the decoding of the general structure of the nervous system to find invariant elements. Seen with Cajal's eye, the nervous arabesque acquired a geometrical harmony, whilst in Golgi's perspective it dissolved in an undefined nebula. Cajal emphasized regional neuroanatomical differences; Golgi minimized their importance. The prototypical example of this is provided by the studies on the architecture of the cerebral cortex. Where Golgi found no regional differences, Cajal and all those who followed in his wake had been able to identify a number of structural peculiarities in the different areas of the cortex, providing the foundation for modern cortical cytoarchitectonics.

The theory of the neuron reconciled the structure of the nervous system with the general paradigm of the cell theory, which had already been successful for other tissues. The enormous wealth of data that electrophysiology and neuromorphology had produced in the previous decades could finally be interpreted within a coherent framework. In addition, the theory of the neuron, along with the law of dynamic polarization, provided an orienting influence for future neuroanatomical research.

The Golgi−Cajal controversy is a remarkable example of how a theory is itself also a research tool, a research strategy that can be applied to concrete problems, a sort of 'filter' that allows one to see more clearly. Of course, in any type of research, there are better theories and worse theories. Different theories lead to different interpretations of the same observation, but a theory can also 'distort' the experimental data, especially when the latter are ambiguous. Golgi was led to see nets and anastomoses where there were only illusory images. But Cajal also in some instances did violence to the experimental data to fit them to his theory.

One of the organs that the Spanish scientist investigated with the greatest passion was the retina ('The retina has always been generous to me.'[2]) Being composed of layers and organized according to a precise cell architecture, the retina lends itself perfectly to the study of the relationships between the various components of nervous tissue. Furthermore, it allowed physiological inferences because the direction of the nerve impulse could be determined a priori. Cajal gave masterful descriptions of this organ, but encountered some difficulty in interpreting the horizontal and amacrine cells.[3] In most vertebrates, there are two main categories of horizontal cells: those with and those without axons. Many anatomists before Cajal had described the second type but Cajal described only those with axons and considered the cells in which the axon was not visible as partial impregnations (he believed that he had glimpsed the presence of the axons in some short filaments). This allowed him to confirm the law of dynamic polarization, which required the presence of axons, even in this special case. With an analogous technical argument, Golgi had attempted to explain away the apparent lack of anastomoses in the plates drawn from Cajal's preparations.

Cajal also had to explain the fact that the horizontal cells appeared to be connected by anastomoses, as suggested by studies of Krause and Dogiel. Applying Golgi's method to the retina for the first time, Tartuferi observed a syncytium ('sub-epithelial net') formed by the anastomoses among the horizontal cells and the terminations of the photoreceptors.[4]

Furthermore, following the introduction of staining methods for neurofibrils, it was possible to obtain clear syncytial images, including numerous horizontal cells, mostly without axons. Despite this experimental evidence, Cajal rejected the existence of the anastomoses. His explanation for what he considered pseudo-anastomoses was that the preparation had been excessively exposed to the staining medium, an explanation peculiarly discrepant with the one he had proposed to explain the apparent lack of axons in some of the horizontal cells. In both cases, the evidence against his theory was attributable to the shortcomings of the staining method.

Electron microscopy has shown that horizontal cells are connected by gap junctions, which in fact establish a certain degree of anatomical continuity. Also at the physiological level, the fundamental unit has to be found more in the syncytium than in the single cells.

The syncytial nature of the horizontal cells in the lower vertebrates is clearly indicated by the terminal fusiform expansions of their axons. In preparations with the black reaction these terminal structures give the appearance of a plexus. Because the fine and long axon that connects them to the cell body is almost never stained, even when using Golgi's method, the terminal expansions had been interpreted as autonomous cells. Some researchers, such as Paul Schiefferdecker, emphasized instead the lack of a nucleus and called them 'concentric cells without nucleus'.[5] Cajal, in contrast, maintained that the nucleus was present and considered them as a particular type of horizontal cells ('internal horizontal cells') and explained away the plexus-like structure as the consequence of artifactual impregnation.

Cajal thought that the general manner of connection of the retinal neurons consisted of a neuronal chain with minimal convergence and no lateral transmission of the signal. The spatial disposition of the horizontal and amacrine cells indicated a structural organization suitable for the flow of signals perpendicular to the main visual axis. The horizontal cells, for example, clearly established a connection between distant photoreceptors. However, Cajal was inclined to exclude a lateral loss of energy that in his model would have progressively reduced visual acuity.[6] Thus he had to invoke an interpretation that distorted the objective data to make them consonant with his theoretical model, maintaining that the visual signal was transmitted from cell to cell without lateral dispersion, in agreement with the law of dynamic polarization.

There is no doubt that in some cases even the very collection of data by Cajal was filtered through the distorting lens of his theory, allowing him to make his observations compatible with the theory of the neuron. Indeed, this was the case with his work on the structure of the retina. Obviously, this does not detract from the great achievements of Cajal, whose unitary and dynamic conception of the nerve cell has provided the basic conceptual framework for the development of modern neuroscience.

The controversy between Golgi's reticularism and Cajal's neuronism can be considered one of the great clashes of ideas in the evolution of biological thought at the turn of the century. Indeed, the experimental data remained inconclusive for many years (even though a number of theoretical considerations and numerous cases of indirect morphological evidence predisposed most neurohistologists to accept the neuron theory), leading the two opposite sides to fight a long and spirited battle. Although the Golgi–Cajal controversy was one of the most dramatic aspects of this battle, other actors participated in the drama. After a first direct challenge between the two champions, which saw the theory of the neuron prevail, the following decades were characterized by the contraposition between neuronists and neo-reticularists. Cajal, who was becoming more rigid and dogmatic with the passing of time, fought hard against the theories put forward by Apáthy, Bethe, Held, and Nissl,[7] who held that the continuity among neurons took place at a structural level lower than the intracellular reticulum of Golgi or Gerlach, that is, at the level of the neurofibrils, as hypothesized by Max Schultze. After 1903, especially thanks to Bethe's work, 'the contagion of reticularism' (to use Cajal's words) spread. Waldeyer wavered momentarily; van Gehuchten accepted that during nervous regrowth the cylindraxis could originate from a chain of neuroblasts (and not from a single cell); and Georges Marinesco, who had once been an ardent advocate of the neuron, temporarily defected to the opposite side.[8] Obviously, Cajal remained the indefatigable champion of the neuronal theory as indicated by a series of masterful studies on the degeneration and regeneration of nervous tissue.[9] Of course, in the end the theory of the neuron prevailed over neo-reticularism, but its definitive triumph had to wait for the advent of electron microscopy in the 1950s, when the physical existence of synapses was finally demonstrated.

There were also some who tried to keep a middle ground. After Golgi's death, for example, Antonio Pensa embraced a weak version of the neuron theory, maintaining that the connection among cells did not always occur through synapses, and that the law of dynamic polarization was not necessarily valid in all cases.[10]

Overall, this controversy was central to modern neuroscience in the same way that the controversy between classical physics and quantum physics was central to nuclear physics, or that between essentialism and evolutionism was central to biology. It had implications for many disciplines associated with neuroscience, from pharmacology to the clinic, from psychology to information sciences.

The debate between neuronists and reticularists reflected two antagonistic models of the cellular organization of the nervous system. For the former, nervous matter was distributed in elementary packages, whilst for the latter it was continuous. In certain respects, it reflected the antinomy between the reductionistic and holistic approaches to the nervous system. The two champions of this challenge endorsed the most radical versions of the opposing conceptions. One can empathize with Golgi's intellectual drama. Although belonging to the holistic side, he had provided the experimental tools for the reductionist programme, which he would call a 'generalized individualizing tendency' and would perceive as insufficient to explain the complexity of the nervous system.

At least initially, however, Golgi's approach was a legitimate attempt to formulate a heuristic model of nervous activity. If one thinks of the state of the field in the early 1870s, it is clear that Golgi's reticular model was as substantial an improvement over earlier conceptions (by emphasizing, for the first time, the role that a ramified axon has in connecting nerve cells) as Cajal's theory of the neuron was over Golgi's reticularism.[11]

Unfortunately for Golgi, his theory became widely known only when it was already partly obsolete. Furthermore, he found himself obliged to defend his theory at a time when, as we shall see, the little time he had left for research was dedicated to the study of malaria and to the investigation of the internal structure of the nerve cell. Once the theory of the neuron had been proposed, Golgi continued to defend reticularism, partly for psychological reasons, but possibly also because he thought his model was better at explaining the functional complexity of the nervous system than a 'rigid' model based on the mere algebraic addition of the activities of single cells. Golgi's stubbornness was also fed by the absence of definitive morphological evidence in favour of one theory or the other.

In any case, even if ultimately proven 'wrong', Golgi's theory had an important heuristic function.[12] Spurred on by the impossibility of performing the 'crucial experiment',[13] neuroanatomists engaged in a colossal 'hunt' for morphological findings in the hope of tipping the balance in favour of one theory or the other, which had a positive influence on the development of neurobiology.

The original version of Cajal's theory of the neuron has undergone repeated transformations, having incorporated elements of the reticular theory and acknowledged the exceptions to the law of dynamic polarization.[14] For example, it is now known that some neurons and astrocytes are connected through 'gap junctions';[15] that some dendrites can have a synaptic output; and that axons can receive impulses from other axons (axo-axonic synapses), as proposed by Golgi. Finally, the neuron is no longer regarded as the only functional unit in the nervous system, being positioned in the middle of a hierarchical scale including subcellular structures (synapses, dendritic tree, etc.) at one end and multi-neuron complexes at the other. The presence throughout the cortex of columnar units consisting of thousands of interconnected neurons that can be activated simultaneously is consistent with some of the 'holistic' aspects of Golgi's model.

The original concept of the neuron fitted very well with the classical computational models in fashion in the 1940s and 1950s. However, recent advances in neurophysiology and artificial intelligence, together with the developments in neuronal network and parallel processing, have rekindled interest in the notion (which has never actually died) that the brain or large parts of it could function also in a holistic or global manner. Golgi appears to have foreshadowed such conceptions by positing that the activity of the nervous system was due 'not to the isolated action of individual cells but to the simultaneous activity of large groups of cells'.[16] What he didn't realize was that 'the isolated action of individual cells' was not incompatible with 'the simultaneous activity of large groups of cells'; that is, that the theory of the neuron could also support a holistic model of neural activity. The 'flexibility' of neuronism, however, was not immediately obvious; on the contrary, at its inception it appeared to be a mechanistic and rigid theory, not very different from the repetitive simplicity of the electric circuits that were becoming popular at the end of the nineteenth century. Furthermore, the limited number of connections that appeared to be possible in Cajal's diagrams reinforced Golgi's impression that the neuronal model could not account for the simultaneous activation of large areas of the nervous system. Finally, Golgi found it difficult to explain how a model based on physically separated cells could account for the phenomenon of recovery of function, which instead could be readily explained by reticularism.

It has recently been proposed that in addition to the neural transmission based on synaptic connections ('wired transmission') it is possible to have the diffusion at a distance of chemical and electrical signals ('volume transmission').[17] Electrical signals can diffuse in the intercellular fluid for short distances (0.1–0.2 mm) whereas chemical signals can diffuse longer distances (some millimetres). Furthermore, chemical signals can also diffuse through the cerebrospinal fluid. One of the main features of 'volume transmission' is the diffuse activation of entire pools of neurons, and thus of large regions of the central nervous system, a phenomenon somewhat related to what was implied at the functional level by Golgi's reticular theory.

Paradoxically, Cajal's neuronism developed in peculiar and elegant symmetry with Golgi's reticularism.

As we discussed in the previous chapters, the 'implicit initial assumption' in Golgi's model was that the brain functioned, according to Flourens' model, in a holistic manner[18] that required the 'continuity' of intercellular connections, although he accepted the possibility of a discontinuity between nerve cells (even before the formulation of the theory of the neuron).

When Cajal began his investigation of the nervous system using the black reaction, reticular models were still prevalent, but the new ideas of His Sr and Forel (about which the Spaniard must have heard in Madrid) were making inroads. It was natural that a young and enthusiastic neophyte would align himself with the New Histology, and that this would become his 'implicit initial assumption'. Cajal maintained from his first study with Golgi's method that he had never seen an anastomosis among the ramifications of cylindraxes. In both cases, therefore, we find 'implicit initial assumptions', almost interpretative theories;[19] 'globalist' for Golgi, and 'individualist' for Cajal.[20] An early series of observations combined with an 'initial assumption' produced two antagonistic theories: the 'diffuse neural net' on one side; the 'theory of the neuron' *cum* 'law of dynamic polarization' on the other. At this point, in the words of Albert Einstein, 'It is the theory that decides what we can observe.' When Cajal observed a preparation, he knew how to draw a nervous circuit according to the law of dynamic polarization and very soon explanatory arrows began to pop up in his diagrams indicating the direction of nerve impulses. He drew 'contacts' between the terminal expansion of the axon and the somato–dendritic complex, even though the optics of the time could not demonstrate the presence of synapses, because the theory demanded their existence. Golgi interpreted as diffuse neural net illusory images produced by the overlapping of neurons located on different planes; for him, too, only what fitted the framework of the theory made sense.

It is legitimate to ask what would have happened to the development of neuroanatomy and thus of neurosciences if Golgi had not discovered the black reaction. The time that elapsed between the moment of this discovery and that of the international diffusion of the method suggests some answer. As we have seen, in that time span some progress in the study of the structure of the nervous system was made. The chemical industry of Germany was producing a great variety of new chemicals, which were then tested as dyes for histological preparations, and several new staining procedures were introduced in that period: Weigert's stain for studying the myelin sheath; Nissl's stain based on aniline; and Ehrlich's 'vital' stain based on methyl blue. Each of these methods, however, stained only some structural aspects of the nervous tissue, without demonstrating the relationships between the elements. Before the black reaction, for example, it was thought that dendrites had no free terminations and that axons had no ramifications. It was impossible, therefore, to understand the architecture of the nervous system and the topographical relationships among groups of cells and bundles of fibres.

The black reaction solved in a single stroke an enormous number of neurobiological problems and provided a formidable research tool for an entire generation of neuro-anatomists. It was so innovative that when it began to be used, it didn't seem possible that this method could stain only a few of the hundreds or thousands of cells present in the microscopic field. And, in fact, Rossbach and Sehrwald immediately hypothesized that the stained images corresponded in reality to lymphatic spaces.

From a certain point of view, the development of new histological methods was 'just a matter of time', but certainly the same cannot be said for the black reaction. As we have seen, Golgi probably developed the method after observing some traces of metallic impregnation during his first studies on the 'lymphatics' of the nervous system. His entire scientific career is a testimonial of his oracular ability to exploit in the most complete and effective way all promising avenues and to extract from them the largest possible number of 'facts'. But if Golgi had desisted from pursuing those vague silver-stained images, would someone else have achieved something comparable? The lapse of time before the importance of the method was widely acknowledged tells us that black reaction was not 'in the air'. Certainly, dozens of histologists were hunting for new methods all over Europe. The progress in histological technique, however, was only in part determined by the introduction of new dyes. An important role was played by empirical elements that could not be decided a priori. It was similar, in a certain sense, to *haute cuisine*, in being based more on the creative intuition of the researcher than on the rigorous application of specific scientific knowledge. On the other hand, no theoretical consideration could have predicted the amazing result of the combination of potassium dichromate and silver nitrate in stain-ing the individual nerve cell in its entirety, including all its processes. With the discovery of the black reaction, Golgi made a unique contribution to the history of neuroscience, as Kölliker acknowledged when he wrote to him: 'I consider you as the first to open the path for a true understanding of such a complex structure as the brain.'[21] One cannot underestimate how difficult it would have been to describe projections, contours, and ramifications of cellular groups without the view *d'ensemble* allowed by the black reaction.

From a historical point of view, Cajal emerges as the scientist who, having realized the potential of Golgi's method, contributed more than any other scientist to the laying down of some of the fundamental concepts that still dominate modern neurosciences. Golgi's contribution was of a different kind: with the discovery of the black reaction, he made a unique contribution that changed the very evolution of neuroanatomy, determining in this way the future direction of neuroscience. Without Golgi, there would not have been a Cajal.

Notes

1. Cajal (1891). The idea of a directional flow of nerve currents was hinted at in 1880 by William James in an address to the Boston Society of Natural History. In his masterpiece *The principles*

of psychology, published in 1890, he developed the law of 'forward' direction according to which the paths of instinctive reaction 'all run one way, that is from 'sensory' cells into 'motor' cells and from motor cells into muscles, without ever taking the reverse direction' (James 1890, pp. 581ff.; see also Berlucchi 1999; Shepherd 1991, p. 196). In a footnote, James quoted Golgi and his theory of the diffuse neural net without commenting on it.

2. Cajal (1917, p. 121).
3. Piccolino (1988); Piccolino *et al.* (1988).
4. Tartuferi (1888).
5. Schiefferdecker (1886).
6. Piccolino (1988, pp. 522ff.); Piccolino *et al.* (1988, p. 23).
7. Beccari (1944–45).
8. Cajal (1917, p. 265).
9. DeFelipe and Jones (1991).
10. Pensa (1961a, p. 447).
11. Jacobson (1993, p. 209).
12. See Cimino (1995, pp. viiff. and xxivff.).
13. Cimino (1995, p. xxviii).
14. See Calligaro (1994, p. 71) and Shepherd (1991, p. 290).
15. Raviola and Gilula (1973).
16. Golgi (1885, p. 43).
17. Fuxe and Agnati (1991).
18. Shepherd (1991, p. 266).
19. Pera (1982, pp. 137ff.; 1986, pp. 76ff.).
20. Cimino (1984, p. 376; 1995, p. xxiv).
21. Letter No. 17 from Kölliker to Golgi, 15 July 1896 (Belloni 1975, p. 178).

17

A tranquil laboratory life

Between 1889 and 1891, the threat posed by the theory of the neuron had compelled Golgi to focus his research on the nervous system. But his interest in infectious diseases, in particular malaria, had continued unabated and his collaborators, particularly Monti, were very active in this field.

There was a continuous turnover of researchers in Golgi's laboratory. Grassi, who had by now become an authority in zoology, left the laboratory in the early 1880s (and as we have seen, would later find himself engulfed in a bitter scientific controversy with Golgi); Rezzonico had moved to the Institute of Forensic Medicine; Fusari went as post-doctoral fellow to Messina in 1887 to work in Nikolai Kleinenberg's Laboratory of Embryology; and Clivio was about to specialize in obstetrics. At the same time, attracted by Golgi's scientific celebrity, new interns were lining up to cram into the small laboratory like worker ants. All looked to Golgi for inspiration. In 1890 Fabrizio Maffi, a pupil of the Collegio Ghislieri who had just joined the Institute of General Pathology, wrote to his father that the Director was 'an ideal type of scientist'.[1]

In 1889 Luigi Sala became Golgi's Assistant. Sala had been introduced to the black reaction by Mondino in Turin, and after graduation in 1887 followed Mondino to Palermo to be his Assistant. In Palermo, Sala also obtained the *Libera Docenza* in histology. He was small and slender, well dressed, with well-tended hair and beard, even tempered, self contained, methodical, and orderly. By contrast, his fellow student Monti was always ruffled, goofy, badly dressed, and with an impetuous and arrogant character (he later earned the nickname 'Ebullient'). The two young scientists rapidly attained a high standing in the laboratory. In 1890 Monti began teaching a *corso libero* of general pathology and the following year Sala began teaching histology. Another pupil who rapidly acquired international renown was Carlo Martinotti, who worked in the laboratory in the second half of the 1880s. After graduating from the University of Turin in 1885, he did post-doctoral studies in Italy with Golgi and in Germany at the University of Leipzig. Martinotti's research on the structure of the cerebral cortex was featured in neuroanatomy texts for many years thereafter. Apparently cold, indifferent, and misanthropic, he was actually 'timid by character, introverted by nature; reserved by personal inclination; a loner out of wisdom rather than because of his mood; restrained in his social relationships because of nobility of sentiment and an absolute lack of vanity.'[2] He had a hypercritical and self-critical attitude toward research.

Many things that he had completed were never published because he did not believe they were sufficiently interesting or adequately demonstrated; and what he did publish was reported, despite the immense work required to achieve it, with such an excessive sobriety that one is led to think that his shyness and modesty bordered on irresolution; something that turned to his disadvantage, as in the case of the rabies bodies which he may have seen before Negri.[3]

At the 15 June 1889 meeting of the Società Medico-Chirurgica, Martinotti presented an important paper on the architectonics of the cerebral cortex[4] which he published in German the following year.[5] In this work, he described axons coming from the deep layers of the cortex and ascending vertically to the superficial layers, where they bent horizontally or divided, in the form of a 'T', and travelled a great distance tangentially. Martinotti did not specify the type of cell from which these axons originated. At first, Cajal used 'Martinotti's cells' to refer to the fusiform cells in Layers III to V of the cortex. This eponym was later used for all non-pyramidal cells with axons ascending to Layer I. Currently the term refers to small multipolar nerve cells scattered throughout the cortex, with short ramified dendrites and an axon that extends toward the superficial layers. However, given its imprecise meaning, the term is now used less and less in studies of cerebral architecture.[6]

Another scientist endowed, like Martinotti, with 'an excessive hypercriticality, especially toward himself' was Emilio Veratti, who entered the laboratory in the early 1890s as an internal student. Golgi, who was 'far from being easy in authorizing the publication of works' nevertheless repeatedly 'incited Veratti to move on and publish the results of some studies that had been conducted with the scruple and exactness that were innate to his personality' but 'the latter successfully continued to resist'.[7]

In 1892 Eugenio Medea, whom Golgi had already met in Varese, came to the laboratory as a second-year student in medicine. Graduating that year were Luigi Villa, who would soon after become Golgi's Assistant, and Giovanni Marenghi, who left immediately for two years' military service. Both Villa and Marenghi led tragically short lives: the first died of a glanders infection contracted while at the Istituto Sieroterapico Milanese; the second returned in 1895 to Pavia as an assistant to Golgi and died of meningoencephalitis. In 1892, the two co-authored an article on the structure of myelin that was widely cited by Cajal and others. Other students conducting remarkable research in the same period were Cesare Sacerdotti and Raffaele Vivante, who carried out important studies on the histology of blood and bone tissue.

Golgi actively encouraged his collaborators to spend periods of study abroad. Sala carried out specialization studies in embryology at the University of Berlin in the Institute of Anatomy directed by Oskar Hertwig, and Monti also spent time in German universities.

Golgi also cordially welcomed foreign scientists who asked to visit his laboratory. In 1891 Léonidas Blumenau from St Petersburg visited Pavia before going to Paris to work with Charcot. Soon after, C. L. Herrick arrived from the University of Cincinnati and it was probably in this period that Golgi received a visit from the noted German anatomist Theodor Boveri, expert in the morphological problems associated with cell division.

A deep emotional link connected Golgi and his students, and he fought tooth and nail to help them obtain university and hospital appointments. Unfortunately, he did so even with individuals who were not outstanding.[8]

After increasing in size from one to four rooms, Golgi's laboratory did not change much over the years. According to Antonio Pensa, who began as an internal student in October 1893 and who left a vivid description of the Institute,[9] the laboratory consisted of the office of the Director and three large rooms facing onto the Botanical Gardens. Those who entered were struck by an odorous 'mixture of oil of turpentine, carnations, bergamot-orange, and oregano'. The largest room was occupied by Sala, a few post-doctoral fellows, and about ten medical students. The second, and smaller, room was occupied by Monti, assisted by a couple of senior and experienced internal students. Finally, there was a small room devoted to bacteriology and animal experimentation. This room and its access corridor were crammed with laboratory ovens, sterilizers, and cages for guinea pigs and rabbits. The water supply consisted of a large zinc container filled daily by the janitor. Large experimental animals, such as dogs, were temporarily housed in small out-houses on the ground floor of the western wing of the building of the Botanical Gardens. Guinea pigs were also kept there, for the experiments by Oehl, Golgi, Sala, Monti and, for a brief period, Nansen.

Golgi's personal study was a room approximately three metres wide and four metres long, with a large window facing onto the Botanical Gardens:

Here a magnificent disorder reigned, an evident sign that a prohibition was in force that no one should touch anything. On the floor, in the corners, and along the walls were jars containing liquids of the greatest variety of colours in which various specimens were conserved, scarcely recognizable; spinal cords or brains, whole or in pieces. Against one of the side walls was a portable specimen cabinet and on the other side was a filing cabinet and a small cupboard with glass doors containing bottles of various sizes and colours; in the middle of the study was a table scattered with papers, books, and magazines. Near the window was a work-table with a microscope, a small microtome, and the most bizarre and disordered collection of objects, which made it look like the table of a house painter or varnisher more than that of a pre-eminent scientist. There were cardboard slide holders, slides of microscopic specimens already mounted or in the process of being mounted, vials filled with liquids of various colours, among which prevailed the chrome-yellow of potassium dichromate, the blackish grey of silver nitrate, the deep green of copper acetate, and the greenish blue of sulfate; and then, scattered around, there was a great number of the characteristic glass jars of the Leibig meat extract, now blackened by silver nitrate, which Golgi used to test the procedures for his black reaction; paper sheets with drawings clearly sketched at the microscope; hanging from a nail stuck into one side of the table was an ignominious rag stained by all colours and fouled by all the injuries it had suffered.[10]

The laboratory was an island, impermeable to the events of the surrounding world. All who entered left behind whatever was extraneous to the duties of research. The dignified and somewhat solemn shadow of Golgi wafted over the laboratory. His time was entirely dedicated to research, teaching (which was heavy because it included lecturing in both general pathology and histology), and managing the laboratory over which he maintained complete control. He frequently made the rounds to look at the pupils' preparations, 'often mute; sometimes he would suggest modifications of technique', but he liked to point out 'details that had escaped us and that his eagle eye had caught'.[11] He commanded great awe from the inexperienced students and when he approached a student at the microscope the latter was taken by 'a distinct panic, despite his [that is, Golgi's] affability and kindness'.[7] Pensa recalled that 'Not always did I have the courage to show him some of my preparations because they did not appear sufficiently well done, and I remember sometimes escaping from the laboratory before he arrived at my work place.'[11] The students had to show great dedication and strong motivation in order to maintain their spot; 'the materials (alcohol, ether, celluloid—which was fairly expensive—paraffin, stains) were all supplied by the student. The laboratory provided only the microtome.'[12] Those who thought they had concluded their research and were impatient to publish their findings quickly learned 'how difficult it was to obtain the maestro's authorization to publish, and how many times a work that in the mind of a young scholar appeared to be completed would have to be re-examined from a new point of view before obtaining the authorization to conclude it.'[13]

A colourful aspect of the management of the laboratory concerned the supply of experimental animals, which since the second half of the 1700s had been in great demand in the biological institutes of the University. These animals were not provided by breeders but rather were caught in the surroundings by people who eked out an income by selling them to the scientists. Spallanzani, for example, had his own suppliers of frogs and salamanders, and of caterpillars of white butterflies. At the end of the 1800s some of these picturesque individuals were still in business. There was, for example, Scola, a clandestine catcher of stray dogs, who would arrive in the early morning at the biological laboratories with a few dogs who were then sold after exhaustive haggling over the price. Another individual provided frogs, toads, salamanders, garden snakes, and vipers, which he handled skilfully after removing their poisonous fangs. In the winter months this individual disappeared from circulation and checked himself into the hospital for scabies in the Clinic for Dermatological and Venereal Diseases (which at that time housed mostly syphilitic patients). There was also a guard at the public slaughterhouse who provided the laboratories with fetuses and embryos of various mammals, with normal or infected internal organs. Veratti was particularly appreciative of livers infected by distoma, while Sala was interested in the intestines of horses infested with live worms of the genus *Ascaris*.[14] In the Institute of General Chemistry was Carlo Mangini, a janitor with unusual technical ability. He had been hired as a low-ranking staff-member, but quickly became the man to see for every problem concerning the machines and technical apparatuses of the various institutes, including General Pathology. If there was something wrong with a microtome or microscope a call would go out to Mangini, who would delicately dismantle the instrument, clean it, and return it to working order again. Some years later he founded a large factory producing scientific and sanitary equipment.

Of course, the reagents in common use in the laboratory had to be purchased commercially. In the early 1890s many of these products were provided by the pharmacy owned by Golgi's sister, Maria Teresa, the widow of the pharmacist Campagnoli. Special reagents were purchased from the chemical company Erba or, more rarely, from Merck or Grübler.

Golgi was approaching the age of 50, and 'he revealed, in his appearance and feelings, the character of an austere person'.[15] He was a man of few words, punctilious, obstinate, and a bit pedantic, and was fond of repeating the old adage: 'I have never felt regret for having been silent; only for having spoken.' However, despite being distant, inaccessible, and reserved, he was endowed with a placid and patient temperament. Behind this cold demeanour he hid strong emotions, which he sometimes allowed to surface, particularly when he was speaking at ceremonies in his honour.

Stocky and not very tall, with dark chestnut hair that was beginning to grey, 'a characteristic head of a thinker, two long moustaches, deep and thoughtful look; a vast forehead that his incipient baldness extended up to the crown of his head; two small hands with measured but expressive movements, those small hands that knew how to perform the most delicate manoeuvres of microscopic technique.'[16] And when a visitor lingered in his office too long, the same hands were used to guide the guest towards the door in a characteristic gesture that said 'the conversation is finished, go away and leave me in peace.'[17] In his countenance there appeared sometimes a characteristic tic, a slight lifting of the moustache on the left. For the preparations of his histological specimens, 'he favoured aromatic substances: oils of cedar, oregano, bergamot-orange, and carnations; he made such extensive use of these reagents that he always carried a characteristic mix of these perfumes on his person and on his clothes.'[18] In addition to his passion for science, he loved music, art, and poetry. He was also fond of physical activities, taking long walks on the plains and riding a bicycle.[19]

He had a unique ability to

look for new methods or procedures of investigation and each of his works included some degree of technical novelty. This ability, which seemed miraculous, was in truth nothing more than the fruit of keen observation which, together with a powerful memory, allowed him to catch and retain the smallest differences in the results of a long series of attempts and therefore to follow step by step the development of a new method.[20]

His legendary powers of observation allowed him to recognize truly important findings with great confidence. He often said that, 'a good preparation is a gold mine; it is certain that when the mine had been explored by him, there was no hope of others finding anything important that had escaped his attention!'[21] Speaking about Golgi, Pietro Grocco said that 'whatever he touched was turned to gold';[22] all in all, he was a true wizard of observation.

His non-scientific writings were usually opaque, meticulous, boring, and often repetitive. He came from a generation that had participated in the *Risorgimento*, for whom the idea of *duty* had an almost religious significance. Consequently, he conceived his scientific and pedagogical activity as a social mission and a contribution to the civil and cultural growth of Italy.

He had a proverbial ability to subdue students' unruly behaviours. He was benevolent and often welcomed their requests (integrative courses of study, some supplementary exam sessions, etc.). But he was severe and authoritarian in the moments of disorder when his presence alone and his fulminating look was sufficient to command respect and awe. At the cry 'Golgi is coming' the spirits were calmed. It was easy for him to receive expressions of deference outside the laboratory as well:

At sunset on a foggy November day, I was walking with a small but lively and noisy group of students, along that street which I always remember with a sense of nostalgia and which, in Pavia, takes one from the Botanical Gardens, where the Institute of General and Histological Pathology was housed at the time, to the University. Suddenly the youthful voices and laughter ceased, and the group moved to the side in respectful greeting. He came down the street with short quick steps, on his way to the laboratory; cloaked in fur, his head covered by a large-brimmed hat, slightly tilted on the side, he appeared solid and strong, with a virility already subdued and made sombre by the early signs of ageing; he answered our greetings promptly and cordially by lifting his hat. I saw a high and powerful forehead unlike any I had seen before, extended in the back by the remarkable baldness dividing his greying hair, two deep and intense eyes that looked at us as if able to read our minds, the lower part of his face slightly smiling, adorned by his full grey moustache.[23]

His face and his glance 'even when expressing modesty ... demanded respect, even from those who didn't know him, so the signs of deference that he received everywhere arose from an almost instinctual feeling rather than from well thought out reasons.'[20] His powerful personality imposed itself like a force of nature. In it lay the mystery of a man who attracted despite his aloofness, who fascinated despite his indecipherability, and who beguiled despite his inaccessibility.

In Pavia, the thickset silhouette of Golgi was known to all; he could be seen walking daily on his way from home to the laboratory, and from there to the University, or going to visit his sister and his elderly father. 'He never considered moving [away from Pavia], despite enticing, honorific, and also remunerative offers that he often received.'[24]

In exam sessions Golgi was exacting but fair.[25] A graduate from the Pavian Medical School, recollected that during a one-hour oral exam in general pathology he was asked by Golgi to explain 'the difference between the respiration in frogs and humans and to identify a number of preparations: tumours, inflammations, etc.'[26] In the academic year 1893–94, 25% of those taking the exam in general pathology passed with full marks (none with honours); 58% passed with an 'adequate' grade and 16% failed. The hardest and most dreaded exams were those in chemistry and in comparative anatomy and physiology, where the numbers failing that same year were 31% and 20%, respectively.

Golgi's lectures on histology were held in the lecture hall of the Botanical Gardens; those of general pathology in the hall called 'V bis' of the main University Hall. He never asked his assistants to fill in for him. From Monday to Saturday he lectured for one hour in the morning, usually from ten to eleven, alternating histology and general pathology. He would enter and sit at the lecture desk, organizing his notes. Then he would begin, 'sometimes with a sort of timidity'; even after many years of teaching he was still 'somewhat hesitant in voice at the beginning of his lesson.'[27] When he had to discuss his own findings, he did so in an impersonal manner, never citing himself directly; in contrast, the contributions of his pupils were emphasized in great detail.[28] His voice was a bit nasal and monotonous, and he spoke slowly, repeating the same concepts many times until he had reached the most precise formulation, often bordering inadvertently on using scientific jargon, as if he wanted 'to avoid in his description the deforming influence of language'.[29] Not surprisingly, given the slow and repetitive manner of his exposition, the lessons were boring and students, even some of the interns, often walked out. Then one day the following warning appeared on the notice board of the Institute:

The interns with a position in this laboratory, who are enrolled in the courses of Gen. Pathology and Histology have the obligation to attend the lectures; they will be considered to have renounced their position in the laboratory if they are absent from class three times in a row without written justification.
The Director of the Institute will decide if the vacant position will be assigned to other aspirants.

C. Golgi.[30]

Despite the apparent coldness, the students who had earned his trust could count on him. They were often invited to his home, as recalled by Medea:

I shall always remember the evenings in which Signora Lina, the kind and precious companion of the Maestro, received us with great courtesy in her beautiful house. Golgi was not very talkative but participated with pleasure in the conversation, intervening from time to time with interesting observations . . . With Signora Lina and her nieces, we used to go skating along the Ticino; thus the life of the laboratory continued somewhat at Golgi's house.[31]

Even students who had left the laboratory could always count on his support; in 1889, for example, Marchi won the Fossati Prize of the Istituto Lombardo with Golgi as Chair of the awarding committee.[32]

And of course there were the letters of recommendation for the students who wanted to visit foreign laboratories. These letters were like a passport, as Medea remembered, thinking of the warm welcome he received in Berlin from Hermann Oppenheim thanks to Golgi's glowing endorsement.

The year 1890 was full of polemics and recognitions. Around the end of the year important news was travelling around the world. As already mentioned, Koch had just announced that he had discovered a cure for tuberculosis, news that was the centre of attention at the Berlin Congress. Until the beginning of 1891, however, Koch refused to provide details about his therapy, which, in fact, was simply an extract of cultured tuberculosis bacteria in glycerin. Naturally the hope of an effective therapy attracted the attention of doctors and patients world wide.

The first Italian who, through the good offices of a German friend, was able to obtain a sample of the preparation ('Koch's lymph'), was a certain Bosisio, whose son had tuberculosis. On 27 November 1890 his physician, Romeo Mongardi, tried it first on himself and the next day on his patient. A vial of the precious medicine arrived the same day to Baccelli, sent personally by Koch.[33] In the following weeks, bottles containing the mysterious preparation began to be received all over Italy, in particular by physicians of the Ligurian Riviera, some of whom knew the German bacteriologist personally. By the end of the year Golgi had also received a certain quantity of the extract, sent to him by Koch himself, probably in response to arrangements made at the Berlin Congress. The San Matteo Hospital decided to carry out clinical trials in two wards, the first one being mostly for poor patients, while the second was a 'special ward for paying patients, devoted exclusively to the Koch cure'.[34]

Golgi availed himself of the collaboration of Monti, who examined the bronchial secretions, and of Bernardino Silva, a 'small man, but with a fine brain, quick-witted and a
tease'.[35] On 10 December 1890 they administered Koch's preparation to three tuberculosis
patients, two men and one woman. The following day they repeated the treatment on two
patients with tuberculosis of the joints.[36] On 1 February 1891 Golgi gave a preliminary
account of the new cure to the Società Medico-Chirurgica,[37] followed by a more complete
report written in collaboration with Silva.[38] While emphasizing that the degree of efficacy
of the treatment would be known only after many years of testing, the two physicians gave
a positive evaluation of the cure: of 29 patients treated repeatedly with the 'lymph', 10 were
apparently cured (7 had been affected by pulmonary tuberculosis and 3 by cutaneous
tuberculosis), and another 10 showed substantial improvement.

In reality, the efficacy of the new cure, which had been adopted by all the major hospitals
of Europe, remained controversial and endless arguments concerning Koch's 'lymph' or
'tuberculin' continued to rage in international conferences and scientific journals for many
years. In the patients affected by tuberculosis the preparation provoked, after some hours,
local and general reactions and very high doses could produce a rapid worsening of the
clinical condition or even the death of the patient. In the end, the vaunted therapeutic
properties of Koch's tuberculin turned out to be illusory, although the local immune reaction produced by its subcutaneous injection became a precious tool for diagnosing latent
tubercular infection.

Although in this period Golgi's activity focused mostly on infectious diseases, he had not
stopped his neurohistological research. He continued to fine tune the mercury dichloride
method, which had already been improved by Mondino. He presented details of the newly
perfected reaction to the Società Medico-Chirurgica,[39] which was by now his preferred
outlet for the preliminary report of his findings. Furthermore, in another attempt to
re-establish his scientific pre-eminence in neurohistology, he published a substantial
German summary of *Sulla fina anatomia* in 1891 in *Zeitschrift für wissenschaftliche Zoologie*.[40]

Golgi and Kölliker continued their correspondence. On 11 March 1891 Kölliker asked his
colleague if he had received the latest work by Retzius on the nervous system of crusta-
ceans, adding 'Very important'.[41] Golgi had undoubtedly read it, but obviously had not
shared its neuronistic position. Kölliker was particularly obsessed with the problem of the
nervous connections in the olfactory bulbs (in particular in the glomeruli) about which, as
we have seen, he had already requested Golgi's explicit opinion. If one accepted, as Cajal
had suggested, that the nerve impulse is transmitted to the dendrites of the mitral cells
from the fibres arising in the olfactory mucosa, it would be easy to explain the particular
relationships between nerve cells at the level of the glomeruli. On the contrary, to explain
how the nerve signals could pass from the olfactory fibres to the higher nervous centres,
Golgi would have to invoke (on the basis of axonal anastomoses) the existence of ascending collaterals arising from the axons of small periglomerular cells and from the fibres
arising in the olfactory tract. But Kölliker maintained strong doubts about the existence
of these collaterals that had been described only by Golgi. The connections within the
glomeruli, like those of the basket cells of the cerebellum, became the critical test of the
explanatory power of the diffuse neural net theory versus the neuron theory. Thus Kölliker

questioned Golgi 'on the critical point':[42] if, as maintained by Golgi, the connections by continuity within the glomeruli were assured on one side by fibres coming from the olfactory mucosa and on the other by ascending axon collaterals, then what function could the mitral cells have? We do not know Golgi's answer. The discussion demonstrates how Kölliker probed Golgi with pertinent questions formulated in such a way as to highlight incongruities of the reticularist theory. But, as far as one knows, Golgi never showed any softening of his position against the theory of the neuron. His conceptual framework could not move beyond the theory of the diffuse neural net.

During brief interludes in his neurohistological studies, Golgi also investigated the structures of other tissues. Indeed, he had realized many years before that the range of applications of the black reaction extended beyond neurobiology. For example, he had used it to stain hepatic preparations for his histology classes. The black reaction allowed the visualization of the network of biliary intralobular canaliculi. In the early 1890s, after the extraordinary results obtained with the nervous system, researchers began to use the black reaction on other tissues: Cajal and Retzius studied liver, salivary glands and pancreas; Fusari, Sala, and van Gehuchten investigated the structure of some types of glands; Carlo Martinotti demonstrated elastic fibres; and Vitige Tirelli studied the structure of the bone. Since the black reaction revealed the details of the excretory ducts of some exocrine glands, Golgi decided to use it on the glands of the rabbit stomach. In the external portions of the cytoplasm of the parietal cells of the stomach he discovered an extraordinary reticular system of canaliculi, which converged in an excretory duct. In some preparations Golgi found 'formations that make me think that the reticular apparatus occupies the entire cell body, with the sole exclusion of a region immediately around the nucleus.'[43] The degree of dilation of this canalicular system was maximal during digestion. Golgi 'was already for some time in possession of preparations demonstrating this delicate uniqueness of structure but had put off publishing these findings, aspiring to obtain always greater perfection.'[44] Just as he was about to publish a brief report with seven drawings (two by Luigi Villa), he became aware of a recently published work by the Swedish scientist Erik Müller, who had obtained analogous results applying the black reaction to the peptic glands. Since Golgi's research had the added feature of demonstrating modifications in the size of the canaliculi in relationship to digestion, he decided nevertheless to publish it. On 25 February 1893 he presented his findings and demonstrated his preparations to the Società Medico-Chirurgica.[45] The day before, he had received a letter from Retzius full of compliments.[46] He thanked Golgi for having sent him the work on the olfactory bulbs and added: 'You already did everything in 1875!' And then he gave his Pavian colleague full credit for having produced, with his work on the central nervous system, 'a revolution in this extremely difficult field of biology', which had not yet received proper recognition and still found strong opposition. Then Retzius continued, 'From now on you are the winner' and thanks to your method 'victorious; science will certainly be able to progress for a long time.'

But this revolution bore perverse fruit that greatly worried Golgi. On 11 June 1892, Golgi presented a brief paper on rabies to the Società Medico-Chirurgica.[47] In examining the brain of a patient who had died of rabies, he found in the mesencephalon an area with nerve cells lacking dendrites. These cells were globular, roundish, and fusiform with a granular cytoplasm and a nucleus that was displaced toward the origin of the axon, which presented circumscribed swellings. This region, which some ascribed to the descending root of the fifth cranial nerve (trigeminal) was instead, according to Golgi, the nucleus of the origin of the fourth (trochlear). The cell types that he described are, however, typical of the mesencephalic nucleus of the trigeminal nerve and it is possible that he was fooled by the complexity of the region he was studying.[48] In fact, the nucleus of the mesencephalic root of the trigeminal is composed of pseudo-unipolar neurons that are similar in appearance to those of the sensory dorsal ganglia. This is probably the only case in vertebrates in which sensory proto-neurons are found within the central nervous system.

The observation of the lack of dendrites in these cells was not discussed in this paper on rabies because Golgi decided that it deserved a separate study. The following year he used this finding in a heavy attack on the theory of the neuron and the law of dynamic polarization.

After reiterating his ideas on the functions of the protoplasmic processes, which for Golgi were implicated in the nutrition of the nerve cells, he continued:

So far, no one has demonstrated that my arguments are groundless or that my findings are illusory; despite this, there is now strenuous opposition to my hypothesis, which, in my judgement, is based more on doctrinal conceptions than on new proven facts.[49]

And what these doctrinal conceptions might be was clarified by him soon thereafter:

These conceptions have been summarized by Ramón y Cajal under the name of the theory of dynamic polarization of nervous cells. According to this theory, the protoplasmic processes would form the apparatuses of perception or reception, and the cylindraxis processes [would form] the apparatuses of transmission of the nerve excitation.[50]

Instead,

even in anatomical studies, given a series of new well-established data, it is not only opportune but also necessary that the researcher try, by analysing them in a synthetic manner and correlating them with other findings, to formulate laws and doctrinal conceptions of general value; however, a fundamental and absolutely necessary prerequisite for all this is that the laws formulated and the doctrinal conceptions elaborated be in harmony with facts, or a true emanation of them.[51]

And he continued, almost in a fit of rage:

But when I see that, through a completely inverse process, one creates a theory to fit the anatomical data; when I observe that, in the service of the theory, one even modifies the facts that have already been demonstrated and that, with little effort, one could verify; when ... it is affirmed that the most typical cylindraxes of the nervous fibres are nothing but protoplasmic processes of exceptional length, daring to identify in these same cylindraxes the morphological characteristics of the protoplasmic processes [Golgi is referring here to studies attributing a dendritic nature to the peripheral branch of the 'T' cells of the dorsal sensory ganglion]: and all of this because according to the theory, the cylindraxial processes, having only *cellular–fugal* conductivity, could not be the apparatuses of *reception*, while one cannot avoid attributing a conductivity in the opposite direction to those nervous fibres, because they are sensory; when, I say, I find myself faced with this behaviour, then for the respect that I owe the methods and criteria of the science of observation, I must ask if this is really doing anatomy or rather exercising imagination.[51]

And finally, considering the cells without dendrites:

if they lack the apparatus of reception, indispensable for the theory [of the neuron], one doesn't understand how, by means of these cells, the cycle of the cellular–petal and cellular–fugal nervous currents can be carried out.[52]

Quod erat demonstrandum.

Golgi then raised another argument against the idea of nervous transmission by contact. For several years he had been proposing that nerve cells could have a neurokeratinic sheath, characterized by a substance that could be stained with the same procedure used to stain horny tissues.[53] Now he returned to the fray, sustaining that such a sheath, by isolating the cell, would impede the passage of the nerve impulse required by the theory of contact.

Then, he couldn't help but make a cutting remark against Obersteiner's statement that he had used the black reaction but could not identify the axon with precision. 'That only proves' wrote Golgi, 'that Obersteiner has not yet managed to obtain good preparations.'[54]

Golgi's criticism of the law of dynamic polarization, although apparently convincing, was easily countered. Both Cajal and van Gehuchten considered the cell body to be part of the reception apparatus of the nerve impulse, even though in their earliest formulation of the law of dynamic polarization they had not stated this explicitly. Thus, even in the absence of dendrites, *contact* could occur on the cell body. Subsequent studies have demonstrated that the cells of the mesencephalic roots of the trigeminal nerve connect both with the periphery and with neighbouring cells in a manner similar to the 'T' cells of the dorsal sensory ganglia.

Golgi reported his findings to the Società Medico-Chirurgica on 29 April 1893,[55] but wishing to give a greater exposure to his argument decided to communicate them also to the Academia dei Lincei;[56] then he also published a French version in the *Archives Italiennes de Biologie.*[57]

Meanwhile, the file on malaria was still open. At the beginning of 1892, Pietro Albertoni, a physiologist at the University of Bologna and Golgi's friend, asked him to test the therapeutic properties of phenocoll hydrochloride in malaria because it had been suggested that this antipyretic medication might have therapeutic properties in this infection. Golgi was the best person for this kind of study, not only because he was able to carry out clinical trials in his ward but also because he had the equipment and knowledge to study the developmental cycle of the *Plasmodium* in the blood of the patients. He began to administer the drug to seven patients in his and Silva's wards. Phenocoll hydrochloride proved to have no anti-parasitic action even in high doses, although its antipyretic effect was confirmed. As usual, Golgi presented the results to the Società Medico-Chirurgica, on 28 May 1892.[58]

Golgi's clinical–haematological characterization of tertian and quartan malarial fevers and of their combinations was in accord with a vast international consensus. However, there were many clinical forms of malaria that did not match these classical schemes. Golgi had already interpreted some of them as malarial fevers of long intervals characterized by the presence of crescents. But the Roman School of Marchiafava had underscored the atypical clinical and parasitological features of the fevers that predominated in the summer and autumn months in and around Rome, compared to the classical forms described by Golgi. In these areas the infection often consisted of febrile cycles similar to the tertian form but with a more severe course; the paroxysms tended to worsen and increase in frequency in such a way as to produce in many cases a continuous fever; moreover, the parasites were smaller, less mobile, and less pigmented than in classical tertian and they were rarely found in blood during their reproductive phase. Sometimes one could observe the crescents in the blood smear. Marchiafava believed that among the summer–autumn fevers there was a variant with daily attacks and so he named the two putative forms of the parasite *Amoeba febris quotidiana* and *Amoeba febris tertianae aestivo autunnalis*, respectively. The blood of these patients contained few parasites and, only rarely, segmentation forms in the red cells. Sometimes, in the blood of patients affected by summer–autumn tertian, one could see brass-coloured red blood cells, that is, wrinkled red cells having an 'old gold' colour (whereas in the classical tertian the red blood cells are swollen and pale). To explain the small number of segmentation forms, Marchiafava suggested that during the repro-duction of the parasite, the red blood cells, for purely mechanical reasons, remain trapped and sequestered in the capillaries of the internal organs. In conclusion, Marchiafava thought that the developmental cycles of the two types of parasites occurred in the red blood cells, as in the classical forms described by Golgi, whereas the reproduction cycles occurred in the internal organs.

The existence of atypical quotidian and tertian clinical forms of the summer–autumn fevers was contested by Baccelli, who questioned the periodicity of 24 and 48 hours and maintained that the course of the fever was entirely irregular. His own clinical studies in-dicated that there was no relationship whatsoever between the febrile bout and the number of micro-organisms in the peripheral blood; sometimes the patient even died without any *Plasmodium* in the blood at all. On the contrary, for the classical tertian and quartan forms, in 1892 Baccelli had, by inoculating healthy subjects, experimentally confirmed Golgi's theory that the different types of fevers corresponded to different parasitic varieties. Baccelli injected one individual with the blood taken from a patient with the quartan fever and another with the blood of a patient affected by double tertian; both donors under-went a detailed haematological examination that confirmed the clinical diagnoses. In the first recipient, a classical quartan fever developed after 12 days; in the second, a double tertian developed after 7 days. In both cases the blood examination confirmed the clinical form.

In Pavia, Golgi saw almost exclusively classical forms of tertian, quartan, and their combinations, but he was extremely interested in learning more about the fevers prevail-ing in the surroundings of Rome and therefore requested the hospitality of Baccelli at Santo Spirito Hospital. And thus, eight years after his first trip to Santo Spirito to visit Marchiafava and Celli, he returned for a period of study in the Capital, guest of Baccelli, who was also an influential politician. Golgi's stay extended into the summer–autumn of 1893. It is certain that Golgi was in Rome in the second half of July and then in the month of September. He had as collaborators the internists Rossoni and Taussig, and Giuseppe Bastianelli for autopsies.

Golgi decided that the malarial fevers could be subdivided into: (1) fevers associated with parasites that develop mainly in the blood; and (2) fevers caused by parasites that develop mainly in the internal organs.

In the first category he included the classical tertian and quartan forms plus their combinations, which, as we know, are caused by parasites that complete their developmental cycle in two (*Amoeba febris tertianae*) and three (*Amoeba febris quartanae*) days. In the second category he included irregular fevers caused by the localization of the *Plasmodia* in the internal organs, where they can be found in different phases of development and from which arise the few parasites found in the blood. Independently of the haematological findings, the splenic biopsy in these cases demonstrated the presence of parasites in more or less advanced stages of development. In cases in which the patient had died, the post-mortem examination showed also intestinal and cerebral localization. Relative to the classical tertian and quartan forms, these forms were associated with a developmental cycle localized exclusively to internal organs and very resistant to quinine. This group also included the forms characterized by long intervals between fever bouts and by the presence of the crescents. Such forms were (and in some parts still are) characteristic of the areas where 'during the hottest months . . . malaria has its greatest intensity and virulence (Roman countryside, pontine marshes, Maremma Toscana, some areas of Apulia, Basilicata, Sicily, Sardinia, Algeria, Caucase, many regions of America, etc., etc.)'. Naturally, even in the regions 'in which malaria is usually mild, it cannot be excluded that, under special circumstances, forms that belong to this group can appear.'[59] And in fact, even in Pavia, where classical tertian and quartan forms prevailed, one could sometimes observe irregular forms with crescents. In this way Golgi provided a pathogenic interpretation of Baccelli's clinical observations; in the summer–autumn forms, the development of the parasite occurred in the internal organs (primarily in the spleen and bone marrow); sometimes a modest quantity of these parasites could invade the circulatory blood stream, hence their rarity in the blood and the lack of correlation with the clinical symptoms.

As soon as he got back in Pavia, Golgi wrote an extensive paper, completed in October 1893 and titled 'On summer–autumn malarial fevers of Rome', with the subtitle 'Letter to Prof. Guido Baccelli'.[60] With this work Golgi concluded his investigations on the clinical pathology of malaria. However, the problem of the relationship between the disease and the environment of swamps remained unresolved and the route of transmission of the disease was also still unknown. Golgi was undoubtedly interested in these problems, 'possibly he also conducted some experiments, without telling anyone about them',[61] but the solution arrived some years later, thanks especially to Giovanni Battista Grassi, Golgi's first pupil in the Laboratory of General Pathology.

Notes

1. Detti (1987, p. 39).
2. Tirelli (1918, p. 188).
3. *Ibid.* (p. 186).
4. Martinotti (1889).
5. Martinotti (1890).

6. DeFelipe and Jones (1988, pp. 587ff.).
7. Medea (1966, p. 4).
8. Golgi and Bizzozero were important players in the committees for the appointment of Professors in General Pathology, Histology, and Pathological Anatomy (and to a lesser extent of Hygiene, Forensic Medicine, Pharmacology, and Neuropsychiatry) and in the choice of members of the High Council for Public Education and of the High Council for Public Health. Golgi, who was Chief Physician *ad honorem* in the San Matteo Hospital was also a member of the committee for the appointment of the chief physicians. The letters from Bizzozero to Golgi in the MSUP contain (in passing) frequent references to competitions, with requests for help in supporting a certain candidate, discussion of feuds and alliances in Italian academia, etc. The two scientists almost always agreed on which candidates deserved their support. Golgi was less diplomatic and perhaps less even-minded than his Turin colleague, as indicated by letters kept in the MSUP. An example is the following passage from a letter that Bizzozero wrote on 10 June 1897: 'Dear Camillo, I have written to some colleagues about the committees for [the appointment of Professors in] Forensic Medicine, Anatomy, Hygiene, and Pharmacology, of which you have provided me with the names of the members. In Pharmacology you have provided me with two less than what is needed, and I put down for one of these the name of [Piero] Giacosa. As for Pathological Anatomy, I could not approve [your list], because from my perspective this list has two defects: it contains my name, and I do not intend to join the committee, because in this periods I feel more than ever the need to rest, and in the second place in the committee [list you proposed] the majority [of names are those of] Professors of General Pathology, and this I find to be an excess that will damage the success of the committee, and it will not look good among colleagues. Two years ago we complained because the anatomo-pathologists had tried to rule in our committee [that is, the committee appointing professors in General Pathology], and now we don't want to commit the same sin'.
9. Pensa (1991, p. 67).
10. *Ibid.* (p. 65).
11. *Ibid.* (p. 69).
12. Medea (1966, p. 3 *bis*).
13. Medea (1918, p. 453).
14. Pensa (1991, p. 70).
15. Arcieri (1952, p. 189).
16. Pensa (1991, pp. 64ff.).
17. *Ibid.* (p. 66).
18. *Ibid.* (p. 160).
19. *Ibid.* (p. 174).
20. Veratti (1926, p. 3).
21. *Ibid.* (p. 4).
22. The comments of Grocco are taken from the *Gazzetta Medica Lombarda* (Anno LXVI, 6 January 1908, p. 2).
23. Pensa (1926, p. 13).
24. Rossi (1927, p. 17).
25. *Ibid.* (p. 16).
26. Cited in Cosmacini (1989, pp. 104ff.).
27. Medea (1918, p. 454).
28. For some testimonials to this tendency see, for example, Perroncito (1926, p. 38) and Rondoni (1943, p. 544).

29. Rossi (1927, p. 15).

30. The original draft is in the author's possession (a gift of Dr Giuseppe Raimondi).

31. Medea (1966, p. 5).

32. *Rendiconti R. Istituto Lombardo di Scienze e Lettere* (1890, **23**, pp. 53–7). The Commission, composed of Biffi, Zoja, and Golgi (who was Chair), awarded the first prize of 2000 lire to Vittorio Marchi. A cheque of encouragement of 500 lire was awarded to the second-place winner Giovanni Mingazzini.

33. *Gazzetta degli Ospitali* (1890, **11**, pp. 783–4).

34. Golgi and Silva (1891, pp. 11ff.).

35. Pensa (1991, p. 71).

36. *Gazzetta degli Ospitali* (1890, **11**, pp. 805–6). The reference to the experiments of Golgi, Silva, and Monti is on p. 807. See also *La Provincia Pavese* (21–3 November 1890; 17 December 1890; 4, 6, 11, 18, and 22 February 1891).

37. Golgi (1891h).

38. On 12 July 1891 Golgi and Silva reported on 'Eight months of experience in the antitubercular cure with the linfa of Koch' to the Società Medico-Chirurgica. *Bollettino della Società Medico-Chirurgica di Pavia* (1891) No. 2, p. 59. The text, distributed to the members, was not published in the *Bollettino* but it was printed in the *Riforma Medica* with a slightly different title (Golgi and Silva 1891).

39. Golgi (1891).

40. Golgi (1891i).

41. Letter No. 10 from Kölliker to Golgi, 11 March 1891 (Belloni 1975, p. 170).

42. Letter No. 11 from Kölliker to Golgi, 14 April 1891 (Belloni 1975, p. 171).

43. Golgi (1893; *OO*, p. 615).

44. Veratti (1926, p. 10).

45. Golgi (1893). The work was then translated into French (Golgi 1893a).

46. Letter from Retzius to Golgi, 24 February 1893 (MSUP-VII-III-15).

47. Golgi (1892d).

48. Golgi's error was revealed in the scientific literature in the following years. See for example Marinesco (1909, p. 459).

49. Golgi (1893b; *OO*, p. 637).

50. *Ibid.* (*OO*, p. 638).

51. *Ibid.* (*OO*, p. 639).

52. *Ibid.* (*OO*, p. 639ff.).

53. Golgi (1885, p. 178).

54. Golgi (1893b; *OO* p. 636).

55. Golgi (1893b).

56. Golgi (1893c).

57. Golgi (1893d).

58. Golgi (1892c).

59. Golgi (1893e; *OO*, p. 1234).

60. Golgi (1893e). The work was then translated into French (Golgi 1894) and summarized in German in the *Deutsche Medicinische Wochenschrift* (Golgi 1894a). The latter edition was the object of two handwritten letters to Golgi from Albert Eulenburg, editor of the journal. They are kept in MSUP (Belloni 1978b, p. 38).

61. Veratti (1942–43, p. 102).

18

The threat from Milan

On 4 November 1893, Golgi read the official opening address for the academic year 1893–94, as the new Rector of the University of Pavia. His election had been bitterly opposed by the members of the old guard, such as Sangalli, who were jealous of their power and prerogatives. Golgi was the leading exponent of that generation of 'progressive' middle-aged academics who were called 'Young Turks' by the students[1] because of their aggressive assault on the key positions within the University.

But Golgi had his eyes on other sources of power as well. In the municipal election of 17 December 1893 he was elected to the City Council of Pavia on the moderate slate. From this position he could manoeuvre to further the interests of his beloved University.

In 1893 Pavia was a drowsy city of about 38 000 inhabitants, in a province of about 500 000. Among the 900 workers who participated in the foundation of the local trade union in 1893 were 113 porters (the most numerous category) and 104 bakers. The most important industrial plant was that of the Genio Militare [Army Corps of Engineers], which employed 120 workers. There was also the mechanic shop of Ambrogio Necchi, which would later grow into an important maker of electromechanical appliances.[2] Agriculture was the main economic activity of the province. Every now and then the turmoil of national politics would reach Pavia, but the absence of a true industrial workforce shielded it from the most violent forms of social unrest. The most important newspaper was *La Provincia Pavese*, founded in 1880 as the official organ of the Republican Party in Pavia; after 1893 its orientation moved leftward. Despite the small number of factory workers, the Socialist Party was an important political force in the City and in the province. In 1893 the Pavian Socialists presented an independent ticket in the municipal elections (which they did not win), and in 1890 they founded a newspaper, *La Plebe*, which three years later became their official organ. The Socialists found support among the peasants, artisans, progressive bourgeoisie, and young academics. Two of Golgi's Assistants, Monti and Sala, were members of the Socialist Party, and they were often visited in the laboratory by two influential comrades, Luigi Majno, Professor of Criminal Law in the University of Pavia Law School, and his wife, Ersilia Bronzini.

Pavia had two theatres: Teatro Fraschini, for the Opera, and Teatro Guidi, for lighter forms of entertainment. Although plagued by audiences of rowdy students, the Guidi boasted among its artists such celebrated actors as Ermete Zacconi and Eleonora Duse.

A number of inexpensive restaurants and cafes provided other popular hangouts for the students. The meeting point for the Pavian upper class was 'Demetrio', an elegant café with grand mirrors in gilded frames, coloured stucco decorations, and red velvet couches. It was located near the University, and in the afternoon and evening it became the meeting point for local dignitaries, professionals, and academics. There one might meet the eccentric explorer−ethnologist Luigi Robecchi-Bricchetti and his pet lion cub, in the company of Mabruc, the African youth he had freed from slavery and adopted.

The fraternities of university students ('goliardic groups') were very active, involved in the most reckless pranks and buffoonery. An accessory in the escapades of the 'goliards' was Luigi Violini, who was known as Professor Roma after his participation in a carnival parade on the theme *The Triumph of Rome*. Although completely illiterate, he used to attire himself in the guise of a university professor: hat, black suit, bow tie, and a pile of books and newspapers under his arm. He made a somewhat precarious living by selling lecture notes, falsifying class attendance records of the students, procuring lodgings, lending money with interest, etc. One of the preferred pranks of the students was to introduce him at scientific meetings as an 'illustrious professor'; he was once passed off as a physician and paraded through the wards of the hospital to visit the patients. For this he was charged by the authorities but not prosecuted.

The University, with its central position, dominated the life of the city. In the academic year 1893−94 there were 1245 students distributed among the various schools. As Rector, Golgi threw himself wholeheartedly into reorganizing the curriculum and giving more prominence to the institutes that were carrying out high-level research.

When Golgi took over the Rectorship a sword of Damocles had been hanging over the University for some months. On 2 March 1893 an engineer named Siro Valerio had died, leaving his estate to the City of Milan to constitute a 'fund to serve for the foundation or transfer to Milan of a university for the study of science, or at least of some of its branches, and in the first place, preferably, of a Medical School that, in my opinion, could find in our hospitals more receptive, diversified and numerous facilities for teaching and for clinical and anatomical studies.'[3] With lightning speed, on 8 March Luigi Mangiagalli, Chief Gynaecologist of the Ospedale Maggiore, the largest hospital of Milan, called for an assembly of the Medical Association of Lombardy, which he chaired, to approve a resolution in favour of the rapid 'establishment of an Institute for advanced biomedical studies, or of clinical institutes, or of clinics that complement medical−surgical specialties'.

The news threw the University of Pavia into a panic. The creation of a second university at a distance of a few tens of kilometres was bound to weaken the University of Pavia or even threaten its very survival, not just because of the predictable siphoning off of students, but also because the richer and politically powerful Milan would inevitably devour its lesser neighbour. Indeed, the news was immediately perceived as a threat by the professors, such as Golgi, most solidly rooted in the Pavian academic tradition; on the contrary, it was welcomed with some satisfaction by those who had strong links with Milan. Carlo Cantoni, who was Rector at the time, called for a meeting of the faculty Senate to approve a resolution arguing that without the approval of an ad hoc law, one could not establish a university school having the right to confer academic degrees, and that the establishment of isolated schools was always damaging to the progress of scholarship. This resolution received ministerial approval, and the crisis appeared to be averted. But soon after Golgi became Rector, he rekindled the concern for the creation of a university in Milan, stating that although the issue had been momentarily resolved, it 'could easily arise again as a *fait accompli*' because of a 'change in material conditions' (such as, for example, additional funding for the establishment of a university in Milan)'. To avert the occurrence of events that could represent a threat to our University', he thought that the University needed 'to be watchful and prepared', increasing its level of scientific output, and providing 'sufficient means for the study of all scientific disciplines',[4] thus making the creation of another academic institution unnecessary.

From this point of view, the strengthening of the University touched upon the prickly problem of Palazzo Botta, a problem that Golgi had inherited from the previous Rector. On 26 December 1886, the national Parliament had passed a law providing for the relocation of the Institute of Anatomy and Comparative Physiology and the Institute of Human Anatomy into this grand historic building, which had hosted Napoleon, among others. The vast halls of Palazzo Botta were perfectly suited to housing these Institutes' important collections of specimens and other scientific materials, some of which dated back to the time of Scarpa. But the sheer vastness of Palazzo Botta stimulated the appetites of many institute directors, including Golgi, whose laboratories were in a sorry state. Thus, despite Cantoni's efforts, the reorganization of the new building was hampered by countless squabbles among the professors fighting for the lion's share of Palazzo Botta. Moreover, there were a number of problems with the contractors carrying out the renovation. The Minister of Public Instruction had established that the University could take possession of the building only after a successful technical inspection. However, owing to a combination of bureaucratic and legal complications the contractors were delaying completion of the work. When Golgi became Rector, the situation had come to a standstill because it was clear that 'having the matter now enter a legal phase, no amount of pressure [on the contractors] would abbreviate the period of time [allowed for the law suit] before the government mandates that the work be completed.'[5]

These matters were heatedly discussed by the students and faculty alike. In addition, just before the Christmas vacation, the buildings of the Botanical Gardens ran out of heating fuel. The dominant feeling was 'Enough is enough! We need to begin the transfer to Palazzo Botta; all the rest will be achieved later'.[6] Some professors, such as Zoja of Anatomy and Leopoldo Maggi of Comparative Anatomy and Physiology, pushed hard for the move, maintaining that the 1886 law gave them pre-emptive rights, and invited the students to plead their cause before the Rector. When the student delegation, of which Pensa was a member, sought an audience with the Rector, they discovered that Golgi had unexpectedly left for Rome to seek the necessary authorization for the transfer. Before leaving, however, he had dropped several hints that a move on the sly wouldn't surprise him or be unwelcome. And so his Assistants decided to confront the authorities with a *fait accompli*. On a snowy night in early January 1894, a few young men, hired by Monti at the local trade union headquarters, loaded all the apparatuses, furniture, and materials of the Laboratory of General Pathology onto carts under the uncertain light of acetylene lamps, and moved into Palazzo Botta. The next day, in Rome, Golgi received a telegram from Pavia announcing the coup. Probably 'he did not lose his composure or show surprise and . . . he probably smiled to himself'.[6] The next day he showed the telegram to the Minister of Public Education, beseeching him to approve the relocation of his laboratory and of the other institutes. Finally, and most importantly, he asked for additional research funding. An investigating commission, led by Bizzozero, who in 1890 had become Senator, regularized the move.

Meanwhile, in the enormous rooms of Palazzo Botta the occupants were freezing; there was no water, electricity, or gas. It took several days before the taps finally began to spit intermittent jets of murky water. Soon thereafter two large heaters and the gas furnace were turned on, and a technician from the Institute of Physics began wiring the building. Palazzo Botta was buried under the unrelenting snowfall; but in its large rooms the new Institute of General Pathology and Histology was being born.

Golgi returned from Rome, charged by the Ministry of Internal Affairs and by the Department of Health to organize in his Institute one of the first Italian facilities for the production of anti-diphtheria serum. He accepted this burden because he saw in it an opportunity for new funding from the State and other sources.

At the end of January he was able to subdue a student uprising that had degenerated into such serious riots that the University had to be shut down temporarily. Not for the first (or last) time, the students were protesting against provisions to reduce the number of exam sessions during the year. Golgi's ability to find a way out of situations of this kind would become legendary.

The cunning with which Golgi's associates had effected the move into Palazzo Botta and the subsequent approval of the move by the Bizzozero Commission obviously triggered Maggi's resentment. He thought that he had been defrauded, and with good reason. Not only had the Laboratory of General Pathology preceded all others in the transfer, but it had occupied parts of the building that the initial plan had assigned to his Institute of Comparative Anatomy and Physiology. And now there was word that the Institutes of Hygiene, Pharmacology, and other institutes, would transfer ahead of him. His heated protest was printed and delivered to the Minister of Public Education, the Rector, and various provincial and municipal authorities.[7] He hoped to elicit a favourable reaction, but 'there was no response' to his denunciation, which was met with a 'sepulchral silence'.[8] Golgi was sufficiently discerning to understand that rather than dealing directly with Maggi's protest, it was better to let the matter dissipate by itself.

On 8 December 1893, Kölliker wrote to Golgi that the University of Würzburg Medical School had unanimously awarded him the prestigious Rinecker Prize. The Prize was dedicated to the memory of Franz Rinecker, an influential member of the medical faculty of Würzburg, and had been established by his son a few years before. It was awarded every three years to a pre-eminent scientist in the biomedical field; Koch had been the first recipient in 1891. For 1894 the Prize was supposed to go to an anatomist and, as Kölliker wrote to Golgi on 8 December 1893, 'we found no one worthier than you, my dear friend, who contributed so very much to the progress of fine anatomy of the nervous system with your discoveries and your work.'[9] The Prize consisted of 1000 silver marks and a medal with Rinecker's profile. Golgi was officially informed of the honour on 2 January 1894 by Adolf Fick, Dean of the Medical School and Professor of Physiology. Kölliker sent the anatomist Giulio Chiarugi, Director of *Monitore Zoologico Italiano*, a note to inform Italian biologists of the news.[10] Golgi replied to Kölliker, thanking him ('I have no doubt that your initiative and your vote had the greatest weight in those deliberations') and the medical faculty of Würzburg for the honour received, which 'for me represents the greatest of the honours and the most important prize to which a scholar might aspire'.[11] He also expressed his gratitude for the great prominence given to his work in the second volume (dealing with the nervous system) of the sixth edition of Kölliker's handbook of histology.

At about the same time Golgi received an important recognition for his studies on malaria. On 5 January 1894 the prestigious Riberi Prize was conferred on him by the Academy of Medicine of Turin,[12] to which Golgi had sent his first communication on malaria describing the correlation between the bout of fever and the 'segmentation' of the plasmodium. The prize of 20 000 lire (a magnificent sum at the time) had been established to honour the Torinese surgeon Alessandro Riberi, who in 1847 had been the first in Italy to use ether anaesthesia, followed by Porta in Pavia. The Prize, which had been given seven times previously, was intended for a scientist who had done outstanding work on the nature and prophylaxis of human infectious diseases. Golgi had participated in the Riberi competition at the request of Bizzozero. Among the members of the adjudicating commission was Mosso, who had a chance to make up for his superficial criticisms of Golgi's pathogenic theory of the malarial bout. There were eight other contestants, among which the most dangerous was Laveran. In the end Golgi prevailed thanks also to a stipulation of the Riberi Prize that only research done after 1886 would be considered. Laveran had in fact made his discovery of the aetiology of malaria in 1880 and his work after 1886 was certainly less important than Golgi's. Thus, in the same year, Golgi's work on both neuro-anatomy and malaria received prestigious international recognition. There is little doubt that, besides the honour, Golgi appreciated the monetary aspect of these prizes, which was quite an financial boost for a physician who refused to have a private practice and lived only on his faculty salary. Another recognition of great international prestige came from the United States: the Medical School of Harvard University awarded him the Elizabeth Thompson Grant for 1893–94.[13]

The controversy between neuronism and reticularism, and Kölliker's solicitations to make his work better known abroad, had convinced Golgi to publish a comprehensive treatise of his neuroanatomical and neurohistological work in German. In early 1894 the enterprise was almost completed. Kölliker wrote Golgi that Fick and the entire Medical School 'would be very proud if you would mention it [the Medical School] in your preface'.[14] Golgi went well beyond this modest request and dedicated the entire treatise to the Medical School of Würzburg. The book consisted of a comprehensive collection of Golgi's papers on the structure of the central and peripheral nervous systems, translated by R. Teuscher. It included also the work by Rezzonico on the horny funnels and was complemented by a rich atlas of 30 plates.[15]

In March, Marchiafava and Amico Bignami published an article on the summer–autumn fevers in the journal *Il Policlinico*, containing a blistering attack on Golgi. Marchiafava claimed priority for most of the observations contained in Golgi's 'letter' to Baccelli and argued that the difference between their studies concerned some clinical–pathological interpretations. He had been stung by the fact that the most important fruits of his work on malaria would be harvested by Golgi. As we have seen, it was in fact true that Golgi had begun his research on malaria in Marchiafava's laboratory in Rome. Owing in part to the prevalence of simpler and more regular forms of malaria in Pavia, Golgi had been able to make fundamental progress in clarifying the aetiopathogenesis of the disease. And now, after having been in Rome and having studied those complicated forms of malaria that Marchiafava had investigated for many years, Golgi was asserting that Marchiafava's identification of two clinical–pathological varieties (quotidian and tertian) of the summer–autumn fevers was a fluke. It is not surprising that Marchiafava was incensed by Golgi's 'impertinence'.

In the spring of that year, the Italian medical establishment was electrified by a yearly event that monopolized the attention of the world's physicians and biologists. In the week between 29 March and 5 April the Eleventh International Medical Congress was held in Rome. Kölliker had initially considered participating in order to 'be able to greet my numerous Italian friends and colleagues, especially you [that is, Golgi] and Bizzozero' but because of his poor health, including an attack of gout some months before, in the end decided not expose himself 'for an entire week to the inconveniences and fatigue of the sessions, workshops, dinners, suppers, shows, etc., etc.'[16]

Rome had been previously proposed as the site for the Second International Medical Congress in 1869, but because of the opposition of the Holy See, which had feared the political implications, it was held instead in Florence. This time it was finally Rome's turn. Baccelli, who was also a powerful politician and minister in the government of Francesco Crispi, was designated President of the Congress; Bizzozero was one of the three Vice-Presidents, and among the members of the executive committee there were Golgi, Marchiafava, Celli, and Mosso. The Congress was organized into sections. Golgi participated in the sections of General Pathology and of Anatomy, chaired by Bizzozero. The official opening ceremony was held in the Costanzi Theatre on 29 March in the presence of Their Royal Highnesses, with speeches by Crispi, Baccelli (in Latin), the Mayor of Rome, and Virchow, who had been the President of the previous congress in Berlin, and who read a speech of welcome in Italian, to the applause of the audience.[17]

There were a number of invited lectures, including the celebrated lecture by Bizzozero on the classification of tissues into stable, labile, and everlasting; a memorable one by Virchow on Morgagni; and one by Cajal on the morphology of nerve cells. The Spaniard was on the committee of the anatomy section chaired by Francesco Todaro. We do not know whether he and Golgi met, or, as is more likely, ignored one another. (A few weeks later Kölliker wrote Golgi to thank him for dedicating his book on the nervous system to the Medical School of Würzburg and asked about the Congress and about Cajal: 'Was Ramón in Rome, did he speak?',[18] but there is no record of a reply from Golgi. Cajal himself, so detailed in describing anecdotal aspects of his life in *Recuerdos*, barely mentioned the Congress in Rome.)[19]

On 3 April, Golgi participated in the discussion following Charles Marie Debierre's presentation on the anatomy of the limbic lobe,[20] in which Golgi's observations of a decade before were fully confirmed. But his interest was focused on Marchiafava's presentation on the summer–autumn fevers planned for the next day in the general pathology section. In his presentation,[21] Marchiafava toned down his criticisms of Golgi. Indeed, he admitted now that the summer–autumn fevers were never completely regular. He maintained, however, that behind the apparent irregularities it was possible to identify two types of febrile course: quotidian (24-hour cycle) and malignant tertian (48-hour cycle); he then confirmed the accumulation of the parasites in the internal organs during the reproductive phase. At the end of the presentation Golgi took the floor and pointed out how, according to Marchiafava, 'the parasites that we find localized in various organs (spleen, intestine, bone marrow, etc.) appear to be parasites that, having completed their cycle in the circulating blood in a period of 24 or 48 hours, ended up in these organs, where they rapidly carry out their cycle up to reproduction.' Instead, according to Golgi, the parasites that are found 'in the different phases of development within the internal organs are found there because that is where they primarily complete their cycle'.[22] In this way he was able to explain why severe cases of malaria could be coupled with the presence of few parasites in the blood.

Golgi's presentation to the Congress concerned the pathological histology of rabies,[23] a topic on which he had been working for some years and about which, in that same April, he had published a full report in a German journal.[24] He maintained that this disease leaves histopathological signs that, if correctly investigated, are very indicative: a structural alteration of the nucleus, modifications in the shape of the nerve cell body, and alterations of the fine structure of the intervertebral ganglia. His insistence on this topic demonstrated his evident desire to discover something of real pathognomical significance in the disease. Interestingly, Golgi published his last work on rabies in the same year that Konrad Zenker and Gustav Mann, respectively, developed the fixative (liquid of Zenker) and the staining method (Mann's methyl blue-eosin method) that, as we shall see, allowed Golgi's pupil Adelchi Negri to characterize in the infected brain the peculiar formation that carries his name.[25]

Back in Pavia, Golgi had to deal with his many duties. First, there was his laboratory, which, was as usual crowded with students and post-doctoral fellows pursuing the most varied research interests. The most brilliant among the students was Veratti, a student in the fourth year of medicine; he assisted Monti in studying pollution in the sewage system of Pavia, the cause of frequent typhoid epidemics in the city. Among the post-doctoral fellows were Rosolino Colella, who was ostracized because of his reputation as a jinx, Carlo Ceni, nicknamed Schwarzemann because of his moustache, black complexion, and introverted character, and Angelo Bettoni; each of them was able to publish some work in the academic year 1893–94. Others active in the Laboratory of General Pathology in that period were Cesare Staurenghi, Amilcare Bietti, and Francesco Radaeli, whose interests were osteology, ophthalmology, and dermatology, respectively.

In addition to teaching, Golgi also had to find time for the faculty meetings of the different schools, for managing the bureaucratic–administrative machine of the University, and for supervising the interminable reorganization of Palazzo Botta. Of course, this left almost no time for research, and it is not surprising that his scientific productivity declined in this period. Nevertheless, he still found time to prepare an entry on the spinal cord for the *Enciclopedia Medica Vallardi*, in which he continued the controversy with Cajal.[26] Against the generalizations and simplifications of the latter, who derived the general plan of the nerve connections from his law of dynamic polarization, Golgi warned:

It is indeed a still prevailing habit, even among anatomists, to substitute rigorously anatomical descriptions with schemas.

 We think that schemas are not only unsuitable to the spirit of anatomy, which requires the naked description of facts; they also more explicitly and directly damage the progress of anatomical disciplines insofar as they divert from research and lead one to accept as established [certain] relationships that are grounded only in hypotheses. In fact, [even] if they sometimes correspond to the results of physiological observation, ... more frequently they represent instead the hypothetical correlates of theoretical preconceptions.[27]

 Golgi considered Cajal's approach methodologically erroneous because his *diffuse neural net* was inconsistent with such generalizations: for him, the reality of the anatomical relationships between the nerve elements had to be much more complicated than the ones described by the neuronists. And therefore it irritated him to see the complicated weft of the nervous structure in schemas that were too simple to be true. Even worse, they were based on the concept of functional polarization of the nerve cell; a concept that he considered a *bad* anatomical hypothesis. He was annoyed that this concept was used as the basis for a theoretical model that purported to provide a functional interpretation for the supposed concatenation of the elements of the nervous mosaic.

 A critical point in the controversy between neuronism and reticularism concerned the anatomy of the olfactory bulbs, about which, as we have seen, Kölliker had asked Golgi in a previous letter. Cajal's notion that the glomeruli contain only fibres from the olfactory mucosa and dendrites, primarily from the mitral cells, put in question the existence of the interaxonal anastomoses, which were required by Golgi's model of the transmission of nerve impulses from the nasal cavity up to the higher centres. Golgi maintained the possibility of anastomoses between fibres coming from the olfactory mucosa, and collateral branches coming from the axons of the periglomerular cells and from the olfactory tract, but these notions were refuted by Cajal in 1890 and immediately thereafter by other histologists. Thus, the neuroanatomy of the olfactory bulb was obviously very important for Golgi, but after 1890 his multiple duties hindered his personal involvement in this research. Antonio Pensa, who was then a second-year medical student, claimed that he began work on the anatomy of the olfactory bulb at that point and obtained preparations that seemed to support Golgi's ideas. From the deep medullary strata of the olfactory bulb he saw the collaterals that come from the axons of the mitral cells climb back to the glomerula and fuse with the fibres arriving from the nasal mucosa. Golgi often passed the desk of the young pupil and followed 'with interest and also with some expression of approval and encouragement' the results of his experiments. According to Pensa, however, 'a person of a certain authority in the laboratory appropriated my most important findings and made them the object of a publication.'[28] The 'person of a certain authority' may have been Monti, who the following year published a work on the neuroanatomy of the olfactory bulbs supporting Golgi's reticularist theory.[29]

 Pensa continued to believe strongly that some collaterals of the mitral cells arising from the olfactory mucosa climbed back to the glomerula and fused with the fibres arriving from the olfactory mucosa, thus establishing an interaxonal continuity. Even in the 1961 new revised edition of his *Trattato di istologia generale* (Treatise of general histology), he still maintained this interpretation.

Golgi was confirmed Rector also for the 1894–95 academic year. On 4 November 1894 he gave the traditional inaugural address.[30] The question of Palazzo Botta was still the centre of attention and Golgi addressed the question head on in his speech. The day before, the University had finally taken formal possession of Palazzo Botta and the Ministry of Public Instruction had allocated the funds for a steam heating plant, research laboratories, and a laboratory for the practical training of the students. It is worth noting that the firm in charge of completing the installation of electrical lights by the middle of the next year (Ditta Einstein e Garrone) had been founded by the father of Albert Einstein, Hermann, and by his brother Jakob, who had moved to Pavia a short time before because of the failure of their electrotechnical shop in Munich.[31]

Confident that he had Bizzozero and Baccelli's support, Golgi left nothing undone to reorganize the biomedical institutes (especially his own), and to complete their relocation in Palazzo Botta.

Although he participated infrequently in the sessions of the City Council, he used these rare occasions to further the interests of the University. On 7 November he managed to obtain a grant of 1500 lire to establish an institute for 'anti-diphtheria serotherapy', which had been in the planning stages for several months.[32] Stables were then built for the horses Linda and Pippo, who would provide the serum. Monti was charged with supervising the preparation of the serum, assisted by Veratti, who was already an able bacteriologist, and by some first-year students such as Pensa.

Despite his shyness, Golgi had by now learned to move himself with a certain degree of boldness in the corridors of power and from all he sought to obtain something.

Among the new professors who had joined the Medical School that year was Luigi Mangiagalli, who succeeded Alessandro Cuzzi in the professorship of Obstetrics and Gynaecology. After graduating from Pavia in 1873 Mangiagalli had taught in Catania and Sassari and then directed the Gynaecology ward of the Ospedale Maggiore of Milan. He was a strong-willed, smooth-talking, eloquent but somewhat pompous, academic, whose lectures were 'very clear, elevated, and well-sculptured'.[33] He didn't shy away from complex surgical operations lasting many hours, from which he emerged as fresh as a rose ready to take his lunch at the nearby restaurant, La Croce Bianca. He would enter the restaurant at a fast pace, greeted by a deferential staff, and head for the last table on the left on the ground floor, where he would join other professors. His assistant Giuseppe Resinelli would arrive a while later, pale and tired, and sit at the same table. One could easily guess the condition of the patient from Resinelli's expression in response to a questioning glance from Mangiagalli.

Despite being a graduate from Pavia and now a professor in the same University, Mangiagalli had Milan's interests at heart. He had promptly recognized the potential implications of the Valerio bequest and within a few years would throw himself headlong into the task of establishing the Milanese university so feared by Golgi. The clash between the Pavian histologist and Mangiagalli (nicknamed appropriately '*MangiaGolgi*'; that is, 'Golgi Eater') lasted for more than two decades, ending with Golgi's defeat and the birth of the Università Statale (State University) of Milan.

In 1895, Monti and Sala left the Institute. New career opportunities had opened up, in part thanks to the good offices of their maestro. Monti moved to Palermo as Professor of General Pathology, along with his Assistant Davide Fieschi, a former intern of the Laboratory of General Pathology. Monti's promotion was not without some unpleasant after-effects. Golgi defended him tooth and nail in the competition for the professorship, but unbeknownst to him, Grassi had made a merciless criticism of Monti's works.[34] When Golgi learned of this, he wrote to Grassi asking why Monti should be considered unworthy of the professorship, adding ironically that 'Unfortunately . . . the matter can only have a retrospective value because the commission has already finished its work; but I have no doubt that even you will agree that the desire to correct my erroneous opinion is a sufficient motive to justify the present [letter]'.[34]

Sala was appointed Professor of Anatomy in Ferrara, a position previously held by Fusari who had now moved to Bologna as Professor of Microscopic Anatomy. Veratti had followed Fusari to Bologna to prepare his doctoral dissertation. Veratti's primary reason for this move was the fear of being a target of the vengeful Sangalli. Veratti, who had passed all exams with high marks, didn't want to compromise his final grade because of this bizarre and unpredictable academic.

Marenghi, who had recently finished his military service, and Francesco Radaeli were called to succeed Monti and Sala, respectively. Marenghi also assumed the direction of the sero-therapeutic unit assisted by the veterinarian Elia Garino.

On 7 April 1895 there were new municipal elections, with a moderate–clerical platform, which included Golgi, and a democratic platform. The moderates won and Golgi ranked third, with 1328 votes[35] out of 2512 voting. The winner was the lawyer Carlo Belli, who was elected Mayor.

During that year Pavia hosted a congress on malaria to which Minister Baccelli was invited. Wanting, naturally, to use the occasion to plead before his colleague for administrative and financial help to solve the lingering problems of the University, Golgi took care to organize a particularly warm welcome for Baccelli. In general, Baccelli was quite popular with the students; having been a teacher most of his life, he understood their problems and as a minister he had passed many provisions in their favour. The goliardic organizations, however, had decided to greet him with hostility. Among their complaints was a new provision barring additional exam sessions (other than those in the summer and autumn) because they 'interrupt the regular courses of lessons and distract the youth from their studies'.[36] Golgi sensed this subterranean mood and decided to take a pre-emptive measure by casting his students in the role of cheerleaders at the official welcome.

But the goliards were determined to make their rage felt on the opening day of the Congress. Most of them gathered around the entrance to the University, whereas a smaller group waited near the Rectorate. When Golgi left his office to greet Baccelli at the main entrance of the University, the students followed him with cheers, which lasted until Baccelli's carriage arrived. As the minister exited the carriage, he was buffeted by an avalanche of whistles, shouts, and insults of every type. Under a rain of whistles, a pale and worried Golgi and an Olympian Baccelli entered the Aula Magna. At this point, Golgi intuited that the students were about to explode in violent disturbances, and to avoid a catastrophic retaliation by the police he made a 'subtle but timely and efficacious intervention'. Instead of addressing Baccelli as the Minister of Public Education, he referred to him as a great man of science, 'the greatest expert of malarial problems',[37] allowing the student leaders to break into an ovation.

Golgi discussed again the problem of the Palazzo Botta with Baccelli. Bureaucratic impasses were delaying the transfer of the Institutes of Hygiene, Legal Medicine, and Pharmacology. So Golgi decided to 'ask His Excellency the Minister to exonerate me from the charge of Rectorship if during the new academic year I am unable to carry out the move of at least four of the Institutes.'[38] The intervention of Baccelli was decisive and all difficulties were rapidly overcome. Furthermore, the National Office of Civil Engineering was brought in to complete the renovation of Palazzo Botta, bypassing the inertia of the previous technical office and the contractors. The premises were then readied for the transfer of the Institutes of Human Anatomy and Comparative Physiology. Finally, Baccelli provided the funds required to complete the building's heating plant.

On 20 September Golgi went to Rome to participate in the celebration for the 25th anniversary of the entry of the Italian troops into Rome, which completed the process of national unification. He was accompanied by a group of students who participated in the parade carrying the banner of the University of Pavia. Golgi considered the conquest of Rome to be 'the greatest event of this century', 'the result of a scientific revolution that has created a superior consciousness in the nation'. For Golgi, to commemorate this event was to celebrate the 'triumph of modern scientific thought',[39] interpreting a historical–political event in the framework of his positivistic ideal of scientific evolution. Both enterprises, the 'heroic one of the *Risorgimento*', which was crowned by the conquest of Rome and the demise of the anachronistic institution that was the Church States, and the scientific one, were simply two aspects of the war waged by humanity against the forces of ignorance and superstition.

In the academic year 1895–96 Golgi was reconfirmed Rector for the third time. The transfer of a number of institutes to Palazzo Botta had freed up space in the Botanical Gardens and in other parts of the University, with great benefit for the Institutes of Botany and Pharmaceutical Chemistry, and even for the Law School. Golgi could now turn his mind to another ambitious project, the creation of a new University *Policlinico*.

After an initial period of adjustment, the institutes in Palazzo Botta began to be productive again, and it was now possible to hold lectures in the new premises. Among those who attended Golgi's lectures were the brothers Arturo and Enrico Gilardoni. Excellent note-takers, they decided to put their skills to good use by preparing lecture notes for purchase by the other students. Arturo prepared the notes for the histology course, which were edited by Radaeli; Enrico prepared the notes for general pathology, which Monti edited. For some years these lecture notes almost had the status of official readings for Golgi's courses.[40]

The Laboratory of General Pathology could now accommodate more interns, amongst which were Adelchi Negri, Carlo Moreschi, Guido Sala, and Panizza's nephew, Alfonso

Zoja.[41] Veratti, having graduated from Bologna, away from Sangalli's clutches, returned to Pavia to replace Radaeli as an assistant in histology. Among the students preparing their dissertations was Antonio Carini, who went on to discover the protozoan *Pneumocystis carinii* in 1910, Angelo Maj who studied the histology of tubercular lesions, and Antonio Pensa, whose dissertation concerned the innervation of glands. Among the students pursuing specialist studies was Giovanni Malfitano, who studied the effects of high-pressure gas on the behaviour of micro-organisms. He later became Chief Scientist at the Pasteur Institute of Paris. Probably in early July 1896, Golgi's Institute played host to the Romanian Georges Marinesco, a former pupil of Charcot at La Salpêtrière.[42]

In May 1895 Cajal published a very speculative paper in the *Revista de Medicina y Cirugía Prácticas*.[43] In 1891 he had designated the pyramidal cells of the cerebral cortex as 'psychic cells',[44] with a boldness similar to that exhibited by Golgi in his classification of nerve cells as motor and sensory. In this new paper he proposed a theory of the 'anatomical mechanism' underlying psychic processes such as association, ideation, and attention. He argued that these processes depended on the state of 'contraction' of the neuroglial cells of the grey matter, which would thereby influence the level of isolation and transmission of the currents in the nervous centres. Obviously Kölliker was wary of such speculative conjectures, and in a letter to Golgi on 16 January 1896 he wrote of Cajal:

Concerning S. Ramón, I think that he is indulging in extravagant ideas, and I cannot follow him in his physiological expositions. I am not at all in agreement with him when he maintains that the conduction [of nerve impulses] in *all dendrites* is directed towards the cell, but I believe that he is right about the dendrites of the mitral cells of the Olfactory Bulb, which project to the Glomeruli; *not for the others* [dendrites] *or for many others as well.*[45]

Once again, the solution to the problem of the transmission of nerve impulses within the olfactory glomeruli was seen as a way to settle the controversy between reticularism and neuronism.

One week after writing this letter, Kölliker participated in the famous meeting of the Physikalisch-medicinische Gesellschaft of Würzburg, at which Wilhelm Konrad Röntgen stupefied the audience with an x-ray film showing Kölliker's right hand, an image that became the symbol of a new era in physics and medicine. The dream of seeing through matter had become reality. Now as never before, science seemed on the point of fulfilling all its promises.

On 19 February 1896 Golgi's father died. The elderly physician had spent his last years in Pavia being cared for by his daughter Maria Teresa 'with great compassion and affection'. 'Since he was a very cultured person and very conversant with Latin literature, he followed the studies of his grandchildren' and, even though sick, 'translated, at sight, their Latin homework'. Golgi was heartbroken and remained at his bedside until the end, holding him in his arms. At the death of his beloved father 'Camillo cried, perhaps for the first time, cried without knowing how to restrain himself.'[46] The old physician had had the satisfaction of seeing his shy, quiet, and introverted son become a famous scientist and Rector of the same University where he had been a student more than 50 years before.

A few months later, on 17 June, Luigi Villa died in Milan, victim of glanders contracted in the laboratory of the Istituto Sieroterapico of Milan. He was one of the most devoted pupils of Golgi, who commemorated him in an obituary for the Bulletin of the Società Medico-Chirurgica of Pavia.[47]

In the fall of 1896 the mathematician and physicist Carlo Formenti was elected Rector; Golgi was thereby relieved of the burden of University administrative duties and was ready to make new scientific discoveries. His status as standard-bearer of the new neuro-histology was further enhanced in the second part of the second volume of Kölliker's Handbook of histology, which he had just received. Kölliker of course had been all too 'happy to have contributed . . . to make your name known to foreigners'.[48]

Notes

1. Pensa (1991, p. 77). Named in analogy to the political movement that opposed the Ottoman autocracy and whose programme was the secularization of the State.
2. Milani (1985, p. 269).
3. Quoted in Zanobio (1992, p. 25).
4. Golgi (1894b, p. 16).
5. *Ibid.* (p. 14).
6. Quoted in Pensa (1991, p. 78).
7. Maggi (1895).
8. Maggi (1899, p. 7).
9. Letter No. 12 from Kölliker to Golgi, 8 December 1893 (Belloni 1975, p. 172).
10. Letter No. 13 from Kölliker to Golgi, 24 February 1894 (Belloni 1975, p. 174) and *Monitore Zoologico Italiano* (1894, **5**, p. 48).
11. Letter No. 12 *bis* (draft) from Golgi to Kölliker, undated (Belloni 1975, pp. 173ff.).
12. Report on the works presented for the eighth Riberi Prize (Italian £20 000), approved during the 5 January 1894 session (*Giornale della Regia Accademia di Medicina di Torino*, 1894, **42**, pp. 69–70). See also the report published in *Archives Italiennes de Biologie* (1894, **20**, pp. 334–6).
13. During the first half of the 1890s Golgi had conferred on him honorary memberships in a number of scientific societies. The most prestigious of these was in the Royal Microscopical Society of London. He was also elected Honorary Member of the University of Dublin and Corresponding Member of the Academy of Medical Sciences of Palermo (1891); Member of the Society of Science of Göttingen (1892); Corresponding Member of the Academia Scientiarum Instituti Bolognensis (1893); Honorary Member of the Lombard Medical Association and of the Medical Association of Genoa (1894); Corresponding Member of the Physikalisch-medicinische Gesellschaft of Würzburg and Physikalisch-medicinische Gesellschaft of Erlangen, of the Society of Internal Medicine of Berlin (1895); Honorary Member of the Neurological Society of London, the Academy of Sciences and Letters of Padua, and the Italian Society of Sciences (1896); and Corresponding Member of the Society of Biology of Paris (1896). In 1895 he received from King Umberto I the title of *Commendatore* of the Ordine dei Santi Maurizio e Lazzaro. In 1896 he even received honorary membership in the Comizio Agrario of Pavia (an agronomic society). Another indication of Golgi's grow-ing international reputation was his appointment as editor of the annual reviews of neuro-anatomy for the prestigious *Verlagsbuchhandlung* (Golgi 1891j; 1892e; 1893f; 1894g; Golgi and Fusari 1895).

14. Letter No. 14 from Kölliker to Golgi, 15 March 1894 (Belloni 1975, p. 175).
15. Golgi (1894c).
16. Letter No. 13 from Kölliker to Golgi, 24 February 1894 (Belloni 1975, p. 174).
17. *Ricordo dell'XI congresso internazionale di medicina,* March–April 1894 (Rome: Edoardo Perino, 1894, p. 25).
18. Letter No. 15 from Kölliker to Golgi, 23 April 1894 (Belloni 1975, p. 176).
19. Cajal was made Honorary President of the Section of Anatomy (*Atti XI Congresso Internazionale di Medicina. Sezione di Anatomia;* Turin, 1894, p. 9). It is not certain whether Cajal actually participated in the Congress. In his autobiography he wrote of having sent a communication to Rome: 'My first work of a theoretical nature was one which bore the title *General Considerations on the Morphology of the Nerve Cell* and which was sent to the International Medical Congress held in Rome in 1894' (Cajal, 1917, p. 187). It is possible, however, that his communication was read by one of his Spanish colleagues. According to Cannon (1949, p. 169), Cajal did go to Rome for the Congress. Even if he was present, he does not seem to have met Golgi personally. In his autobiography he stated that he had met Golgi for the first time in December 1906, just before the ceremonies for Nobel Prize (Cajal 1917, p. 280).
20. *Atti XI Congresso Internazionale di Medicina. Sezione di Anatomia, quinta seduta, 3 aprile 94.* (Turin, 1894, p. 61).
21. Marchiafava (1894).
22. *Atti XI Congresso Internazionale di Medicina. Sezione di Patologia Generale ed Anatomia Patologica, quinta seduta, 4 aprile '94* (Turin, 1894, p. 231).
23. Golgi (1894d).
24. Golgi (1894e).
25. Belloni (1978b, p. 46); Mann (1894); Zenker (1894).
26. Golgi (1894f).
27. *Ibid.* (p. 213).
28. Pensa (1991, p. 81). Concerning the collateral fibres of the mitral cells, Pensa wrote: 'Furthermore, I must say that here, in some fortunate cases, I could observe—Achille Monti has also described it—a direct continuation of these fibres into the olfactory fibrils' (Pensa 1961a, p. 447). See also the note of Prof. Bruno Zanobio in Pensa (1991, p. 81).
29. Monti (1895).
30. Golgi (1895).
31. During the meeting of the City Council of Pavia of 15 December 1894 (concerning the 'Project of illumination of the peripheral parts of the City'), Golgi expressed his conviction 'that it will not be long before the system of electrical illumination will be installed, because the Hainstein [that is, Einstein] and Garrone firm pledged to complete the illumination of Palazzo Botta within six months' (*La Provincia Pavese*, 19 December 1894). The firm 'Officine Elettromeccaniche Nazionali in Pavia, Ing.ri Einstein Garrone & C.' had its offices in a building (currently deserted) at the intersection of Viale Partigiani and Viale Venezia, a representation in Milan, and a branch in Turin. In 1894 the Officine Elettromeccaniche Nazionali began producing electromechanical apparatuses (arc lamps, dynamos, and the like). Initially the firm was very successful, thanks also to a new model of arc lamp that was cheaper and more efficient than its predecessors, but closed in 1896 because of mismanagement.
32. See *Atti del Consiglio Comunale di Pavia* for the ordinary sessions 1894–95 (Pavia: Premiata Tipografia Fratelli Fusi, 1895, p. 31). See also *Atti del Consiglio Comunale di Pavia* for the ordinary sessions 1895–96 (Pavia: Premiata Tipografia Fratelli Fusi, 1896, pp. 90–1 and 120).
33. Pensa (1991, p. 103).

34. Draft of a letter from Golgi to Grassi, 21 October 1895 (MSUP-VII-III-5).

35. *La Provincia Pavese* (10 April 1895). See also *Atti del Consiglio Comunale di Pavia* (Pavia: Premiata Tipografia Fratelli Fusi, 1895, pp. 123–5).

36. Decree of the Ministry of Public Instruction No. 90, 25 July 1894, signed by the Minister, G. Baccelli.

37. Quoted in Pensa (1991, p. 83).

38. Golgi (1896, p. 11).

39. *Ibid.* (p. 22).

40. 'Outlines of General Pathology', from Golgi's lectures, were already in circulation in the academic year 1882–83; a copy is conserved at the Istituto Lombardo-Accademia di Scienze e Lettere (Villa 1984, p. 313). In the Institute of General Pathology of Pavia are copies of the outlines for subsequent years; in 1885–86 they were edited by A. Cattaneo and R. Fusari; in 1888–89 by D. Cattaneo; in 1901–02 by the students Bassi, Carpi, Rosa, and Sabbia (further edited by Marenghi); the editors for the years 1892–93 and 1907–08 are not known. The 'Outlines of Histology' were edited by G. Marenghi and L. Villa (in 1889–90), by A. Moschini and A. Perroncito (in 1904–05), and by E. Veratti and Vincenzo De Dominicis. A treatise of histology (*Trattato di Istologia*), illustrated with histological plates, was also compiled from Golgi's lectures.

41. On 26 September 1896, at the end of his first year as intern, Alfonso Zoja froze to death, along with his brother Raffaello who was an Assistant of Anatomy and Comparative Physiology, during an excursion on Mt Gridone in Val Vigezzo. This dramatic event was recounted by Filippo De Filippi, who accompanied the Zoja brothers on their tragic excursion. Reproduced in Mosso (1897, pp. 111ff.).

42. See letter from Marinesco to Golgi (12 June 1896) and the draft of a response to the letter (MSUP-VII-II-M). Marinesco recalled his visit to Golgi's laboratory in *La cellule nerveuse* (Marinesco 1909, p. 15).

43. Cajal (1895).

44. Cajal (1917, p. 124).

45. Letter No. 16 from Kölliker to Golgi, 16 January 1896 (Belloni 1975, p. 177).

46. Quoted in Bianchi (1973, p. 14).

47. Golgi (1896a).

48. Letter No. 17 from Kölliker to Golgi, 15 July 1896 (Belloni 1975, p. 179).

19

The Golgi apparatus

During his three years as Rector of the University, Golgi had been occupied primarily with bureaucratic and administrative issues, even if every now and then he was able to return to the laboratory to carry out some experiments. He had resolved to his advantage the problem of the Palazzo Botta (and had cut a few corners in the process) and now his Institute occupied a vast wing of this building. In 1894 he had set up the section for the production of the anti-diphtheria serum and now, three years later, he added a section for anti-smallpox vaccine.

Starting at the end of 1896, Golgi no longer had any administrative duties within the University, but he still had political responsibilities. And in his capacity as a member of the City Council he had entered into a controversy with Tullio Brugnatelli, Professor of Chemistry at the University and Alderman for Public Hygiene. Golgi opposed the projects for the new sanitation system and the new sanitation code, both advocated by Brugnatelli, because he felt that they did not take into account the most recent scientific findings. This was a very serious accusation and on 27 September 1897 Brugnatelli resigned his post, officially for 'reasons of health', but most likely because Golgi had the majority of the City Council on his side. Indeed, at the end of the following October Golgi became the new Alderman for Public Hygiene (with 18 out of 22 votes).

Golgi was now 53 and could have contented himself with supervising the work of his collaborators, but his passion for doing research personally was too strong.[1] And once again his uncanny instinct led him to another outstanding discovery, which he communicated to the Società Medico-Chirurgica on 19 April 1898.[2] In 1897, while studying the spinal ganglia using the rapid procedure for the black reaction, which was widely used by Cajal and others, he observed an intracellular filamentous and convoluted apparatus, arrayed in such a way as to form a cytoplasmic network. The only parts of the neuron free of the apparatus were an area around the nucleus, the periphery of the cell, and the axon. Initially Golgi wasn't able to 'establish with precision the procedure to follow for its reliable demonstration',[3] and he decided therefore not to report the observation. But when Veratti was able to observe a similar formation in the cells of the fourth cranial nerve in the early months of 1898, Golgi took up the study of this formation again, and found it also in Purkinje cells; it did extend for a brief distance into the dendrites. In the words of the discoverer, this unique structure consists of a fine and elegant reticulum hidden in the cell body, having such a unique appearance that, when the reaction is incomplete, even its small filaments can be recognized with certainty as belonging to this intracellular apparatus . . . The characteristic appearance of this internal reticular apparatus derives from the prevalence of ribbon-like threads, from their manner of dividing and anastomizing and their course (particularly in the large cells where one sees a distinctly tortuous course), and from the presence within it of faint plates or disks, roundish and transparent in the centre, which appear as nodal points of the reticulum, and finally from the peculiar yellowish colour that the filaments assume as an effect of the reaction. But the most characteristic mark of the apparatus results from its physiognomy—that is, while its external boundaries are clearly limited, such that . . . the area of cellular substance [that is, protoplasm] between it and the surface of the cell appears perfectly free and in the form of a regular clear rim, toward the interior, instead, the filaments of the reticulum penetrate to different levels.[4]

Golgi recognized the novelty of his observation:

[This structure] is completely different from anything heretofore described in the structure of the nerve cell; it has nothing in common with the classic description [of neurofibrils] by M. Schultze and his school; it has no connection with the well-known images that one obtains with Nissl's stain; no correspondence is offered with the interesting reports that we owe to Apáthy on invertebrate nerve cells.[5]

When Cajal read of Golgi's new discovery he was understandably upset. According to his own account, a few years earlier (in 1891 or 1892) he had prepared some pieces of young rabbit brain with a mixture of equal parts of dichromate of potassium (3%) and chloro-gold (1%), and had obtained splendid images of an intracellular structure similar to the apparatus just described by Golgi. His further attempts to reproduce it, however, had been unsuccessful; 'it refused to appear again'. Being uncertain about its reproducibility and 'excessively rigorous and restrained', he decided not to publish his observation. When he saw Golgi's report, which described the internal reticular apparatus obtained 'certainly by means of a procedure well known for its unreliability' (in reality, Golgi published his finding only after becoming confident about its reproducibility), he regretted that his prudence had deprived him of a discovery that would otherwise have been 'to my credit and in my name'.[6]

But even before this (assuming that Cajal's vague recollection refers to the same structure characterized by Golgi), Adolph von La Valette St George and then other researchers had observed cytoplasmic structures that could be identified as an internal reticular apparatus.[7] In any case, it was Golgi who defined it morphologically as a structural component of the cell and differentiated it clearly from other cytoplasmic elements, providing a reliable histological procedure for highlighting it.

In the same meeting of the Società Medico-Chirurgica at which he presented the discovery of the internal reticular apparatus, Golgi also reported that on the surface of the cell he had previously observed another structure: 'a special very delicate covering, made of a substance clearly differentiable from that of the cell body'.[8] He had spoken of this regularly in his histology course and he had referred to it on several occasions: in the article on the spinal cord for the *Enciclopedia Medica Vallardi*, in the work on the origin of the fourth cranial nerve, and in the German version of his works on the nervous system.[9] Golgi had attached a certain importance to this finding, even if he had not been able to dedicate a systematic work to it. In this covering he saw a proof against the possibility of nervous transmission 'by contact' as claimed by the neuronists. If the nerve cell is covered by a membrane that could act as an insulator, how would it be possible to ensure the passage of nervous information from a nerve process to the soma of another nerve cell?

A similar membrane on the surface of the cell had already been described in 1895 by Ernesto Lugaro, who, however, did not cite Golgi's earlier observations. He described it as a brown homogenous 'shell' riddled with small holes. Being a good neuronist, he assumed that the 'contacts' between axons and the surface of the soma occurred through these holes.[10] Golgi, who never passed up an opportunity to point out experimental evidence incompatible with neuronism, attacked Lugaro, not just because he had ignored his previous findings ('to such neglect, and this is a minor case, I am accustomed!'), but also because:

Possibly it is more worthy of attention that Lugaro had never again mentioned such coverings in his subsequent publications, especially since his theorizing has often provided an opportunity for it.—But any reason for surprise, even concerning this point, disappears when one considers that the finding represents somewhat of a hindrance to the theory, all the more so because in many categories of cells the covering has no holes, but appears to be a continuous layer: What is important above all is the theory; the facts not only must take second place, but can also be twisted or suppressed if they have the pretension of not fitting well-designed theoretical structures.[11]

That the existence of this 'isolating' covering was at odds with 'the theory of contact' had been pointed out also by Martinotti in 1897.[12]

Golgi attempted to demonstrate the supposed 'neurokeratinic' nature of the covering (Kühne had shown, in fact, that this substance was present also in the central nervous system) by trying to break it down using tripsin and gastric juices, but the results were inconclusive.

Golgi then emphasized that:

I must say the same about the insulating properties that I and others have thought reasonable to attribute to the supposed neurokeratinic layer: this interpretation has never ceased to be an hypothesis! You are aware, however, how this finding represents only one of the arguments among others of other types, which in my opinion stand against the theory of transmission by contact or the theory of dynamic polarization.[13]

The cytological structures that Golgi characterized using the rapid method could be observed at different times after the beginning of the reaction. Thus he recommended that 'repeated testings be conducted at brief intervals on a series of small pieces prepared with the rapid method'. The superficial covering of the cell was stained first, 'usually immediately before the black reaction stains the nerve cells and their processes'. Then, when the cell body is not yet stained, 'the black reaction begins to diffusely stain' the dendrites and the reticular apparatus.[14] The staining of the reticular apparatus was facilitated by hardening the pieces in an osmic–dichromate mixture (the best dichromate being rubidium), and then immersing them in an acid solution. In contrast, the staining was hampered by immersion in an alkaline solution.

Lugaro read about Golgi's communication in a critical review that appeared in the *Monitore Zoologico*. He responded immediately, sending a note to a new journal, the *Rivista di Patologia Nervosa e Mentale*. Rejecting Golgi's 'acerbic reproach', which he thought was completely unjustified, Lugaro noted that 'an insulating covering would appear to be completely unnecessary according to the hypothesis of transmission by continuity; if one denies the possibility of a transmission by contact, what purpose would be served by the presence of an isolation apparatus?'[15] He pointed out that the presence of an insulation does not constitute an impediment to an interaction via 'contact', not even when the covering was a continuous layer on the cell soma, because the nerve terminations often make contact on the dendrites. Then Lugaro asked, 'Why should I support the theory of contact to the detriment of the facts?' Perhaps because of 'the attraction exerted by new ideas when they come to upset the old way of seeing things? No, because today the theory of contact represents the opinion of the majority; it has passed into didactic treatises, and is an emblematic expression of our current state of knowledge.'[16] Finally, Lugaro began a devastating critique of Golgi's empiricism which, he said, emphasized the importance of 'facts' while exhibiting an 'aversion for every hypothesis, not just the ones that could appear adventurous or ungrounded, but also well-designed theoretical structures.' On the contrary:

A theory represents at every moment the synthesis of our knowledge, it only shows us which conclusions we can draw from facts, which possibilities should be regarded as likely. [A theory] always guides research, opens the path to experiments; it is the ferment that attacks the unknown and transforms it into new knowledge that widens our intellectual horizon. Without theory, scientific research would be a futile practice, tantamount to counting the grains of dust on the road or recording the history of the flights of flies.

Theories per se can do no harm to science; what is harmful is only the stubbornness with which they are often advocated against the mounting wave of new findings, only the delusion, from which one sometimes suffers, that they are not theories but rather demonstrated facts.[17]

Lugaro concluded by recalling how there was no one who 'had left his mark in science who had not made abundant, courageous use of theories'. And he prodded Golgi by reminding him that it had been he who had given 'the example of bold and innovative hypotheses, which, even if they had not been completely confirmed by subsequent research, [nevertheless] stimulated an enormous number of studies that have led to an undreamed-of progress in neurology.'[18]

Golgi did not let this controversy with Lugaro distract him from his interest in the internal reticular apparatus, 'which I had the fortune to place in evidence',[19] indicating that he fully appreciated its importance. Indeed, in the following months he plunged head-long into an investigation of the unique features of the internal reticular apparatus, 'with a persistence deriving from the conviction that I was not making a vain effort.'[20] On 15 July 1898 he was ready to present his new findings to the Società Medico-Chirurgica.[21] In this study he examined the spinal ganglia (ganglia of the posterior roots) of dogs, cattle, rabbits, and particularly kittens, 'specimens that, during this period, were available to me in great abundance'.[22] In the neurons of the spinal ganglia, the apparatus appeared to be somewhat different than in the Purkinje cells (more filamentous and less reticular), but he confirmed its main characteristics and its independence from other cytological structures, such as the fibrils described by Apáthy in invertebrates. He also noticed that in the adult animal it occupied a larger portion of the protoplasm than in the young animal. Golgi would return to this issue in a communication delivered on 20 January 1899 to the Società Medico-Chirurgica in which he noted some variations of the reticular apparatus related to age.[23] In the adult animal, the apparatus was often detectable with partial reactions; Golgi attributed this to the accumulation of pigment 'that is rarely absent from the cells of old individuals'.[24]

Remarkably, neither his work nor that of his collaborators appeared to suffer from the grave political–social events that were troubling Italy at the time.

'A spectre is haunting Europe—the spectre of Communism.' The phrase of the 1848 *Manifesto of the Communist Party* retained all its cathartic and terrorizing power in 1898. It was a bugbear for the bourgeoisie and nobility and an article of faith and inspiration for the thousands of workers and political agitators who were preparing to celebrate its fiftieth anniversary.

On 1 March 1896 the traumatic defeat of the Italian Army in Adua led to the fall of the Crispi Cabinet, and eventually precipitated the end of the Italian colonial adventure in Ethiopia. This provoked fiery demonstrations throughout Italy and particularly in Pavia, where groups of rioters removed the sleepers (railway ties) from the rail line and pitched them into the Ticino River to impede the Army convoys leaving for Africa. The entire country was thrown into a state of intense general turmoil. The malcontent of the populace mounted on the wave of a grave economic crisis.

On 7 March 1898 Pavians learned of the death of Felice Cavallotti, the 'Bard of democracy' and champion of the radicals. He had died on the previous day from a sabre wound to the carotid artery received during a duel with Deputy Ferruccio Màcola, who had been incensed by a violent article by Cavallotti in a Milan newspaper. The grief was immense. Cavallotti had been elected in the district of Corteolona, near Pavia, and was extremely popular in the entire province, where there were impressive demonstrations in his honour.

That spring, an increase in the price of bread provoked riots around the country, which were violently repressed. In Pavia, where the price increased from 46 to 48 centimes per kilo, significantly more than the national average of around 40, the popular discontent became uncontrollable. The students were, as usual, at the forefront of the protest. The evening of 5 May on Via Mazzini near Palazzo Mezzabarba (then the seat of the munici-pality) the demonstrators, primarily women, confronted a squadron of mounted cavalry called in by the authorities. When a group of students tried to join the mass of demonstra-tors around nine o'clock, an 'ominous trumpet call' gave the order to shoot. The hail of bullets left Muzio Mussi, a third-year law student, on the ground, his cranium shattered. He was the son of Giuseppe Mussi, Vice President of the House of Parliament, a radical member elected in the district of Milan and friend of Turati and Kuliscioff. The students held a wake over his coffin for three days while the riots were suppressed; political organizations were dissolved, the *Camera del Lavoro* was shut down, and *La Provincia Pavese* and *La Plebe* were ordered to suspend publication. But even more powerful commotions occurred in Milan between the 6th and 9th of May, prompting a state of siege under the command of the ill-famed General Bava Beccaris. His orders led to the use of artillery on a rioting crowd, causing the death of over one hundred people. Severe measures were enacted to restrict political liberty and dissolve political associations. Radical newspapers were suppressed and republicans and socialists, including Anna Kuliscioff and Filippo Turati, were arrested.

In that period of political repression, the Institute of General Pathology was frequently visited by Ettore Ciccotti, who spent long hours working in the library. He was obliging and friendly, and 'despite a prevalently humanistic attitude and culture, he exhibited an extremely intelligent interest in our research activities, in the equipment, and in the experimental procedures and techniques.'[25] He was a contributor to the socialist daily *Avanti!* and a former teacher at the Accademia di Scienze e Lettere of Milan. He kept out of sight in the Institute, where he was provided with a comfortable bedroom to which he could escape in the case of an arrest order. He was protected by some assistants who were sympathetic to socialism, but certainly all of this occurred with the consent of Golgi, who had absolute control over his Institute and therefore could not have been unaware of his presence.[26] Politically, Golgi was a moderate but evidently he also had some sympathy for the left (possibly a legacy from earlier times).[27] As a member of the Disciplinary Committee of Collegio Ghislieri, which was considered by many to be a dangerous 'hotbed of socialism', he opposed those who suggested that attendance in the College was incompatible with political militancy.[28]

One of Golgi's pupils who distinguished himself in political activities was Edoardo Gemelli. He was present the night Mussi was killed and participated in the three days of vigil over the corpse.[29] A contributor to the newspaper *La Plebe*, he held political rallies for the socialist candidates and was one of the speakers at the celebrations for the 50-year anniversary of the *Manifesto of the Communist Party*. He had been admitted as a pupil in the Collegio Ghislieri on 24 March 1898, while a second-year student in medicine. He was physically robust and of impetuous temperament, cordial, expansive, and loud. 'When he entered the refectory, always at the end of the meal, he was greeted with a general cheer in response to his customary shout, *oè! oè! oè!*'[30] To keep awake while studying he often injected himself with caffeine. 'His exuberance sometimes induced him to questionable actions that occasionally got him in trouble.' In College, 'he earned frequent reprimands and finally was severely punished for a flagrant violation of the disciplinary code, exploding a fire-cracker in the corridors.'[31] His reckless and quarrelsome behaviour and his verbal and physical intemperance were directed particularly against the Catholics in the University. Indeed, he professed an atheistic credo that was reinforced by the anti-metaphysical and scientific atmosphere of the Institute of General Pathology, and by his faith in socialism. His unruly behaviour, however, subsided when he was in the laboratory; under the influence of Golgi's personality, he became a disciplined and methodical researcher.

Meanwhile, new events had occurred in Golgi's otherwise quite uneventful personal life. Sometime in the early 1890s, he had adopted his niece Carolina, orphan of his brother

Giuseppe. The girl came to be considered by Camillo and Lina as their daughter. Even if Golgi was a non-believer, he was very attentive to her religious education, making sure that she followed the rigorous precepts of the Catholic Church.[32] This speaks volumes about Golgi's attitude toward religion. Around the same time, the Golgi household was joined by Maddalena 'Ciccia' Bizzozero, and in 1899, by Aldo Perroncito, who enrolled in the Medical School.

Important changes were also occurring in the academic environment of the University of Pavia. In 1897 Sangalli had died and Monti had immediately expressed his desire to return to Pavia, passing from the professorship of general pathology to that of pathological anatomy. But many at the University of Pavia were against the transfer, and the other Italian anatomo-pathologists, who saw another of 'their' professorships slipping away, were also dead set against it. Even Bizzozero was opposed. Finally, there were objections in the High Council of Public Education, which would have to give the final approval. However, Golgi saw in Monti the possibility of having one of his faithful (and meritorious) pupils occupy an important professorship through which he could increase his power in the University. 'Golgi had to conduct a difficult campaign but in the end he prevailed'[33] and Monti was able to transfer from Palermo to Pavia.

After receiving the final confirmation of his transfer, Monti suddenly changed his attitude toward Golgi. 'Not only did he demonstrate that he felt no gratitude for him, gratitude that he owed him for having been a precious mentor and for having helped him effectively in his career, he also proved to be an enemy, and even caused him annoyance and displeasure.'[33] In part, the disagreement had been caused, or at least exacerbated, by personal events: Monti's sister Rina, a noted scholar of zoology and comparative anatomy, had recently broken off her engagement with Marenghi, who then became engaged to one of Golgi's nieces in Varese. The disagreement between Monti and his old maestro was then transformed into a political opposition.

The souring of the friendship with Monti was not the only disappointment suffered by Golgi that year. In 1898, Casimiro Mondino was allowed to transfer his professorship of neuropsychiatry from Palermo to Pavia. In this case, too, Golgi's efforts and influence were instrumental in getting things moving, but yet again he had the misfortune to back the wrong horse.[33] Although Mondino exhibited some administrative abilities, which were put to good use during the process of reorganizing the Clinic of Neuropathology as an autonomous entity, he greatly disappointed Golgi's expectations 'especially because of his poor scientific, clinical, and didactic performance'. He was also a despotic and vindictive man who indulged in 'jokes, pranks, and frivolous company, and long coffee breaks at the café Demetrio, which was the heart of the city at the time.'[34] At first, Golgi thought he would be able to influence Mondino, either directly or indirectly, by placing some of his disciples at his side. But his attempt to convince Pensa to become Mondino's Assistant failed. Medea also declined:

One day . . . in a period in which, while still working at the Ospedale Maggiore, I was not neglecting to frequent, though sporadically, [Golgi's] laboratory, who came to see me in Milan when I was in bed for a appendicular indisposition? None other than the Professor [that is, Golgi].

He came to ask me to become an assistant at the Neurological Clinic directed by Mondino. I thanked him warmly for his demonstration of faith, but, having little sympathy for that person and not wanting to leave Milan, I begged the dear Maestro to allow me not to accept his proposal. He insisted, hinting that in that case I would soon become a *Libero Docente* and acquire a position of considerable importance in the Clinic. But fortunately I refused; otherwise I would have found myself in a sorry situation when, years later, a serious rift developed between him and his old pupil and protégé.[35]

In the end, Guido Sala agreed to work with Mondino, but the differences between the two led to Sala's departure a few years later.

After the bitter disappointments suffered with Monti and Mondino, Golgi finally saw the arrival of a colleague in whom he could place absolute trust. In 1899 Giovanni Zoja died, opening a professorship of anatomy in Pavia. Luigi Sala, who was still in Ferrara and the most obvious candidate, naturally aspired to this position, and in 1900 he won the competition. Another academic success of Golgi's anatomical school came with the appointment of Fusari as Professor of Anatomy at the University of Turin, after the death in 1898 of Carlo Giacomini. One by one, Golgi was installing all his former pupils in the most prestigious professorships.

In the months following the events of May 1898, the political situation had become so volatile that on 25 November Mayor Carlo Belli, unable to maintain control, resigned along with the councillors of the moderate coalition. The final blow had been dealt by the eruption of a popular uprising when the moderates in the Communal Council rejected a petition to drop the charges against those who had been implicated in the May riots. And so the zealous Royal Commissioner, Adami Rossi, arrived in Pavia to govern the city with an iron fist, based on a rigorous application of laws and governmental directives.

Thus, at the beginning of 1899 a deep rift separated the moderates, consisting of Catholics and Liberals, from the democrats, which included Socialists, Republicans and radicals. This situation reflected at the local level the national opposition between the authoritarian and reactionary Luigi Pelloux (who, after the bloody events of Milan, had succeeded Antonio Starabba, Marquis of Rudinì), and the extreme left.

On 25 June 1899 the polls opened in Pavia for the election of the City Council. The moderates had 32 candidates, 29 Liberal and 3 Catholic. Golgi was one of the 29 Liberals. Among the progressives there were 3 Socialists, including Monti.

The moderates had agreed secretly on a political platform, the contents of which demonstrated yet again how distant Golgi's attitude toward religion was from the radical anticlericalism typical of many of his University colleagues.[36] The platform was articulated in nine points, including 'the duty to guarantee religious instruction and the Catechism; to offer no help to the 'work of Masonry and Socialism'; to erect a cross in the cemetery'.[37]

The electoral forecasts were all in favour of the 'clerical-moderate clique' (as it was called by the opposition newspapers, such as *La Provincia Pavese*), because of the support from the organizations of the Catholic Church. But unexpectedly the left triumphed in a number of municipalities of northern Italy, including Pavia, and all 32 progressive candidates, led by the ophthalmologist Roberto Rampoldi, were elected. Monti came in 18th, with 1524 votes (of 3743 registered voters in the electoral lists); Golgi, with 1003 votes, was not elected.[38]

In the following months, taking advantage of their majority status in the City Council, the political organs of the Republican and Socialist parties launched a violent attack against the moderates. In a series of articles entitled 'La Camarilla' ('The Clique'), *La Provincia Pavese* singled out Golgi, who was considered the ring-leader of the 'clerical-moderate cabal'. The newspaper accused Golgi of having committed two improprieties during his tenure as City Councillor. The first was alleged to have occurred in the summer of 1897 when, during a session of the 'Provincial Health Council the Prefect read a letter sent by an *illustrious professor and City Councillor* to complain about the management of the Municipal Medical Office and to invoke the necessary remedy'.[39] The Health Council concurred with the accusation and sanctioned Cesare Cazzani, the physician responsible for the office, and one of his administrative clerks. 'Incensed by such an admonishment after so many years of service, the chief physician preferred to ask for retirement rather than stay in an office in which he felt barely tolerated'.[39] *La Provincia Pavese* explicitly denunciated Golgi as the author of the letter read by the Prefect (who had omitted the name of the sender). Golgi was accused of having bypassed the ordinary procedure that demanded the initial involvement of the Alderman for Public Hygiene, who at the time was Brugnatelli. Brugnatelli, however, 'was too kind-hearted and in addition was also a friend of Cazzani; and therefore it was unlikely that he would be severe with him. Thus an indirect way to strike was found and the hit did not miss its target'.[39] In sum, Golgi was accused of having behaved improperly in order to punish a physician whose only fault, the article insinuated, was not being liked by Golgi. Golgi was then accused by the newspaper of having shamelessly sponsored one of his protégés for the position of Chief Municipal Physician after Cazzani's retirement, an office under Golgi's control now that he was Alderman for Public Hygiene. According to *La Provincia Pavese*, Golgi had manipulated the competition to favour Egidio Perini, with great prejudice against more worthy candidates, first among whom was Costantino Gorini, *Libero Docente* of Hygiene and former assistant to Sormani, who had withdrawn his name after he found out the names of the members of the reviewing committee.[40]

Golgi answered dryly that he had never written a letter to the Prefect of Pavia 'concerning the management of the health services of this municipality or about the work of the late Dr Cazzani and of his co-workers'. He then haughtily rejected the accusation of having exerted his influence 'on the advertisement and on the requirements for the competition for the position of Chief Physician of the Municipality of Pavia'. Finally, he concluded that 'what is printed in the aforementioned two issues of *Provincia Pavese* concerning the presumed letter, which never existed, is a daring lie.' The newspaper published his statement in its issue of 6 August 1899.

At the end of July, Golgi, who was very worried about the political situation in Pavia, wrote to Baron Sidney Giorgio Sonnino, the conservative statesman who advocated a 'strong', *dirigiste* and authoritarian state. Golgi lamented to him that 'in this hour, characterized by a certain moral relaxation', the Liberal–Monarchist Party, 'while numerically prevalent, is overwhelmed by the Republican–Socialist Party'. And desiring to see the presence of the central government strengthened at a time when the city was in the hands of the left, he inquired about the new Prefect, who some thought was 'inclined to the motto of *laissez faire*'.[41] Sonnino answered reassuringly that he had 'heard good things said of' the Prefect who certainly would hold high 'the prestige of the [national] government' in Pavia.[42]

At the end of May, splendid news arrived from England. Michael Foster, the deacon of physiologists at Cambridge, informed Golgi that Cambridge University would bestow upon him a degree *honoris causa* in science during the Fourth International Congress of Physiology to be held in Cambridge from 22 to 26 August.[43] Golgi shared the honour with, among others, Kühne from Heidelberg, Dohrn from the zoological station of Naples, Henry Bowditch from Harvard, and Haeckel, the prophet of Darwinism. The degrees were conferred in the Senate House of Cambridge on the afternoon of Thursday, 25 August.[44] Golgi prepared a brief speech for the social events that followed the ceremony. He remembered 'the great Darwin' who, enlightened by the 'light of morphological studies', had 'provided the thread of Arianna which has brought about the modern renewal of biological knowledge.' And then he criticized the philosophical tendencies that were proclaiming the 'failure of science',[45] and that unfortunately were also affecting the world of science. Later, during a reception in the hall of Trinity College, Kühne launched another ferocious attack against the neo-vitalistic tendencies that were re-emerging in some sectors of biology.

Among the Italians participating in the Cambridge meeting was Mosso, who was nominated President of the International Committee for the next congress, planned for September 1901 in Turin.

On 11 June 1898 Kölliker wrote Golgi a letter in which he hinted that Pavia was under consideration as the site of the Fourteenth Meeting of the Anatomische Gesellschaft planned for 1900. He emphasized that 'the majority of the members of our society have a great desire to come to Italy' and added, 'I am certain that if we received an invitation from you, it would be accepted unanimously with great pleasure.'[46] In response, Golgi sent a letter of invitation to the organizing committee, which included Retzius, Waldeyer, Merkel, and Walther Flemming.

Probably in early August, Golgi received official confirmation from Waldeyer that Pavia would be the site of the Congress.[47] On 20 August, Kölliker wrote from Grünau that 'the decision has been made to come to Pavia in 1900; nevertheless it will be for us a great pleasure if at Tübingen [site of the Thirteenth meeting of the Anatomische Gesellschaft] *you*, or *another member of the Medical School* or of the City of Pavia—that is of the *academic body*—would have the goodness to repeat the invitation already made by you.' Kölliker was then 81 years old, but still extremely active; the day before he had participated in an 'expedition in the mountains, hunting for chamois'. He planned to go to Partenkirchen in Bavaria and then to Vahrn, near Brixen, where he would meet Ebner. Since Golgi, as usual, was spending part of his vacation in Varese, Kölliker inquired how long he would remain there because 'if the weather isn't too hot' he would be able to 'find my way to Varese, around the middle of September', adding[47]

I am very fond of grapes, fish, figs, and other good products of Italy, especially when they are accompanied and made sweeter by the society of friends like you, dear Signor and Signora Golgi, and Bizzozero, whom I don't yet know.[48]

This is indicative of Kölliker's extraordinarily lively personality: friendly, expansive, good-humoured. The letter probably arrived in Pavia when Golgi was at the meeting in Cambridge. On 2 September, Bizzozero's sister, Maddelena, wrote to Kölliker to inform him of the dates of Golgi and Bizzozero's vacation in Varese.[49] Unfortunately, the letter was greatly delayed in reaching Kölliker, and he missed the chance to meet with his Italian friends.[50] In the meantime, Golgi sent him his work on the internal reticular apparatus, which Kölliker read, 'with a lively interest'.[51]

In May 1899 Golgi went to Tübingen to finalize the decision to hold the next meeting in Pavia.[52] On his return, Golgi resumed his studies on the reticular apparatus, and as usual presented his findings to the Società Medico-Chirurgica, at the 14 July session;[53] these findings were also included in an anniversary publication of the Société de Biologie of Paris.[54] The study described the development of spinal cord nerve cells and contained a number of argumentative remarks against researchers who had criticized the black reaction. Indeed, since its triumphal adoption by Cajal, Retzius, Kölliker, and van Gehuchten during the first half of the 1890s the black reaction had become the target of severe criticisms, based on the work of Apáthy, Nissl, and Bethe, which had opened the door to the development of the neo-reticularist theory.

In 1897, Apáthy, working at the zoological station of Naples, had published a large monograph[55] containing a wealth of illustrations and descriptions 'which challenges the patience of the most willing reader'.[56] This work dealt with the structure of the ganglia of the ventral chain in invertebrates, using new methods based on chloro-gold or methylene blue. Apáthy strongly criticized Golgi's black reaction, which according to him did not reveal the basic morphological element responsible for the conducting properties of the nervous system: 'the neurofibril'. He was convinced that this would also hold true for vertebrates. In 1898 Bethe extended Apáthy's criticisms of the black reaction, maintaining that it was responsible for propping up the theory of the neuron, which they deemed completely flawed. Sarcastic remarks were made about 'black silhouettes that had invaded Italy'.[57]

Obviously, their criticisms elicited conflicting sentiments in Golgi.[58] On the one hand, as the creator of the black reaction, he had to defend it; but at the same time, as the leading anti-neuronist, he welcomed the criticisms of the theory of the neuron, even if he did not share their rationale.

For Golgi, the attacks by Apáthy and Bethe against the black reaction were understandable in the light of the distorted use of the method by the supporters of the neuron theory, for which he did not feel responsible. In fact (emphasis added):

Insofar as that response [that is, the attacks of Apáthy and Bethe] has been able, in some way, to personally implicate me, it doesn't seem to me superfluous to emphasize that I cannot accept in any way being considered responsible for the accusations made against the method and against the scholars who have worked with that method, because I have *always and with all my strength opposed the tendency that has led to excessively adventurous*, however genial, interpretations [that is, the theory of the neuron].[59]

Poor Golgi! *Vox clamantis in deserto.*

Then Golgi described in detail the best techniques for demonstrating the intracellular reticular apparatus, based on modifications of his rapid method, including the so-called 'Veratti formula', which specified the addition of a small amount of platinum chloride to the osmium–dichromate mixture.

Finally, Golgi dealt with the fact that some preparations might give the impression that his reticular apparatus was a homologue of the neurofibril. But Golgi 'after having looked at Bethe's preparations' maintained that it 'has nothing to do with the fibrillary structure described by Max Schultze and demonstrated by Bethe with the new methods.'[60]

In the following months another threat to the structural uniqueness of Golgi's apparatus came from Emil A. Holmgren. In a study published in the 5 July 1899 issue of *Anatomischer Anzeiger* the Swedish histologist reported on, to use the words of Kölliker in a letter to Golgi, 'marvellous things, found in the gangliary cells; lymphatic canals, partly equipped with walls and that he [Holmgren] compares to the reticuli found by you'.[61] Holmgren himself suggested that what he had observed was analogous to the structures described by Golgi. These 'canaliculi', according to Holmgren, were interconnected, forming a dense network communicating with another system of canaliculi located around the cell. But Golgi rejected Holmgren's suggestions, and maintained that the internal reticular apparatus was completely independent of the system described by the Swedish scientist. Subsequent studies proved Golgi to be right.

The evidence that the internal reticular apparatus was present in all eukaryotic cells, which suggested that it played a fundamental role in cell physiology, came from Golgi's laboratory. Pensa, who had just graduated in 1898, identified Golgi's apparatus in the cells of the surrenal capsule and Negri, then a sixth-year student of medicine, found them in the cells of the pancreas, salivary glands, thyroid, and in the epididymis and ovarian follicles.[62]

Golgi's laboratory was never short of outstanding pupils and collaborators. Good results on the study of the nervous system of worms were obtained by Giulio Ascoli, using the methods described by Apáthy. Pioneering research on the regeneration of peripheral nerves was conducted by Francesco Purpura, and Giovanni Laboranti worked on developing serological diagnostic tests for typhoid. Another newcomer in the laboratory was Aldo Perroncito, who immediately distinguished himself with his skills, diligence, and great passion for research. Pensa was invited by Golgi to collaborate in the preparation of a chapter for the *Trattato Italiano di Chirurgia* (Italian treatise of surgery), an unusual honour since this is one of the few instances in which Golgi co-authored a book chapter or review with one of his associates.[63]

As usual, Golgi's laboratory continued to be visited by foreign researchers. An interesting episode occurred in the summer of 1898. In August Koch visited Pavia, presumably to meet Golgi and be shown the developmental cycle of the *Plasmodium*, but all biological institutes were closed except that of Pathological Anatomy. The only person in the laboratory was Antonio Mariottini from the University of Siena, who was visiting Monti's Institute that summer to study infantile malaria.

[Mariottini] was perhaps alone in the laboratory—the only laboratory open in that torrid Pavian August—when Robert Koch appeared ... to see fresh malarial parasites. It was Mariottini who showed Koch various cases of tertian and demonstrated Golgi's cycle to him.[64]

In the spring of 1900, Serge Soukhanoff of the Psychiatric Clinic of Moscow arrived. He was a kind of itinerant scientist who moved indefatigably from one European laboratory to another. Soukhanoff was particularly interested in the internal reticular apparatus, on which he would become an expert. Then it was the turn of F. Ris, the Director of the Mental Hospital of Rheinau. Initially, both Soukhanoff and Ris were 'very reserved and circumspect', but later they acclimatized perfectly to the Pavian environment.[65] Other foreign visitors in those years included Hans Ziemann, a physician and Captain in the German Navy, and a certain Alloch from New York.

In the second half of 1899, new administrative work was piling up on Golgi's desk. In addition to his duties as Dean of the Medical School, he was responsible for organizing the celebration for the centenary of the invention of the electric battery by Volta.[66] Golgi participated in these festivities as an official representative of Minister Baccelli and as the President of the Medical Executive Committee of Como, the birthplace of Volta.

Golgi's moderate political ideas, based on the idea of unending civil progress and far removed from the political radicalism of the turn of the century, were articulated clearly in his speech honouring Volta. 'The philosopher who considers the world with a synthetical mind perceives a continuous evolutionary flow, constant though slow, which, having human perfectibility as its foundation, pushes for progress.'[67]

Golgi was also busy organizing the Congress of Anatomy planned for 18–21 April 1900. It was probably the main subject of conversation with Bizzozero, who had invited Golgi to his home in Turin for the New Year's celebration.[68] This would be the first time that the Anatomische Gesellschaft had met in Italy and Golgi wanted to make a good impression before such an important international audience; he therefore looked forward to the event with great trepidation. He was thrilled that the most important anatomical society in the world would be meeting in Pavia; but at the same time he was afraid that he might not be able to organize the meeting adequately. Funds were scarce: he had received little financial support from the central government and from the other Italian universities. Of this he lamented to Bizzozero, who in turn wrote to his niece Lina:

it doesn't surprise me, the attitude of the Government and that of the University towards the Anatomical Congress. And the Municipality, what does it do? If it doesn't unfasten the purse strings of the treasury, and states in black and white that it doesn't want to do so, I would not hesitate from proposing another site for the coming Congress. But naturally Camillo would not consider giving so deserved a lesson to his beloved Pavia![69]

Traces of Golgi's preoccupation can also be found in a letter that Kölliker wrote on 12 February 1900:

I have no doubts about the success of the Congress and I don't want you to worry about that. We will be contented with everything and the most important thing will be to meet our Italian colleagues, who I expect will attend in great numbers.[70]

Another source of worry for Golgi was the news from Manfredi that Monti, during a recent visit to Guglielmo Romiti, Professor of Anatomy in Pisa, was trying to organize, with Maggi's help, a 'separate Committee to welcome the anatomists with the latter as

Chair'.[71] In the end, Golgi managed to defeat these naive cabals and obtained adequate financial and logistic support for the Congress.

Kölliker asked Golgi to reserve two hotel rooms, one for himself and the other for Ebner and his wife, near the site for the Congress. 'Given my 82 years of age I don't walk much, especially when the weather is bad.'[61] In fact, the Swiss scientist stayed with the Golgis.

The Congress was a noteworthy success, even if there were fewer foreign scientists than Kölliker had predicted.[72] Because of his mother's illness, Retzius, President of the Anatomische Gesellschaft, could not attend, but Vice Presidents Waldeyer and Merkel were there, as was the Secretary Bardeleben. Among the foreign participants were His Sr, Obersteiner, Ebner, Apáthy, Julius Tandler, Ludwig Stieda, Auguste François d'Eternod, Claude Regaud, Ivar Broman, Joseph Eismond, Fritz Frohse, F. K. Studnicka, and H. Eggeling. There were many Italians, including Bizzozero, Todaro, Emery, Fusari, Mondino, Marenghi, Martinotti, Monti, Ruffini, Rina Monti, Luigi Sala, Giuseppe Levi, Guglielmo Romiti, Ercole Giacomini, Gemelli, Negri, Guido Sala, and Enzo Bizzozero. There were over 30 presentations and numerous demonstrations of microscopic preparations.

The Congress was officially opened on Wednesday, 18 April with a meeting of the officers in Golgi's home, followed at 9 p.m. by a stately welcome hosted by Mayor Pietro Pavesi at the Municipal Palace. The Mayor, who was Professor of Zoology at the University of Pavia, read a welcoming address in German to the participants and then gave a lecture on the history of anatomical studies in Pavia. Then it was Waldeyer's turn, 'a man with a long patriarchal beard, of genial demeanour, with the liveliest eyes shining behind the lenses of his glasses', who also celebrated the Italian anatomical traditions that had been revived by Golgi, Todaro, and Romiti. After the speeches there was a reception, which lasted until midnight.[73]

The first session of the Congress was held the following day in the amphitheatre of the Institute of General Pathology.[74] Kölliker introduced the session, 'greeting the participants' and offering regrets for the absence of Retzius who had sent a message containing great praise for Golgi's scientific work. A telegram of greetings was sent to the Swedish anatomist at the suggestion of Todaro. The speakers at this session included His Sr, Marenghi, and Tandler. In the afternoon, the proceedings were dedicated to microscopic demonstrations.

The next day was organized in a similar manner, with lectures in the morning and demonstrations in the afternoon. In the evening a banquet was held in the refectory of Collegio Ghislieri . The newspaper *La Provincia Pavese* described the event as follows:

In the seat of honour was the venerable Kölliker, [Honorary] President of the Congress, and at the same table were Mayor Prof. Pavesi, University Rector Prof. [Pasquale] Del Giudice, Professors Golgi, Todaro, His Sr, Waldeyer, and a number of their wives.

At the end of the meal, the first speaker was Prof. Merkel, who addressed in German the Mayor of the City and the Rector of the University; then Kölliker, in Italian, and Prof. Pavese, in French, greeted the guests, and Prof. Del Giudice inopportunely toasted the King. There followed Golgi, Todaro, Romiti, and [Giulio Luigi] Sacconaghi, a graduating medical student, who, speaking in German, brought the salute of the students of the Collegio to the illustrious guests. Last to speak were Profs. Nicolas and Bardeleben, the latter reading a telegram from Retzius and one from Oxford University to Golgi.[75]

Golgi's presentation was given on Saturday morning during the third and last session. His speech was followed attentively because it concerned the internal reticular apparatus, the centre of a scientific controversy because of its presumed links with Holmgren's canalicular structures (which were subsequently shown to be an artifact), and Apáthy and Bethe's neurofibrils. Golgi emphasized the unique characteristics of the apparatus (such as its perinuclear disposition and the presence of a free zone between it and the cellular membrane) that distinguished it from both canaliculi and neurofibrils. But just prior to the Congress, he had observed, using an acidic osmium–dichromate fixative mixture, 'another special finding concerning the structure of the nerve cells'.[76] In the zone between the internal reticular apparatus and the cell membrane, that is, in the peripheral zone of the nerve cell, he saw 'fibrils of extreme fineness, which exhibit at brief intervals tenuous swellings, which follow and conform to the curves of the cell body, and which continue into the protoplasmic processes.'[77] This fibrillary structure, unlike the internal reticular apparatus, continued into the axon. Golgi did not advance any interpretation of his findings, maintaining that they required a 'suspension of judgement'.[78] The text of the speech was published in the proceedings of the Congress, accompanied by two drawings by Veratti obtained with an Abbe–Zeiss *camera lucida*.

In addition, Golgi communicated Negri's important findings on the presence of the internal reticular apparatus in non-nervous cells.

The Congress was officially closed by Kölliker. After lunch, the participants boarded a special train provided by the Municipality of Pavia to go to the Certosa of Pavia where the Italian scientists, led by Romiti, offered refreshments to their foreign colleagues. Further speeches were given by Waldeyer, who thanked the organizers for their hospitality and 'Extolled—to great applause—the triumphant art of the Certosa and the internationality of science', and by Alderman Luigi Credaro who 'improvised a very felicitous response. Saluting the participants of the Congress, he spoke of the arts and of their educational purpose, of science without boundaries, and broke into an anthem of good omen for social pacification and fraternity amongst all peoples.'[75]

The Congress was a personal success for Golgi, who had had another chance, after the Berlin Congress of 1890, to met the most important anatomists.

At the end of the month, he allowed himself a well-earned vacation in Naples accompanied by his wife, his mother-in-law, and d'Eternod. On his return to Pavia, he found the following letter of thanks from Bizzozero:

A letter from Ciccia [that is, Maddalena Bizzozero] tells me that you had a good time in Naples, and this makes me happy. You really needed some diversion after the enormous exertion of the Congress in Pavia. As for me, even if I participated almost passively, I felt very strongly the need to return to a condition of absolute calm, and I assure you that on my return to Turin I spent many hours alone recovering from the excessively vivacious social life in which I was engulfed for four days. The longer I live, the more imperious becomes the need to stay away from my fellow humans.

Of the days passed in Pavia, however, I conserve a very dear recollection, which reflects especially on you and your affectionate hospitality. The older one gets the more one appreciates these demonstrations of affection, which perfume one's life, and which are like so many life-boats that survive the shipwreck of infinite illusions![79]

Bizzozero's letter suggests a sad and disillusioned man, perhaps feeling that he had been unable to realize more than a part of what his early promise had led him to hope for.

Kölliker, on his return to Würzburg, also wrote Golgi to thank him for his hospitality: 'In truth, I felt at home, and that's all there is to say', adding that, 'I shall never forget this beautiful time when I was also able to get to know the merits of your relative Bizzozero.'[80] Kölliker decided to draft a report on the Congress for the Physikalisch-Medicinische Gesellschaft of Würzburg and asked Golgi for some details, primarily concerning the talks by the Italians. Revising the report kept him busy for several months[81] and the final result was a detailed chronicle[82] containing a summary of the principal presentations and other information, such as the text of the telegram sent to Minister Baccelli, Golgi's political patron in Rome.

On 14 June 1900 splendid news came to Golgi. King Umberto I had appointed him Life Senator for high scientific merits,[83] a great honour that was ratified by the Senate on 27 June with 71 in favour and 3 against. On 2 July a banquet, organized among others by Mangiagalli and Forlanini, was held in Pavia to fête Golgi. Bizzozero, who had been invited but was unable to attend, wrote to Forlanini that he 'concurred wholeheartedly … in honouring a man who is endowed with perhaps a more unique than rare combination of superiority of intellect, strength of temperament and goodness of the soul'.[84] On 11 July Golgi was sworn into office. So far, he had been engaged only in local politics but now he entered the national political arena, at a time when the country was still agitated by social unrest. The events in Milan had created a gulf between the monarchy and large sectors of the Italian people. Certainly the King had become the symbol of oppression for the most radical elements. On 29 July, while Golgi was pleading in the Senate for the construction of a new Psychiatric Clinic in Pavia,[85] the King was assassinated by the anarchist Gaetano Bresci. This dramatic event did not keep Golgi from attending the Thirteenth International Medical Congress in Paris, from 2–9 August, at which he talked about the internal reticular apparatus.[86] Although Golgi 'was unable to take part in the grand commemoration' by the Parliament, he sent a message of condolence in which he declared that he 'concurred unreservedly with the deliberations of the Senate'.[87]

In 1900, Golgi once again spent the summer vacation with Bizzozero in Varese, where they were joined by Kölliker. On this occasion, the 18-year-old Aldo Perroncito snapped the famous photograph, reproduced innumerable times, showing the three colleagues. As usual, Kölliker was overwhelmed by the solicitude and kindness of the Golgis, who made sure he had an abundance of 'grapes, peaches, figs and other good products of Italy'. It was on this vacation that he met Countess Amalia Carandini, who flattered him by requesting his autograph. He reciprocated, requesting in return a photograph of her Ladyship. Back in Würzburg, he wrote to Golgi on 7 November:

I was so happy to have been able to enjoy such a tranquil and beautiful family life, with your Mamma and the dear Carolina and all the relatives, that I suffered a real pain when I was obliged to leave. And you, my dear friend, and the excellent Giulio [Bizzozero] have treated me like a member of the family and it was very hard to leave you. I cannot express in Italian all that I would

like to say and I pray that you believe me if I say to you that I would never have thought it possible
to find so many friends in Italy.[88]

Kölliker also wrote to Bizzozero, in particular to ask his opinion about possible
nominees for the Nobel Prize. Bizzozero answered initially that 'many of his colleagues
speak of Grassi' who had recently discovered the insect vector of malaria. But on 7 November Kölliker received a defamatory pamphlet *Unicuique suum, Prof. G.B. Grassi,* by Salvatore
Calandruccio, in which Grassi was viciously attacked and accused of having understated
the contributions of his collaborators.[89] Calandruccio had been an Assistant to Grassi in
Catania and had published some scientific work with him. To better understand the aetio-
pathology of malaria, he had inoculated himself subcutaneously with the blood of a patient
with quartan and had contracted the disease. The results of this human experiment were
described in a note by Grassi and Feletti in 1891. In 1898 and 1899 Calandruccio unsuccessfully participated in two competitions for professorships; in both cases, Grassi had been on
the evaluation committee. Feeling robbed of his due, and enraged by the reasons given for
his exclusion, he published several pamphlets in which he emphasized the importance of
his own contributions to the study of malaria. It was one of these pamphlets that reached
Kölliker at an important stage in the process of evaluating the respective merits of those
who had investigated the mechanism of transmission of malaria. And in fact the libel had
its desired effect. Kölliker, asking Golgi for his opinion on possible Nobel nominees,
wrote that Calandruccio's pamphlet 'makes me think that perhaps Grassi is not entirely as
worthy as many think, and I beg you therefore to tell me the truth in this matter.'[88] Kölliker
did not immediately consider Golgi as a viable candidate for the Prize because he thought
initially that the recognition was reserved only for those who had made recent discoveries.
And in fact in a subsequent letter of 25 December 1900 Kölliker wrote to Golgi:

I have also thought of you, dear friend, but it seems to me better to wait one more year when you
will have completed your observations on the nerve cell [referring here to the internal reticular
apparatus] and published a more extensive review on this topic.[90]

As for Grassi's nomination, Bizzozero was indecisive. In the end, the Swiss scientist
intended to propose the name of Retzius, suggesting also the possibility of a shared Prize
between him and 'a clinical physician, such as Grassi'. But Kölliker asked his two Italian
colleagues for their explicit sponsorship of Grassi: 'If you two are for Grassi then I will also
propose and support your nomination.'[90] Unfortunately for Grassi, Bizzozero, who had
ultimately decided in his favour, was unable to send his proposal to the Swedish Committee.[91] Golgi responded on 23 January 1901, taking a position in favour of Retzius and
suggesting as alternatives the names of other researchers on malaria such as Patrick
Manson, Ronald Ross, Grassi, and Robert Koch. And, referring to these four researchers,
'certainly benefactors of humanity', he added:

The difficulty lies in determining their respective merits. I must confess, however, that considering the nomination, after having thought over the contents of the polemical publications that
have appeared recently, I feel myself inclined to place higher the names of those I have indicated
first, Manson and Ross . . . In terms of the application of the knowledge and the development
given to the studies, also with respect to prophylaxis, the work of Grassi and of Koch have

certainly more weight; but since the initial discoveries in these, as in other fields, always have major value, if we have to make a ranking perhaps I would place those 4 names in the same order as I have listed them above! Manson—Ross—Grassi—Koch.

In conclusion, I will propose [to the Nobel Committee] definitely the name of Retzius and I will probably place the names of Manson—Ross—Grassi and Koch—in this order, for their discoveries about malaria, in case others might be of the same opinion.

Finally, Golgi added:

You have also let me know a thought made in my favour . . . Not even in my dreams have I considered the possibility of being nominated for such a high prize . . . I consider that eventuality always as a dream. However, it is already for me a grand and inspiring prize that you, Kölliker, the most eminent man of our epoch, have thought of me in this sense![92]

So it appears that Golgi's opinion was strongly influenced by the controversy on the priority of the discoveries on the transmission of malaria. Manson had demonstrated that the parasite of filariasis in humans (*Filaria bancrofti*) could pass into the mosquito when it was sucking the blood of an infected individual, and develop in its tissue. It was the first evidence that parasites could be hosted by an insect. He then hypothesized in 1894 that mosquitoes could play the same role in the transmission of malaria. However, his theory, despite having the merit of focusing attention on this insect, was wrong insofar as it considered the mosquito as a passive vehicle of infection. After having ingested the malarial parasite with the blood, Manson claimed, they would lay eggs and then die; the malarial parasite released by their decaying bodies would then pollute the environment, in particular in swampy areas, from which it could re-enter humans through an oral route. Manson, however, did not carry out any experiments to prove his theory. And on the other hand, the idea that the mosquito could play a role in the transmission of malaria had already been proposed (although in a contradictory manner) in 1717 by Giovanni Maria Lancisi and then taken up again by Laveran and others. Ross had defined the modality of transmission of malaria in birds (the protozoan of which had been discovered by Vasili Iakovlevich Danilewsky in 1886 and shown by Grassi to be related to the human *Plasmodium*) and had hypothesized, on the basis of some experiments, that the human disease was transmitted by a similar mechanism. Koch, in the course of two lavish research expeditions in Italy in 1898–99 (funded by the same Italian government that was shamefully stingy with Grassi) made a series of inconclusive experiments; only after the discovery of the mosquito anopheles was he able to confirm the modality of transmission of the disease. In contrast, Grassi, owing to his profound entomological preparations (for which he had received the Darwin Medal from the Royal Society in 1896), had been able to prove the transmission of human malaria by mosquitoes, to define clearly the vector species of the disease, and to characterize its biological aspects. But Grassi was ill-tempered (as had been obvious even in his student years when he was expelled from the Collegio Ghislieri) and had made many enemies both in and outside Italy. His contemptuous and sarcastic remarks about Ross and Koch, who had no entomological knowledge whatsoever, alienated the opinion makers who influenced the assignment of the Nobel Prize.

As we have seen, Golgi, too, was blinded by the venomous polemical atmosphere and unable to appreciate that Grassi's contribution placed him on a level of merit substantially comparable with that of Ross. And the opinion of a world renowned expert on malaria, such as Golgi, certainly affected the Nobel Committee[93] in its decision to award the Prize to Ross alone in 1902. Bizzozero himself did not agree with Golgi's opinion on the role of Grassi in the discovery of the malarial vector:

I cannot share fully your opinion on the role of Grassi in the discoveries about malaria. If the problem had been dealt with by Ross alone, very probably it would not yet have been resolved, since he had no idea which species of mosquito was to be incriminated, and, in consequence, he was in no position to ascertain through his investigations that malaria is propagated only by means of the mosquito. We would therefore still lack the notion that is the foundation of the current prophylaxis.[91]

We don't know if Golgi's opinion might have been a personal idiosyncrasy. One must keep in mind that Grassi initially discounted the idea that protozoans could be an aetiological factor in human diseases in general and malaria in particular. Later, when he changed his mind, he presented a detailed description of the nucleus of the malarial parasites without mentioning that this had already been vaguely reported by Golgi. Grassi had further irritated Golgi by criticizing Monti's work. But it seems unlikely that these slights alone could have been sufficient to produce a permanent attitude of hostility against Grassi. After all, hadn't he humbled himself before his former professor? And when he passed through Pavia, didn't he always go to 'pay his respects to Golgi',[65] remaining in Golgi's laboratory 'for advice or to complete some research'? After 1895, their correspondence had been characterized by extreme respect, with Grassi always showing the greatest deference toward his old teacher.

Retzius, meanwhile, had asked not to be nominated and requested that Kölliker drop his name. He also informed Kölliker that, for the first time, the Prize could be given on the basis of work done even six to ten years earlier.[94] As Kölliker described in a letter to Golgi, he decided to nominate 'only one and this *is my friend, the great Camillo Golgi!*' whose 'discoveries on the anatomy of the nervous system I have put in the most exalted relief, especially on the basis of [Golgi's] great publication in German, which everyone knows' adding that 'Even v[on] Ebner, His, [Friedrich Daniel von] Recklinghausen, have proposed Golgi, and thus my friend Golgi can see that he has nothing more to do than wait.'[94]

But Golgi responded with great modesty to Kölliker's letter:

What you had the kindness to say to me in your last letter concerning the Nobel Prize, is nothing but another manifestation of your personal benevolence. That you felt like proposing my name is for me a prize so great that I cannot imagine any higher. I see the material prize as too much above my merit; nor can I believe there are many persons who can evaluate me with a degree of benevolence comparable to that used by you!

For your very good opinion for which I feel extremely moved, I offer you the warm expression of my deep gratitude.[95]

Others were less restrained than Golgi and boldly emphasized their own worthiness for the Nobel Prize. Cajal had the Medical School of Madrid print a detailed curriculum of his scientific activities, which was sent to various pre-eminent scholars, including Kölliker and Golgi. But Kölliker did not appreciate this excessive vanity and furthermore was annoyed by the attacks that Cajal had made against Golgi in recent publications, for instance the accusation that his writings were not in favour of truth but rather 'in defence of a particular School'. And so Kölliker, wrote to Golgi:

Have you read in what insolent manner Ramón has expressed his opinion on your observations and conclusions and those of your students in his recent book *Textura del sistema nervioso* 1900 pg. 146?

I find that in such a difficult matter it would be better to abstain from expressing so secure an opinion and to wait for new observations.

But it seems to me that Ramón believes himself the foremost histologist and the only one allowed to have an opinion on the structure of the nervous system, especially when I take into account his newest production, which he must also have sent to you, entitled *Relacion de los Titulos, Méritos y Trabajos cientificos del Dr S. Ramón y Cajal, con el retratto del Autor* [Report of titles, honours and scientific works of Dr S. Ramón y Cajal, with a portrait of the author], Madrid 1900, containing a list of 117 articles by the author.

If one considers how many repetitions one finds in these articles, their number diminishes considerably and one sees that *'multa non prova il multum'* [quantity is no evidence of quality]. It also displeases me that this *'Relacion'* has been prepared *only in view of the Nobel Prize*, and it seems to me that it is not proper to put oneself in evidence in such a manner.[96]

In January Kölliker wrote to Golgi expressing his intention to visit him in Pavia in April, 'if you allow me and if I do not disturb you'.[97] The news was received by the Golgis with 'expressions of great contentment! It will be a real celebration for our family and for Pavia! We shall come to meet you!'[93] Kölliker had intended to go first to Turin to meet Bizzozero. But on the morning of 5 April 1901 he received a letter from Erminia Brambilla, Bizzozero's wife, telling him that Giulio had been stricken by a serious pneumonia. He immediately sent a telegram asking for further news, to which he received the following response:

Pneumonia rather extensive; up to now a regular course, we hope a good outcome, greeting and thanking you E.B.

Golgi had meanwhile just returned from an anatomical meeting in Lyon held between 1–3 April. On the 6th, Kölliker wrote Lina that he was now planning to skip the stopover in Turin and would arrive in Milan on the 11th or 12th of April, adding that 'If Camillo is at home and if it doesn't disturb him, I shall come immediately from Milan to Pavia.'[98]

Bizzozero died on 8 April after a week's illness. The news spread quickly around the scientific community and telegrams of condolence arrived from everywhere, including one from Rudolf Virchow. Golgi and his family attended the funeral and memorial service in Varese, where the scientist was buried in the family tomb. On 12 April Golgi gave a commemorative speech on the personality and scientific work of his friend and teacher.[99]

We do not know for certain if, despite Bizzozero's death, the planned meeting between Golgi and Kölliker ever occurred. From one of Kölliker's later letters, it seems that it did. Since Golgi had decided to participate in the annual meeting of the Anatomische Gesellschaft, which that year was held in Bonn between 26 and 29 May, Kölliker wrote to remind him to bring to the congress 'your preparations and drawings on the axonal net which you told me about in Pavia', and added,

My son and I invite you for dinner Monday evening. My wife will stay in Bonn for three weeks, but I shall return with you and I hope you will stay in my home in Würzburg as long as possible before going to Munich. Ebner too will stay at least two days with me and all is ready to receive my friends.[100]

In April Golgi gave another commemorative speech in honour of Bizzozero at the Istituto Lombardo, of which the late pathologist had been a Corresponding Member,[101] and prepared an obituary for publication in the *Archivio per le Scienze Mediche*.[102]

At the Bonn meeting Golgi presented a series of preparations by Pensa (on the reticular apparatus of the hyaline cartilage), by Guido Sala, about to graduate in medicine (on Herbst's corpuscles), and by Aldo Perroncito (on the demonstration of the ultraterminals of the nerve fibrils with chloro-gold).[103]

On 7 June Golgi participated in a session of the Senate concerning a law on the 'Provisions to reduce the causes of malaria', which he supported. Because of the recent discoveries on the aetiology of the disease, this law included malaria among infectious diseases and therefore extended to it a number of legal provisions established in 1888 for the protection of health and public hygiene.

After Bizzozero's death, the Medical School of Turin repeatedly invited Golgi to accept the vacant professorship and academics and students alike signed a petition to this effect. Enzo Bizzozero wrote to Golgi that when he learned that the latter might accept the professorship of his late father, 'it seemed to us that a ray of light would come to break through the darkness that surrounds us . . . And it would appear to us that our Papa would live again through you; and you would certainly be a father for us, who are now without support or guidance, and who, alone here, feel all around us a deeply oppressive sense of emptiness.'[104] In the meantime, the anatomo-pathologist Foà, who in recent years had had a stormy relationship with Bizzozero, let it be known that if Golgi declined the offer, he would apply. The news upset Erminia Bizzozero, who knew how much her husband detested his old pupil. So she wrote to Golgi that only he could 'stop such an enormity' from occurring, and she implored him 'for the memory of poor Giulio, to prevent this' and wrote that 'the salvation of all of us is in your hands'. She added that the feared event 'would be a terrible blow for me, for my children and for all of poor Giulio's pupils.' And she ended with an appeal 'to your good and sincere heart, to the sincere affection that ties you to the dear departed because you appreciate the grave consequences that your refusal would bring.'[105] Golgi's family was in also favour of the transfer, especially because of the family ties with the Bizzozeros. Against these forces trying to draw Golgi away there were strong pressures from Pavia to stay, including a petition signed by professors and over 250 students of the Medical School, begging him to remain. After a period of agonizing indecision, Golgi decided against cutting his umbilical cord with Pavia and declined the invitation in a dignified formal letter, and in more private correspondence.[106] However, the designs of Foà did not succeed. It is likely that Golgi used all his power to block the event so feared by Erminia. Bizzozero's professorship was temporarily entrusted to Cesare Sacerdotti, his last assistant, and in 1903 was permanently assigned to Benedetto Morpurgo.

At the end of June, Golgi was elected Rector again with 25 votes, against 20 for Mangiagalli and 19 for Vittore Bellio, of the Faculty of Letters and Philosophy.

In the second half of September 1901, he participated in the 5th International Congress of Physiology in Turin, presided over by Mosso. During the meeting, he was shown preparations of neurofibrils by Arturo Donaggio, who had characterized them in 1896, and who recalled the meeting many years later:

At the International Congress of Physiology in Turin in 1901, he looked at the preparations on which I based my report concerning the fibrillary net that I had found in the nerve cells of vertebrates. It was the first time that I met Golgi, and I can still see before me that vast and strong forehead, bent over the microscope, his face concentrated; I remember the long pause, and then the words that he pronounced with that singular voice of his, a deep voice, calm and yet suffused by a subtle vibration, which infused that man, strong and with an iron will, with some kind of a sense of sweetness and almost shyness.[107]

During the autumn Golgi suffered from an annoying 'suppuration of the foot caused by a wound sustained during the bathing season',[108] which kept him in bed.

The Nobel Prize was awarded to Behring for the development of the anti-diphtheria serum. To Kölliker's dismay, Anatomy would have to wait.

Notes

1. On 17 April 1897 Bizzozero wrote to Golgi from Turin: 'I hear with pleasure that you resumed working with great intensity; take care, however, that you do not let your passion for research overwhelm you. Remember that we are no longer in our prime, and that it is better to work with moderation for many years, than breathlessly for a few years. Listen to the advice on this matter that your Lina will not neglect to give you—for some time I have been putting this rule of life into practice and I find it serves me well.' (MSUP-VII-III-1.)

2. Golgi (1898; see also 1898a and 1898b). Golgi wrote on many occasions that he presented his communication on 19 April 1898, but according to the minutes published in the *Bollettino della Società Medico-Chirurgica di Pavia*, **13**, III–IV, the communication occurred on 22 April.

3. Golgi (1898; *OO*, p. 647).

4. *Ibid.* (*OO*, pp. 645ff.).

5. *Ibid.* (*OO*, p. 651).

6. Cajal (1917, p. 311).

7. Trautmann (1988, pp. 42ff.).

8. Golgi (1898; *OO*, p. 643).

9. Golgi (1894c, p. 261).

10. Lugaro (1895).

11. Golgi (1898; *OO*, pp. 648ff.).

12. Martinotti (1897).

13. *Ibid.* (*OO*, p. 650).

14. *Ibid.* (*OO*, p. 652).

15. Lugaro (1898, p. 268).

16. *Ibid.* (p. 269).

17. *Ibid.* (p. 270).

18. *Ibid.* (p. 271).

19. Golgi (1899; *OO*, p. 667).
20. Golgi (1898c; *OO*, p. 656).
21. Golgi (1898c). Also translated into French (Golgi 1898d).
22. Golgi (1898c; *OO*, p. 657).
23. Golgi (1899). Also translated into French (Golgi 1899a).
24. Golgi (1899; *OO*, p. 670).
25. Pensa (1991, pp. 106ff.).
26. That Golgi was aware of Ciccotti's presence in his Institute is confirmed by a letter that Ciccotti wrote to him on 30 May 1917 in which he recalled 'my always vivid memory of the well-wishing benevolence [you] exhibited to me during my brief stay in [that] University' (MSUP-VII-I-3).
27. In an article published in *La Provincia Pavense* of 28 June 1899 is a phrase that hints at a 'leftist' past of Golgi, before becoming a moderate: 'Afflicted by the socialism-phobia, *L'Aevenire* [misspelling of *L'Avvenire*] denounced the socialist danger—quite surprisingly, considering that its patrons, like Golgi, once felt quite differently.'
28. Bernardi (1967, pp. 118ff.).
29. Cosmacini (1985, p. 15).
30. See Cosmacini (1985, p. 33) for Eugenio Medea's recollection of the reunion of the ex-Ghisleriani in 1960.
31. Pensa (1991, p. 99).
32. As reported by Golgi's niece Carolina, to Prof. Bruno Zanobio. Subsequently reported by Prof. Bruno Zanobio at the memorial meeting on Golgi organized on 28 March 1994 by the Società Medico-Chirurgica di Pavia.
33. Pensa (1991, p. 121).
34. Savoldi (1990, p. 264).
35. Medea (1966, p. 4 *bis*).
36. Gemelli recollected that: 'in the first surgery lecture, Bottini, then in decline but still celebrated, presented us with an unfortunate priest who carried in his body the consequences of his misbehaviour [syphilis]. Thus in Bottini's classes one sneered at the priest's frock, while in the Institute of Comparative Anatomy [directed by Leopoldo Maggi] one learned that religion is the fruit of ignorance.' Quoted in Cosmacini (1985, p. 29).
37. Tesoro (1981, p. 120).
38. *La Provincia Pavese* (28 June 1899).
39. *La Provincia Pavese* (30 July 1899). Cazzani's retirement was decided by a deliberation of the Municipal Council of Pavia on 12 October 1897 (*Atti del Consiglio Comunale di Pavia* for the ordinary sessions 1897–98 (Pavia: Premiata Tipografia Fratelli Fusi, 1898, p. 18).
40. *La Provincia Pavese* (2 August 1899).
41. Draft of a letter from Golgi to Sonnino, 20 and 22 July 1899 (MSUP-VII-III-17).
42. Letter from Sonnino to Golgi, 1 August 1899 (MSUP-VII-III-17).
43. In the same period, Golgi received honorary memberships in the Regia Taurinensis Academia, the American Neurological Association, the Regia Romanae Medicorum Academia (1898), and in the Imperial Academy of Medicine of St Petersburg (1899).
44. Franklin (1968, p. 261).
45. Transcript of Golgi's speech with a partial translation in French (MSUP-III-II-4). See also MSUP-III-II, 1–3.
46. Letter No. 19 from Kölliker to Golgi, 11 June 1898 (Belloni 1975, p. 180).
47. Letter No. 20 from Kölliker to Golgi, 20 August 1898 (Belloni 1975, p. 181).

48. Some biographies of Bizzozero report that, soon after his graduation, he spent some months in various laboratories of central Europe, including that of Kölliker (see for example Gravela 1989, p. 18), but this seems improbable since the two were not acquainted at the time.

49. According to Pensa (1991, pp. 116ff.), Edoardo Perroncito and his son Aldo were also present during Golgi and Bizzozero's holiday at Varese in the summer of 1898.

50. Letter No. 20 *bis* from Kölliker to Maddalena Bizzozero, 13 September 1898 (Belloni 1975, p. 182).

51. Letter No. 21 from Kölliker to Golgi, 12 October 1898 (Belloni 1975, p. 183).

52. *Verhandlungen der Anatomischen Gesellschaft* (Supplement of the *Anatomischer Anzeiger*, 1899, **13**, p. 138).

53. Golgi (1900).

54. Golgi (1899b).

55. Apáthy (1897).

56. Beccari (1944–45, p. 52).

57. Golgi (1900; *OO*, p. 678).

58. Golgi wrote: 'Concerning the critical reaction that, as mentioned above, has recently arisen with regard to the methods of black staining, a critical reaction in which even scholars who have used that method have participated, I don't have difficulty recognizing that some of the notes voicing that reaction might appear not entirely unjustified, if one takes into account the one-sidedness with which some have interpreted their results and if one considers that, in the hands of scholars who have subordinated too easily the fact to the theory or who, on the basis of incomplete facts [Golgi is referring here to incomplete staining], sometimes incompletely studied, do not hesitate to formulate laws and doctrines of an high order—actually, with regard with certain issues, the methods based on the silver-chromate reaction might have even represented a pernicious role in the progress of the studies!

'The most celebrated among the modern theories that have pretended to explain the specific functions of the nervous system in their biomechanical bases, a theory that, because of its apparent anatomical basis, has managed to impose itself almost as a principle of faith, perhaps includes one of the arguments, which better justifies that form of critical reaction. But it is important to make distinctions between the facts that are well-demonstrated and that, as such, are enduring, and the interpretations [of such facts], which are always of subjective value; and I have already been obliged to point out how the best arguments against that doctrine are derived from the applications of that very method; of course, I am not referring to the imperfect findings obtained with a hasty application of the method, but to those findings that are the result of quite long work and of innumerable tests, counterproofs, and verifications!' (Golgi 1900; *OO*, p. 682).

59. Golgi (1900; *OO*, p. 682).

60. *Ibid.* (*OO*, p. 693).

61. Letter No. 22 from Kölliker to Golgi, 8 February 1900 (Belloni 1975, p. 184).

62. Negri (1900).

63. Pensa collaborated with Golgi in the drafting of a chapter for the *Trattato Italiano di Chirurgia* (Golgi and Pensa 1900). Among others, the following spent time in the Istituto di Patologia Generale, with various titles, in those years: Giuseppe Moriani, Alfredo Corti, Mauro Jatta (who was also Golgi's Assistant in 1893), Romano Maggiora, and Giuseppe Tricomi Allegra.

64. Monti (1935, p. 80).

65. Pensa (1991, p. 135). Soukhanoff's research interests focused on neuroanatomy, clinical and experimental neurology, and military psychiatry (of which he received first-hand experience

during the Russo-Japanese War). See the *Rivista di Patologia Nervosa e Mentale* (1916, p. 448). One of his letters to Golgi, dated 5 January 1900, in which he announces his intention to spend some time in the Laboratorio di Patologia Generale, is kept in the MSUP (partially reproduced in Pensa, 1991, p. 262).

66. Golgi gave two speeches during the celebrations in Volta's honour for the centenary of the invention of the electrical cell. The first speech was given at the opening of the First Italian Congress of Electrobiology (Golgi 1899c); the second at the opening of the Congresses of Hygiene and Veterinary Medicine (Golgi 1899d).

67. Golgi (1899d, p. 9).

68. Letter from Bizzozero to Golgi, 19 December 1899 (MSUP-VII-III-1).

69. Letter from Bizzozero to Lina Golgi, 5 February 1900 (MSUP-VII-III-1).

70. Letter No. 23 from Kölliker to Golgi (Belloni 1975, p. 185).

71. Letter from Manfredi to Golgi, 6 January 1900 (MSUP-VII-I-8).

72. Letter No. 24 from Kölliker to Golgi, 4 April 1900 (Belloni 1975, p. 187).

73. *La Provincia Pavese* (20 and 21 April 1900).

74. As recorded in a memorial plate: 'IN THIS HALL / FROM 18 TO 21 APRIL 1900 / THE INTERNATIONAL ANATOMICAL SOCIETY / HELD ITS XIV MEETING / HON-ORARY PRESIDENT A. v. KOELLIKER / PRESIDING PRESIDENT G. RETZIUS / VICE PRESIDENTS / W. WALDEYER F. MERKEL / W. FLEMMING / SECRETARY K. v. BARDELEBEN'.

75. *La Provincia Pavese* (22 April 1900).

76. Golgi (1900a; *OO*, p. 713).

77. *Ibid.* (*OO*, p. 714).

78. *Ibid.* (*OO*, p. 715).

79. Letter from Bizzozero to Golgi, 1 May 1900 (MSUP-VII-III-1).

80. Letter No. 25 from Kölliker to Golgi, 14 May 1900 (Belloni 1975, pp. 187ff.).

81. See also letters from Kölliker to Golgi, Nos. 25–30, written between 14 May and 19 June 1900 (Belloni 1975, pp. 187ff.).

82. Kölliker (1900).

83. The same year he was also made Honorary Member of the Medical Society of Gand, Cor-responding Foreign Member of the Neurological Society of Paris, and Foreign Member of the Medical Academy of Paris and the Society of Psychiatry and Neurology of Vienna.

84. Letter from Bizzozero to Forlanini, 30 June 1900 (MSUP-VII-III-1).

85. Golgi (1915, p. 2).

86. Golgi (1900b).

87. As reported in the parliamentary proceedings.

88. Letter No. 34 from Kölliker to Golgi, 7 November 1900 (Belloni 1975, p. 200).

89. A copy of Calandruccio's libel was also sent to Golgi and is held in the *Golgi Collection* of reprints of the Istituto di Patologia di Pavia.

90. Letter No. 35 from Kölliker to Golgi, 25 December 1900 (Belloni 1975, p. 203).

91. Letter from Bizzozero to Golgi, 3 February 1901 (MSUP-VII-III-1).

92. Letter No. 35 *bis* (draft) from Golgi to Kölliker, 23 January 1901 (Belloni 1975, p. 205).

93. From a letter from Golgi to Kölliker, we know that Golgi's opinion was posted to the Com-mittee. Letter No. 36 *bis* from Golgi to Kölliker, 8 February 1901 (Belloni 1975, p. 209).

94. Letter No. 36 from Kölliker to Golgi, 26 January 1901 (Belloni 1975, p. 207).

95. Letter No. 36 *bis* (draft) from Golgi to Kölliker, 8 February 1901 (Belloni 1975, pp. 208ff.).

96. Letter No. 37 from Kölliker to Golgi, 24 February 1901 (Belloni 1975, p. 210). A copy of Cajal's scientific curriculum was also received by Golgi and is currently held in the *Golgi Collection* of reprints of the Istituto di Patologia Generale (No. 229-5).

97. Letter No. 36 from Kölliker to Golgi (Belloni 1975, p. 208).

98. Letter No. 37 *bis* from Kölliker to Lina Aletti Golgi, 6 April 1901 (Belloni 1975, p. 211).

99. Golgi (1901a).

100. Letter No. 38 from Kölliker to Golgi, 16 May 1901 (Belloni 1975, p. 212).

101. Golgi (1901b).

102. Golgi (1901).

103. *Verhandlungen der Anatomischen Gesellschaft* (Supplement of the *Anatomischer Anzeiger*, 1901, **15**, pp. 205–6).

104. Letter from Enzo Bizzozero to Golgi, 10 April 1901 (MSUP-I-II-1).

105. Letter from Erminia Bizzozero to Golgi, 15 April 1901 (MSUP-I-II-2).

106. Pensa (1991, p. 137).

107. Donaggio (1926, p. 13).

108. Letter from Romeo Fusari to Golgi, 8 December 1901 (MSUP-VII-III-4).

20

The laboratory where a discovery is made every day

By the end of the century, the Laboratory of General Pathology had became an institution of world-renown and was considered the most important centre of biological research in Italy. In its new location in Palazzo Botta it was better equipped than ever and could host a considerable number of researchers.

In March 1901 Pensa had become Assistant to Luigi Sala in the new Institute of Anatomy, also located in Palazzo Botta, next door to the Laboratory of General Pathology. The relationship between Golgi and Sala was extremely friendly, and there were intense interactions among the personnel of the two laboratories, which were connected by a passageway. Marenghi continued to be Golgi's Associate; the Assistants were Veratti and, from 1900, Negri. There were also many bright students, including an extremely young Perroncito, who already, in 1901, had published a brief paper 'On the terminations of nerves in the striated muscle fibres', which according to Golgi represented 'a line of resistance against the transcendental school of Apáthy',[1] as he sarcastically called the Hungarian scientist's generalization of the neurofibrillar hypothesis. Also in evidence was Guido Sala, who even before graduating had concluded important studies on the sensitive corpuscles of Pacini and Herbst.[2]

And then there was Gemelli. The stern 'Temple of Science' environment of the laboratory in Palazzo Botta constrained his exuberance and channelled it into scientific research. Golgi was like a bottle cork on this ebullient personality.[3] Research became the dominant interest of the young socialist militant who in June 1900, while still a fourth-year medical student, had already presented a paper to the Societá Medico-Chirurgica on the structure of the pituitary gland, in the cells of which he had identified the internal reticular apparatus.

Joining the Laboratory of General Pathology had, however, confronted Gemelli with a dilemma. As a socialist militant and contributor to *La Plebe* he propounded political ideas opposite to those of his scientific master who, as leader of the 'clerical−moderate alliance', was vilified by left-wing newspapers. Gemelli, under Golgi's influence, began to substitute for socialism the ideal of science, in Golgi's meaning of the true 'coefficient' of human progress and development. But among his fellows at the Collegio Ghislieri were many left-wing students, who, with the intransigence typical of young radicals, did not bother to distinguish between the merits of the scholar and his questionable political opinions, and Gemelli's idealization of Golgi the scientist was the object of sharp criticism. So Gemelli was accused of having opportunistically betrayed the socialist ideal in order to advance his career in Golgi's laboratory. Of course, being labelled a careerist incensed Gemelli and turned him into a loaded spring ready to uncoil at the least provocation. As Medea would later recall at a meeting of alumni of the Collegio Ghislieri in 1960:

It happened that in the local newspaper [*La Provincia Pavese*] a fellow student wrote an article against Golgi, the great Master. Gemelli, who worked in Golgi's laboratory, and was under his spell, quarrelled bitterly with the writer of the article. The latter answered immediately with an even more critical article. Gemelli was blind with rage: entering the dining hall, he slapped the offender . . . This behaviour was condemned by the directorship, which severely censored Gemelli.[4]

The writer of the article was Eugenio Bravetta, an intern in Monti's laboratory.

A lawsuit followed the physical attack almost immediately. Bravetta brought Gemelli to court but the latter, 'thanks to the good offices of the judge, expressed his utter regret for having debased himself with such violent behaviour against his fellow student, and begged Bravetta to accept this declaration and to forgo the lawsuit, of which he agreed to pay all expenses. Bravetta, commendably, accepted Gemelli's offer and forgave him.'[5]

But such a volcanic temper was always likely to erupt again and in 1902 Gemelli was expelled from the Collegio Ghislieri because of his recidivism.[3]

On 4 November 1901 Golgi gave the opening speech for the solemn inauguration of the 1901–02 academic year. He was back at the helm of a university with 1329 students, of which 553 were enrolled in the Medical School. To them, he addressed his positivistic credo.

We, who have grown up in the faith of infinite progress, but who have been educated by experience and disciplined by scientific logic, look confidently upon you, on whom rests the task of consolidating and widening acquired knowledge, to participate, by spreading intellectual education with a mind free from political prejudice, in transforming of society, which we believe will be achieved, not through political commotions and revolutions, but because of the inescapable law of evolution.[6]

The University had to solve a number of problems dating from Golgi's first Rectorship, among which was the reorganization of the clinics. For Golgi, the modernization of the University of Pavia was the only way to ward off the creation of a second university in Lombardy, a possibility that was constantly on the horizon because of the power and wealth of Milan.

Pavia should not delude itself with historical and juridical considerations, or with the richness of its glorious past and splendid traditions. Pavia will overcome its fears only by providing the necessary means for the study of all branches of science and by becoming a true academic magnet because of the excellence of its institutions and faculty.[7]

The financial autonomy of the University, however, had been strengthened a few months earlier when the Consorzio Universitario Pavese disbanded,[8] to be resurrected on

11 September 1901 as Consorzio Universitario Lombardo. The meaning of this modification was to emphasize the Lombardian spirit of the University of Pavia with the inclusion in the new alliance of the other provincial administrations of Lombardy. Among the aims of the new consortium was that of 'supporting the most needy university institutions, funding those lacking financial aid from the national government, and augmenting the number of professorships of high scientific relevance.'[9]

Around the middle of December, Golgi received a letter from Kölliker, who commented on the awarding of the Nobel Prize to Behring for his introduction of passive immunization therapy. The Swiss histologist believed it was 'not right' because 'men, who had worked all their lives to enlarge our knowledge of the anatomy of the human body, are worthier of esteem than those who have obtained without effort and fatigue one finding, which although useful to human society, cannot be compared with the discoveries of others.[10]

On 21 January 1902 Golgi intervened at the National Senate during the debate of the law on the 'suppression of the Municipality of San Giovanni and its annexation by Sestri Ponente'. He knew these two municipalities 'like the back of his hand' (he had studied the hygienic aspects of the sewer system of Sestri Ponente) and he argued in favour of their unification particularly because this would allow a more efficient management of their sewer systems with less hindrance by bureaucratic red tape.

In February, the students began to agitate against rules that kept them from taking the same exams at different times during the year. Golgi had to intervene to calm the waters. Because of the 'unlimited trust that on that occasion the students placed in the Rector', it was sufficient that he guaranteed that he would 'defend the interests of the youths, to restore the status quo'.[11] Golgi skilfully found a solution by retrieving a regulation that allowed extra sessions of exams to be held for those students who had been unable, for a justifiable reason, to take the regularly scheduled exam.

During that winter Kölliker's health began to deteriorate. In March he wrote to Golgi that he was suffering from a respiratory insufficiency which, according to his physician, was caused by 'a certain plumpness and by excessive development of fat tissue'. Then he added that 'you will understand that I need the climate of a country warmer than Germany.'[12] He planned to spend some time in Lugano the following April, and from there to join his friend in Pavia and stay with him between 18 and 20 April.[13] Meanwhile, Golgi, fully aware of Kölliker's fondness for the 'good products of Italy', sent him a barrel of wine as a gift.[14]

Kölliker's sojourn with his Italian friends was, as usual, extremely pleasant.

The days I spend with your dear family are always festive and incomparable [sic; he obviously meant 'comparable'] only to those which I have spent with my children, that is to say, that I feel like a member of your family. A thousand thank-yous for your amiability and solicitude, which you have bestowed on my health and my well-being.[15]

The older Kölliker became, the more attached he became to the Golgis, 'who have had such a great influence on my life'.[12]

With the royal decree of 1 May 1902 Golgi was appointed Cavaliere dell'Ordine Civile di Savoia.[16] The honour surely gave him a great satisfaction and despite his modest and reserved personality he sent the news to his Swiss friend. The latter wittily complimented him (in an awkward Italian):

Dearest friend!
Today I received here [Jena] your letter of 28.IV. which gave me great pleasure for the news that the cross for civil merit has been conferred to you, a cross that has such a great value that I see the good Lina smile with all her amiable person at the thought of the benefits associated with it. We have nothing that could be compared to that cross, unfortunately.[17]

Probably on 10 May the Golgis were hosts to Kölliker's son, Konrad Alfred Oskar Kölliker, who was returning from a vacation in Capri.[18] A few weeks earlier he too had received a barrel of wine as a gift.

With the work carried out by Golgi, Bethe, Apáthy, Donaggio, Nissl, and Holmgren, the structure of the nerve cell had become much more complex. Luigi Luciani, Professor of Physiology of the University of Rome, asked Golgi to explain the relationship between his cytological discoveries and those of other histologists. The answer, in the shape of a letter, was sent on 30 May 1902 and Luciani published it in an abridged form in his handbook *Fisiologia dell'Uomo* [Human physiology].[19]

Concerning the functional meaning of the internal reticular apparatus, Golgi took no position and simply discussed the morphological 'facts'. He then emphasized the nervous nature of the fibrillary structure located in the periphery of the nerve cells (the description of which he had given at the meeting of the Anatomische Gesellschaft held in Pavia), which was indicated by its continuity with the axon. This was a confirmation of the neurofibrillary nature of the nerve cell, in line with the 1871 studies by Max Schultze and with the more recent work by Bethe (whose overall theoretical interpretations were, however, rejected by Golgi) and Donaggio.

As we have seen, four years earlier Golgi had, in the same paper in which he announced the discovery of the internal reticular apparatus, reported on 'a covering of reticular nature' on the surface of the nerve cells. He had suggested that it was an 'insulating shell' of neurokeratinic nature and considered it a further problem for the 'contact' hypothesis, that is for the theory of the neuron. Bethe, who had called this structure *Golgi-Netz* (Net of Golgi), attributed to it a great relevance for his reticular theory, which resuscitated Apáthy's notion that the neurofibril was the conductive element in the nervous system. According to Bethe, on the surface of, and among, the nerve cells, there was a continuous neuro-fibrillary reticulum. The part of this reticulum lying against the cells was the *Golgi-Netz* (which in turn was continuous with the intracellular neurofibrils), whereas the part located among the cells was a 'fundamental intercellular reticulum'. For Bethe, the neurofibrils in the afferent nerve fibres continued into the *Golgi-Netz* and via the latter the nerve impulse could travel through both the fundamental intercellular reticulum and the neurofibrils of the efferent fibres. Therefore the *Golgi-Netz* would play a pivotal role in ensuring the continuity between the afferent and the efferent sides of the nervous system.

All in all, it was an overly convoluted theory, even more complex than that of the diffuse neural net. Predictably, Golgi rejected Bethe's interpretation of the pericellular 'covering of reticular nature' and continued to consider it a neurokeratinic 'shell'.

In concluding his letter, Golgi restated his antineuronist position.

During an anatomical meeting, I was especially commended for having never adhered to the neuron concept: I accepted that compliment and still now I pride myself on never having used that word even in my lectures, except for historical reasons. Neuron is a word that became successful especially because of the authority of the individual who introduced it (Waldeyer), but it cannot claim any well-grounded right to citizenship in science.[20]

Cajal, in his *Textura del sistema nervioso*, had accused the Pavian School of partisanship. Now Golgi struck back by attacking the initial observation upon which the Spaniard had built his 'theory of the contact': that is, the baskets around the Purkinje cells.

As is well known, Cajal had the bright idea for that theory from the observation of the anatomical relationship between the vertically descending collaterals of the nerve process of the small nerve cells of the molecular layer (cells described by me back in 1873, and well drawn by Fusari in one of his papers published in 1887), and the body of Purkinje cells. Having observed that those vertical collaterals give rise to short ramifications at the level of the Purkinje cell, ramifications that adhere to the contour of the said cells, he thought that such ramifications represented true terminations on the body of the nerve cells, and compared them to the motor plate of muscles. And it is indeed from this comparison with the motor plate that he got the idea of naming what he believed were the terminations of the nerve fibres on the surface of the ganglion cell bodies, as 'plaques of the soul' (*placas de l'alma*).[20]

These structures, which had now become 'a sort of anatomical gospel in the service of physiological interpretations' were, according to Golgi, nothing more than 'the expression of incomplete reactions, which are easily produced by staining the cerebellum with my methods of the black reaction.'[21] On the contrary,

the best and most successful reactions, which to tell the truth can be obtained only with great effort and then by hammering again and again on the same point, show that the nerve fibres, which form the well-known baskets, continue in the granular layer, where they branch in the most complicated manner, taking part in the formation of the diffuse neural net of the said layer.[22]

It was the usual accusation of not having worked in the best manner and having achieved imperfect impregnations.

The internal reticular apparatus continued to attract considerable interest. Kölliker asked Golgi to provide him with some preparations, which he wanted to show to Philipp Stöhr, his successor in the Chair of anatomy at the University of Würzburg. The latter was preparing a new edition of his handbook of histology and, wishing to deal with the internal reticular apparatus, wanted to observe it '*in majorem Golgii gloriam*'[23] in a preparation obtained directly from the discoverer. Reciprocating, on 19 June Kölliker sent to his Italian colleague a selection of his preparations of various tissues obtained by his technician, Georg Peter Hofmann, and by some assistants at the Institute of Anatomy of Würzburg.[24]

After the discovery of the internal reticular apparatus, another crucial cytological discovery (although acknowledged as such only many years later) came out of Golgi's laboratory, this time at the hand of Veratti. Because of his extremely strong background in fields ranging from bacteriology to histology, and his excellence as an experimenter, Veratti had emerged as one of the leading figures in Golgi's group. He was always very generous in helping anyone who sought his advice and many had availed themselves of his expertise, beginning with Golgi, for whom Veratti also drew fine morphological figures from histological preparations. We have already mentioned how Veratti's hypercritical attitude tended to hinder his scientific activity. Nevertheless, he had many important papers under his belt. In 1902 he published a study on the structure of the muscle fibre in which he described a unique structure, which had been partially described in 1895 by Romeo Fusari in two short papers published in *Archives Italiennes de Biologie*. By using the black reaction on different types of muscles, he discovered a series of transversal reticular systems, which followed the architectonic disposition of the bands of the muscle fibre and which were connected by longitudinal bridges.[25] Reticular structures in the muscle fibre had already been glimpsed by some authors, in particular Cajal and Retzius, who, however, had not appreciated the most important morphological peculiarities and the regularity of their distribution. Initially, Veratti emphasized the morphological similarities with the internal reticular apparatus of Golgi, but later it became clear that the endoplasmic reticulum of the muscle fibre had unique characteristics. Until the introduction of electron microscopy, Veratti's reticulum (later called sarcoplasmic reticulum) was accorded little functional significance. Many even thought that it was an artifact caused by a reaction of the chemical reagents used for the staining. Modern physiology has unveiled the role of the sarcoplasmic reticulum in the transmission of action potentials and in the storage and release of Ca^{2+} (responsible for the contraction of the muscle fibres).

On 9 July Gemelli graduated, before a beaming Golgi. He defended a complex experimental dissertation on the embryology and anatomy of the hypophysis, which would later be the subject of a communication to the Societá Medico-Chirurgica. Golgi ensured that the young scholar would receive the Harnack microscope, which the University awarded 'to the student who had given the highest evidence of preparation and competency in histological studies'.[26] From the Army hospital of Milan, where he was doing his military service, Gemelli thanked the master 'for his goodness' of which he felt 'so unworthy' and expressed gratitude 'for the inspiration to love positive sciences and for the even too-benign indulgence towards my escapades', and concluded with the assurance that he would remain 'loyal to the teachings' of his professor.[27] Everything indicated that he was on his way to a successful academic career under Golgi's protective wing.

But his restless personality would once again surprise everybody. He had been a materialist, a socialist and a *mangiapreti* ['priest-eater'], and so no one could have expected his sensational conversion to Catholicism, much less a religious vocation. In November 1903, after an existential crisis lasting several months and in which a failed romantic relationship had probably played a role, Gemelli became a Franciscan novice in the monastery of Rezzato, and then entered the order with the name of Agostino. The news caused a stir in the local press, and was also taken up by the *Corriere della Sera*, the most influential national newspaper. Naturally, this news raised some eyebrows at Palazzo Botta where everybody knew the young histologist as a boisterous materialist and positivist.

Among the anonymous essays that Golgi evaluated at the end of 1903, in his capacity as the committee Chair of the Cagnola Prize, was a monograph of 371 pages and 27 tables, concerning the histology of the hypophysis. It was obviously written by Gemelli. The committee concluded that, although the study was a 'thorough monographic study on the hypophysis' with 'original contributions in all chapters', it couldn't win the Prize insofar as the author had not been 'able to provide the critical contribution that is necessary in this kind of investigation'. Furthermore, the methodology used in the study was accused of 'eliciting doubts about its scrupulosity'.[28] It is probable that his unseemly philosophical treachery had alienated Golgi and the other members of the committee (which also included Forlanini). Certainly, his religious vocation struck Golgi as a betrayal of the positivistic credo that was supposed to inspire all serious scientists.

On 11 July 1902 Golgi read a report on the state of the university institutes before the Council of the Consorzio Universitario Lombardo, of which he was President.[29] The situation he described was quite depressing. The Institute of Chemistry did not have enough laboratory space for chemistry and pharmacy students; the Institute of Physiology consisted of four rooms 'in which there was insufficient space for the equipment, let alone the students',[30] and its director, Oehl, had stated in a letter that he was 'unable to buy equipment because of the lack of space'; the Institute of Physics lacked the laboratories for the training of senior students and the lecture hall could not accommodate all students. But the most catastrophic situation was that of the clinics, except for the Surgical and Gynaecological Clinics, the conditions of which were considered satisfactory by their directors Bottini and Mangiagalli. The Clinic of Dermatology and Venereal Diseases and the Clinic of Ophthalmology were in abysmal conditions. The Psychiatry Clinic was virtually non-existent, consisting simply of some patients from the mental hospital of Voghera who were brought in to be shown during the lectures in a 'circus-like' atmosphere.[31] Paediatric clinics had been established in many Italian universities (Padua, Bologna, Rome, Naples), but Pavia continued to be without one. And then there was the situation of the Medical Clinic. The new director Carlo Forlanini described it in these words:

The Medical Clinic of Pavia is nothing but a ward from a medieval hospital dedicated to educational purposes. Of the radical changes that progress has produced in hospital treatment, and in the organization of university clinics, there is no trace whatsoever . . .

For Pavia, the need to create completely new clinics is urgent and vital. Not doing so would unavoidably lead to decadence and abandonment: And there are signs that the latter have already begun and progressed.[32]

In a deliberation about two months earlier the Medical School had requested that 'the Consorzio Universitario Lombardo sponsor an initiative for the creation of new clinics with an attached Institute of Pathological Anatomy, in agreement with the needs of modern science, and to this end that it request the support of the State, and of the provinces and municipalities of Lombardy.'[33]

In reviewing this disheartening situation and interpreting the wishes of the Medical School, Golgi sowed the first seed for the future *Policlinico Universitario*. But, reading between the lines, his initiative was nothing more than an attempt to defend the University of Pavia from the threat from Milan, which as we shall see was becoming ever more concrete.

During the first six months of 1902 Lina Golgi had been in poor health. When the news reached Kölliker, he wrote to his Italian friend (again in his clumsy Italian syntax):

In this letter of mine I am concerned above all that your very dear Lina has not been in very good health for the greater part of the year. I have to say however that I didn't notice that she wasn't in good health when I lived [sic—he meant 'saw'] her in Munich. Then she was in an extremely good mood, ate and drank beer with great pleasure, and was as active as a young lady of 16 years of age. It is possible that at home she had some disturbances that might have worried you. But now, as you tell me, she is much better because of the climatic therapy and the rest that she has found in the mountains, and I hope that this state of good health will last, especially if she avoids fatiguing herself with the minor tasks in the home.[34]

And then, addressing Golgi's apologies for not having written with greater frequency, he added:

I know how many things and preoccupations weigh on you, and I am always happy to receive letters from you even though they do not arrive regularly like the letters of a lover to his mistress.

Kölliker intended to spend most of the winter on the Italian Riviera, and planned to visit the Golgis in October for the celebration of their Silver Anniversary and Camillo's academic jubilee. But given his age, he would not be travelling alone:

I am bringing with me one of my servants as an aide, and I beg you to let me know if you could provide a room for her when I come to visit in October. I am too old to travel alone and I prefer a female to a male servant.[35]

Although 85, he was still quite a lively fellow.

In fact, Golgi's actual professorial jubilee for 25 years of teaching had been the year before, but his students and admirers had decided to wait until his 25th wedding anniversary on 28 October 1902 to celebrate simultaneously and in the most solemn manner the two milestones of his academic and private lives. His disciples, Fusari, Marenghi, and Luigi Sala, collected Golgi's scientific articles in three volumes, which were published with the title *Opera Omnia* by the publisher Ulrico Hoepli of Milan, who covered the considerable printing expenses with his own money. Although the 325 copies of the *Opera Omnia* would be printed only in 1903,[36] a copy was ready to be offered to Golgi during the ceremony.

The lecture hall of the Institute of General Pathology was 'filled with ornamental plants, crowded with academics, physicians, and authorities, and presented a solemn appearance'[37] compounded by the presence of Kölliker, the 'Nestor of histologists', who had come to pay homage to his Italian friend. 'The illustrious old man, entering the lecture hall of the Institute of General Pathology and climbing with Golgi to the podium, was greeted by a warm and prolonged ovation, a testimonial to the sympathy and respect that also surrounded his name in Italy.'

Fusari placed on the podium the three large volumes, embossed in gold. Speaking 'in the name of all fellow students from the glorious School of Histology and General Pathology', he congratulated Golgi on his quarter century of university teaching and matrimony. With great emotion, he recalled that the Institute of General Pathology 'is our pride, and to it alone most of us owe the position that we now have in the world of science', adding:

You, who admirably persevere in studying and research, and your worthy and kind companion, who has surrounded you with the greatest affection, sweetening your life with the most delicate attention, exhorting to be calm in days of sadness, with the joyous expansiveness of her soul and taking an interest in the rigour of scientific research, sometimes even helping you in your strenuous work, both of you can now claim to have succeeded.[38]

He then remembered Golgi's studies collected in the *Opera Omnia* as 'a most worthy and enduring monument erected in celebration not only of this day but of an entire epoch in the history of biology.'

After Fusari, it was the turn of Nicolò Manfredi, an old friend since the happy times in Bizzozero's laboratory. Manfredi thanked Golgi and the organizing committee 'for not having forgotten to invite me as your oldest collaborator in that now historical Laboratory of Experimental Pathology',[39] as 'your most loyal friend and admirer', as the person who 'always kept his heart open for you, even when occasionally there was a divergence of opinion.'[40] Following the brief speech, 'accompanied by applause, the two friends, repeatedly and affectionately embraced'.

Then it was the turn of Ulrico Hoepli, who recalled the important role of his publishing company in promoting culture and stated his pride in 'having been the godfather of three splendid volumes, which the disciples have edited with patient, indefatigable, almost filial dedication.'[41]

Finally, Golgi spoke. First, he thanked Kölliker for his presence at the ceremony, 'another manifestation of the friendship with which he has honoured me since our first encounter' and indicative 'of the sympathy and affection he has always demonstrated, since his youth, for our country and its scholars'. Here Golgi was alluding to the ties of friendship and collaboration that Kölliker had with Corti, De Filippi, and other Italian scholars. He concluded by thanking Hoepli, the municipal authorities, and, finally, his disciples. And to the latter:

With an affectionate and delicate thought you arranged that this ceremony would coincide with the 25th anniversary of a date dearer to me than any other one, but that so far I have celebrated only in the intimacy of the home, the only true festive day in our family, and I cannot imagine anything that could have been more pleasant to me than this thought of yours, of associating in the ceremony me and the companion of the best years of my life. To her, who has made my home cheerful, who has shared with me happy and sad hours, who has helped me and heartened me in my work . . . the simple flower that, with a brief note, every year without exception, I sent to her from near and far, to show her all my gratitude, has transmuted in the splendid celebration of which 'the two of us together' are the object.[42]

On this moving occasion, the usually introverted Golgi opened up, and rhapsodized about his relationship with Lina. Without any reticence, he told everybody of his habit of sending her every year a fragrant flower of *gaggia* on the occasion of their anniversary.[43]

Then, with customary modesty, he decidedly declared that he did 'not deserve the exceptional demonstrations of which I am today the recipient: they are, to say the least, disproportionate to what my efforts, my attitude, and the circumstances under which I spent most of my life, have allowed me to achieve for the benefit of science and scholarship.' In his speech, repeatedly interrupted by applause and delivered with a lump in his throat, he then restated what had always been his methodological philosophy in scientific research:

The most solid scientific knowledge . . . is never conquered with flights of fancy, which can only lead to an appearance of progress, but with minute, methodical, daily work, which, leading to the solid acquisition of a single fact, creates the unshakeable knowledge of the laws of life.

Here is a manner of conducting research that makes one think of long and snowy winter months and of the slow rhythm of daily life in the mountains from which he came.

At the end Kölliker spoke a few words of congratulation to the applause of the crowd, and then the two friends hugged and kissed. In the following weeks, Kölliker described the celebration in an affectionate tone in the *Anatomischer Anzeiger*.[44]

Golgi received 170 congratulatory telegrams from disciples, colleagues, and politicians, including the Minister of the Interior, Giovanni Giolitti, Baccelli, Mangiagalli, Bassini, Sertoli, Martinotti, Mosso, and Nansen. The Medical School of the Imperial University of Charkoff sent a telegram announcing Golgi's election to honorary membership of the University.[45]

In the meantime, the news of a project to create 'Clinical institutes for specialist studies of young physicians' in Milan had become public. The establishment of a large Obstetrical–Gynaecological Clinic and a Clinic for Occupational Diseases were also rumoured. The concern that these institutions could be the core of a future Medical School in Milan was voiced by Golgi on 10 November in his Rectorial address inaugurating the 1902–03 academic year. He realized that he could not oppose the creation of a Gynaecological Hospital, insofar as 'in a city as densely populated as Milan, it corresponded to a real necessity that had to be met as soon as possible'. However, the rumoured idea of a Clinic for Occupational Diseases was an entirely different matter. Indeed, Golgi noted that 'from one point of view or another, most if not all diseases, regardless of their nature . . . could be considered as work-related . . . In reality this could be only a prelude to a new University *Policlinico!*'[46] And almost as if to exorcise this idea, he added:

I am far from suspecting that someone is planning to establish a true university in Milan, or to establish there a complete course of medical studies. Milan's exuberant activity can be channelled in other ways than by taking away some of the scientific institutes of Pavia, or competing in any other way with our Medical School.[47]

He warned, however, that

the day when Milan will have clinical institutes of the quality that can be easily obtained with the plentiful means available to her, while Pavia's medical institutes will be barely surviving amongst all kinds of difficulties, that day the idea that medical research should move where there are adequate means will fatefully prevail; nor would any historical and juridical reason be sufficient to save Pavia from this danger.[48]

Hence the call for a greater involvement of the Consorzio Universitario Lombardo in the modernization of the Pavian facilities.

But Golgi had to watch his back. Some of the most active advocates of the Milanese cause were in fact in Pavia. The idea of a Clinic for Occupational Diseases, for example, had been launched by Luigi Devoto, Professor of Medical Pathology at the University of Pavia since 1899. Pragmatic and skilful in obtaining funding, he had quickly managed to improve the state of his Clinic considerably. In 1901, besides teaching medical pathology, he offered a *corso libero* in occupational diseases, the first of its kind in Italy. He also founded a journal of occupational medicine, *Il Lavoro*. In its first issue he published a paper on the diseases of workers in the rice fields, which was received enthusiastically by Ersilia Brønzini, an active promoter of feminist initiatives linked to the movement Unione Feminile. And in 1902 Devoto published a piece titled 'Concerning occupational medicine' in the official journal of the Unione Feminile. Devoto's activism was openly opposed by Forlanini, who resented his *modus operandi*. Only with great difficulty, and thanks to the pressure that Luigi Majno (husband of Ersilia Bronzini) exerted on Nunzio Nasi, the Minister of Public Education, did Devoto succeed in obtaining tenure in 1902. Obviously, the natural outlet of his project could only be in a big industrial city like Milan, and this explains his close ties with Mangiagalli.[49]

The war with Milan was about to start and Golgi was ready to throw all his political weight into the battle to defend the University on which 'I focus all my aspirations and ambitions'.[50]

Within ten days of Golgi's speech, the plans for a Medical School in Milan became a reality. On 20 November the city council of Milan approved the establishment of the 'Clinical institutes for specialist studies of young physicians'. A number of clinics were envisioned, including the one most dreaded by Golgi: a Clinic for Occupational Diseases.

The individual who would become the main promoter of this project was about to arrive in Milan. On 8 July 1902 the Director of the School of Obstetrics of Milan, Edoardo Porro, had died and Mangiagalli was called to replace him. On the surface, it seemed to be a step backwards in his career, but in reality, by gaining a foothold in Milan, he was now able to throw himself into the project body and soul, beginning with the creation of a great Obstetrical–Gynaecological Clinic. The foundation of a new Medical School in Milan was on the horizon. In November, after a few hesitations (probably more of appearance than substance), Mangiagalli decided to move to Milan. The swords were out of their scabbards, and the two duellists ready.

Golgi was so engulfed in his administrative and didactic duties that he had little time to conduct research personally. He continued, however, to advise and direct the research in progress in his laboratory, with an apparently detached attitude but actually with sincere interest. A topic in which he periodically took an interest, with modest results, was the pathological anatomy of rabies. Back in 1897, G. Daddi had reported, at a meeting of the Societá Medico-Chirurgica, on the inflammatory lesions of the nervous system in three patients who had died because of this disease.[51]

The studies on the histopathology of rabies that had been published in the following years had given the impression that the problem of the aetiology of rabies could not be solved at that time. But Golgi, whose morphological studies had contributed to the solution of the pathogenesis of malaria, persisted in this task despite the meagre results obtained so far. In 1902 he gave Negri responsibility for resuming the research on the histopathology of rabies, and with verifying a recent report on the alterations of the cells of the spinal ganglion of animals that had died from the disease. Negri 'accepted the advice of his Master without enthusiasm, because at that time the topic of the aetiology of rabies had been put aside, as often happens when there is a conviction that a problem cannot be investigated with the means available.'[52] But even with the earliest preparations, especially those obtained using the staining method of Mann, 'Negri noticed the presence in the nerve cells of corpuscles having characteristics that led him to believe that they could be sporozoites.'[53] He showed the preparations to Pensa, who was astonished. However, the two researchers still had lingering doubts about the interpretation of this finding. Negri extended his research to the nervous system of dogs that had died of rabies (provided by Daddi, then director of the Centre against Rabies in Florence), of a cat experimentally infected by subdural inoculation, and finally on pieces of cerebellum, which had been kept for years in the laboratory, from a woman who had also died from rabies. With great satisfaction, he was able to find similar (although more complex) corpuscles in several areas of the central nervous system, and particularly in Ammon's Horn. It is clear that 'the staining method used in the early phases of his research had surely contributed' to Negri's success 'although it was later found that the corpuscles could be identified and studied also in fresh preparations or following fixation [with Zenker's fixative] without staining.'[52] Naturally, the fact that the corpuscles could be observed even in fresh preparations excluded the possibility that they were simply artifacts induced by the reagents.

The peculiar regularity and consistency of these corpuscles and their structural complexity reinforced Negri's conviction that he had identified the micro-organisms responsible for rabies. These considerations overcame the reluctance of the cautious Veratti, who was initially somewhat perplexed about this aetiological hypothesis.

Once confident about his discovery, Negri 'plucked up his courage' and showed his preparations to Golgi, who 'had no doubt that those formations were parasites'.[54] It was, however, necessary to confirm this verdict by consulting an expert parasitologist, such as Grassi, who often visited the Laboratory of General Pathology. Grassi fully corroborated the idea of a pathogenic micro-organism, and thought that the mystery of the aetiology of rabies had been solved.

The discovery was announced at a meeting of the Societá Medico-Chirurgica of 27 March 1903, chaired by Luigi Sala and attended by numerous Pavian academics, among which were Golgi, Veratti, Pensa, Gemelli, Medea, Aldo Perroncito, Monti, Sormani, and Marenghi. The interest in the disease had been rekindled in Pavia a few weeks earlier by a communication of Sormani, Professor of Hygiene, who believed that he had identified the aetiological agent in the schizomycete Coccus polimorphus lissae.

In presenting his findings, 'not without a certain trepidation', Negri, who was not yet 27 years old, expressed the hope 'that we have finally found the path leading to the solution of the problem concerning the nature of the specific agent of rabies.' And with great confidence he stated that he had demonstrated 'the presence, in the brain of rabid animals, of a special micro-organism, all the characteristics of which lead us to believe that it should be classified among the protozoans.'[55] Clearly, Negri was impressed by the resemblance of his corpuscles to the endoglobular forms of the malarial parasite, which he had seen many times in Golgi's laboratory, and by the fact that intracellular phases in the cycle of protozoan parasites had been previously demonstrated. At the end of the presentation, Monti intervened, pointing out the similarities between the corpuscles of rabies and the endocellular bodies of Guarnieri, which were found in smallpox; putting aside for the moment the aetiological interpretation given by Negri, Monti underscored the novelty of the observation from an anatomo-pathological point of view. It was then the turn of Sormani, who pointed out that in his recent research he had not observed anything comparable. 'Nothing was said by Golgi, always very economical with his words, because his approval was implicit.'[56]

The following day, Golgi wrote to the editor of *Zeitschrift für Hygiene und Infections-krankheiten* sponsoring the publication of Negri's paper in German. He emphasized that 'It concerns very detailed and interesting observations and, if you allow me to recommend the acceptance of the work . . . I take upon myself all the responsibility for this recommendation.'[57] The paper was immediately accepted,[58] and on 16 April was also presented at the Istituto Lombardo.

Negri continued to believe that he had discovered the protozoan responsible for rabies, even when the following 28 June Alfonso Di Vestea reported to the Medical Academy of Pisa the transmissibility of the infection by material that could pass through porcelain filters. And Negri's opinion was shared by illustrious microbiologists such as Gary Nathan Calkins, who called the putative parasite *Neuroryctes hydrophobiae*. In addition, Negri thought that he had identified an endocellular cycle of growth and a phase of sporulation of the parasite, which would give rise to a new generation of parasites, small enough to pass through the filters that blocked protozoans and bacteria. Independently of his specific aetiological hypothesis, which was later demonstrated to be erroneous, Negri had made a discovery of great practical importance as it allowed the rapid identification of infected animals and therefore the immediate treatment of a person who had been bitten. As Veratti remarked later, even if 'only this remained of Negri's work, he would have the right to be numbered among the benefactors of humanity.'[59]

Negri's achievement was immediately recognized. He was awarded the Cagnola and Secco Comneno Prizes from the Istituto Lombardo (Golgi was on the committees for both), and a special medal that was conferred every three years by the Societá Italiana delle Scienze (also called 'Society of the Forty').

Besides rabies (or possibly thanks to it), there was also romance in Negri's life. At the turn of the century women had began to enrol in medical school in ever greater numbers and to attend 'the laboratories where the camaraderie between the male and female students often ended in love stories and marriages.'[60] One of these was Lina Luzzani, who collaborated with Negri right from the beginning of his research on rabies. In 1904, Luzzani published two papers on the diagnosis of the disease, the second of which was translated into German and published in 1905 in the *Zeitschrift für Hygiene und Infections-krankheiten*. From collaboration to marriage was but a short step: the two were married in 1905.

Golgi's time was now almost completely absorbed by the plans for the renovation of the University, with the Milanese threat looming in the background. Some progress, however, was in sight. The beginning of the construction of the new Psychiatric Clinic (which would later be renamed the Neuropathological Clinic) was scheduled for the spring. On 10 February 1903, the technical committee sent to the Consorzio Universitario Lombardo a set of plans (with projected costs of 2 500 000 lire) for the construction of a *Policlinico,* and for the building *ex novo* of a number of scientific institutes and the renovation of others. On 20 February, Golgi sent the conclusions of this technical committee to the Minister for Public Education, soliciting the participation of the national government in the enterprise. The project was also illustrated in a meeting of the Consorzio held on 11 March.[61] Three days later the Minister answered this request with an official statement of support for the efforts of the Rector to reach an agreement between national and local administrations 'in allocating a fund of 2 500 000 lire for all the works required by the plans for the renovation of the clinics and of various scientific institutes'.[62] The national government would provide about half of this amount, while the rest would have to be shared among the Municipality and the Province of Pavia, the Collegio Ghislieri, and the Consorzio Universitario Lombardo. In April, the administrators of the Collegio Ghislieri stated their intention to contribute a sizable sum and on 16 May the Municipal Council of Pavia pledged to allocate the sum of 500 000 lire. On 23 May the representatives of the Lombard provinces, meeting in Milan, decided to double for twenty years the funding to the Consorzio Universitario, to participate in the modernization of the University.

Sometime during the spring, Golgi must have unburdened himself to Kölliker about the troubles with the new *Policlinico.* The latter answered that he found it natural 'that your government tries to make use of a man as distinguished as you', and that 'the great progress that your University has made in the process of renovating the clinics and the other scientific institutes, must be of great comfort to you.'[63]

Despite all his commitments Golgi maintained a steady flow of correspondence with his Swiss friend. Kölliker had decided to participate in the 17th Meeting of the Anatomische Gesellschaft, to be held in Heidelberg between 29 May and 1 June 1903. He planned to participate with a presentation on the development of the vitreous body. Golgi sent him some Italian papers on the subject that could not be found in Germany. In thanking him, Kölliker noted that even in this area of anatomy 'the Italians had made a great number of discoveries, and one realizes the pre-eminence of your researchers in science.'[64]

On 5 April 1903 Eusebio Oehl died. He had been responsible for the resurgence of experimental studies in Pavia around the middle of the nineteenth century. By a trick of fate he died of cancer of the skin, that is, of the tissue that he had investigated with great dedication and of which he had first described the *stratum lucidum*, which is still sometimes called Oehl's layer. After his wife's death, he had fallen into a state of melancholy, which sapped his scientific activity; the thought of his wife obsessed him to the point that he saw 'the image of the companion of his life looking down at him from the celestial spheres' and inviting him 'to keep his promise'. Golgi, in commemorating him before the Istituto Lombardo, thought that this emotional weakness was in contradiction to the rigour of the scientist, but he justified it, saying that even scientists 'while guided by logic to the extreme in their scientific investigation, in the affective or moral sphere, especially when

it concerns the most intimate family matters, cannot defend themselves from their instinctive repugnance at the thought of *nothingness* (emphasis added). [65]

In August Cajal visited Italy as a tourist, accompanied by his wife. He stopped in a
number of cities, including Pavia. We don't know if he met any scientists in Pavia. At any
rate, Golgi was on vacation elsewhere. It was during this vacation that Cajal conceived a
new method for staining the neurofibrils. Back in Madrid, he put his intuition to work,
and in a rush of feverish activity developed the important histological method that still
carries his name, a method based on the reduction of silver nitrate with pyrogallic acid.
He immediately published two technical notes in Spanish journals, and sent some preparations to Retzius for evaluation. He might also have been thinking that the Swedish
scientist could exert a certain influence on the awarding of the Nobel Prize. But Retzius
had resigned from the Medical School of the Karolinska Institute in 1890 and so was not
among the professors who assigned the Prize for Medicine and Physiology; furthermore,
he was not on good terms with those who did. Ironically, as a member of the Swedish
Academy of Sciences and as a modest poet, he was on the committees that awarded the
Prizes for Chemistry, Physics, and Literature. [66]

Golgi's vacation was interrupted at the end of August by sad news. Giovanni Marenghi,
while visiting his fiancée, Golgi's niece, had been stricken by a fulminating meningoencephalitis, and died on 26 August near Varese. He had been suffering for a while
from otitis and mastoiditis, which seemed to have healed following repeated surgeries.
Marenghi's death was a great loss for Golgi. [67] The young academic had been teaching a
corso libero in bacteriology and histopathology for the last six years, and had had a good
chance of being appointed Professor of General Pathology at the University of Ferrara.
Among his scientific achievements were the discovery of special retinal cells (often called
'cells of Marenghi'), which were discussed by Kölliker in his histological treatise; the
demonstration that a dog could survive following bilateral section of the vagus nerve, an
experiment later replicated by Ivan Petrovich Pavlov; and the remarkable discovery, made
just before his death, that the bilateral removal of the adrenal glands produced a compensatory hypertrophy of the adenohypophysis. [68]

Despite the grief from Marenghi's death, the activity in Golgi's laboratory continued
apace and foreign guests continued to arrive, among them the Dutchman Cornelius Ubbo
Ariëns Kappers. [69] Marenghi's position was taken over by Veratti, and Saverio Verson took
over the position of Assistant. To Veratti fell the job of managing the laboratory and maintaining contacts with the suppliers of laboratory material. [70] He was also in charge of the
Istituto Sieroterapico Provinciale, which produced and distributed the anti-diphtheria
serum, and which analysed the fragments of tonsils sent by municipal doctors for the
microscopic assessment of diphtheria.

On 9 November 1903 Golgi gave the traditional Rectorial lecture for the inauguration of
the 1903–04 academic year. [71] He reviewed the various administrative problems of the
previous year, beginning with that of the funding for the new *Policlinico*. Unfortunately,
the lack of action by the Province was dooming 'the plans, so promising, to a discouraging
standstill'. [72] Golgi's interest in this project must have been incredibly strong since because
of it he was neglecting scientific research right at the moment when the discovery of the

internal reticular apparatus was raising his laboratory to world heights. Furthermore, the race for the Nobel Prize was still open, and certainly some new findings could tip the balance in one direction or the other, as Cajal knew very well. But notwithstanding Golgi's effort, the negotiations were proceeding slowly because of the difficulties in forging an agreement among so many disparate institutions. And then there were the political difficulties. Many of Golgi's enemies, especially the radical Member of Parliament Roberto Rampoldi,[73] were in a position to undermine his efforts, and they did so using the most underhanded methods.

At the beginning of April, Golgi probably received news of Kölliker from Giuseppe Mantovani, President of the administrative council of the San Matteo Hospital. Mantovani was a prominent politician in Pavia and the publisher of the newspaper *L'Avvenire*, the organ of the moderates. Given his position, he was frequently in contact with Golgi 'who kept him on a leash' and used him to facilitate 'the difficult relationship between University and Hospital'.[74] Mantovani and Kölliker met in Pavia in 1900 during the congress of the Anatomische Gesellschaft.[75] The two men had met again in Rome and together toured the City,[76] and were received at the Vatican, possibly owing to connections between Mantovani and members of the Curia.

On 7 April Golgi was elected Honorary President of a special committee for the celebration of the 40th anniversary of Angelo Scarenzio's innovative treatment of syphilis with hypodermic injections of calomel (a mercury compound). In his speech, Golgi went back to the years, 'deeply engraved in my soul', when 'as young assistant under your supervision I took the first steps of my scientific career'.[77] And then he presented to his former professor the volume written in his honour by friends and colleagues. On 12 May 1904 Kölliker wrote to Golgi that during the 18th meeting of the Anatomische Gesellschaft, held in Jena between 18–21 April, the participants had been 'disappointed that you were not among them' and that 'your [Italian] language is most appropriate for a toast'. Then he added:

Retzius, who was present with his wife, would have loved to talk with you about the new research by Ramón, which you certainly know. Both of them showed excellently the fibrils drawn and described by Ramón, and I believe that the method described by R. merits all our confidence. Stöhr and I are busy at this moment testing this method, and we feel that it is much better than that of Bethe, but I would like to know your opinion on these matters.[78]

In contrast to Dohrn's theory, according to which a number of nerve cells would merge in a chain to give rise to a nerve fibre, the following statement by Kölliker must certainly have irritated Golgi [emphasis added]:

Thus, the fibres originate each from a single cell. And it appears to me that it has been proven by your and Cajal's observations that the terminal ramifications of the central fibres are not connected with the cells, *but are only in contact with them*.[76]

For Kölliker, Dohrn's theory was disproved both by Cajal, who denied the presence of fusions between the terminations of the fibres and the cell body, and by Golgi, who supported the notion that occasionally the fibres barely touched the cell body (as, for example, the baskets around Purkinje cells), before ending in the diffuse neural net.

Whichever of these last two positions was the right one, both of them contradicted Dohrn's theory.

Golgi's plans for the renovation of the University of Pavia continued to be hindered by innumerable uncertainties and difficulties. Under the indefatigable stewardship of Mangiagalli, the buildings for the clinical institutes in Milan were now at an advanced stage of construction. But Mangiagalli was very cautious in calling openly for the creation of a Milanese university. He was aware that from his seat in the Senate Golgi was pushing for the approval of laws that would block the creation of new medical schools. For the moment, he was focusing on building a large hospital, the rest would arrive with time. Therefore Mangiagalli was sending conciliatory and cooperative messages to Pavia.

The new foundation . . . far from threatening in any way the University of Pavia, is destined to be an institution complementary to it, a fact that could benefit the very University of Pavia, and which also Pavia should support, joining Milan in this effort.[79]

Notwithstanding these diplomatic overtures, however, Mangiagalli's designs were followed with suspicion by Golgi, who certainly would have agreed with the old Pavian proverb: 'lümlin, tira l'acqua al so mülin' (the person from Lomellina [the geographical region of Mangiagalli's birth] always channels the water to his own mill).[80]

Making an exception to the custom of rotating the Rectorship every two or three years among members of the different schools, Golgi was reconfirmed Rector for 1904–05. Golgi's long stay at the helm of the University had created some mild discontent, which was reflected in a number of jokes. One of the more vicious was a pun on the Pavian vernacular for male Rector (retur) and female Rector (retrice). Lina had adopted the habit of calling Golgi 'el me retur' ('my Rector') and when the two of them appeared together they could be pointed at as 'el me retur' and 'la me retrice' (which means 'my female Rector' but sounds like la meretrice, that is, 'my meretrix').[81]

In the course of his inauguration speech, Golgi emphasized his efforts to 'fend off the danger of decadence for the University, and ensure its progressive enlargement'.[82] Unfortunately, these efforts continued to encounter enormous difficulties because of the ongoing feud between the various institutions involved in funding the project. The 2 500 000 lire of 1903 had now become 3 000 000 lire , and although the Province had finally allocated 200 000 lire (which, when added to the amount allocated by the Municipality and the Consorzio, came to a grand total of only 961 000 lire) there were now problems with the Collegio Ghislieri. The distribution of Provincial funding was in fact subordinated to a change in the constitution of the Collegio Ghislieri, in a direction more favourable to the Province and this precondition brought the bureaucratic procedures to a halt. The enterprise, which had appeared to be well on its way in 1903, had now become a Sisyphean effort.

But Golgi was not disheartened and continued in his efforts. He managed to unblock the funding from the Province, and to secure the availability of the Cassa di Risparmio di Milano to lend 1 500 000 lire to the national government (to cover its part of the funding) with interest set at 3.5%, repayable over 40 years. He also hoped to involve to a greater extent the other Lombardian provinces and the Banca Popolare-Agricolo-Commerciale of Pavia.

Although Golgi had virtually given up scientific research, his laboratory was more than ever at the centre of international attention, especially because of the discovery of the characteristic bodies of rabies by Negri. Negri and Luzzani, in collaboration with Domenico Pane and Alfredo Macchi, continued their work on rabies; other lines of research were pursued by Ottorino Rossi, Mondino's assistant who attended the lab in his spare time; by the students Domenico Cesa Bianchi and Corrado Da Fano; and by Gaspare Alagna, Carlo Bezzola, and Celestino Gozzi.

But beginning in 1905 it was the work of Perroncito on nerve regeneration that began to attract the greatest interest. In Golgi's laboratory this problem had already been attacked by Marenghi and Purpura. The former had suggested in 1897 that the regeneration of a nerve following its section did not depend on the restoration of the anatomical continuity of the nerve through the scar, but on the growth of collateral pathways.[83] But Purpura demonstrated, using the black reaction, the anatomical continuity of the regrown nerve, which crossed the scar to continue in the distal stump. Unfortunately, Purpura's findings were valid only for non-myelinated fibres, the only ones stained by the black reaction (and even these were stained with great difficulty). However, the new reduced silver method of Cajal, the importance of which had been emphasized by Kölliker in his letter to Golgi, suddenly opened new perspectives in this kind of research. 'Perroncito intended to attack the problem on a large scale from both an anatomical and physiological point of view, and devised a grandiose research programme, which he carried out over a period of almost five years of uninterrupted activity, obtaining results that allowed him to put this century-old problem to rest'.[84] In particular, Perroncito confirmed that

new nerve fibres originate from the central stump of the sectioned nerve, travel toward the peripheral stump, penetrate it and, using the degenerating fibres as a guide, reach the periphery. In addition he was the first to demonstrate that also in the central stump, a brief ascending tract of the cylindraxis of the fibre degenerates, with newly formed fibres originating above this degenerated tract. While it was believed that the regeneration of nerves was a slow process, he demonstrated the presence of changes in the central stump of the cylindraxis, which could be interpreted as the beginning of the regenerative process, as little as three hours after the cut; he followed the newly formed fibres in their trajectory through the connective tissue of the scar and among the various surviving elements in the peripheral stump, demonstrating a number of interesting characteristics concerning the behaviour of these fibres, such as terminal platelets and rings, [and] spiral-like formations [spirals of Perroncito].[85]

He then carried out a series of experiments on the collateral regeneration of nerves, describing its fundamental mechanisms. Independently, Cajal and Marinesco made similar experiments at about the same time, with results that agreed with those of the Italian scientist. Perroncito, however, was the first to study the initial phases of the process in a thorough manner, as indicated by the fact that Cajal proposed to refer to the division of the fibres of the central stump in the first hours following the cut as the 'phenomenon of Perroncito'.[86] The work of Perroncito, Cajal, and Marinesco finally put to rest the poligenetic theory of Bethe, according to which the distal stump could regenerate independently of its connection with the proximal neuron.

Perroncito, who was then only 25, immediately received important international recognition for his work. The Boston Medical School awarded him the Warren Prize in 1907 and the Academy of Sciences of Paris gave him the Lallemand Prize in 1910 and granted him an honorary degree.

In less than ten years a number of important discoveries had been made in Golgi's laboratory, among the most important of which were: the internal reticular apparatus (Golgi apparatus), the sarcoplasmic reticulum, Negri's bodies, and the mechanisms of nerve regeneration. As never before, one could appreciate the appropriateness of Mantegazza's comment that there was in Golgi's laboratory 'every day a new discovery'. On 27 March 1905 Kölliker, who had spent a period of convalescence in the mild climate of Nervi on the Italian Riviera, wrote to Golgi: 'Concerning the Nobel Prize, I have not received any news from Stockholm, but I shall write to you immediately if I learn something.'[87] From this one can deduce that he continued to pressure the members of the Swedish Committee in favour of his Italian friend.

After his return to Würzburg, Kölliker's health continued to worsen : 'I had never thought that my sojourn in Nervi could be so bad for me.'[88] On 2 May he received from Golgi another copy of the *Opera Omnia* (he had donated his complimentary copy from the publisher Hoepli to the local medical society). The possibility of a Nobel Prize for Golgi was still open, but Kölliker was disheartened and wrote to Golgi that he didn't know 'yet anything about the Nobel Prize, but Retzius tells me that there are people in Stockholm who are considering *Bethe*! and *Apáthy*, and we [that is, Retzius and Kölliker] are both scandalized by such a stupid idea. I hope that what these half-wits have the intention to do will not come to pass.'

This was the last letter of Kölliker to Golgi. The death of the elderly deacon of histology interrupted a beautiful friendship that had been based on scientific esteem and personal sympathy. It is interesting to notice the similarity of this friendship to the one a century earlier between the Swiss biologist Charles Bonnet and another giant from Pavia, Lazzaro Spallanzani.

That year, the Nobel Prize was assigned to Koch; yet again a histologist had been excluded. The savants of Stockholm had decided to wait before honouring a morphologist, and in some ways this was fortunate because in the meantime the infatuation for Bethe and Apáthy was evaporating; new evidence obtained with Cajal's method for demonstrating neurofibrils was showing more and more clearly that the physiological hypotheses of Bethe and Apáthy were plainly wrong.

The academic year passed without great problems. On 25 March 1905 the 8th Italian Inter-University Congress was held in Pavia under the auspices of King Vittorio Emanuele III; delegations from French universities also participated. Golgi, in his capacities as Rector and Senator, opened the proceedings with a brief speech. Among the points to be debated were the international equivalency of academic titles and the reduction of train fares for students. The latter point was warmly supported by Golgi, who emphasized that 'the greater facility of travelling is one of the most efficacious educational tools, and the best remedy against the regional chauvinism that prevents us from knowing and thoroughly evaluating what is good and beneficial to progress in other countries.'[89] In April, Golgi participated in the Congress of General Pathology in Rome, and participated in the discussion that followed a presentation by Donaggio concerning the alterations of the neurofibrillary net.

As Rector, he had to deal with a 'strike', by the students enrolled in the fourth year of medical school protesting against the fact that the exam of topographical anatomy had been made mandatory. He had also to mediate between the hospital administrators and the national government, which were in eternal strife over the contracts for the management of the clinics.

Golgi wanted to be elected Rector once again, to continue his close supervision of the plans for the new *Policlinico*, to which he had dedicated so much time and energy. And as expected, the appointment arrived in time for the traditional opening ceremony of the academic year 1905–06.

On 13 March 1906, on the portal of the Institute of Chemistry, the students found the following sign:

Owing to the absolute lack of financial means, insufficient numbers of assistants and janitors, and the extreme disproportion between the wages and the backlog of work, the Laboratory of General Chemistry will remain closed to all students who wish to carry out experimental exercises, or research of whatever nature.[90]

The note had been posted by the new Professor of Chemistry and Director of the Institute, Giuseppe Oddo, who had also sent a copy of the notice to Golgi, in his capacity as Rector. The most penalized were the students of chemistry and pharmacy who had to prepare a dissertation based on laboratory research before graduating. The sudden and unforeseen decision by Oddo jeopardized the possibility for many of graduation at the end of the summer term. The students immediately gathered in an assembly, approved a deliberation of protest against the situation, and began to boycott their classes. On 15 March Oddo sent a harsh letter to Golgi in which he not only defended his behaviour but threatened to keep the Institute shut 'until appropriate measures have been taken'. The next day Golgi presented a strongly worded petition to the Minister of Public Education in which he requested rapid provisions for the immediate reopening of the Institute of Chemistry and defended the protests of the students. He pointed out that Oddo's Institute had enough financial resources to permit the regular laboratory schedule and that the renovation of the Institute of Chemistry had been planned but could not be realized 'with the wave of a hand'. The intervention of the Minister, who telegraphed Oddo ordering him to reopen the Institute, brought the stand-off to an end.

At the end of spring, all the funding for the reorganization and modernization of the University appeared to be finally in place. The funds allocated by the Municipality, Province, and Consorzio Universitario brought the amount of money allocated for the year 1906 to 1 010 000 lire. Furthermore, the Collegio Ghislieri had allocated 200 000; the Banca Popolare–Agricolo–Commerciale etc., 40 000 lire; the Cassa di Risparmio di Milano, 140 000 lire; and the seven Lombard provinces, 160 000 lire. The total was now 1 550 000 lire. And the Cassa di Risparmio delle Provincie Lombarde was available to make a loan to the government for the remaining sum (that is, 2 000 000 lire). In June 1906 Golgi presented to the Ministry of Public Education a document in which he solicited the government to remove the last obstacles. But the government was now being recalcitrant in accepting the loan from the Cassa di Risparmio delle Provincie Lombarde.

Besides the University, there were other things on Golgi's mind. On 15 August he asked the Prefect to issue special provisions to fight malaria, which had made its appearance in the region around Pavia.[91] Between 1 and 4 October, Pavia hosted the 4th Meeting of the Italian Society of Pathology. Golgi, as President of the organizing committee, gave a brief speech at the opening of proceedings, concluding with a 'thought in memory of our master Giulio Bizzozero, whose spirit is always alive in this University, where he began his work for renewal of medical studies in Italy'.[92] Sometime in October a gas pipe broke, causing a fire in the laboratory, which 'although not of great magnitude, produced considerable damage'. The losses included an Arsonval thermostated oven 'with all its contents of glass tubes and flasks', and an enormous closet full of graduated pipettes and burettes; the damage totalled 1500 lire.[93] A few days later, Golgi participated in the Meeting of the University Professors of Milan, in which he strongly supported the increase in wages for professors, both as a form of economical justice and to avoid that 'owing to depressed economic conditions, the University cease to be a centre of attraction for the best forces, with consequent scientific decay of the nation itself'.[94] Between 27 and 29 October he participated in the 3rd International Congress of Rice Agriculture held in Pavia 'to accommodate the kind request' of the organizing committee, and made a controversial speech. The subject, 'The physical condition of the farmers in the rice-growing regions',[95] was at the centre of a political debate between the socialist left and the more or less reactionary right. The former emphasized the unhealthy conditions of the rice fields; the latter tended to minimize them. Golgi accepted the invitation to speak on this theme 'with a certain degree of satisfaction, and with a firm will that I always put into carrying out all my duties', even when 'absorbed by many other preoccupations'.[96] He limited his analysis to an evaluation of the health problems of rice workers, with special reference to the problem of malaria. Was the rice field, as many suggested, a condition favouring the transmission of the disease, or did such an idea represent an 'unwarranted prejudice'? The side that Golgi was on was immediately clear:

The truth is that there are really impressive statistics in support of the notion that the influence of rice fields [on health] is not so deleterious as it was once thought.[97]

And finding support also in other studies, Golgi cited the indices of annual mortality per 1000 inhabitants, which suggested that the rice fields had positively influenced public health by reducing the incidence of malaria. In addition, Golgi found evidence that the rice growing had improved the 'physical constitution of the youth', both in the numbers of people who had been medically exempted from military service and in the differences in life expectancy among the various provinces. He concluded that 'the rice growing industry is no less nor more healthy than any other of the best industries.'[98] Golgi then took a position on another controversial issue: the duration of the working day for rice workers (who, incidentally, were almost all women, the so-called *mondine*). On the basis of empirical data, it was believed that the air in rice fields was particularly unhealthy at dawn and dusk because it was at these times that the 'so-called miasmas' made their appearance, to the great detriment of human health. On the basis of Grassi's discoveries about the mechanism of malaria transmission, Golgi was able to conclude that 'delaying the beginning of work one hour after dawn and stopping before sunset would be useless';[99] on the contrary,

everything that gets in the way of the rapid harvesting of the rice (such as a provision to begin the work in the rice fields one hour after sunrise and to end it one hour before sunset; limitation of the working day to eight or nine hours) could have serious health consequences because this would prolong the harvesting well into the hot month of July, not only exposing the rice workers to worse working conditions . . . but also increasing the probability of contracting malaria.[100]

Thus, for Golgi, *from a scientific point of view* the health of the rice workers was better protected by working 13 to 14 hours a day. Fortunately, 'rice workers younger than 15 years' could be exempted from this working schedule because of their 'scarce stamina'.[101]

The speech was violently attacked by exponents of the left. Nino Mazzoni declared that it was at the service of the rice field owners, and an anonymous critic in the newspaper *Il Secolo* accused Golgi of having implied that 'the rice field was a holiday resort'. Gaetano Pieraccini, a socialist academic, attacked Golgi in an article on occupational diseases published in the medical magazine *Il Ramazzini*, maintaining that the mortality indices on which Golgi had based his argument were of little value. Pieraccini objected that to make valid statistical deductions, it would be necessary to compare homogenous regions, but Italian provinces 'are so different, from geological, geographic, ethnographic, anthropological, psychological, hygienic, economic, and sociological points of view, that it is sufficient to mention this fact to invalidate the statistical basis of Golgi's reasoning.' So according to Pieraccini, if the mortality in the provinces with rice fields was lower than in others without rice fields, this was due simply to the fact that in the latter there were even more serious pathological factors.

Once again Golgi was elected Rector, and on 5 November he gave his usual inauguration speech.[102] The time for the greatest honour was finally approaching and he continued to receive recognition from all over the world.[103] Within a few weeks he would see Stockholm in all its December glory.

Notes

1. Letter No. 35 *bis* (draft) from Golgi to Kölliker, 23 January 1901 (Belloni 1975, p. 206).
2. Savoldi (1990, p. 263).
3. Quoted in Cosmacini (1985, p. 35).
4. Quoted in Cosmacini (1985, pp. 33ff.).
5. *La Plebe*, 22–3 June 1901. Also in Cosmacini (1985, p. 34).
6. Golgi (1901c, p.15).
7. *Ibid.* (p. 10).
8. Vaccari (1957, p. 274).

9. Golgi (1901c, p. 7). Golgi received separate grants from the Consorzio Universitario, one for the Laboratory of Histology and one for the Laboratory of General Pathology. For example, in 1902 he received a grant of 550 lire, which he used to repair microscopes and microtomes, and to buy books 'of particular relevance to research and to complete existing collections'. Another grant was used 'for laboratory materials, such as laboratory animals, gas, glassware), of which unfortunately large amounts are broken because of the great number of students I must accept in my laboratory' (letter to the President of the Consorzio Universitario, 30 May 1902, in possession of Dr Giuseppe Raimondi).

10. Letter No. 39 from Kölliker to Golgi, 12 December 1901 (Belloni 1975, p. 213).

11. Golgi (1903a, p. 11).

12. Letter No. 40 from Kölliker to Golgi, 13 March 1902 (Belloni 1975, p. 215).

13. Letter No. 41 from Kölliker to Golgi, 10 April 1902 (Belloni 1975, p. 217).

14. Letter No. 43 from Kölliker to Golgi, 28 April 1902 (Belloni 1975, p. 219).

15. Letter No. 42 from Kölliker to Golgi, 22 April 1902 (Belloni 1975, p. 218).

16. In 1901 he became a member of the Societá Medica di Batavia (a colony of the Netherlands) and in 1902 Honorary Member of the Societá di Neurologia e Psichiatria of Kazan.

17. Letter No. 44 from Kölliker to Golgi, 4 May 1902 (Belloni 1975, p. 220).

18. Letter No. 43 from Kölliker to Golgi, 28 April 1902 (Belloni 1975, p. 220).

19. Luciani (1905, pp. 213ff.).

20. Golgi (1903b; OO, p. 727).

21. Ibid. (OO, p. 728).

22. Ibid. (OO, pp. 728ff.).

23. Letter No. 45 from Kölliker to Golgi, 9 June 1902 (Belloni 1975, p. 222).

24. Letter No. 46 from Kölliker to Golgi, 19 June 1902 (Belloni 1975, p. 222).

25. Veratti (1902).

26. In Cosmacini (1985, p. 45).

27. Letter from Gemelli to Golgi, date unreadable (MSUP-VII-I-6).

28. In Cosmacini (1985, p. 64).

29. This presentation was partially reported in a footnote to the transcript of Golgi's speech for the inauguration of the academic year 1902–03 (Golgi 1903a), and later published in full (Golgi 1903c).

30. Golgi (1903a, p. 37).

31. Pensa (1991, p. 103).

32. Golgi (1903a, p. 39).

33. Ibid. (p. 41).

34. Letter No. 48 from Kölliker to Golgi, probably at the end of summer 1902 (Belloni 1975, p. 227).

35. Ibid. (p. 228).

36. Golgi (1903d). A fourth volume was added after Golgi's death (Golgi 1929).

37. Gazzetta Medica Lombarda (1902, p. 434).

38. Ibid. (pp. 434ff).

39. Ibid. (p. 435).

40. Ibid. (p. 436).

41. Ibid. (p. 437).

42. Ibid. (p. 438).

43. Bianchi (1973, p. 15).

44. Kölliker (1902).

45. The telegram from Prof. N. Kultschitzky (who had visited the Laboratory of General Pathology) read: 'Dear professor, I am extremely happy to inform you, on the same day as your academic jubilee, that, because of your glorious merits in science, the Medical School has decided to elect you Honorary Member of the Imperial University of Charkoff. Please, accept the expression of my sincere and deep esteem and present to your kind family my most admiring congratulations for the 25th anniversary of your marriage.' The telegram from the Rector Prof. Koplewasky read: 'The Imperial University of Charkoff salutes you in the solemn day of your academic jubilee and wishes sincerely that you might continue your glorious scientific work for many more years for the benefit of humanity.' (*Gazzetta Medica Lombarda*, 1902, p. 439).

46. Golgi (1903a, p. 23).

47. *Ibid.* (p. 24).

48. *Ibid.* (pp. 24ff.).

49. See Majno (1984), Pensa (1991), and Zanobio (1992) for information about Devoto's role in founding the Clinic for Occupational Diseases of Milan and about Golgi's opposition to it.

50. Golgi (1903a, p. 6).

51. Daddi (1897).

52. Veratti (1953, p. 2).

53. Pensa (1991, p. 144).

54. *Ibid.* (p. 145).

55. Negri (1903, pp. 88ff.).

56. Veratti (1953, p. 5).

57. The letter is reproduced in Belloni (1978b, p. 47).

58. Negri (1903a).

59. Veratti (1953, pp. 5ff.).

60. Pensa (1991, p. 155).

61. Golgi (1903e).

62. Golgi (1904, p. 32).

63. Letter No. 50 from Kölliker to Golgi, 10 June 1903 (Belloni 1975, p. 230).

64. Letter No. 49 from Kölliker to Golgi, 19 April 1903 (Belloni 1975, p. 228).

65. Golgi (1903, p. 493).

66. Afzelius (1980, p. 691).

67. See Golgi's commemoration of Marenghi before the Societá Medico-Chirurgica on 22 January 1904 (Golgi 1904a).

68. These studies were partly published in 1903 in *Rendiconti dell'Istituto Lombardo*, and after his death were communicated by Golgi at the Second Meeting of the Italian Society of Pathology, held in Florence in 1904.

69. As recalled by Medea (1966, p. 4). See also the letters by Kappers (MSUP-VII-II-K).

70. Among the supplier of Golgi's laboratory were Attilio Filippini of Genoa, G. B. Rossini, Prospero Erba and Ettore Grasselli of Milan, Pietro Bellati of Florence, Augusto Tartagli of Brozzi (Florence), A. G. Cavallo of Turin, Francesco Motti of Reggio Emilia, Soffieria Monti of Sesto San Giovanni (Milan), Heinrich Mayer of Berlin, and Carl Zeiss of Jena.

71. Golgi (1904).

72. *Ibid.* (p. 34).

73. Golgi's relationship with Rampoldi had deteriorated because of a letter in which Golgi had made harsh comments on Rampoldi's position on the renovation of the University of Pavia and the creation of a university in Milan. The letter had been sent to three influential persons

and was not intended for public consumption, but unfortunately it ended up in the wrong hands and was reproduced on posters and newspapers to embarrass Golgi. This episode is recalled by Pensa (1991, p. 140).

74. Pensa (1991, p. 113).

75. Kölliker had cited him in his report at the Congress in Pavia (Kölliker 1900, p. 3).

76. Letter No. 51 from Kölliker to Golgi, 12 May 1904 (Belloni 1975, p. 233).

77. The quote is taken from Golgi's dedication in *Ad Angelo Scarenzio, in occasione del XL anniversario della prima iniezione di calomelano, Colleghi e Discepoli* (Milano: Tipografia degli Operai, 1904, pp. 7–9).

78. Letter No. 51 from Kölliker to Golgi, 12 May 1904 (Belloni 1975, p. 232).

79. In Golgi (1906a, p. 14).

80. Terni (1925, p. 22).

81. This pun has been reported to me by a reliable source.

82. Golgi (1904b, p. 6).

83. Marenghi's hypothesis of collateral pathways also puzzled Bizzozero, to whom Golgi had written to recommend Marenghi for the exam of *libera docenza*. Golgi emphasized the novelty of Marenghi's findings but anticipated the scepticism that it would trigger. Indeed, in his typewritten reply Bizzozero wrote: 'Concerning Marenghi's work, you have perfectly understood our feelings. The novelty of his results in an area so important and so well investigated has elicited not only our interest but also the desire to carry out some experiments to verify them. I must tell you in fact that I have arranged to have some animals operated on and I have re-examined numerous preparations I have kept from [Guido] Tizzoni's work on nerve section. Obviously, we won't have the results of these experiments for a few months. If you do wish that Marenghi obtain his *docenza* during the fall session of the Council, I have so much trust in your good judgement and fairness that I will underwrite your opinion blind-folded. If instead it is possible to wait, the experiments in progress will allow me to reach a personal opinion, the importance of which is indisputable . . . since the dissertation submitted by the candidate is the only scientific work that will be considered . . . Returning, with a digression, to Marenghi: In your letter of yesterday, which I shall share with Foá today, you inform us that when we visit [your laboratory] we will assist in an experimental demonstration of the conclusion reached by the candidate. This is an excellent idea, but I am afraid that it will not be definitive. E.g., to solve this puzzle, I would like to know the effects of the simultaneous section of the crural and sciatic nerves on motility. When one considers the slowness with which the peripheral stump regenerates, don't you think the suspicion arises that the functional recovery observed by Marenghi after only 20 days could depend not on the functional reinstatement owing to the regeneration of the nerve, but rather on vicarious compensation, as suggested earlier on by Van Lair?' Letter from Bizzozero to Golgi, 10 June 1897 (MSUP-VII-III-1).

84. Veratti (1929, p. 152).

85. *Ibid.* (pp. 152ff.).

86. DeFelipe and Jones (1991, p. 21).

87. Letter No. 52 from Kölliker to Golgi, 27 March 1905 (Belloni 1975, p. 235).

88. Letter No. 53 from Kölliker to Golgi, 3 May 1905 (Belloni 1975, p. 236).

89. Golgi (1905a, p. 7).

90. Session of 16 March 1906 (*Atti parlamentari del senato*, Roma: Tipografia del Senato, 1906); also in Goldaniga and Marchetti (1993, pp. 201–3). See also Zanobio and Armocida (1994, p. 618).

91. Letter to the Prefect (MSUP); also in Goldaniga and Marchetti (1993, p. 192).

92. Golgi (1906b, p. 6).
93. In a letter dated 30 October 1906 Golgi requested (in the draft there is no addressee, but it was probably addressed to the Consorzio Universitario) the extraordinary amount of 700 lire to repair the damage (draft in possession of Dr Giuseppe Raimondi).
94. Golgi (1907, p. 11).
95. Golgi (1907a).
96. *Ibid.* (p. 4).
97. *Ibid.* (p. 7).
98. *Ibid.* (p. 16).
99. *Ibid.* (p. 17).
100. *Ibid.* (p. 18).
101. *Ibid.* (p. 20).
102. Golgi (1907).
103. In 1903 he became Honorary Member of the Medical Society of Erlangen, Member Emeritus of the Medico-Surgical Academy of Naples, and Corresponding Member of the Imperial Academy of Sciences of Vienna. In 1904 he became Honorary Member of the Imperial Society of Physician of Vienna of Vienna, Foreign Honorary Member of the Royal Academy of Medicine of Belgium, and Member of the University of Karkegy. Soon afterwards he became Corresponding Member of the German Neurological Society and Honorary Member of the Royal Society for Tropical Diseases of London.

21

Siamese twins joined at the shoulder

On 26 October 1906 Golgi received the following telegram from Emil Holmgren, Professor of Histology in Stockholm:

Flueckwuensche nobelpreis sie und cajal—Holmgren.[1]

He was going to share the Nobel Prize for 'Physiology or Medicine' with Cajal.

Golgi immediately responded with the following telegram of thanks, stating that he was honoured to share the Prize with the 'celebrated scholar Cajal':

Prof. Holmgren, Stockolm
Gerührt unervartete Nachricht, erfreut Vereinigung mit berühmtem Gelehrten Cajal, danke herzlich schnelle liebenswürdige Mittheilung.[2]

The official announcement arrived in Pavia in a letter from Count Karl Axel Hampus Mörner, President of the Karolinska Institutet, sent on 26 October. That year, 191 840 francs had been set aside for the Prize in Medicine, and half of this would go to the Italian researcher. The recognition had been motivated 'in appreciation of your work on the anatomy of the nervous system'. Mörner asked Golgi if he intended to take part in the awards ceremony planned for 10 December, and if so, whether he would be accompanied by some members of his family.[3] Golgi was then informed that it was customary for the laureates to give a lecture and was asked to keep the notice of the conferring of the Prize secret; but in fact the news was already in the public domain. On 2 November Golgi sent to Mörner a telegram thanking him for 'the great unexpected honour', and stated that he would participate and would be accompanied by his wife and an assistant.

After these telegrams, Golgi sent more formal letters of thanks to both Holmgren and Mörner. In the letter to Holmgren, he also expressed regret that the news was by now widely known, 'though I'm not responsible for this. I believe that this occurred because [as soon as] the telegram was received by the Post Office it quickly made the rounds of a small town like Pavia, and from here to all of Italy.'[4] But since it seems unlikely that the personnel of the post office could read German, it is probable that the news passed around in the small circle of his collaborators and colleagues and from there to the general public.

In his letter to Mörner on 7 November, Golgi thanked the Karolinska Council for 'having considered me worthy' and stating 'my satisfaction at finding myself accorded this honour together with such a scholar as Mr Ramón y Cajal'. He then asked for more information about the ceremony and the language to be used for his lecture.[5]

The response from Mörner was dated 15 November and arrived in Pavia three days later, informing Golgi that the lectures usually lasted 45 minutes and should preferably be given in French, German, or English, the languages best known to the Swedish audience. And then he added:

Mr Ramón y Cajal has written that his health does not permit him to make the voyage at this time (I think that he will not come); on the other hand he intends to come here next spring and to give a lecture on that occasion.[6]

Golgi and Cajal were the first histologists to receive the Nobel Prize. But the battle to recognize their merits had been stormy and lasted from 1900 to 1906. Golgi's candidacy had been consistently supported by Kölliker, Retzius, and Carl Magnus Fürst; against Golgi were, among others, Bror Gadelius. Those who supported only Cajal pointed out that Golgi's discovery of the black reaction, though a great one, occurred too long ago, while his doctrine of the diffuse neural net, which he continued to propound even in his most recent publications, was shared by almost no one outside his sphere of scientific influence. The battle, therefore, was rather bitter and in fact it continued even after the news of the Prize was unofficially known.[7]

In the end, the proposal to divide the Prize garnered the majority of the votes of the committee for Medicine; certainly, one of the two anonymous votes, favourable to Cajal alone came from the Professor of Histology, Emil A. Holmgren. In 1904 he had supported both researchers but later shifted his support in favour of the Spaniard. In 1906, in a written report to the Nobel Committee, he considered Cajal 'far superior to Golgi'. It is also possible that he was irritated at Golgi's firm refusal to identify his internal reticular apparatus with the hypothetical 'canalicular' system communicating with the exterior of the cell. The Italian must therefore have received supporting votes from Mörner (Professor of Clinical Medicine), Carl Sundberg (Professor of Pathological Anatomy), John Berg (Professor of Surgery), and Johan Gustaf Edgren (Professor of Internal Medicine).

The other scientists receiving the Prize that year were Ferdinand Frédéric Henri Moissan for Chemistry, and Joseph John Thomson for Physics. Italy celebrated the contemporaneous success of Giosuè Carducci, who won the Prize for Literature but whose poor health prevented him from attending the ceremonies in Stockholm.

Toward the end of November, an 'indisposition' kept Golgi at home for 'a few days'. Meanwhile, he was preparing for the trip to Stockholm, with some uneasiness. In a letter to Grassi on 30 November he confided in fact that 'My main wish would be to stay hidden!!'[8]

But eventually the moment for departure arrived, and Golgi and his wife began the journey to Stockholm accompanied by Veratti. They had a stopover in Berlin where they met Medea who was doing his specialist studies in Oppenheim's clinic. The pupil tried his best to show them 'something of interest' but the weather 'was terrible, snowy, and windy'.[9] They boarded the ferry at Sassnitz where the sea was 'raging'; the crossing was dreadful. Then, disembarking at Trelleborg, Lina slipped on the frozen ground and suffered a fall 'like those that one makes in the skating rink, nor could I get up because my foot could not get a hold on anything'. The evening of 6 December was spent in Malmö, 'a beautiful city of more than 50 000 inhabitants' where it was decided to stopover for one day because they were 'not feeling very well'.[10] On their arrival, they were met by Fürst (with whom Golgi had been corresponding) who offered to accompany them the following day to Lund for a brief tour. In this 'well-built and elegant' town, accompanied by the 'very kind' Fürst, they met 'a number of academics and their wives'. Then they returned to Malmö, where they spent the night. Finally, on the morning of the 8th they left for the elegant *belle époque* Stockholm.

Golgi had not told anyone about his arrival plans because 'he was rather nervous and wanted to remain incognito so he could go to the hotel to revise and rehearse the French text of his lecture'.[11] But evidently Fürst or one of the professors they had met the day before had sent news of their train schedule to the capital. And so when Golgi arrived at the Stockholm station on the evening of the 8th he was flabbergasted to be met by Mörner, Retzius and his wife, many professors and, completely unexpectedly, his magniloquent and prolific antagonist, Santiago Ramón y Cajal.

There was no better occasion to put a cap on the past and acknowledge the merits of both of them, those merits that the *Synedrion Carolino* had so objectively and lucidly appraised! And it would have been truly agreeable if a gesture of reconciliation had originated from the older of the two, because Cajal, with his presence [at the station], had in a certain way encouraged him to do so. But the ice was not broken either that evening or in the subsequent unavoidable encounters during their stay in Scandinavia.[11]

The Golgis had sumptuous accommodations at the Grand Hotel of Stockholm:

Our room, which had already been booked, was on the second floor with two windows opening over the most beautiful square of Stockholm, right in front of the Royal Palace; there are mirrors, plush carpets, elegant couches and divans—a bathroom with unlimited hot and cold water, and a walk-in closet. Poor purse, how it would become empty! Believe it or not, there's a telephone in every room to call the chambermaid or manservant etc.! On the stairs, in the vestibule, on the terraces, are very rich empire carpets. Heating by steam—In the room there are electric chandeliers with lamps on the night stand and on the writing table; thermometer, warning card in case of fire, etc. etc.[9]

This letter from Lina Golgi to her mother reveals her simplicity and her marvel at the extraordinary adventure she was living.

In the hotel

(the grandest and most beautiful of Sweden and Norway) we found invitations to lunch, concert, and dinner—We saw newspapers with portraits of all the *Nobél* (here it's pronounced like that) laureates and articles about all of them—Finally, we understand very well that the awarding of this prize assumes the proportions of a *national festivity*! Later we're going out, accompanied again by the student [met at the train station] who will take us to see the most beautiful part of the city.[9]

Golgi was very nervous. He had decided to focus his lecture on a critique of the theory of the neuron. But in the last few years he had substantially suspended his research activity and he was probably not entirely up to date on the most recent scientific literature.

Certainly he had been struck by the work on neurofibrils, which seemed to have dealt a decisive blow to the theory of the neuron. Perhaps he wanted to use the Nobel lecture to claim priority for a theory that appeared to him to be supported by recent research. Indeed, the reticularist theory, which had seemed to have been utterly defeated a few years earlier, was now being revitalized in a new guise. But Golgi was aware that he would be speaking before the greatest champions of the rival theory. Retzius had been a convinced neuronist for a long time, and his and Cajal's latest research, using the silver nitrate method, was exposing the vacuousness of Bethe and Apáthy's speculations.

Golgi may also have been uneasy because he knew that the topic he had chosen for his lecture was destined to fuel a controversy, which contrasted dramatically with the festive atmosphere of the Nobel ceremony. Or, perhaps, he feared an attack from Cajal, and wanted to deal a pre-emptive strike.

There was also another reason to be agitated: the lecture, written in French, needed to be retouched and completed, but almost all his time was being eaten up by parties, meetings, and other social activities. On 9 December, Golgi and Veratti were breathlessly engaged in working on the text of the lecture in Golgi's hotel room.

Lina Golgi, still sore from her fall on the ice, described the situation to her mother:

Dear Mother,
I begin by apologizing if I write in a disconnected way, because I am always being interrupted by Camillo who with Dr Veratti is going over his lecture, and who is having me correct or transcribe phrases, and is making me do research in Dr Sala's *infamous* French dictionary. And it is necessary that I jump to my feet and run at his behest because Camillo, while feeling physically well, is rather nervous; the turn that the events are taking here is terrorizing him, and I think that if he could, he would bolt for home like a race horse.[9]

It is likely that Golgi's panic only increased with the passing of the day. They were interrupted first by Retzius carrying flowers, then by the secretary of the Italian legation, by journalists, and by the writer Astrid Ahnfelt, who had lived in Italy for many years and who offered to guide them around Stockholm. Other untimely visitors were Erik Müller and Salomon Eberhard Henschen, who 'speaks Italian a bit badly, but he wants to speak it'. Finally, it was the turn of a 'reporter' who came to interview Golgi and then 'a lady . . . I think a writer, who wanted to hear *what was going on*.' 'In sum, it is a serious affair, more serious that one could have imagined. Oh, poor us!'[9] This phrase conveys all her preoccupation with their being inadequate and out of tune with the situation. Golgi's state of mind was clearly making everyone around him anxious, especially his poor Lina.

That evening they were guests of Retzius for a dinner at the Grand Hotel. The next day, Monday the 10th, Golgi and the other laureates participated in a banquet provided by the King, while Lina, 'in the company of the wives of *two other laureates,* Mrs Thomson and Mrs Moisan [sic.]'[12] went to the Opera, where they saw Wagner's *Der fliegende Holländer*.

Now, on our return, I realize that the *half-full* bag of sweets that from time to time we are offered has been secretly introduced into the pocket of my, or rather your fur coat! The last straw!— I don't know how to render even an inkling of the kindness that they are bestowing on us: it is a true competition of who can bestow the most, and it is not an expression of my arrogance if I say that the three of us have elicited the greatest sympathy.[12]

At 7 p.m. the laureates, accompanied by Count Mörner, gathered in the grand salon of the Royal Academy of Music, and at 7.30 the ceremonies began. Mörner read his lecture praising the laureates in the 'Medicine or Physiology' section. Golgi was hailed as the pioneer of the modern investigations of the structure of the nervous system, Cajal as the one who had built on these studies and shaped the outlook of modern neuroscience. Then the King presented the laureates with the diploma and medal, addressing a few words of congratulation to each of them; with Golgi he spoke in Italian. After a brief musical inter-mission, the laureates went by carriage to the Grand Hotel for an official banquet. Count Mörner presented Lina Golgi, who was fluent in French, to Prince Eugene, son of the King, who was designated as her escort for the evening. Golgi escorted Mrs Retzius.

Lina Golgi experienced it all as a fairy tale:

The conferring of the prize by the King was solemn—then there was a grand banquet—Can you imagine your Lina on the arm of a royal prince, then seated at the table between two princes, talking to them most cordially as if they were friends? And after the meal to receive the con-gratulations of the hereditary princess and to converse with her?—I'm telling you that all in all our life here is like a dream: I would never have imagined that I would have experienced so many satisfactions.[13]

During the banquet toasts were offered by various participants, including Mörner and the Ambassadors of the laureates' countries, France, England, and Italy (the Spanish Ambassador could not attend). Golgi's toast was given in Italian. According to Cajal, Golgi 'displayed ... Olympic pride and pretentious mien',[14] but it is possible that he may have been misinterpreting as haughtiness Golgi's shyness and nervousness in the face of so much honour and attention. It is not unusual for an introvert to erect around himself a defensive barrier that makes him seem distant, antisocial, arrogant.

The three Italians returned, exhausted, to their rooms after 2 a.m. The crucial moment came the next day, Tuesday 11 December. At noon Golgi read his lecture 'The doctrine of the neurone. Theory and facts', with the goal of systematically demolishing Cajal's theory.

Golgi began by pointing out how it might seem strange that he was talking about the theory of the neuron just 'when this doctrine is generally recognized to be going out of favour';[15] here he was referring to the neoreticularist studies of Bethe and Apáthy, which sharply contradicted the position of Cajal and the neuronists. And then he added:

Despite these signs of decline, this topic is still very important and of current relevance because the majority of physiologists, anatomists, and pathologists still support the neuron theory, and no clinician could think himself sufficiently up to date if he did not accept these ideas as articles of faith.

Golgi's criticism began with the concept of the neuron as initially formulated by Waldeyer:

At the moment when the method of the black reaction was just beginning to spread, a diffusion that took place when I had, already for a decade, been obtaining results of much greater detail than those that were then attracting attention, the idea that nerve cells and fibres could form an anatomical unit was becoming evident in a far more objective way than had been made possible by previous studies. The concept then developed that the cell body and all its processes make up one independent elementary unit that is not connected to others but merely contiguous with them; to such a unit, as it was perceived, Waldeyer gave the name *neuron*.[16]

This concept implied:

(1) embryological unity (every neuron derives from a single embryonic cell);

(2) anatomical unity (body, dendrites, and axons constitute a single cell);

(3) physiological unity (the neuron is the fundamental functional element of nerve activity).

The first point derived from the histogenetic investigations of His Sr. Contradicting the concept of embryological unity, Golgi cited the studies supporting the multicellular origin of the nerve cells, and those by Bethe and Dohrn (among others) who advocated that nerve fibres originated from chains of cells. But then he underscored how these studies were not definitive and instead recalled how Aldo Perroncito had demonstrated 'that the fibres of a new structure always derive from pre-existing nerve fibres connected to the cell of origin, and not from putative peripheral cell chains.'[17] Thus he concluded that the current state of knowledge did not allow definitive conclusions on this point. Many of Golgi's reservations against the asserted embryological unity of neurons were overcome in following the two years with the decisive experiments of Ross Granville Harrison on the mechanisms of growth of the axon from the cell body.[18]

On the second point, Golgi was his own authority. He confirmed point-by-point his reticularist credo, reviewing all his objections to Cajal's theory. The theory of the neuron could not be true because it was incompatible with the concept of a diffuse neural net, which was 'formed by filaments that were demonstrably nervous because of their origin from the nerve processes of Type I and Type II cells, and from fibres demonstrably identifiable as nerve fibres.'[19] And the net was 'a distinct anatomical entity and not . . . a simple hypothesis'.[20] He then returned to the idea, to which he had already alluded many times, that anatomical continuity was not required for the transmission of nerve impulses from one fibre to another. And on this last point he cited Forel (chief advocate of neuronism). He claimed that the modality of formation of the diffuse neural net 'demonstrates the anatomical and functional continuity between nerve cells',[21] a fact that indicates how little weight he gave to the idea of intercrossings without anastomoses. The net, according to Golgi, was diffuse throughout the grey matter of the nervous system as indicated by his own studies on the dentate gyrus, published more than 20 years earlier.

On the concept of the neuron as an independent physiological unit, Golgi placed himself in direct opposition to Cajal. While adorning his words with laudatory remarks towards Cajal, the substance was mercilessly hostile to his theories. Golgi made a frontal attack on the law of dynamic polarization, Cajal's most beloved physiological inference.

This theory . . . cannot be considered an essential part of the neuron theory. In fact it only expresses one interpretation of the functioning of nerve cells, whereas it is not possible to exclude the possibility of others. Thus I believe that it is beyond the task I set myself to continue to discuss it. I shall therefore confine myself to saying that, while I admire the brilliancy of this theory which is a worthy product of the high intellect of my illustrious Spanish colleague, I cannot agree with him on some points of an anatomical nature which are of fundamental importance for his theory.[22]

He then recalled his studies on cerebral localization which, in his opinion, did not support the notion of an absolute functional autonomy of the neuron. He also mentioned his discoveries concerning the structure of nerve cells and, arguing against Holmgren's hypothesis that his system of canaliculi (Trophospongium) was identical to Golgi's internal reticular apparatus, stated that

in my opinion, the two structures do not coincide; I remain convinced that we are faced with different findings and I am also sure that my eminent colleague, continuing his research, will join me in this opinion.[23]

He then pointed out to Holmgren, present in the audience, the difference between their cytological positions.

The conclusion of his lecture was indicative of Golgi's holistic model of the nervous system and particularly his fundamental 'neurophilosophical' assumption (emphasis added):

Until now, I had no reason to depart from the idea, which I have repeatedly stated, that nerve cells, rather than working individually, act together, so that we must think that several groups of elements exercise a cumulative effect on the peripheral organs through whole bundles of fibres. It is obvious that this concept implies another regarding an action in the opposite direction insofar as sensory functions are concerned. No matter how opposed this may seem to the prevailing tendency to individualize nerve elements, *I cannot abandon the idea of a unitary action of the nervous system, and I don't mind if this brings me closer to an ancient theory.*[24]

Here he was clearly referring to Flourens' concept of an unitary action of the nervous system, an idea rooted in the old conception of the structural continuity of the brain mass as the morphological basis of nervous function.

Golgi ignored even the contributions of scientists such as Kölliker and Retzius; essentially, he remained attached to his research of 20–30 years before. Cajal was incensed and consumed by a desire to intervene. In the *Recuerdos* he wrote that:

The noble and most discreet Retzius was in consternation; Holmgren, Henschen, and all the Swedish neurologists and histologists looked at the speaker with stupefaction. I was trembling with impatience that the most elementary respect for the conventions prevented me from offering a suitable and clear correction of so many odious errors and so many deliberate omissions . . . What a cruel irony of fate to pair, like Siamese twins joined at the shoulders, scientific adversaries of such contrasting character![25]

On the contrary, according to Retzius:

I met Golgi several times personally at the Anatomical Congress and on his visit to Stockholm, when, together with Cajal, he received his (half) Nobel Prize. He was a noble, friendly and agreeable personality, who gained everyone's sympathies and esteem. He also behaved extremely nicely and with dignity to Cajal, although they had rather opposing views on important scientific issues, and in his official lectures in connection with the Nobel banquet in Stockholm he openly expressed these widely different views.[26]

After the lecture, Golgi and Lina

were abducted by Count Mörner, the Countess, and their daughters . . . and taken to Skansen— This is a hill that overlooks Stockholm, entirely surrounded by a palisade—on this hill there are sparse residences, in antique Swedish style. And also scattered here and there [are] grandiose cages, enclosures, ponds, etc. with various animals, all the fauna living in Sweden—Meanwhile it was snowing and becoming dark . . . we got into sleighs and away . . . We arrived at a grand house, rustic (in appearance), where a rich lunch [in English in the original] had been prepared—there were fruits, smoked reindeer, preserves—all excellent Swedish stuff—We returned at half past three, perhaps four o'clock, when it was completely dark and we had beneath us the spectacle of the illuminated city—Splendid! The city is a Venice, larger and cleaner, certainly because it is newer—.[12]

That evening, Golgi participated in a second banquet hosted by the King for the laureates and Lina was taken to the Opera.

At noon the next day Cajal spoke on the structure and connections of neurons. His lecture was calm and relaxed, aimed at demonstrating his discoveries and those of other supporters of the theory of the neuron such as Retzius, van Gehuchten, and Kölliker, rather than arguing with Golgi. There was, however, a critique of the neoreticularist position, clearly perceived as much more dangerous than that advocated by Golgi, and he also admitted, as a hypothetical possibility, that some 'enigmatic' system of filaments could interconnect neurons. Part of the lecture was dedicated to his recent studies on the regeneration of nerves and he cited also Perroncito, a fact that Lina Golgi pointed out with pleasure in one of her letters to her mother.

At 2.30 p.m. Golgi attended Moissan's talk and at 6 p.m. he participated in another banquet put on by Count Mörner with the academics of the Karolinska. In all there was about 30 guests invited. Mörner gave his arm to Lina Golgi, Camillo to the Countess.

The meal splendid, the house very beautiful, the kindness peerless—We were told that the father of the Countess possesses 10 millions and that the Count himself has 100 000 lire of private income. The family is composed of two very beautiful girls and four boys, also very good-looking—all the family very kind and affable—There were also toasts to Camillo and Cajal, and even to me—Camillo and Cajal responded.[12]

Thursday the 13th was very cold; there were 'coachmen with fur coats and large berets, every hair of which was white with frost'.[12] In the morning they visited the museum of antiquities; at noon Cajal exhibited some histological preparations and at 7.30 in the evening there was a meeting of the Concordia Society at the Grand Hotel, during which Henschen gave a speech in honour of the laureates, followed by a concert and dinner.

Friday was 'very grey and a bit wet, but it allowed us to go for a sleigh ride with Mrs Retzius.'[27] The next day, which was splendid, they went to visit Uppsala, guests of the University. On Sunday they strolled around the environs of Vaxholms, took a boat trip, and then were guests of Erik Müller for lunch. On Monday the 17th, they departed from 'Stockholm, with sorrow, where we have left many dear memories'[28] and travelled to Christiania (Oslo).

Our new friends have treated us with great kindness all the time, actually Retzius telegraphed to one of his local friends so he could be our guide on our arrival—in fact we found him at the station and today he took us to see various curiosities—among others an unearthed boat over 1000 years old, apparently belonging to ancient Norwegian pirates who, it is said, ventured as far as Sicily.[28]

On the 19th they were en route for home via Copenhagen and Frankfurt.

The news of the Nobel Prize had been announced in a few lines in the national press. It has often been recounted that when Golgi arrived in Pavia a band was playing near the railway station. Naturally Golgi thought that the celebration was in his honour, but he was dumbfounded when he realized that all the commotion was instead for Giovanni Rossignoli, a champion bicyclist who was returning home on the same train after a great performance in an important race.[29]

In Pavia, the students took it upon themselves to organize celebrations for the victory of the Nobel Prize.[30] At 2 p.m. on 23 January 1907 Golgi made his triumphal entrance into the *Aula Magna* of the University, where the academic body was gathered along with a crowd of students and numerous authorities including the Mayor.[31] The first to speak was a student, Ernesto Brugnatelli, whose speech was applauded enthusiastically. Then Golgi was presented with a parchment in Latin signed by the students. In his acceptance speech, Golgi regretted that he did not possess 'the gift of an easy and ornate word' and of not being able to express adequately the feelings that he felt. With great modesty he confessed that the awarding of the Nobel Prize, 'the greatest honour for a scholar', seemed to him 'enormously disproportionate' with respect to his merits. All he had achieved was 'without any other aspiration than of being of some utility: to scholarship, to my country, to the University', and should be considered 'a solemn affirmation of the anatomical thought that has guided us to the most definitive conquests of biology.' Golgi also mentioned his satisfaction at seeing 'the name of a modest researcher of tiny morphological particularities, such as I am . . . appear beside the glorious name of Giosuè Carducci', establishing a 'reconciliation of two so diverse and distant expressions of the human mind'.

The words of the Rector were followed by a 'triplicate salvo of applause'; a speech by the Mayor of Pavia brought the ceremony to a close.

In the late afternoon the students celebrated Golgi's triumph again by gathering in the street 'below the windows of Prof. Golgi, who made an appearance among the cheers'.

Two days later, Father Agostino Gemelli, in order to point out that there was something else beyond the agnostic and atheistic science celebrated in Stockholm, read a lecture at the Circolo Cattolico, titled 'From microbe to man'. The *Provincia Pavese,* in a venomous biographical note, recalled how, as a Ghislieri student, 'he [that is, Gemelli] had been renowned among his fellow students as a fanatic' and that 'neither the tears of his old father nor the love of a beautiful woman of our city were sufficient' to divert him from his intention of becoming a friar.[32]

Notes

1. MSUP. Reproduced in Calligaro (1994, p. 69). See also Zanobio (1978a, p. 144).
2. Undated note in pencil by Golgi (MSUP), in Zanobio (1978a, p. 144).

3. MSUP. Reproduced in Zanobio (1978a, p. 145).

4. As deduced from a rough copy (MSUP). Reproduced in Zanobio (1978a, p. 144).

5. A copy of the letter, stained at the moment of signing (MSUP) is reproduced in Zanobio (1978a, p. 146).

6. Letter from Mörner to Golgi (MSUP). Reproduced in Zanobio (1978a, p. 147).

7. Zanobio (1986a, p. 48).

8. Letter from Golgi to Grassi (Library of the Institute of Comparative Anatomy of the Università 'La Sapienza' di Roma).

9. Letter from Lina Aletti to her mother, 9 December 1906 (MSUP). Reproduced in Zanobio (1978a, pp. 153–4).

10. Postcard from Lina Aletti to Aldo Perroncito, 7.X [sic] 1906 (MSUP). Text in Zanobio (1978a, p. 152).

11. Riquier (1952, p. 72).

12. Letter from Lina Aletti to her mother, written on 11 and 12 December 1906 (MSUP). Reproduced in Zanobio (1978a, pp. 154–7).

13. Postcard from Lina Aletti to her mother, sent from Stockholm on 12 December 1906. Text in Zanobio (1978a, p. 152).

14. Cajal (1917, p. 283).

15. Golgi (1906; OO, p. 1259).

16. *Ibid.* (OO, p. 1260).

17. *Ibid.* (OO, p. 1266).

18. Shepherd (1991, p. 260).

19. Golgi (1906; OO, p. 1277).

20. *Ibid.* (OO, p. 1273).

21. Golgi (1906; OO, p. 1274).

22. *Ibid.* (OO, p. 1262). Then, Golgi continues: 'For example, I believe it is absolutely to be rejected that the peripheral branch of spinal ganglion cells must be identified with a protoplasmic process and that the presence of the myelin sheath must be considered as an absolutely secondary phenomenon required by the length of the process. Similarly, I could not accept as a conclusive argument in support of the theory the observation, which, however, represented its starting point, that the processes of the cells of the molecular layer of the cerebellum form terminations on the bodies of the Purkinje cells, for I have demonstrated that the fibres coming from the nerve process of the cells of the molecular layer only pass near the Purkinje cells to continue into the rich and characteristic net existing in the granular layer.' (OO, p. 1262.)
    And then: 'As for the new formulation of the theory of dynamic polarization, I have not been able to agree with my illustrious colleague about the direct passage of the nerve current from the peripheral branch to the central branch of the T division in the spinal ganglia, because it is not difficult to show that at this point the [neuro]fibrils of the peripheral and central cylinder axis change their course and turn towards the cell body, while there is no direct passage of [neuro]fibrils from the peripheral branch to the central branch.' (OO, p. 1263.) A fundamental role in the transmission of the nerve signal was in fact attributed to the neurofibrils. The fact that the neurofibrils always originated in the cell body and then distributed themselves in the two branches of the T axon led Golgi to suppose that the impulse could not skip the cell body.

23. *Ibid.* (OO, p. 1284).

24. Golgi (1906; OO, p. 1290).

25. Cajal (1917, p. 282).

26. Retzius (1948, p. 245). Translation by Professor Gunnar Grant; see also Grant (1999).

27. Postcard with a view of Uppsala, 15 December 1906. Text in Zanobio (1978a, p. 157).

28. Postcard with a view of Christiania, 18 December 1906. Text in Zanobio (1978a, p. 157).

29. The anecdote has been told to me many times. It is also reported in the text of Pavian folklore, *Fà e däsfà l'é tut laurà* (Pavia: Luigi Ponzio e figlio, 1990, Book I, pp. 77–8). I have been unable to verify its accuracy.

30. *La Provincia Pavese* (23 January 1907).

31. *La Provincia Pavese* (25 January 1907). *La Provincia Pavese* (27 January 1907).

32. *La Provincia Pavese* (27 January 1907).

22

Back to research

Now back in Pavia, Golgi was elected President by acclamation of the Società Medico-Chirurgica. But he already had too many engagements and decided to decline the honour. At Pensa's suggestion he was made Honorary President of the Società.

He used the prestige associated with the Nobel Prize to further his efforts for the renovation of the University and to ward off the Milanese foe. Meanwhile, in July 1905 the Parliament had approved a law that allowed the creation in Milan of Clinical Institutes for Specialist Studies, which it endowed with a modest State contribution. In December a non-profit organization was created to manage the Clinics of Obstetrics and Gynaecology, of Occupational Diseases, and of Infectious Diseases. The courses would be taught by instructors equivalent in status to university professors. The Clinic of Obstetrics and Gynaecology was inaugurated in 1906 while the Clinic for Occupational Diseases was in advanced stages of construction. The new Milanese institutions were configured to complement those in Pavia, and the tension between the two great antagonists, Mangiagalli and Golgi, appeared to subside. In a much more relaxed climate, Golgi was invited to give a lecture in the Clinical Institutes for Specialist Studies.[1] However, he continued to be suspicious about the intentions of the Milanese, despite their apparent spirit of cooperation. In January 1907 Mangiagalli proposed that he form a committee, which would include Devoto as well, to create a Cancer Institute in Milan, under the aegis of the Clinical Institutes for Specialist Studies.[2] It is easy to imagine Golgi's circumspection in evaluating the proposal. He must certainly have considered as hypocritical the stated intention of seeing 'Pavia and Milan united in this noble and high-minded initiative' because it was obvious that it favoured the latter at the expense of former by moving toward the creation of a true University in Milan.

The Nobel Prize winner had not yet been adequately celebrated by his own Medical School. In February, Arturo Marcacci, Dean of the Medical School, established a committee for the creation of a Camillo Golgi Foundation, which would award a scholarship bearing the name of the laureate. Among those who immediately supported the proposal were the most important names of Italian science and some of the most prominent Italian and Lombard politicians, including Rampoldi, who in the past had repeatedly been at loggerheads with Golgi. Naturally, there was also Mangiagalli, who in March established a similar committee for Milan.

At the end of May a letter arrived from the Institute of Tropical Medicine of the University of Liverpool announcing that Golgi had been awarded the prestigious Mary Kingsley Medal, bearing the name of a famous explorer of Africa who had died in 1900. Previous recipients of the Medal had included the most outstanding experts in infectious diseases, such as Koch, Laveran, and Manson. In mid-July, he received congratulations from Ronald Ross and at the beginning of October the Medal was given to Golgi by the Minister of Public Education, who had received it from the British Embassy in Rome.[3]

A few months later, despite the offer of collaboration and proffering of adulation, Mangiagalli's true designs came into the open, with all their threatening consequences for Pavia. On 14 November 1907, during his speech at the inauguration of the academic year of the Clinical Institutes for Specialist Studies, Mangiagalli did not hide his intention to create 'a great Medical School for Specialist Studies'[4] and thereafter to reunite all institutes for scientific research and higher education, 'in a great Politechnical University'.[5] For the moment, he contented himself with creating the largest possible number of specialist courses. Serafino Belfanti of the Istituto Sieroterapico Milanese taught Infectious Diseases, whereas the course of Occupational Medicine was entrusted to Devoto,[6] and other pre-eminent academics were appointed to teach a number of other courses.

Meanwhile, the plans for the renovation of the University of Pavia were enlarged to include a grandiose project for the construction of a new Policlinical Hospital and the buildings for the Institutes of Physiology, Physics, and Chemistry. The cost had now risen to 5 250 000 lire with a State contribution of 2 200 000.

After winning the Nobel Prize, Golgi recovered his appetite for research. The internal reticular apparatus was still at the centre of attention of histologists world-wide. Friedrich Kopsch, Waldeyer's assistant in the Institute of Anatomy in Berlin, had managed to demonstrate it with a simple immersion of pieces of tissue (specifically spinal ganglia of rabbit) for about eight days in a 2% solution of osmic acid.[7] The fact that it could be demonstrated with techniques very different from those initially proposed by Golgi was further evidence that it was a real structure and not an artifact. Following the studies of Pensa, Negri, and Gemelli, who had observed the apparatus in non-nervous tissue, more and more confirmations of its existence were coming from a number of laboratories and it was beginning to assume the status and importance of a true intracellular organelle. There were, however, dissenting voices and some continued to regard it as an artifact without functional significance. Others attempted to equate it with other intracellular structures. In particular, Holmgren, in Sweden, published a series of works on certain intracytoplasmic particularities that led him to elaborate a comprehensive theory of the functional organization of the cell's nutritional system. He observed a canalicular structure communicating with the extracellular environment, which he called 'Trophospongium'. According to Holmgren, it derived from the intracytoplasmic invagination of processes originating from neighbouring cells, and ensured cell trophism. He did not hesitate to identify it with Golgi's internal reticular apparatus, an opinion shared by Cajal who began to call it the Golgi–Holmgren apparatus (although the Spaniard denied that this system of intracellular canaliculi could be in communication with structures outside the cell). Others called it instead the Golgi–Kopsch apparatus. In 1910, Carlo Besta referred to the structure as the 'Golgi apparatus', but this term entered the international literature only after the influential paper by Józef Nusbaum in 1913. Even in his Nobel lecture Golgi rejected its identification with the Trophospongium. At any rate, he was eager to return to research and this controversy was at the top of his agenda.

And once again he succeeded. At the beginning of 1907, he found an easy way to stain the internal reticular apparatus using a modification of the reduced silver method, which Cajal had been using since 1903, to demonstrate the apparatus in invertebrates and in the epithelial cells of young mammals. Golgi's modification (which he described at the 31 January 1908 meeting of the Società Medico-Chirurgica)[8] consisted of adding arsenous acid as fixative, thus allowing for consistent and reproducible impregnations of the apparatus.

All through this period Golgi had continued to maintain close ties with his home town. Beginning in the 1880s, his summer vacations were divided between Aprica, Varese, and the Ligurian Riviera. And since 1905 he had taken an interest in the ferruginous springs of the Val di Corteno, and had unsuccessfully attempted to promote a spa there. He was therefore well known in the valley, where he could be seen hiking each August. He would walk from Corteno to Aprica Pass along the old 'Napoleonic' road, a journey of some days, and having arrived in Aprica Pass would take lodging in the Negri Hotel or the Aprica Hotel, stopping at the ferruginous spring *dei Camizzù* in San Pietro of Corteno on the way. He had kept close ties of friendship with the Cortenese, in particular with the schoolteacher Antonio Stefanini. After the awarding of the Nobel Prize to Golgi, the Municipal Council decided to organize appropriate celebrations. Of course Golgi was flattered, and he thanked his old friends for the honour which was 'no less appreciated than that received in Stockholm!' because 'the memory of my native town is deeply engraved in my mind.'[9] On 26 July the Mayor of Corteno distributed an invitation to the entire citizenship for the party for Golgi to be held on 9 August 1907. The Cortenese organized the event in grand style. Everyone participated in the preparations for the celebration, and in front of the City Hall the town erected a grandiose platform from which the standard of Corteno and the national flags waved. By 21 July a celebratory plaque had been cemented onto the front of the City Hall, to be unveiled by Golgi during the celebrations.

August 9 was beautiful; the mountains surrounding Corteno were shimmering in the blue sky, and while the sun was hot there was a fresh cool breeze. The central square was crowded by the Mayors from the towns of Val Camonica, clad in their municipal sashes with national colours, and a brass band came from Edolo. Golgi, who was vacationing in Aprica, arrived with his wife in a carriage drawn by four horses. At the entrance to the town he descended to receive the homage of the Mayor and the other town officials, the Archpriest, and Stefanini. Stefanini's two daughters offered a bouquet of flowers to Lina, and recited a poem. From the podium, Stefanini welcomed the participants and then the plaque was unveiled, to warm applause. This was followed by an official speech by the lawyer Giuseppe Rodondi. And finally it was the turn of Golgi, who, visibly moved, spoke a few simple words. Another child offered a large bouquet of edelweiss to Golgi and his wife. At the end of the ceremony, everyone participated in a banquet in the court-yard of the parish rectory.

Golgi did not expect such a warm celebration, and he decided to reciprocate by provid-ing free medical visits to the Cortenese during his summer vacations in Aprica, and indeed he continued this tradition until the summer of 1912, his last visit to his home town.[10]

Golgi was again unanimously confirmed Rector of the University, and on 4 November 1907 he made his usual inaugural speech to open the new academic year.[11] After seven years of Rectorship, the plan for the new *Policlinico* had finally reached the operational phase.

His scientific prestige, suffused in the halo of the Nobel Prize, had reached its zenith. The Lithuanian histologist Dogiel expressed his great admiration by dedicating to him, Cajal, and Retzius his monograph on the spinal ganglia of humans and animals.[12]

In January 1908 he received a letter from the Harvard embryologist Charles Sedgwick Minot, secretary of the Elizabeth Thompson Science Fund of Boston, who invited him to prepare a report on his studies on malaria, which had been supported since 1893 with their grants. But Minot added that no studies supported by the Fund appeared to have been published. A very embarrassed Golgi answered that he had sent regular reports and a copy of the *Opera Omnia*, and that he did not understand what else he needed to do 'to satisfy the obligation deriving from the grant'.[13] Evidently the Americans wanted to see publications in which the support from the Elizabeth Thompson Science Fund was acknowledged. But this practice was not the norm in Italy, and besides, Golgi had not published anything important on malaria after 1894. The matter ended there and his justifications appear to have been accepted. At any rate, in 1908 the American foundation again provided the Laboratory of General Pathology with 1250 lire for Adelchi Negri as a contribution for the continuation of his studies on rabies. This young disciple of Golgi, who was then teaching a *corso libero* in microbiology, had begun to work on initiating the so-called *bonifica umana* (human bonification) as a weapon in the fight against malaria, a problem that was also dear to Golgi. The *bonifica umana* consisted 'of the radical intensive cure of all malarial patients in a specific area during the intervals between epidemics, with the twofold aim of avoiding relapses and of minimizing, at the beginning of the hot season, the possibility of being infected by the *Anopheles* mosquitoes, and therefore of becoming a carrier of the disease'.[14] Hence it was hoped that the preventive use of quinine on certain individuals during the first half of the year would lead to the magical disappearance of malaria in Italy.

During the winter of 1908, the first campaigns of *bonifica umana* were carried out in seven municipalities (for a total of 1481 individuals) by some municipal doctors under Negri's supervision. The subjects were suspected of being currently infected, or of having been infected during the previous malaria season. The experiment was successful and in the following four years the procedure was extended to a larger area under Negri's direction and Golgi's attentive eye.

Golgi spent the spring of 1908 taking care of bureaucratic and political burdens. The institutional agreement for the *Policlinico,* which was about to be approved by the govern-ment, had been modified at the request of the Administrative Council of San Matteo Hospital, and so at the beginning of April Golgi travelled to Rome to show the Ministers of the Treasury and of Public Education 'a new version of the Draft and related additions and modifications for the required approval'.[15] He then went to Sicily for a few days, returning to Rome to speed up the bureaucratic process.

Finally, the laborious process for the renovation of the University of Pavia was approved on 29 June 1908 with the signing of an agreement between the Ministers of Internal Affairs, Treasury, Public Education, and Public Works. The State participated with a sum of 1 800 000 lire, and the final amount, subdivided among the various Lombard institutions, reached 5 100 000 lire. A supervising committee would oversee the execution of the work. After many years of failed attempts, Golgi had finally succeeded in realizing his dream.

The new method for the ready demonstration of the internal reticular apparatus had triggered a great deal of research in the Laboratory of General Pathology. Once again, a technical innovation by Golgi was spurring his pupils and collaborators to new discoveries. The method was used immediately by Veratti, Verson, and a student, Ferruccio Marcora, for a study of the organelle in pathological conditions. Aldo Perroncito used the method to differentiate the internal reticular apparatus from the mitochondria and the centrosome, and to study its progressive modification during cellular division. The students Giuseppe Carlo Riquier and Luigi Stropeni successfully applied the method to study the internal reticular apparatus in the corpus luteum and in hepatic cells.

Golgi, anxious to try it on non-nervous tissues, chose the cells of the gastric and intestinal mucosa of vertebrates, and demonstrated the presence of the internal reticular apparatus in the epithelium of the intestinal villi, of the Lieberkühn and Brunner glands, and of the gastric mucosa, and in the non-parietal (but not in the parietal) cells of the gastric glands. He also described the changes in shape and location that the apparatus underwent during the secretory process (in particular, the fact that the apparatus was oriented towards the secretory surface while the nucleus was dislocated at the base of the cell). These findings seemed to suggest an involvement of the apparatus in the secretory activity of the cell.

In September 1908 Golgi presented this study to the 7th Meeting of the Unione Zoologica Italiana, held in Bormio, and along with a critical review of the works of Holmgren, Cajal, Kopsch, and others, to a meeting of the Società Medico-Chirurgica held in 1909.[16]

Golgi was confirmed as Rector for the eighth time, and in the inaugural speech of 4 November 1908 he was finally able to announce the happy conclusion of the saga of the Policlinico.[17]

On 10 December, on the second anniversary of his Nobel Prize award, a committee chaired by Marcacci inaugurated the Camillo Golgi Foundation. The solemn ceremony was held in the Aula Magna of the University. Speakers included Marcacci, the Prefect, the Mayor of Pavia (who compared Golgi to Volta), Pasquale del Giudice as a representative of the entire academic body, the representatives from the Lombard provinces, and a student. Golgi thanked the participants with the usual modesty.[18] Count Mörner wrote a cordial letter of participation and telegrams joining in the celebration were sent by many others including Mangiagalli, Grassi, and Bassini, who apologized for their absence.

The Foundation, a non-profit organization by decree of King Vittorio Emanuele III, had an endowment of 34 000 lire and would award the Golgi Fellowship for two years of specialist studies at the University of Pavia for a newly graduated physician. Golgi offered to cover the expenses for the first year. The first winner was Giuseppe Fiorito.[19] In the following years, the Fellowship was awarded to Cesare Frugoni and Antonio Gasbarrini, who spent part of their two years in the Laboratory of General Pathology,[20] and later became Professors of Clinical Medicine in Rome and Bologna, respectively.

At the end of the year Golgi took part, as a volunteer, in the national rescue efforts in response to the catastrophic earthquake that hit Messina and Reggio Calabria, causing 150 000 deaths.

In the first months of 1909, he had some health problems.[21] Being compelled to interrupt 'for personal reasons' and 'possibly for a quite a long period, the work in the laboratory',[22] Golgi decided to present the results of his unfinished research on the structure of cortical nerve cells at the Società Medico-Chirurgica,[23] hoping to complete them as soon as possible. The internal reticular apparatus presented some peculiarities that made its identification dubious. Golgi, however, ascribed this to the special silver methods he had used in this study.

By summer he was well again, and on 4 August was hiking in the Corteno Valley, in the company of Father Romolo Putelli.[24] As a sign of gratitude to his home town, he joined the association Pro Valle Camonica of Breno, and, together with the newly elected Member of Parliament Livio Tovini, and Antonio Stefanini, he sponsored an unsuccessful proposal to construct a railroad connecting Edolo, Aprica, and Tirano.

In 1909 Georges Marinesco, who had briefly visited the Laboratory of General Pathology, published *La cellule nerveuse* in which, remembering his time in Pavia, he wrote:

During my brief sojourn in Pavia, I had the honour of visiting the celebrated histologist who kindly showed me a series of his beautiful preparations. I could not be convinced that the net he describes exists. In the same way, I couldn't see the connections between the dendrites and the blood vessels.[25]

The book embraced Cajal's theories completely (Cajal wrote the Preface) and criticized all the physiological interpretations of the Pavian School. Marinesco attacked not only the diffuse neural net but also the functional interpretation (motor versus sensory) of the classification of neurons in Type I and Type II, and the theory of the trophic role of dendrites. But what may have incensed Golgi the most was his reference to a visit to the Laboratory of General Pathology, with the statement that not even a direct examination of Golgi's slides demonstrated his conclusions. This was tantamount to accusing Golgi of being delusional.

The answer to Marinesco's provocations arrived the following year, at the conference on 'Evolution of the doctrines and of the knowledge about the anatomical substrate of psychic and sensory functions', in which Golgi expounded on his neurobiological 'philosophy'.[26]

Since his earliest works with the black reaction, Golgi had attributed to the dendrites a predominantly trophic role, even though he didn't exclude the possibility that they could have other functions as well. Now he toned down this conclusion, stating that

to the protoplasmic processes, taking into account their relationships, it is possible to attribute *also* a trophic function, by this not ruling out that they could participate also in the specific function that is thought to belong to the cell body [with which they] . . . share the same structure.[27]

Thus, Golgi emphasized the possibility that the dendrites had other functions than a purely trophic one, an idea that was strengthened by the documented presence within them of neurofibrils, which had been given a role in the transmission of nerve impulses.

Rejecting the accusation of Marinesco that he had advocated an exclusively trophic role for the dendrites, he added:

I reckon that it is difficult to accumulate so many inexactitudes in so few lines as this author has managed to do in the citation he makes of my works and of those of my pupils on such points![28]

And concerning the visit of Marinesco in Pavia:

I do not remember if on the occasion of Marinesco's very brief visit to my Institute I was able to show him some preparations; but because he states so, I do not dispute it; however, after having weighed the manner with which he appraises, I can understand the negative impression he took away with him; the fact is not less true for this and I can assure that other scientists have not only confirmed the observation [the diffuse neural net], but have also obtained very convincing preparations of their own.[28]

Thus, according to Golgi, Marinesco's statements about the diffuse neural net were not surprising, considering the superficiality of his judgements.

Meanwhile, the feud between Milan and Pavia appeared to have abated. Mangiagalli continued with his velvet glove approach, disguising the real nature of his designs with offers of cooperation and collaboration, and with the deference that he always exhibited for Golgi, with whom he shared the honorary presidency of the 19th Congress of Internal Medicine organized by Devoto in the *Aula Magna* of the Clinical Institutes of Specialist Studies.[29] Also celebrated in Milan was the creation of the National League against Malaria, presided over by Baccelli. Golgi, as President of the local organizing committee, stated that 'the dream of freeing the workers from the diseases of the swamp . . . is no longer a distant utopia: we are calmly and irrevocably marching towards it, sure that our efforts will be crowned by victory.'[30] At another level, the victory he was trying to achieve was that of receiving funding for Negri's projects. Toward this end, he was able to obtain financial support from the Ministry of Public Health by mobilizing the Lombard Committee of the newly born League.

In Pavia, after many uncertainties and negotiations, the site for the new *Policlinico* was finally chosen in the area to the north and west of town. This was the site for which Golgi had fought. He had double lines of linden trees planted along the avenue to the new *Policlinico* (the present-day Viale Golgi). The original project was later modified and this avenue remained a secondary access road to the hospital. At the end of 1909 the mathematician Luigi Berzolari was elected Rector, and Golgi had to give up the helm of the University, probably with a certain amount of regret. The plans for the renovation of the University to which so much time and so many efforts had been dedicated was progressing slowly but surely. Its main promoter was always ready to intervene to overcome a bureaucratic obstacle or to find political support. Ten architectural proposals were submitted in a first competition, but the supervising committee decided that none satisfied the necessary prerequisites. In the end, a new competition took place in 1912 and the project by Gardella and Martini was approved with work to begin in 1913. Golgi, released from rectorial duties, participated more assiduously in the sessions of the Senate. On 9 and 13 March 1911 he intervened during the debate on a law that would have required a medical degree for the practice of dentistry, suggesting instead the creation of dental schools independent from the medical schools as an alternative to the two years of specialization after the medical degree (a proposal that was unsuccessful).[31]

The project of *bonifica umana*, supervised by Negri, was a resounding success. He had created a wide network of municipal doctors who put his instructions into practice in numerous areas afflicted by malaria. In 1911 the programme involved 45 municipalities with therapeutic interventions on 4328 persons, and the results were published by Negri. A certain Giulio Wyler had made available 1000 lire to be awarded to the best applied scientific work concerning the fight against malaria and the committee, which included Grassi, deemed Negri's epidemiological–therapeutic experiments the most deserving. With great philanthropic spirit, the winner ceded the prize to the Lombard Committee of the anti-malarial league.

But a new threat to public health, an epidemic of cholera, was about to hit Lombardy. Negri, who since 1909 had been charged with the teaching of bacteriology, played an important role in analysing the biological samples from patients. He also organized a bacteriological laboratory at the hospital of Bergamo, and from July to October 1911 he single-handedly worked to contain the epidemic with little personal scientific gratification. But the number of analyses to be carried out was so large that he had to spend several nights in the Laboratory of General Pathology.[32] Unfortunately, his health suffered from this strenuous overwork, especially because since 1900 he had been affected by osteo-articular tuberculosis.

The important work done by Negri for the prophylaxis and therapy of malaria and cholera received the enthusiastic approval of Golgi, who while not directly involved in the projects, followed and approved them unconditionally.

Although Golgi had no more scientific work to fill his day, he had still many other activities. He participated in the 1st International Congress of Pathologists held in Turin from 2–5 October 1911; he participated in the session of the Istituto Lombardo, where he occasionally intervened;[33] and he also worked on making nominations for the Nobel Prize, suggesting Forlanini, Grassi, and Edoardo Perroncito.

At the beginning of 1912, Negri's feverish activity was tragically interrupted. His 'truly excessive sense of duty for his obligations' towards society 'pushed him to exaggerate his work to the point of lowering the resistance of his constitution before the insidious disease that threatened his life.'[34] The tubercular process that was lingering in the embers was suddenly rekindled, spreading to the brain and to the meninges with 'catastrophic intensity', causing his death on the morning of 19 February 1912. Like Dieters and Boll, he died in his prime. In the delirium just before his death, 'he hoped to the last to be able to return soon to the Laboratory, and his mind, even if dulled by the disease, continued to plan new studies, new research!'[35]

Golgi was devastated by the pain caused by the death of his beloved pupil. In his honour he wrote a biographic, scientific, and personal testimonial, which he read in a session of the

Società Medico-Chirurgica held on 8 May 1912.[36] In this tribute, Golgi thoroughly analysed Negri's great contributions to microbiology and cytology. He emphasized Negri's great moral and scientific rigour, and his unrelenting reserve, which sometimes led one to think that he 'did not feel that sort of camaraderie that represents one of the main attractions of laboratory life'.[37] Confronted with the disquiet produced by this great loss, Golgi could 'find no comfort other than by doing everything possible to honour his memory and by working to make his work known in all its value.'[35]

Negri's death, like that of Marenghi, was a hard blow for the laboratory. The emerging figure became Aldo Perroncito who had recently returned from a period of study in Berlin and Paris; with Veratti he became the main pillar of the Institute.

The interest of the laboratory in malaria continued even after Negri's death. In November Golgi participated in the 4th International Congress of Rice Agriculture, held in Vercelli. Here, he defended his controversial speech given during the Third Congress six years earlier, accusing his critics of using 'rancorous and vulgar' language to support arguments put forward 'in the most complete disregard of truth'. In substance, he charged them with having distorted his words for political reasons. He then discussed various anti-malarial measures such as mechanical prophylaxis (for example, using nets around houses to keep the mosquitoes away), the quininic prophylaxis on healthy individuals (here he mentioned some results obtained by his pupil Ernesto Brugnatelli on the effects of quinine on dogs and guinea pigs), and expressed his clear preference for the project of *bonifica umana* which he had personally supervised with Negri.[38] Remembering the person who had been for him 'pupil, friend, and colleague', he emphasized the philanthropic aspect of Negri's concept of research as 'science for humanity', as indicated by his anti-malarial campaign.[39]

Italy was enjoying a particularly favourable period of cultural and material prosperity.[40] Wages were on the rise, budgets were in the black, and the entire society was permeated by a climate of freedom and faith in progress. Italian public opinion was focused on the colonial ambitions of a country that was the last to arrive in the rush for Africa. On 27 September 1911 Italy sent an ultimatum to Turkey that it should not resist the occupation of Libya, and two days later Italy declared war, occupying first Tripoli and then Bengasi, and a few months later some islands in the Aegean Sea. The crisis ended with direct negotiations between Turkey and Italy, culminating on 18 October in the Treaty of Lausanne, which recognized Italian sovereignty over Libya. This triggered a disproportionately enthusiastic reaction in Italy, especially amongst those capitalists eager to exploit new markets and among some trade unionists who toyed with the idea of allowing the proletarian and peasant masses to colonize the newly conquered land. The conquest of Libya, in itself a modest enterprise, was a balm for Italian pride, satisfying these expansionist aspirations.

But there were sinister omens of the gloom to come. A general atmosphere celebrating force and aggression was poisoning European society, and Italy in particular. In 1910 the manifesto of the Futurist movement had sung 'the love for danger' and war as the 'only hygiene of the world', and the mystical decadence of the poems of Gabriele D'Annunzio[41] married the mythical past of Italy to the new nationalism. The will to power was contrasted with 'petty Italy, shabby and pacifist'. Even a man with his feet as solidly on the ground as Golgi let himself be transported by the enthusiasm for the 'glorious events in which we have had the privilege to assist during this year' and that had 'enhanced the prestige of our country in the international arena . . . giving to Italy a new consciousness'. Following the example of the Army, which had 'so splendidly fulfilled its own duty' with its 'marvellous collective and individual heroism', even those who, like Golgi, were 'proud to belong to the ruling class' must 'feel an obligation to contribute more energetically to the solution of problems of social life'.[42] He clearly felt this obligation also towards Italians living outside the Kingdom, as indicated by his support for the initiative of the Pavian University committee in favour of the creation of an Italian University in Trieste.[43]

Similar feelings were harboured in other countries preparing for the inevitable catastrophe. On the night of 14 April 1912, in a symbolic representation of the disintegration of the certainties and illusions of *la belle époque*, the *Titanic*, the largest liner in the world, newly built and supposedly unsinkable, went to the bottom of the ocean after hitting an iceberg. Only two years later Europe would plunge into the carnage of the First World War.

On 18 February 1913 Lina's mother, the 82-year-old Maddalena Bizzozero, who had been living for many years with the Golgis in Pavia, died. It was a sad occasion for the Perroncitos and Bizzozeros to meet again. Since Carolina had married an Army officer and left home, Camillo and Lina were now alone.

Between the end of 1912 and the beginning of 1913 Golgi became involved in a bizarre project. An assistant in the Laboratory of Hygiene had taken a fancy to a project for using rice fields as pools for breeding fish. He managed to convince Golgi to support the creation of an aquarium—incubator, where suitable species (such as Gorizia carp) could be bred, before transferring them to the rice fields.[44] Since carp feed on mosquito larvae, the project could help in fighting malaria. Golgi used all his influence as President of the anti-malarial League to finalize this project in record time. A small building was built close to the Palazzo Botta, with tanks, water pipes, and a pool created by diverting a nearby stream. On 18 May 1913 the plant was dedicated with an official speech by Golgi in the presence of local dignitaries and zoologists.[45] Seven days later, Golgi, excited by the project, gave another speech at a national meeting on fishing that he had organized in Pavia.[46]

The infatuation for fish evaporated quickly because breeding carp in the rice fields proved to be unprofitable and ineffective in fighting malaria. On the contrary, the mosquitoes found a favourable environment in the breeding pools and a vicious rumour began to circulate that there were also some *Anopheles* among them. Over a few years the aquarium became progressively neglected and was eventually abandoned.

Golgi, who had been averse to 'grand politics', participated happily in the Parliamentary sessions when they concerned arguments that he knew well and that touched on concrete problems of university life. On 11 June 1913 he was in the Senate to discuss the salaries of high school and university personnel, particularly those of university assistants. In complete opposition to the opinion expressed by Maragliano, for whom 'the assistant should not be independent from the professor . . . he can not and must not have autonomous functions', Golgi maintained that an assistant should represent a 'fellow traveller' who 'must deal with scientific problems in the most absolute freedom and independence of thought'. And, possibly remembering the many assistants and collaborators in his Institute, he recalled how he had always been 'ready . . . to learn from the youth' whose minds were 'more agile, more elastic, more suited to follow the best currents of modernity'. Thus, Maragliano's ideas were, for Golgi, 'incomprehensible' and the 'expression of bygone times'.[47] He then expressed his support for appropriate financial remuneration for assistants, to attract to the university those individuals who are most predisposed to scientific research.

On 17 June he intervened in the discussion of the provisional law to create two new professorships in the Clinical Institutes for Specialist Studies of Milan. Golgi did not oppose the provision, but the leitmotif was always the same: the approval should not be a prelude to an enlargement of the sphere of influence of the *Istituti*, such as might lead to the creation of 'another university 25 to 30 minutes from Pavia', when everybody agreed 'that in Italy there are too many universities!' And then he concluded that Minister Luigi Credaro certainly was not of the opinion to create a new university in Milan, 'notwith-standing the privileged treatment given to the Institutes of Milan'.[48] Any occasion that offered an opportunity for putting obstacles in the way of Mangiagalli's potent machine was to be grasped.

However, he was not involved only in the discussion of university issues. As a member of the 'Central Commission' of the Senate, he signed a report in favour of reducing taxes for phosphorous substitutes in order to enhance their use in the match industry, thus eliminating the use of the dangerous 'white phosphorous' which was responsible for acute and chronic occupational diseases well known to the hygienists.[49]

Notes

1. Golgi's speech concerned the nature of the connections among nerve cells, and was crafted along the lines of his acceptance speech for the Nobel Prize.
2. Mangiagalli's proposal was illustrated in the following letter to Golgi, using the letterhead of the Senate (Mangiagalli had been made life Senator by King Vittorio Emanuele III) and dated 'Milan 11 January '909' (in possession of Dr Giuseppe Raimondi):

   Honourable and Illustrious Colleague
   Italy is the only one among the great nations which does not take an adequate part in the formidable battle against cancer. Under the auspices of the Istituti Clinici di Perfezion-amento I would like to establish here in Milan an institute for research on cancer and I would like again to unite Pavia and Milan in this noble and lofty initiative, by creating a committee composed of you, me and Prof. Devoto, and possibly of other members, and beginning meanwhile to procure the necessary means. There is no lack of accomplished youths whose activity could be useful and productive in the new institute, and I am sure that success will smile upon our effort and our country will bring an important contribution to the solution of a problem that continues to concern science and humanity. I will be grateful to you if you could reply as soon as possible and most grateful if this will be in the affirmative.
   Sincerely, L. Mangiagalli

We do not know Golgi's response to this letter. Although Mangiagalli's proposal had no practical consequences for several years, it was taken up again in 1925, leading to the foundation in 1928 of the Institute Vittorio Emanuele III for the study and treatment of cancer, later renamed National Institute of Tumours of Milan. Concerning the early years of the Institute, see Cosmacini (1989, pp. 131ff.).

3. In the MSUP there are some letters and documents that refer to the Kingsley Medal (MSUP-III-XI- from 1–8).
4. Mangiagalli (1907, p. 23).
5. *Ibid.* (p. 24).
6. Devoto, who had been living in Milan since 1905, obtained the transfer from the University of Pavia to the Istituti Clinici di Perfezionamento di Milano with the Royal Decree of 26 January 1908 (Zanobio 1992 p. 25).
7. Kopsch (1902).
8. Golgi (1908; 1908a).
9. Letter from Golgi to Stefanini, reproduced in Bianchi (1973, p. 18). The details reported here of Golgi's visit to Corteno were communicated by Dr Lino Stefanini, grandson of Antonio Stefanini, who learnt them through the oral tradition of the family.
10. The chronicle of the celebrations is found in Bianchi (1973, pp. 23ff.). See also Goldaniga and Marchetti (1993, p. 287).
11. Golgi (1908b).
12. Dogiel (1908).
13. Golgi sent Minot the following letter (in French) in response to a request by Minot of 27 December 1907:

Esteemed Colleague
The letter of 27 December 1907 in which you call my attention to the necessity of sending to you before next January a report on the progress of the work carried out with the grant 'Elizabeth Thompson' is a source of considerable embarrassment for me.

I had believed that I satisfied the requirements of the grant by sending first reprints of my papers, then an album of photographs, and finally, about two years ago, a letter in which I summarized the results of my work on malaria.

What you write me makes me think that this is not sufficient and my embarrassment comes from the fact that for some time I have not occupied myself with these studies. However, I must add that the volumes entitled 'opera omnia', which I felt the obligation to send to you, contain . . . all my studies on malaria including the ones carried out after the grant was awarded. I might feel somehow justified, therefore, in thinking that the award itself has in part contributed to the publication of the 'opera omnia'.

Given this, I beg that you provide me with some explanation about what else I must do to satisfy the requirements deriving from the award of the 'Elizabeth Thompson' grant.
Sincerely yours, C. Golgi'

The French translation of the letter is dated Rome 26 January 1908. The drafts (in Italian and in French) are in the possession of Dr Giuseppe Raimondi. There are other letters from Minot to Golgi concerning the 'Elizabeth Thompson' grant (MSUP-VII-II-M).
14. Golgi (1912 p. 107).
15. Letter from Golgi to lawyer Buzzi, secretary of the Deputazione Provinciale di Milano, 26 April 1908. In the possession of Prof. Marco Fraccaro.
16. Golgi (1909). The French translation of the work appeared soon after (Golgi 1909a).
17. Golgi (1909b).

18. Golgi (1909c).
19. Information about the ceremony for the inauguration of the Golgi Foundation can be found in the *Annuario dell'Università di Pavia* for the academic year 1908–09 (Pavia: Tipografia Successori Bizzoni, pp. 337–80).
20. In each year during the period 1904–14 the Institute of General Pathology was attended by about 40 internal pupils (students and recent graduates), as can be seen in the requests for admission kept in the Institute. Among the students who were attending the Institute in the first two decades of the century were: Giuseppe D'Agata, Eugenio Morelli, Francesco Maccabruni, Carlo Barinetti, Gian Luigi Colombo, Giorgio Sinigaglia, Carlo Barazzoni, Arnaldo Vecchi, Alessandro (Sandro) Golgi (son of Camillo's brother Giuseppe), and Giovan Battista Stefanini (son of his friend Antonio of Corteno).
21. On a postcard dated 20 February 1909, Benedetto Morpurgo wrote to Veratti: 'I hope that Senator Golgi has recovered: Give him my best regards'. (In the possession of Dr Giuseppe Raimondi.)
22. Golgi (1909d; *OO* p. 1336).
23. Session of 30 April 1909.
24. Putelli (1913).
25. Marinesco (1909, pp. 15ff.).
26. Golgi (1910).
27. *Ibid.* (p. 26).
28. *Ibid.* (p. 73). In 1909 Marinesco and Guido Sala engaged in a lively debate on the problem of regeneration in the central nervous system (see *Anatomischer Anzeiger*, 1909, **34**, pp. 193–9, 443–5, 583–4).
29. *Gazzetta Medica Lombarda* (1909, 68th Year, p. 413).
30. Golgi (1909e, p. 15).
31. Session of 9 March 1911 (*Atti parlamentari del Senato*; Rome: Forsani & C. Tipografi del Senato, 1911, reprint, pp. 3–27). Reproduced in Goldaniga and Marchetti (1993, pp. 204–11). See also Zanobio and Armocida (1994, pp. 611–15).
32. Golgi (1912, p. 115).
33. During the 1st International Congress of Pathologists, Golgi, Felix Marchand, and Gustave Roussy participated in the discussion following the communication by A. Bignami and A. Nazari 'On the anatomical pathology of chorea'. In addition, Golgi presented a communication ('Observations on canine plague') on behalf of one of his disciples, G. Sinigaglia (*Atti del I Congresso Internazionale dei Patologi*; Torino: UTET, 1912, pp. 255 and 256–73). On 9 November 1911 Golgi commemorated the anatomo-pathologist Achille Visconti, who had been a disciple of Virchow and Director of the Autopsy Section of the Ospedale Maggiore of Milan (Golgi 1911).
34. Golgi (1912, p. 121).
35. *Ibid.* (p. 122).
36. *Ibid.*
37. *Ibid.* (p. 120).
38. See also Zanobio (1973) concerning the *bonifica umana* campaign in Lombardy.
39. Golgi (1912a, pp. 41ff.).
40. Salvatorelli (1971, p. 530).
41. Among the cards conserved in the Museum for the History of the University of Pavia, I have found the lyric 'Un ricordo' from the *Poema Paradisiaco* (1893) of Gabriele D'Annunzio. The madrigal, hand-written and signed by the author, is contained in an envelope along with

letters of Edmondo De Amicis, Giosuè Carducci, and other celebrated literati (MSUP-VII-III-21). Unfortunately, there are no clues that allow one to determine the date and circumstances surrounding its composition and why it is among Golgi's papers.

42. Golgi (1912a, p. 56).
43. On 12 December 1912, under Golgi's auspices, an agitation committee in favour of the Italian University of Trieste was created. This committee published a Numero Unico universitario (single issue university magazine) on 5 June 1913.
44. Pensa (1991, p. 155).
45. Golgi (1913).
46. Golgi (1913a).
47. Session of 11 June 1913 (*Atti parlamentari del Senato*; Roma: Tipografia del Senato, 1913, reprint, pp. 5–14). Reproduced also in Goldaniga and Marchetti (1993, pp. 212–13).
48. Session of 17 June 1913 (*Atti parlamentari del Senato*; Roma: Tipografia del Senato, 1913, reprint, pp. 5–18). Reproduced also in Goldaniga and Marchetti (1993 pp. 212–13).
49. Report of the Central Office (with Golgi as chairman) on a draft presented by the Minister of Finance in the session of 6 June 1913, 'Trattamento doganale dei surrogati del fosforo destinati alla fabbricazione dei fiammiferi' (*Atti parlamentari, Senato del Regno*, n. 1075A).

23

The veil of Isis

Golgi's cultural formation was permeated by positivism. For him, science was the supreme ideal, to which one could consecrate one's entire life. Only science could guarantee continuous unending progress for humankind. From this perspective, metaphysical speculations had no relevance for an understanding of the human condition.

But Golgi's positivism was never crassly materialistic; for him that would have been as antiscientific as a dogmatic religious belief. As early as 1883, in his speech at the conference on 'Experimentalism in Medicine', he placed spiritualism and materialism on the same level. Indeed, for Golgi, medical science

vigorously rejects the former [that is, spiritualism] because it would explain everything through the power of a supernatural being whose existence was separate from matter; but [medical science] also considers it unsuitable to the experimental method to submit to the conceptions of the latter [that is, materialism] because it too pretends to consider as already explained what science has been unable to explain so far; it would indeed be the case of one dogma replacing another, something that I maintain must be rejected in the name of experimentalism.[1]

Golgi's positivism consisted above all in extolling the virtues of the experimental method as the only way to establish scientific truth. However, this 'truth' was not absolute but rather could be reviewed and corrected as new facts showed as 'imperfect and erroneous tomorrow what today appears complete and certain'.[2] In this position is a hint of the epistemological approach based on 'falsifiability' of a scientific theory, even though Golgi was actually an inductionist who would have found it impossible to embrace Popper's hypothetical–deductive method.

The second cornerstone of Golgi's positivism was his radical rejection of the *ignorabimus* plea of du Bois-Reymond. Golgi thought that in scientific research one should not attempt to circumscribe or limit a priori the boundaries of what can be investigated, although this did not necessarily imply the possibility of reaching the 'ultimate explanation'.[3] The attitude that shaped his research method can be summarized in what he called the 'psychology of the fortunate traveller':

It happens that in these days, I was reading in the notes of a *simpatico* traveller, who was justly the object of exceptional honours for having triumphed in a long and eventful journey, words having in my opinion a philosophical value well above their literal meaning. 'During the long and eventful itinerary', he wrote, 'we never thought of the remote destination or of the enormous difficulties that would hinder the completion of the journey . . . We only worried about each small daily step, of the modest destination to be reached before night, and of the immediate difficulty to which we could calmly apportion our efforts . . . In this way, almost unconsciously and with less than exceptional means, we were able to accomplish the enterprise that the world now admires!'

Well, allow me to confess that in this psychology of the fortunate traveller I see a perfect analogy with the psychology that has characterized my actions, both in my scholarly life and in the other fields in which I took an interest.

In the fields of science that I have investigated, I followed nothing but the guiding idea of the small steps (which, however, sometimes last for years) represented by tiny, even microscopic problems. And it is the sum of the small steps, coordinated and always proportionate to the strength of the more modest worker, that allowed me to achieve the results that the world has judged worthy of consideration and because of which I too, like the *simpatico* traveller, have become the recipient of exceptional honours.[4]

Golgi's attitude is one of great modesty and concreteness. Scientists must be content to achieve their daily grain of knowledge without imposing a priori limits on knowledge. This 'psychology of the fortunate traveller' who does not rush and who can wait patiently, shaped all Golgi's activities, even the administrative ones. The challenging affair of the *Policlinico*, which demanded his attention for many years, is a perfect example in this respect. Arturo Marcacci could rightly state that the development of Golgi's activity followed the motto 'without repose but without haste'.[5]

Following this approach, Golgi consistently shied away from the grand problems that the extraordinary progress of science of the nineteenth century had posed to the intellectual world. Apart from the above mentioned participation in the 1883 conference, his writing rarely made even indirect reference to speculative aspects of scientific research.

After winning the Nobel Prize, however, Golgi was often asked to offer his opinion on problems of more general interest. While he was hesitant to stray outside the strictly experimental world in which he felt confident, he eventually surrendered to the insistence of the mathematician Vito Volterra and gave a lecture on the 'Anatomical substrate of psychic and sensory functions' before the Italian Society for the Progress of Science. The topic was very speculative but closely related to his scientific activities. Golgi accepted with great reluctance, aware that he had no great aptitude for 'expounding with ornate words',[6] and very apprehensive about speaking to an audience composed of the pre-eminent Italian representatives of all scientific disciplines to whom he could only offer some 'philosophical' considerations. Indeed:

Following what can be rightly considered the highest aspiration of the human mind to know the causes of things, scholars of the moral disciplines, no less than those of the positive disciplines, expect, with some trepidation, the solution of problems concerning psychic and sensory functions based on knowledge about the organization of the nervous system.[7]

But this need, this anxiety to know, could not justify 'the most adventurous doctrinal constructs of a psychological nature' in which philosophers, psychiatrists, and anatomists so often indulge. Indeed, there was an attempt to use neuroanatomical and functional models to explain the 'mechanism by which the nerve cell presides over the elaboration of sensation and movement, ... the manner in which different centres interact in giving rise to thought', and how 'from the infinite complexity of the organizational relationships the unity of consciousness originates!'

Golgi felt that he was too imbued

with the spirit that must dominate the field of experimental disciplines, to accept, for the satisfaction of the postulates of psychology, constructs of a speculative nature, which, far from being grounded in rigorously established facts, have no other status than hypotheses arising from other hypothetical constructs.[8]

Golgi, however, was eager to point out that in principle he was not against hypotheses, and his position in this regard had been often misrepresented.

Many years ago, in talking with a pre-eminent scientist, an advocate of the theory of the neuron, which at the time was at the pinnacle of its prestige [when Golgi gave this lecture, the theory of the neuron was flagging under the violent attack of neuroreticularists], this colleague accused me of having an almost morbid aversion, a true phobia, for hypotheses.

The accusation was not only unjust, but in my case was also strange!

The formulation of hypotheses is not only consistent with the principles of the experimental method, but is in itself a method of research and a guide to activity![9]

But according to him there were 'legitimate' hypotheses (those having a rigorous scientific foundation) and 'illegitimate' hypotheses (those lacking adequate experimental support). The former were working hypotheses, which must 'originate from rigorously established facts'; the second were nothing but 'hypotheses arising from other hypothetical constructs'.

Golgi was an 'inflexible' inductionist (as had been his teacher Panizza), and he thought it was legitimate to formulate working hypotheses only if they emerged directly from the experimental data; otherwise it was necessary to work patiently day after day to accumulate an appropriate amount of 'facts' before attempting a hypothetical explanation. These attitudes are surprising when one considers the number of hypotheses (some of them quite adventurous) that Golgi had advanced during his scientific career. The trophic role of dendrites and the physiological significance of Type I and Type II cells are good examples. The diffuse neural net was for him almost a scientific 'fact'; if one could not demonstrate it then one was not using the right experimental procedure. Golgi did not realize that his hypotheses, which he considered absolutely legitimate, were based on experimental data that had been filtered through the hypothesis that he was supposed to be demonstrated. Unwittingly, Golgi was following the example of Baron Munchausen, who dragged himself out of the swamp by pulling on his own hair.

In his lecture, Golgi completely ignored recent reports of structural differences between different cortical areas and insisted on the validity of his conclusions of 30 years before in which he maintained that he had demonstrated the histological homogeneity of the cerebral cortex. Although he mentioned some recent studies (for example those of Harrison), overall one has the impression that he was no longer well-acquainted with the literature outside neurocytology.

At about the same time, Giulio Ascoli, working in Golgi's laboratory and using a new silver method, had demonstrated an extremely tight reticulum of nerve fibres in the inner core of the ganglia of leeches, the nervous system of which appeared to be syncytium-like. These findings were substantially compatible with a neoreticularist model. Golgi, perhaps trying to come closer to these positions (which still opposed the theory of the neuron with some success), emphasized the great similarity of Ascoli's reticulum and the diffuse neural net. But contrary to the neoreticularist doctrines, which assigned to the neurofibrils the dignity of a fundamental independent nervous element, while the cells were given an auxiliary trophic function, Golgi confirmed the centrality of the latter in specific nervous function.

The conceptual assumption of Golgi's holistic 'neurophilosophy' emerged clearly at the end of the lecture (emphasis added):

Even if my statements clash with the widespread tendency to individualize the nervous elements, *I cannot deflect from the idea of a unitary action of the nervous system*, and I don't mind if this brings me close to an old conception of how the nervous system works.[10]

This idea arose from a deeply rooted conviction, independently of any scientific demonstration (emphasis added):

Besides rigorous scientific thinking, in me there moves an *intuitive form of thinking that has always guided me, without exception.*

This 'intuitive thinking' had led him to make fundamental choices, including the 'holistic' choice.

Of course, there is a contradiction between his 'rigid' allegiance to inductivism, the only guarantee of scientific reliability, and this 'intuitive thinking' which guided him in his scientific practice. But for Golgi this contradiction disappeared when intuition found confirmation in concrete scientific 'facts', which he considered to be neutral and unconditioned. We have seen, however, how the theoretical approach conditioned even the harvesting of facts.

In a period of great advances in immunology, biochemistry, and genetics, Golgi maintained the centrality of the anatomical approach to biology and, citing Dante's invitation to proceed cautiously with 'lead in one's feet',[11] concluded by

restating my unbending faith in the anatomical approach, which is nourished by patient research, by the acquisition of single well-studied and coherent facts that admonish us not to be prey to adventurous syntheses and which has led, at a slow but certain pace, to the marvellous transformation of biology, which is a pride of the modern world.[12]

From Amsterdam, Golgi was asked to give a philosophical lecture on the meaning of his studies as part of a lecture cycle organized by the Société Sections pour l'Oeuvre Scientifique for the benefit of the students of medicine and natural sciences. The series had been inaugurated in 1904 with a talk by the physical chemist Jacobus Hendricus Van't Hoff and Metschnikoff, and had continued with other pre-eminent scientists such as van Gehuchten and the physicist Hendrik Antoon Lorentz in 1905, the chemist Wilhelm

Ostwald in 1907, and Ehrlich in 1908. On 9 June 1909 it was Golgi's turn and he read a paper on the anatomical substrate of psychic and sensory functions, translated into French.[13]

Golgi made an even stronger defence of the histomorphological disciplines four and a half years later in another 'philosophical' lecture given at the Istituto Lombardo on 8 January 1914. Among his listeners was Achille Ratti, the future Pope Pius XI, who was so impressed by Golgi's speech that he remembered it on his death bed.[14] Golgi lectured on 'Modern evolution of the doctrines and the knowledge of life',[15] and discussed the topic from a broad comparative perspective that took into consideration the main currents of turn-of-the-century biological thought, which was based on the cell theory and dominated by evolutionism. He argued that 'Darwin's Law' had such seminal consequences 'on the development of all branches of the natural sciences' that 'Zoology, and Comparative and Human Anatomy, adopted a highly scientific approach, being addressed to one single aim: the knowledge of the origin and the laws of life'.[16] But for Golgi the connection between these disciplines, 'so they could become a single entity, depended on a new science: the science of organization: Histology'. Thanks to this discipline, which allowed the identification of the substantial structural unity among the multiform morphological aspects of life forms, it was possible to find a unifying element linking the different branches of biology. Thus Golgi emerged as the defender of morphological disciplines in a period when they appeared to be relegated to a secondary position by the growth of other disciplines, especially those based on physical chemistry.

For Golgi, the different approaches were not antithetical, 'although they use different research methods'.[17] History had taught him that 'the secure and constant progress of science, which is the main indicator of the ascending path of mankind, is always the result of the harmonious cooperation of all branches of knowledge. Far from pretentious exclusiveness ... all approaches that are based on observation and experimentation are important'.[18] Certainly, the 'refinement of chemical and physical chemical methods of investigation' would lead to fundamental answers to biological problems. It was natural, for example, to expect that immune reactions would be reduced to simple chemical reactions as soon as 'the bodies that are found in the sera or the so-called toxins are chemically characterized.' Golgi insisted on this point because he didn't want to 'reinforce the notion that there are in life forces other than the physical and chemical ones',[19] as was being maintained by the neo-vitalists.

In dealing with the nature of life and psyche, once again the starting point was the 'renowned phrase' *ignoramus ... ignorabimus* formulated by du Bois-Reymond over 40 years before and which was now 'the motto written on the banners of those who consider as vain any human effort to lift the veil with which the ancients imagined that Isis kept hidden the secrets of life.'[20]

Pointing out how these conclusions were a reaction to the 'inadequately supported and rigidly materialistic positions, which had as their main advocates Vogt and Moleschott',[21] Golgi remembered how these two scientists were later criticized because they reduced science to mechanistic knowledge.

Indeed, du Bois-Reymond maintained that

the mechanics of atoms must be the target for the efforts of all scientists [who seek] to understand the universe; all natural phenomena are explained only insofar as they can be reduced to a system of equations based on atoms and the forces that move them. More precisely, according to the *idee fixe* of du Bois-Reymond, to produce a rigorous scientific reasoning, based on the mechanics of atoms, it is necessary to achieve what he defined as 'the astronomical knowledge of material systems', that is, a knowledge of the position and movement of the atoms in any material system such that at any point in time it would be possible to calculate the position and movement of atoms with the same degree of certainty that the position and movement of celestial bodies can be calculated![22]

This kind of knowledge was indistinguishable from what Pierre Simon de Laplace had put at the centre of his deterministic system.

But du Bois-Reymond conceded that even with 'the astronomical knowledge of material systems' (which he considered the most complete form of scientific knowledge) it would have been possible to detect only matter in movement, whatever the object in study, and therefore

no provision, no movement could serve as a bridge to enter into the domain of intelligence: between the molecular movement and intellectual phenomena there would always be something incommensurable![23]

But the new discoveries and theories on the structure of matter (among which Golgi recalled the 'doctrine of electrons', radioactivity, and electrolytic dissociation) relegated to the historical background the concept of scientific knowledge conceived as mechanistic knowledge, and led one to believe that they would shed new light on the fundamental problems of life (which du Bois-Reymond considered insoluble).

Furthermore, progress in the investigation of the nervous system, to which Golgi had given a crucial contribution, suggested that 'some new light has been shed on psychic and sensory phenomena',[24] although he immediately added that he had little 'faith in the complete fulfilment of this task'. Clearly, the morphological indeterminacy of his reticularist model, as an interpretative 'paradigm' in which all nerve cells were in communication with all others through the diffuse neural net, made it conceptually difficult to forecast the thorough neuroanatomical characterization required to achieve this goal. However, even on this point Golgi did not establish a priori limits to scientific knowledge. Truth can be found, and the duty of the biologist is 'to continue the struggle, a struggle not of grand ideas but of facts accumulated with the pertinacity of patient and indefatigable work: He [that is, the biologist] knows that the progress obtained in such a way, even if very small, will be imperishable'[25] and will 'reduce evermore the confines of ignorance'.[26]

In conclusion, Golgi took from positivism the conviction that science, as an accumulation and inventory of 'facts', would provide the pathway to the solution of the great problems of nature. He refused any a priori 'agnostic' approach that would set absolute restrictions on the potential of scientific investigation. On the other hand, he did not have unlimited faith in the possibility that science would one day solve all problems, particularly those of life and psyche. This was exactly the same attitude he had maintained for the past 30 years. Taking into consideration both his scientific activity and its informing principles, the coherence and obstinacy of his position represents one of the fundamental characteristics of the intellectual persona of Golgi.

Notes

1. Golgi (1884, pp. 37ff.).
2. *Ibid.* (p. 37).
3. Cimino (1984, p. 269).
4. Golgi (1909c, pp. 374ff.). Speech at the inauguration ceremony of the Fondazione Camillo Golgi. According to Medea (1918, p. 454), the '*simpatico* traveller' was Luigi Amedeo di Savoia, Duke of Abruzzi, 'the Prince explorer', who had just returned from a sensational expedition in which he had advanced closer to the North Pole than any previous Arctic explorer.
5. Marcacci (1909, p. 363).
6. Golgi (1910; *OO*, p. 1341).
7. *Ibid.* (*OO*, p. 1342).
8. *Ibid.* (*OO*, pp. 1341ff.).
9. *Ibid.* (*OO*, p. 1390).
10. *Ibid.* (*OO*, p. 1418).
11. *Paradiso,* canto XIII, 112–18.
12. Golgi (1910; *OO*, p. 1419).
13. Golgi (1910a).
14. Pius XI considered Golgi a *naturaliter christianus*, in Tertullian's terminology. In a letter addressed to Carolina Golgi on 18 February 1939, and published in Bianchi (1973, pp. 26ff.), Domenico Cesa Bianchi (whom G. Bianchi erroneously referred to as Cesare Bianchi) wrote 'During the last two years, I repeatedly had the good fortune to approach his Holiness Pius XI, who honours me with his esteem and I dare to say with his affection. In many long conversations during his illness, the Pontiff, aware of the feelings of deep gratitude and lively affection that bound me to my great master Camillo Golgi, on a number of occasions recalled the contacts he had with Golgi, especially during the meetings of the Istituto Lombardo di Scienze e Lettere, and the great impression that that [that is, Golgi's] great mind, austere character, and good nature had elicited in him. But particularly moving was our last conversation, a few hours before his death, when his heart was beating at no more than 40 beats [per minute], and the catarrh was making it ever more difficult for him to breathe. Presaging that his end was near, he responded to my attempts to comfort him by talking serenely about the great mysteries of life and said: "I want to recollect a great speech given many years ago by your master Camillo Golgi at the Istituto Lombardo, a speech that produced a great impression on all of us because of the grandness of the knowledge and the serenity of the conception. After exposing the problems concerning the essence of life and discussing Dubois-Reymond's [du Bois Reymond's] proposition '*Ignoramus seu ignorabimus*', that great mind and serene soul concluded in favour of the '*ignorabimus*'. And we have to kneel before this." These are the Holy Father's almost exact words a few hours before his death. You can imagine my emotion in hearing them!' In fact, Golgi did not subscribe to du Bois-Reymond's *ignorabimus* and thought it unacceptable to restrict a priori the limits of human knowledge even though this did not necessarily imply the actual possibility of discovering 'ultimate explanations'.

Cesa Bianchi gave a similar account of his last conversation with Pius XI in an interview published in *Il Popolo d'Italia*, 11 February 1939. Pius XI's esteem for Golgi has been confirmed during the celebration for the 150th anniversary of Golgi's birth (held at the Società Medico-Chirurgica of Pavia and the Istituto Lombardo-Accademia di Scienze e Lettere) by Prof. Bruno Zanobio, on the basis of the personal recollection of Prof. Giulio Cesare Pupilli, and by Carolina Golgi.

15. The text in *Rendiconti del Regio Istituto Lombardo* is slightly different from that reproduced in *Opera Omnia*. The citations are from the *Rendiconti* version.
16. Golgi (1914, p. 61).
17. *Ibid.* (p. 70).
18. *Ibid.* (p. 101).
19. *Ibid.* (p. 73).
20. *Ibid.* (p. 54).
21. *Ibid.* (p. 57).
22. *Ibid.* (p. 55).
23. Quoted in Golgi (1914, p. 56).
24. *Ibid.* (p. 58).
25. *Ibid.* (p. 64).
26. *Ibid.* (p. 103).

24

Working unto death

The last years of Golgi's life were set in a period of dramatic events for Italy and Europe. On 28 June 1914 Archduke Francis Ferdinand of Austria-Este and his morganatic wife, the Duchess of Hohenberg, were assassinated by a Serbian nationalist in Sarajevo. After a century of optimistic faith in technical, scientific, and moral progress, Europe plunged into the abyss of the First World War; a war that was expected to be over in a few months and instead lasted five years, devastating the youth of the continent.

Austria's aggressive reaction to Serbia in response to the assassination of the hereditary prince triggered a chain reaction that immediately involved Germany, Russia, France, and Great Britain. Initially, Italy remained neutral even though since 1882 she had been tied to Germany and Austria by the Triple Alliance. By 1914, however, this treaty was not worth the paper on which it was written. Austrian annexation of Bosnia in 1908 had already stirred a resurgence of irredentist sentiments among the Italian middle-class and intellectuals. Austria's ultimatum to Serbia, without first notifying Italy, and their subsequent refusal of adequate compensation (both required by Article 7 of the Triple Alliance), essentially released Italy from the obligations of the treaty.

But Italy's neutrality was not to last. Like most other European countries and Japan, early twentieth century Italy was swept by virulent paroxysms of jingoism. 'The least of the great powers' had began the new century with great hopes of regaining a 'place in the sun'. The booming economy had fanned delusions of grandeur and an irrational appetite for militaristic adventure, of which the invasion of Libya was only the first act. Italian public opinion was bitterly divided between *neutralisti*, who advocated neutrality, and *interventisti*, who favoured intervention in the war. The *interventisti* included nationalists and republicans, whereas the *neutralisti* included the socialists, the Catholic world, and most liberals. But in such dramatic moments traditional party lines were easily crossed and about-faces were common. The most momentous of such conversions was that of Benito Mussolini, then Editor-in-Chief of the official organ of the Socialist Party, *Avanti!*. After joining the ranks of the *interventisti* and being expelled from the Socialist Party, the future Duce founded the newspaper *Il Popolo d'Italia*, which became the most vehement voice in support of Italian intervention on the side of the Entente. Interventionists were in fact overwhelmingly in favour of fighting against Austria and wresting from her the last irredentist Italian regions, Trentino and Istria.

The academic environment was particularly responsive to interventionist propaganda and many university professors were actively inciting the students to take up arms and bring the *Risorgimento* to its culmination. Once again, the University of Pavia became a hotbed of irredentism and its Hall VI was transformed into the headquarters of Pavian interventionists. In this excited atmosphere Golgi, who had been imbued since his childhood with the most patriotic feelings, could not but be a fervent interventionist. Another sign that the irredentism of his student years was still alive can be found in his membership in the Dante Alighieri Society, which defied Austria by promoting the use of Italian in Trentino and Istria.

Until Italy's entry into the war, however, Golgi continued to fulfil his academic duties. On 13 December 1914, in a speech commemorating the second anniversary of the Neuropathological Clinic, he complained that psychiatry was abandoning the 'positive and experimental' bases that had led to its inclusion in the realm of medicine, to evolve 'in the opposite direction: that is, in the direction of a return to prevalently philosophical-speculative tendencies in the study of mental diseases'. He may have expressed these concerns because of 'a form of pessimism towards the direction taken by medical studies', a pessimism fed by the growing demands 'for separating . . . the study of psychiatry from that of neuropathology'.[1] Golgi was probably referring to the emergence of psychoanalysis and the spreading of anti-reductionism in psychiatry, tendencies that appeared to him as 'metaphysical speculations' devoid of scientific legitimacy.

At the end of 1914 another of Golgi's protégés, the 32-year-old Aldo Perroncito, left the Laboratory of General Pathology. His exceptional scientific work had been rewarded with the professorship of General Pathology at the University of Cagliari.

On 23 May 1915 Italy declared war on Austria and on the following day the Italian Front was opened on the battlefield. From Hall VI of the University the Pavian students left for the front 'chanting motherland and freedom'.[2] The summer examination session was held ahead of schedule and the academic year was brought to an early close.

With the war came severe logistic and sanitation problems. Pavia was declared a 'Hospital City', and university structures, schools, and industrial plants were converted into military hospital wards, with about 2000 beds. Golgi felt duty bound to participate in the war effort. He abandoned the direction of the hospital ward attached to the Institute of General Pathology and was appointed Director (first with the rank of medical Major and then Lieutenant Colonel, as were all other full professors in the army)[3] of the Ospedale Militare di Riserva (Reserve Military Hospital), which was established on the premises of the Collegio Borromeo on 5 June 1915. He took on his duties renouncing 'all economic benefit linked to his rank', which by the end of the war would represent 'a conspicuous amount of money'.[3] Veratti was appointed Director of the military hospital in Collegio Ghislieri.

Despite the obvious problems posed by the transformation of an old building into a modern hospital, the septuagenarian Golgi took up his duties with great energy. With the help of Count Giberto Borromeo, patron of the Collegio, he managed to equip the hospital with two surgery rooms, an enormous kitchen to feed 450 patients, new hygienic services, a pharmacy, and a 137-metre-deep well to provide the hospital with clean water. His organization of the hospital was innovative. In addition to the medical and surgical wards, Golgi created a special neuropathological ward, which became the prototype for other military hospitals. The neuropathological ward was entrusted to his old pupil Guido Sala, who was renowned for his studies on the regeneration of peripheral nerves and who, after many years at the Neuropathological Clinic, had become an expert in treatment of lesions of the nervous system. Furthermore, from February 1916 the hospital was endowed with a Mechano-therapeutic Institute for the rehabilitation of wounded patients who had recovered from the acute phase. This institute was entrusted to Giovanni Verga and was organized in three sections for kinesiotherapy, thermotherapy, and massotherapy.

Golgi was also untiring in his efforts to furnish the hospital with sufficient materials and equipment. Italy had entered the war in a lamentable state of unpreparedness and the military hospitals fared no better than the rest of the army. Among other things, the Ospedale Militare di Riserva lacked machines for electrotherapy and Sala was initially obliged to use his own equipment.[4] Golgi used all his influence, both personal and as the President of the Pro-Pavia Association, to coordinate private and public donors in providing funds for the hospital.

In March 1916 Golgi participated in the meeting of the Italian Society for the Progress of the Sciences, of which he was the President. Before a public that included also the most distinguished member of the Society, Prime Minister Antonio Salandra, Golgi gave an emphatically patriotic but not chauvinistic speech. The country was engaged in a exhausting and bloody trench war against the 'traditional enemy'.[5] The conflict was not only historically necessary, it was a 'holy war' that Italy had the moral right to wage to defend 'sacred national interests'; it was a 'war of civilization, of justice, of morality'.[6] Golgi's anti-Austrian feelings were tempered by his admiration for German supremacy in science and technology. He hoped that Italy would imitate 'Germany in her disciplined perseverance and energy',[7] the only way to take full advantage of Italy's rich intellectual potential. This was in line with Golgi's advocacy of a rapid industrialization of Italy, indicated also by his active support for the creation of a School of Industrial Chemistry in 1916.[8] Golgi's admiration for Germany, however, did not blind him to the danger of German nationalism, which trumpeted the superiority of German race and culture. Golgi remembered that in 1901 the Rector of the Industrial University of Charlottemburg had declared that 'All People of Latin or Roman origin are falling into decadence and Germany is called to walk at the head of the civilized world'.[9] And in 1914 ninety-three German intellectuals, including Max Planck, had declared in a 'manifest to the civilized world' that 'Germany is so superior to all other nations in terms of race, culture, and civilization . . . to derive from it her right or even duty to prevail over all other nations of the world'. For Golgi these ideas were the expression of the dangerous 'collective psychosis' that had engulfed German society and was leading to that 'collective manic exaltation, which, in past centuries, had endowed war-making with a character of religious fanaticism!'[10] He contrasted this with the strongly held belief in Italy that 'civilization was the product not of single nation, but of all nations, and that the intellectual and moral wealth of mankind derived from the concurrence of all forces and from the achievements of the mind and genius of all nations.'[11]

At the end of March, despite some health problems, Golgi gave a commemorative speech in honour of the architect Angelo Savoldi, who had linked his name to various

architectural projects in Pavia and who had founded the Pro-Pavia Association.[12] On
15 April 1916, Golgi became President of an association that represented the interests of
the Army men who had suffered permanent disability because of war-related injuries.
More important was his appointment, after Baccelli's death, to the Presidency of the
National Council of Public Health.

On 20 September 1916 Nicoló Manfredi died at the age of 80. With the death of this
loyal companion of his heroic years in Bizzozero's laboratory a piece of Golgi's youth
disappeared. This must have been a sad reminder of the passage of time for Golgi. He was
now 73 years old and his health was deteriorating.

But there is no trace of slowing down in Golgi's frenetic work in the war years. In
November he established a 'convalescence' ward in the premises of the Pio Albergo
Pertusati, for the patients of his hospital who were recovering from surgery or undergoing
physiotherapy. The presence of a scientist of Golgi's stature and of assistants like Sala, Verga,
and, for brief period, Pensa contributed to the transformation of the Ospedale Militare
Collegio Borromeo into an important centre for the study of war-related pathologies. Sala
and Verga published a number of papers on clinical cases, made original observations
in physiopathology and neuropathology, and developed new diagnostic and therapeutic
protocols. In March Golgi reported on the activity of the neuropathological ward at a
meeting of the Società Medico-Chirurgica of Pavia.[13] Two weeks later, he was in the
Senate to participate in the discussion of a law concerning the 'Protection and assistance
of disabled veterans'.[14] He supported provisions that would compel wounded soldiers to
undergo appropriate surgical or medical procedures. More and more soldiers were in fact
taking advantage of existing regulations (dating back to 1890) allowing them to decline
therapy, which meant that they could avoid returning to the front lines. Golgi argued that
this would result in the swelling of the disabled roll, which would later weigh heavily on
society. His intervention was tactfully criticized by the Minister of Internal Affairs Vittorio
Emanuele Orlando, who noted that 'anyone who, being called to fulfil his Army duty,
presents a deformity or an infirmity that, if operated upon, would heal [for example, a
hernia]' was not obliged to undergo such an operation. Thus, it would not be fair to place
the same obligation on a wounded veteran 'because in the end the latter has already paid a
personal price, and it would appear bizarre to apply a sterner provision against him than
against one who has been called to [but who has not yet fulfilled] his military duty.'[14]
Golgi's proposal was rejected.

In the last months of 1917 the Italian Army, plagued by crumbling morale, suffered a
catastrophic military reverse. Since the beginning of the war Italians and Austrians had
been locked in a bloody stalemate, despite 11 colossal battles fought on the River Isonzo.
But on 24 October 1917, under a joint attack by German and Austrian forces, the Italian
line broke near Caporetto. The battle raged for another three months, taking the lives of
half a million men, before the Italians, with a Herculean effort around Christmas, halted
the invaders on the River Piave. After the collapse of Caporetto the plain of Lombardy
filled with several hundred thousand retreating soldiers and refugees. Pavia was crowded
with the wounded. Among the patients in the Military Hospital of Collegio Ghislieri
Golgi found Aldo Perroncito, who had contracted tuberculosis in the trenches. The disease
had rapidly worsened after the retreat, during which 'he did not panic, and overcoming all

difficulties ensured the orderly functioning of the medical unit entrusted to him and saved it.'[15] As soon as he recovered, he asked to return to the front and only at the insistence of Veratti took a few weeks of convalescence.

In 1917 the second part of Cajal's autobiography, *Recuerdos de mi Vida,* appeared. This was an autobiographical recounting of the author's discoveries, written in a romantic, argumentative, and aggressive but effective style. It was full of egocentric claims of priority, naive philosophical considerations, and pretentious and unsupported assertions, such as that of having invented the disks for phonographic recording before Thomas Alva Edison. He also claimed to have discovered the internal reticular apparatus in 1891–92 and to have been the first to discover the phenomenon of passive immunity.[16] It was the apotheosis of the Dionysian concept of scientific enterprise, where competition reigns supreme; it was a style of research that, in a less extreme form, would eventually become dominant. Trespassing the boundary of a serene and civilized critique, he abandoned himself to heavy personal attacks on Golgi. The book received a favourable review in Italy in *Rivista di Patologia Nervosa e Mentale*, edited by Tanzi. Golgi did not reply; being polemic for the sake of argument was not his style. When he entered a controversy, even a harsh one, he always remained on solid scientific ground. But here there was nothing concrete to argue about. It was a stinging and brilliant story that in many places appeared to have been written more with the hand of an artist than of a scientist, and one in which ostentatious compliments to Golgi were designed to make the harsh attacks appear as fair assessments. Unfortunately, from that moment on, with rare exceptions, Golgi's international reputation rested on the portrait provided by the Spanish anatomist.

In August 1918, the moment most dreaded by Golgi finally arrived: obligatory retirement at the age of 75. The Medical School and later the Ministry of Public Education approved a proposal by Luigi Sala to consider the *Corso Libero* of Histology, which Golgi would teach as Professor Emeritus, as equivalent to an official course. Golgi's retirement weakened considerably the ability of the University to stave off the ever-growing Milanese threat. From the existing regulation it was not clear whether as a Professor Emeritus Golgi could participate and vote in the sessions of the faculty senate. He wrote to ask for clarification from the Rector and from the Ministry of Public Education and even to the Minister himself. Initially he received only ambiguous answers, but later it was established that a Professor Emeritus could participate and intervene but not vote. Golgi was bitterly disappointed by the impossibility of continuing to influence University politics. Some consolation came in the form of a moving and deferential homage written by Medea, which appeared at the end of 1918 in the *Rivista d'Italia*. Medea lamented that his old professor had to retire from teaching 'because of the inexorable rigidity of law' and celebrated his many scientific and social achievements.[17] Another honour was bestowed on him by Donaldson who, as member of the Editorial Board of *The Journal of Comparative Neurology*, sponsored the dedication of the 30th volume to Golgi.

The year 1918 was a sad one for Golgi, not only because of his retirement but also because of the death of two of his oldest friends, Gaspare Emilio Brugnatelli and Carlo Forlanini.[18] The latter had become world famous because of the development of the artificial pneumothorax to treat pulmonary tuberculosis, and had been repeatedly proposed by Golgi for the Nobel Prize.[19] And in March of the following year he learned with consternation that his former pupil Fusari had died.

As usual, Golgi's response to adversity was to immerse himself in his work. For the moment, he was still busy with the direction of the Ospedale Militare Collegio Borromeo. Although at the end of October 1918 the Italians had routed the Austrians in the battle of Vittorio Veneto, ending the war on the Italian Front, the military hospitals in Pavia continued to remain active for a while, in part because the country was now confronted with another deadly emergency: the Spanish flu pandemic. Golgi reported on the functioning of the Italian neurological centres at the conference on the rehabilitation of traumatized veterans organized by the victorious powers.[20] But eventually this emergency passed and the hospital was decommissioned. After many years spent at the head of the Ospedale Militare, Golgi missed the Laboratory and active research, the only thing that could still make him feel alive. Despite his retirement he was able to resume scientific work because the loyal Veratti had been temporarily put in charge of the Laboratory of General Pathology.

And, sure enough, as soon as the old master was back at the microscope, new histological details were observed. Using a new method based on chloro-gold, he was able to visualize a nucleus-like body in the centre of mammalian blood cells. Golgi, however, immediately distanced himself from those who propounded that a true functionally active nucleus persisted in the mature red cell. Among these was Angelo Petrone, who had advocated such a thesis since 1897 on the basis of experiments conducted using his own particular method. However, Petrone's conclusions had been shown to be in error by work carried out in Golgi's laboratory by Adelchi Negri in 1899. Petrone subsequently presented new observations that appeared to confirm his old theory. Golgi's now emphasized that his findings were not supportive of Petrone's claim, but he did not provide any alternative explanation for them. Golgi also discovered the presence of the centrosome in the white cells. In no way did these findings represent an exhaustive body of work and further investigation was necessary. Unfortunately, the Laboratory might be entrusted at any moment to a new Director and in that case Golgi knew that he would be unable to continue his research with the dignity that he demanded. On the other hand, he was afraid that his absence 'could have, as on other occasions, disastrous effects on the specimens'. Thus he decided to report his work in a preliminary report to the Società Medico-Chirurgica on 12 June 1919.[21] In the audience was a young assistant at the Institute of General Pathology, Costanza Boccadoro, who had followed Golgi's work step by step and was attempting to apply his techniques not only in the laboratory but also at the clinical level.

Ever since 1915, the Board of Physicians of Pavia had been wanting to celebrate the 50th anniversary of Golgi's medical degree, but this project had been suspended because of the war. Now the Board and the University decided to celebrate this anniversary jointly with the occasion of his retirement. A subscription was set up, collecting about 44 000 lire from national institutions and private citizens to establish a foundation in his name that would grant scholarships to deserving orphans of physicians.[22] The ceremony was held on 29 June 1919 in the *Aula Magna* of the University of Pavia. The initial official speakers included

Emilio Cornelli, President of the Board of Medical Doctors of Pavia, Oreste Ranelletti, Rector of the University, Innocente Clivio, professor of Obstetrics and Gynaecology, and Luigi Sala, who spoke for all the disciples of the Institute of General Pathology. Then it was the turn of the Mayor, who conferred upon Golgi the honorary citizenship of Pavia, a gold medal from the Municipality, and a lettered parchment. Finally, the old patriarch of Italian histology spoke. 'Visibly moved', he replied with great modesty to the congratulations he had received, and possibly for the first time in his life he let himself indulge in autobiographical recollections. He talked about his youth, the resurgence of Pavian medicine embodied in the figures of Bizzozero, Mantegazza, Oehl, Tommasi and especially in the great Panizza. He remembered his years in Abbiategrasso and the difficulty of working 'in the rudimentary laboratory, set up by me in the kitchen of the small apartment that had been allocated to me.'[23] He defended histology as the 'science of organization', advocating its centrality in biological sciences at a time when it seemed to be pushed to the sidelines by new research approaches. And he publicly acknowledged that Lina had 'supported and directly helped' him in his long scientific career. At the conclusion everybody 'gathered around the podium, surrounding the guest of honour to congratulate him and to admire the artistic album containing the signatures of the subscribers and bearing on an artistically engraved bronze plate the simple words, 'To Camillo Golgi—Pavia—29 June 1919'.[24]

Unfortunately, despite this display of affection, Golgi was becoming more isolated in the University, and some of his enemies, including Monti and Mondino, were now among the most powerful academics in the University; Monti would become Dean of the Medical School in 1919.

On 18 January 1920, Mangiagalli announced, at a meeting organized to promote higher education in Milan, that the project of fusing the University of Pavia and the Istituti Clinici di Perfezionamento had been completed. The intention of the sponsors of the project was to a create a grand hybrid organism (Facoltà Medico-Chirurgica e di Perfezionamento) devoted to drawing together the best of Pavian and Milanese medicine. Golgi was disquieted and embittered by this turn of events. In his view, the University of Pavia was finally capitulating to the mighty Milan.

Once again, he found consolation in research. In the early months of 1920, he completed, with the help of the loyal Boccadoro, a study on the centrosome of red blood cells, which he presented to the Istituto Lombardo on 8 April 1920.[25]

At the beginning of December, Golgi went to Rome to participate in a parliamentary debate on a proposed new law 'in support of fishing and fishermen'. Golgi was very interested in the problems of fresh- and salt-water fishing. For many years he had been taking long vacations on the Italian Riviera, often as a guest of the Perroncitos in Arenzano, and in Pavia he had become Honorary President of an association of Ticino River fishermen. In his speech, Golgi advocated strict and severe application of the laws against the illegal use of explosives for fishing, a practice quite common on long stretches of the coast around Arenzano, 'a notorious centre of smuggling linked to the Genoa Harbour'.[26] He then raised the issue of the Pavian fishermen who were unfairly constrained in their activity by a 'dealer in lumber, wine, and other products, a certain Montemezzani' who held exclusive rights to fishing on 'the entire section [of the Ticino River] that extends from the Pavia bridge to Boscazzo di Bereguardo (over 40 km)'. Montemezzani would fine the fishermen who dared to enter his section of the river and from those who had rented from him a portion of the river front he demanded 'a part of their catch' for a negligible price. He then resold these fish in Milan at a four-fold profit, making a fortune from the practice. Montemezzani had leased that section of the Ticino River from a French firm, the Société des Placers aurifères de la haute Italie (Society of Gold Place Miners of Northern Italy), which, three years earlier, had obtained the mining rights for the river from the Prefect. Golgi contested the legality of the Prefect's decision, and asked for a provision in support of the fishermen. Three days later he was on the attack again, having learned that in Pavia public demonstrations against the Société were in preparation. In the end the draft law under debate was modified to include the possibility of expropriation of the fishing rights 'for reason of public utility', a provision that could nicely fit the Pavian case.

At the end of January 1921 Golgi went to Paris to participate in the Oceanographic-Biological Congress as the representative of the Maritime Ministry, and as President of the Italian Delegation.[27]

The political situation of post-war Italy was meanwhile deteriorating, and ominous signals of social unrest were surfacing. The Peace Conference in Versailles had frustrated the expectations of the Italians. Although Italian casualties were of the same order of magnitude as those of the British, the Allies refused to fully acknowledge Italy's sacrifice. The deep sense of wounded pride and the worsening of the economic situation concurred to create a poisonous climate of ideological radicalization. In March 1919, Benito Mussolini founded the Fasci di Combattimento which after a shaky start began to grow quickly, finding support among veterans, nationalist intellectuals, the urban middle-class, and landowners. Two years later the left wing of the Socialist Party split, giving birth to the Italian Communist Party.

An episode in the spring of 1921 gives an idea of the social and political climate in Pavia. In mid-April, Fabrizio Maffi, a government expert in hygiene in charge of the organization of tuberculosis sanatoria and dispensaries, was in Pavia to discuss with Golgi and Luigi Montemartini the 'problem of the hospitalization of tubercular patients'. Maffi, who had been Golgi's pupil around 1890, was a communist and a Member of Parliament. Besides being a politician, he was particularly active in issues of public health, particularly in the fight against tuberculosis. He had assisted in the early experiments with the 'lymph of Koch' by Golgi and Silva, and had suffered a bitter disappointment when its ineffectiveness had become evident (one of his brothers was suffering from the terrible disease at the time). During his visit in Pavia the unfortunate Maffi underwent a public humiliation at the hands of the fascists. According to a news article in La Provincia Pavese of 24 April, Maffi, after an altercation with fascists at the café Demetrio, was attacked by the local ras Luigi Lanfranconi, who dragged him to a balcony before a boisterous crowd that 'demanded that Maffi be obliged to yell "Hail Italy".' When a pale Maffi, despite being 'surrounded by a threatening group', refused, someone in the crowd 'threw a pair of scissors which fell on the balcony and was picked up by the lawyer Lanfranconi'. After a few moments of indecision, the latter grasped Maffi's beard and 'cut off a clump' while poor Maffi was

'vainly trying to escape from the outrage'. Later the fascists escorted Maffi to the train
station where he remained under the surveillance of the Carabinieri until his departure.
That very night brawls between communists and fascists broke out. The fascists got the
worst of it and one of them was knocked unconscious. The following day the fighting
escalated into armed conflict and one of the communists, Ferruccio Ghinaglia (a medical
student of the Collegio Ghislieri) was killed.

The end of Golgi's life was embittered not only by the war and the grievous post-war
years, but also by a series of events linked to the academic environment of the University
and to the epilogue of his long-standing battle against Milan.

On 31 March 1921, the fusion between Pavia and Milan was approved, to Golgi's dismay,
and few months later, on 7 December, Father Agostino Gemelli inaugurated the Università Cattolica of Milano, which represented another possible nucleus for a Milanese
university. For the moment, however, the Cattolica appeared to be less threatening than
Mangiagalli's project because it included only the Faculties of Philosophy and Social
Sciences.

At the end of 1921, Mondino, probably at Monti's suggestion, proposed the unification
of the professorships of general pathology and pathological anatomy. In this way Monti
would take over the Institute of General Pathology. As in a classic drama, the harshest
blows came from those he had helped most in their careers.[28] Mondino's proposal was
approved by the faculty senate and from that moment Golgi deserted the Institute. However, the fusion of the two professorships encountered the opposition of both general
pathologists and anatomo-pathologists, and a petition asking for its revocation was sent
to the Ministry of Public Education, which eventually invalidated it.

Perroncito immediately asked to be transferred from Cagliari to the professorship of
general pathology in Pavia, but he found an obstacle in Eugenio Centanni of the University of Modena, who also asked to be transferred to Pavia. An official competition was
held and finally Perroncito was appointed. This sad episode had a lasting effect on Golgi,
who afterwards appeared depressed and complained of 'cardiac arrhythmias'. However,
he returned to the Institute, where he secluded himself in a room, continuing to teach
histology and occasionally conducting some experiments.[29]

Around this time Veratti left the Institute of General Pathology (although he continued
to teach bacteriology as Adjunct Professor) and took up the direction of a laboratory in the
Medical Clinic. His academic career had in fact come to a standstill. Some of his former
pupils, such as Perroncito, had already reached the pinnacle of the academic ladder, while
he was still limping along as an Associate. Besides his unrelenting self-criticism, which
paralysed him at the moment of publishing his work, Veratti may have been damaged by
his generosity. Countless times he had helped his students with their research projects,
sometimes suggesting original ideas, without asking for authorship on their publications.

Golgi's opposition to a hybrid Pavia–Milan was soon vindicated.[30] The interests of the
Pavian and Milanese factions turned out to be incompatible, and the continuous frictions
made the management of such an elephantine structure all but impossible. One of the *casus
belli* was the so-called 'Besta' case. On 8 May 1922 a faculty meeting discussed the proposal
to add to the Istituti Clinici di Perfezionamento an institute of neurophysiopathology
under the direction of Carlo Besta. The proposal was rejected because of strenuous opposition

by the Pavians, obviously with Golgi in the lead. This successful blockage was, however, only a temporary setback for the Milanese. A few months later, on 27 December, Bertarelli, backed by Mangiagalli, put the issue of the move to Milan on the table again, and a committee was created to study the problem.

Disappointed and frustrated by the inexorable unfolding of the events, Golgi withdrew from the academic arena. His speech was now hesitant and broken and his walking uncertain, and 'he became conscious, perhaps even overly so, of the deterioration of his health'.[31] He underwent some unsuccessful therapy 'with a docility that was unusual for his character'. He even submitted to a cure by Serge Voronoff, who was then something of a celebrity thanks to his sensational 'rejuvenating' treatments based on implants of monkey genital glands (which purportedly enhanced the 'vital energies' of the patients). While visiting Golgi in Pavia, Voronoff recommended to his ailing host a special diet including cumin, which, however, had no effect.

In the early months of 1922 he reported to the Istituto Lombardo the findings of a study on the globules of the yolk of frog eggs that he had begun ten years earlier. He found that the globules exhibited all the properties of living organisms, including the ability to reproduce.[32] 'The communication was a moving scene: only the spirit of the man was left; his words were disjointed and broken, but concerned new findings and ideas and promised future research.'[33]

Finally, on 19 March 1923, the committee and then the faculty senate approved the transfer of the Medical School to Milan. Among the few who voted against it were Luigi Sala and Perroncito, while Golgi, who could not vote, sent an indignant letter to the faculty senate. The latter, he wrote, had committed in fact a true suicide, suppressing a centuries-old institution with a simple vote.

Golgi's 80th birthday was solemnly celebrated on 9 July 1923, during a ceremony sponsored by the Pavian press. Indeed, since the early 1860s Golgi's official birth certificates reported this incorrect date, probably because of a mistake in the transcription of the parish records. Throughout his life Golgi had made repeated attempts, through his friend Stefanini,[34] to have the mistake corrected, but without success.

At 11 in the morning Golgi's home was full of personalities and dignitaries and he was presented with an album containing messages from thousands of Pavian citizens. Visibly moved, the elderly histologist described himself as a 'lucky man' for the exceptional circumstances of his life: lucky in his studies, lucky for having disciples 'who surrounded him with ... enthusiasm and energy, and whose names are renowned abroad', lucky for having a 'sweet and affectionate companion in his life'.[35] The Minister of Public Education Giovanni Gentile granted a request from the Medical School to have the Institute of General Pathology named after Golgi. Telegrams arrived from all parts of Italy, including one from the head of the Government, Benito Mussolini, which was read by the Prefect to general applause. Mussolini had bestowed upon Golgi the Gran Cordone Mauriziano, an honour of great prestige.[36]

There is some evidence that Golgi had some sympathy for the Fascist Party and for the *Duce*. Of the latter he is reported to have said 'Oh, finally an Italian who does not enrich himself with public money!'[37] On the other hand, fascism attracted even previous radicals and socialist exponents such as Roberto Rampoldi and Achille Monti.

In the evening a crowd gathered outside Golgi's house and the municipal band played in his honour. Golgi appeared on the balcony and with few modest words thanked the citizens for the celebration.

Although the battle with Milan was clearly lost, Golgi was not the type of man to concede defeat graciously. During the summer, although in poor health, he went to Rome to advocate the cause of the University of Pavia at the relevant ministries. He felt that this was mission of duty for him, a burning passion he could not resist, a compulsion lived as a faith that could and should override the very desire of the majority of professors who had voted for the transfer to Milan. In the end, the Gentile Law would dissolve the Pavia–Milan hybrid. From that moment on, the two cities went their separate ways. However, the Law allowed for the establishment of the University of Milan with partial financial support from the National Government. This was the moment Mangiagalli had long awaited: the creation of the Università Statale di Milano.

On 24 November Golgi received an honorary degree from the Sorbonne.[38] Despite his aches and pains, and ignoring Lina's worries about his health, Golgi decided to attend the ceremonies. He had to go 'for the sake of Pavia's honour'. On that occasion, he told Pensa:

I would most gladly renounce because I feel tired but, thinking that this honour bestowed upon me could be of some advantage for the future of the University, I cannot pass up the occasion.[39]

For Golgi, everything that could enhance the image of his University would contribute to warding off the Milanese danger. He went with Lina, Aldo Perroncito, and his pupil Luigi Magnaghi. Among the seven to receive the honour from the Sorbonne were Svante August Arrhenius and Golgi's fellow Nobel laureate, Thomson.

Of course, it would take more than an honorary degree from the Sorbonne to stop Mangiagalli. On 16 October the latter managed to obtain a Royal Decree officially establishing the University of Milan, of which he became the first Rector. Being also the Mayor of Milan, he was in the best position to obtain public support and funding for the project. Furthermore, as a vociferous supporter of fascism,[40] he had all the political backing he needed. On 22 November he gave a speech before academics, professionals, and representatives of the arts and industry, requesting their help in finalizing the convention for the funding of the new university. His appeal was successful. On 18 December a meeting of the Board of the Istituto Sieroterapico Milanese was scheduled, of which Golgi was President, to discuss how to deal with Mangiagalli's request. Golgi wrote to the Director, Serafino Belfanti, that because of his well-known position on the issue, he felt that it would be 'appropriate to abstain from intervening to avoid his presence in any way hindering free discussion and deliberation'.[41] And, not surprisingly, the Board deliberated in favour of Mangiagalli's request. Too many powerful interests were involved; the new university promised new academic positions and career possibilities, and it seemed unfair to continue to deprive Italy's economic capital of its own university. As soon as Golgi was informed of this, he wrote Belfanti that he understood that 'the fatality of things had led the Institute to such a decision', which, however, put him in the 'moral' impossibility of continuing in his 'charge as President of that Institute which he had the honour to hold for many years'.[42] On

5 January 1924 the Board refused to accept Golgi's resignation and Belfanti travelled to Pavia to try to convince Golgi to change his mind, without success.[43]

On 18 June 1924 Mangiagalli wrote to Mussolini about the 'right of Milan' to have its own university and on 28 August the convention was signed.[44] On 8 December Mangiagalli inaugurated the academic year 1924–25. In the space of a few months he had finally obtained what he had been struggling for since the early 1890s.

Golgi's health continued to worsen. Pensa met him in the fall or winter of 1924 and found him aged and aching.

When I called on him at his home, he gave the impression of being an elderly convalescent; on another day, when I went to visit him in his laboratory, I could still detect in him soundness of judgement, technical originality, and sharpness of observation, but I also noticed something that he had never exhibited before: a certain disillusionment and dissatisfaction with his own work and with himself. I felt very sorry for him.[39]

But the elderly histologist, despite all his physical problems, refused to give in. Only by increasing the efficiency and importance of Pavian university structures would it be possible to keep the University of Milan from making the University of Pavia superfluous, and thus at the beginning of December he was in Rome to advocate the cause of the new San Matteo Hospital.[45]

Of course, this trip was hard on him, and at the end of 1924 there was a dramatic worsening of his health, from which he recovered only slowly over the following months.[46] During the celebration held on 21 May 1925 for the 11 centuries of the University of Pavia (which according to tradition was founded in 825), he was still ailing and could not participate in any of the ceremonies. When King Victor Emmanuel III, who was visiting for the celebration, heard of Golgi's precarious condition, he sent his aide-de-camp General Arturo Cittadini, accompanied by General Ambrogio Clerici, to extend to him his personal best wishes. Golgi followed the official parade from the balcony of his house. When the King arrived below the balcony, he waved to the old scientist who was visibly moved.

Golgi spent that summer in Arenzano, recovering on the balmy Italian Riviera. In October he was back in Pavia, where he found a letter from Henschen announcing the possibility of a trip to 'beautiful Italy' and a visit to his laboratory 'renowned throughout the world'.[47] He began to work on a paper concerning follow-up experiments on the structure of yolk, in which he extended his earlier findings to other species including the chicken. He intended to present his findings to the Istituto Lombardo with the title 'Concerning the development of the chicken egg—Note II'. He began with a detailed review of the literature and then a summary of the results.[48] But in the middle of December he contracted severe influenza; his condition became critical for several days and then seemed to improve. When he appeared to have recovered, he received a letter from his former pupil, Corrado Da Fano, of King's College, University of London, informing him that he had been appointed 'Honorary Fellow of the Royal Society of Medicine' and was a candidate for the election as 'Honorary Foreign Member of the Royal Society'.[49] Unfortunately, on Thursday 14 January 1926, 'trismic phenomena localized to the left cheek, due to a phlegmonous form, appeared within his mouth'.[50] His general condition began to deteriorate again and now Lina, helped by Sandro and Carolina Golgi and Aldo Perroncito, was constantly at his bedside. Also helping were many of his disciples, including Veratti and Luigi and Guido Sala. The physician Adolfo Ferrata followed the course of the illness.

Gemelli, who was now a Minor Franciscan friar, tried in vain 'to bring the light of Christ also into the soul of a person who had him [that is, Gemelli] as a beloved disciple'.[51] But Golgi was not a person to convert in *articulo mortis*. Golgi's behaviour during his final hours is perfectly suited to Michel de Montaigne's aphorism 'Every death should conform to life. We do not become different in dying. I shall always judge death from life.'[52]

On 20 January 1926 his condition became critical with the development of septicaemia, and on the following day, around noon, Camillo Golgi's life came to an end.[53]

His body, clad in a black redingote and decorated with the Cross of the Ordine Civile di Savoia, was placed in a casket in the candle-lit reception room of the Golgi home. Four firemen in dress uniform and students with the Goliardic head-dress acted as guards of honour.

The news spread rapidly in a city in which Golgi was held almost as a tutelary deity. Flags were lowered to half-mast at the University, the City Hall, and a number of public and private buildings. As a sign of public grief, classes were suspended until the following Tuesday. A crowd of visitors came to pay their last respects to the great scientist. On the same evening, public obituaries were prepared by the new Rector, Ottorino Rossi, by the Mayor, Pietro Vaccari, by the local section of the National Fascist Party, and by other associations. Condolences from all over Italy began to arrive, including telegrams from the King, Mussolini, the Ministers of Public Education and Finance, and luminaries in politics and science. Golgi's body was encased in a triple casket of spruce, lead, and white maple, and transported on Sunday morning to the *Aula Magna* of the University for a public viewing. The next day, 25 January, one of the coldest days of that winter, a solemn non-religious State funeral was celebrated. In the early afternoon, accompanied by the slow tolling of bells from the University and the City Hall, the students transported the casket to the central court of the University under Alessandro Volta's statue, as requested by Golgi himself,[54] to symbolize his lifelong dedication to the ideal of scientific pursuit, as embodied in Volta. There followed commemorative speeches by the Under-Secretary of Finance, Francesco D'Alessio, representing the Government, an envoy from the Senate, the Rector, the Mayor, and a representative of the student body.

After the commemoration, the coffin was placed on a hearse drawn by four horses and honoured with a military salute by units of the Carabinieri, the Army, and the Fascist Militia. The funeral procession, leading an imposing crowd, followed Corso Vittorio Emanuele (currently Strada Nuova) and Corso Garibaldi. At its head were 12 municipal guards and 12 firemen in full dress uniforms, the representatives of Italian and foreign students, and civil and military organizations, a platoon of Carabinieri, and two military bands. Beside the hearse walked Guido Sala, representing Golgi's disciples, and other authorities. Behind were the relatives, led by Lina Golgi, Aldo Perroncito and his wife, and Giulio Bizzozero's son, Enzo. Then followed Ottorino Rossi, representatives of the Academic Senate, the faculty body, the Federal Secretary of the National Fascist Party, and a multitude of local, provincial, regional, and national delegations, including the

Mayor of Corteno. Along the path of the procession, the shops and entranceways of residences were closed as a sign of respect. At dusk, the imposing procession reached the cemetery where the coffin was again honoured by a military salute before being interred in the tomb of the Magnaghi family, while his marble tomb was being prepared. Golgi's remains were later moved close to the funerary monument of his old teacher, Bartolomeo Panizza.

And thus ended the life of the man who had forged the 'instrument of revelation' and saw for the first time the beautiful silhouette of an entire nerve cell. A complex personality, Golgi was at the same time an academic educated in the rigorous Austrian–Hungarian tradition, admirer of the German culture, and a spirited patriot; an innovator whose discoveries allowed the rise of modern neuroscience and a conservative who never came to terms with the theory of the neuron; an introverted and taciturn man, and a loving husband and mentor; professing agnosticism but respectful of religious tradition. Perhaps the image that best symbolizes Golgi's personality can be found in the mysterious and austere beauty of the beloved Alps from which he came.

Notes

1. Golgi (1915, p. 56).
2. As recorded on a commemorative plaque. Reproduced in Milani (1985, p. 274) and in a note by Prof. Bruno Zanobio in Pensa (1991, p. 165).
3. MSUP-I-I-65. Near the end of the war he became auxiliary medical Colonel for exceptional merit.
4. Golgi (1917, p. 37).
5. Golgi (1916, p. 8).
6. *Ibid.* (p. 7).
7. *Ibid.* (p. 13).
8. Signori (1993, p. 213).
9. Cited in Golgi (1916, p. 14).
10. Golgi (1916, p. 14).
11. *Ibid.* (p. 15).
12. Golgi (1916a).
13. Golgi (1917).
14. Session of 19 March 1917 (*Atti parlamentari del Senato*; Rome: Tipografia del Senato, 1917, reprint, pp. 3–26). Reproduced in Goldaniga and Marchetti (1993, pp. 216–20). See also Zanobio and Armocida (1994, pp. 615–18).
15. Veratti (1929, p. 163).
16. Jacobson (1993, p. 250).
17. Medea (1918, p. 447).
18. Brugnatelli was commemorated in the session of 27 February 1918 by the Council of the Consorzio Universitario (Golgi 1918), and Forlanini in the meeting of the Istituto Lombardo on 6 June (Golgi 1918a).
19. On the candidacy of Forlanini for the Nobel Prize, there exists a rich documentation, kept in the MSUP. See also Introzzi (1961, p. 328).

20. Golgi (1918b).
21. Golgi (1919).
22. *La Provincia Pavese* (26 March 1919 and 2 July 1919).
23. Mazzarello (1993, p. 361).
24. *La Provincia Pavese* (2 July 1919).
25. Golgi (1920).
26. Sessions of 3, 6, and 8 December 1920 (*Atti parlamentari del Senato*; Roma: Tipografia del Senato, 1917, reprint, pp. 3–56). The citations are on pp. 9 and 15.
27. *La Provincia Pavese* (2 February 1921).
28. Pensa (1991, p. 180).
29. I have been told by Prof. Luigi Bianchi that these lectures of the early 1920s were rather boring and attended by only a few students. Golgi arrived accompanied by an assistant (probably Boccadoro) and lectured while following an outline he kept in his hand and pointing with a stick to explanatory drawings mounted on some panels.
30. Pensa (1991, pp. 182ff.).
31. *Ibid.* (p. 181).
32. Golgi (1923).
33. Morpurgo (1926, p. 52).
34. See letter from Golgi to Stefanini. This has been confirmed by Dr Lino Stefanini in a personal communication.
35. *La Provincia Pavese* (11 July 1923).
36. After the Nobel Prize Golgi continued to receive honours from around the world. He received honorary medical degrees from the Fredericiana University of Christiania (former name of Oslo) and from the University of Athens (in 1912). He received honorary affiliations to a number of Italian and foreign scientific societies, including the Society of Biology and the Society of Neurology of Paris, the Society of Exotic Pathology of London, the Society for the Study of Tropical Diseases of London, the Royal Academy of Science, Literature, and the Arts of Modena, the Royal Academy of Medicine of Turin, the Accademia Gioenia of Natural Sciences of Catania, the Imperial Academy of Sciences of St Petersburg, the German Society of Neurologists, the Dutch Society of Sciences, the Swedish Royal Society of Sciences, the Royal Academy of Sciences of Berlin, the Imperial Academy of Sciences of Vienna, the Dutch Royal Academy of Sciences, the Royal Society of Medical and Natural Sciences of Bruxelles. The Italian Government honoured him with the title of Grand'Ufficiale dell'Ordine dei Santi Maurizio e Lazzaro and with the decoration of the Gran Cordone dell'Ordine della Corona d'Italia. He also received the title of Cavaliere dell'Ordine pour le mérite Federico II. Golgi also continued to serve on various committees, including the Committee for the Prevention of Tuberculosis, of which he was appointed President.
37. *Il Popolo-La Provincia Pavese* (24 January 1926).
38. The news was announced at the meeting of the Istituto Lombardo on 29 November 1923. *Rendiconti del Regio Istituto Lombardo di Scienze e Lettere* (1923, series II, **56**, p. 872). Various documents on the conferring of this degree are kept in the MSUP (MSUP-III-V, from 1–26).
39. Pensa (1991, p. 186).
40. In a letter to Mussolini on 23 December 1926, Mangiagalli declared his support of fascism 'perinde ac cadaver' (until death) (Signori 1993, p. 195).
41. Letter from Golgi to Belfanti, 17 December 1923 (in the possession of Prof. Marco Fraccaro).
42. Letter from Golgi to Belfanti, 25 December 1923 (in the possession of Prof. Marco Fraccaro).
43. Letters of 5 and 12 January 1924 from Belfanti to Golgi (MSUP-XXIX-II-22 and 23).

44. See Signori (1993, p. 195) and Pensa (1991, p. 185).
45. See the report on the inauguration of the academic year 1924–25 in *La Provincia Pavese* (3 December 1924).
46. *Il Popolo-La Provincia Pavese* (24 January 1926). It was probably in this period that Golgi wrote a brief introduction to the complete edition of the works of Agostino Bassi (Golgi 1925).
47. Letter from Henschen to Golgi, 14 October 1925 (MSUP-VII-II-H).
48. This part was published in the *OO* (vol. IV, p. 1562), as an appendix to *Intorno alla struttura ed alla biologia dei così detti globuli o piastrine del tuorlo*.
49. In the letter, Da Fano told him also of the election as Honorary Fellow of the Royal Society of Medicine (MSUP-III-VIII-27). See also the letter from the Secretary of the Royal Society of Medicine (MSUP-III-VIII-26).
50. *Il Popolo-La Provincia Pavese* (24 January 1926).
51. *Memoria di Padre Agostino Gemelli dei frati minori* (Milano: Tipografia Bertolotti, p. 126).
52. Essays, Book II, Chapter XI.
53. Officially at 11.30 a.m.; according to some newspapers, at 11.45 a.m.
54. As mentioned by Mayor Pietro Vaccari in his commemorative speech.

Appendix

Years of birth and death

When unknown the presumed period of life has been indicated; b = born; ba = born around; d = death; da = death around; aa = active around; ap = active in the period; sa = still alive at year cited. Contemporary living persons have been omitted from this list.

Adami Rossi aa 1898
Ahnfelt, Astrid aa 1906
Alagna, Gaspare aa 1905
Albertoni, Pietro 1849–1933
Aletti, Giuseppa Evangelina 'Lina' (in Golgi) 1856–1940
Alighieri, Dante 1265–1321
Alloch aa 1900
Amici, Giovanni Battista 1786–1863
Apáthy, István 1863–1922
Arïens Kappers, Cornelius Ubbo 1877–1946
Aristotle 384–322 BC
Arnold, Friedrich 1803–1890
Arrhenius, Svante August 1859–1927
Ascoli, Giulio 1870–1916
Aselli, Gaspare 1581–1625
Avicenna (Abu Ali Hussain ibn Sina) 980–1037
Baccelli, Guido 1832–1890
Balsamo Crivelli, Giuseppe 1852–1874
Barazzoni, Carlo aa1910
Bardeleben, Karl 1849–1918
Barinetti, Carlo aa1910
Bassi (student) 1901
Bassi, Agostino 1773–1856
Bassini, Edoardo 1844–1924
Bastianelli, Giuseppe 1862–1959
Beccaria, Cesare 1761–1835
Beccaris Bava, Fiorenzo 1831–1924
Bechterew, Vladimir Mikhailovich 1857–1927
Behring, Emil Adolf 1854–1917
Belfanti, Serafino 1860–1939
Bellati, Pietro aa 1900
Belli, Carlo 1848–1917

Bellonci, Giuseppe 1855–1888
Belmondo, Ernesto 1863–1939
Berg, John aa 1906
Bernard, Claude 1813–1878
Bernardini, Ciro aa 18878
Bertarelli, Ernesto 1873–1957
Besta, Carlo 1876–1940
Bethe, Albrecht 1872–1954
Betz, Wladimir Aleksandrovitsch 1834–1894
Bezzola, Carlo aa 1905
Bichat, François Xavier 1771–1802
Biedermann, Wilhelm 1852–1929
Bietti, Amilcare 1869–1930
Biffi, Serafino 1822–1899
Bignami, Amico 1862–1929
Bizzozero Maddalena (mother in law) 1831–1913
Bizzozero, Enzo 1882–1975
Bizzozero, Erminia Brambilla ba 1855–sa 1901
Bizzozero, Giulio 1846–1901
Bleuler, Eugen 1857–1929
Blumenau, Léonidas aa 1891
Boccadoro, Costanza 1893–1983
Boll, Franz-Christian 1849–1879
Bonaparte, Napoleon 1769–1821
Bonghi, Ruggero 1826–1895
Bonnet, Charles 1720–1793
Borges, Jorge Luis 1899–1986
Borromeo, Giberto 1859–1941
Boscovich, Ruggero 1711–1787
Bottini, Enrico 1835–1903
Boveri, Theodor 1862–1915
Bovio, Giovanni 1841–1903
Bowditch, Henry 1840–1911

Bozzolo, Camillo 1845–1920

Brambilla, Giovanni Alessandro 1728–1800

Bravetta, Eugenio ap 1900–1926

Bresci, Gaetano 1869–1901

Bright, Richard 1789–1858

Broca, Paul 1824–1880

Broman, Ivar aa 1900

Bronzini, Ersilia 1859–1933

Brown, John 1735–1788

Brown, Robert 1773–1858

Brown-Séquard, Edouard 1817–1894

Brücke, Ernst Wilhelm von 1819–1892

Brugnatelli, Ernesto ap 1906–1925

Brugnatelli, Gaspare Emilio d 1918

Brugnatelli, Tullio 1825–1906

Buchholz, Reinhold aa 1863

Butzke, Victor ap 1870s

Cairoli, Benedetto 1825–1899

Cairoli, Enrico 1840–1867

Cajal, Santiago Ramón y Cajal 1852–1934

Calandruccio, Salvatore 1855–1908

Calkins, Gary Nathan 1869–1943

Campagnoli, Siro aa 1870

Canestrini, Giovanni 1835–1900

Cannizzaro, Stanislao 1826–1910

Cantani, Arnaldo 1837–1893

Cantoni, Giovanni 1818–1807

Cantoni, Carlo 1840–1906

Carandini, Amalia aa 1900

Carcano Leone, Giovanni Battista
    1536–1606

Cardano, Gerolamo 1501–1576

Carducci, Giosué 1835–1907

Carini, Antonio 1872–1950

Carpi (student) aa 1901

Cattaneo, Alfonso aa 1887

Cavallo, A. G. aa 1900

Cavallotti, Felice 1842–1898

Cavour Benso, Camillo 1810–1861

Cazzani, Cesare aa 1897

Celli, Angelo 1857–1914

Celsus, Aulus Cornelius ba 30 BC–da AD 50

Ceni, Carlo 1866–1965

Centanni, Eugenio 1873–1942

Cesa Bianchi, Domenico 1879–1956

Charcot, Jean Marie 1825–1893

Charles IV (Emperor) 1316–1368

Chiarugi, Giulio 1859–1944

Chiodi, Bortolino aa 1843

Chiodi, Pietro aa 1843

Ciaccio, Giuseppe Vincenzo 1824–1901

Ciarrocchi, Gaetano aa 1884

Ciccotti, Ettore 1863–1939

Cittadini, Arturo aa 1925

Clerici, Ambrogio 1868–1955

Clivio, Innocente 1862–1956

Cohn, Ferdinand Julius 1828–1898

Colella, Rosolino 1864–1940

Colombo, Gian Luigi aa 1910

Colomiatti, Vittorio Francesco aa 1876

Columbus, Christopher 1451–1506

Comte, Auguste 1798–1857

Concato, Luigi 1825–1882

Coppino, Michele 1822–1901

Cornalia, Emilio 1824–1882

Cornelli, Emilio aa 1919

Corradi, Alfonso 1833–1892

Corti, Alfonso 1822–1876

Corti, Alfredo 1880–1973

Cosenz, Enrico 1820–1898

Costa, Andrea 1851–1910

Councilman, William Thomas 1854–1933

Credaro, Luigi 1860–1939

Crispi, Francesco 1818–1901

Cruikshank, William 1745–1800

Cuboni, Giuseppe 1852–1920

Cuneo Gabriele ap 1554–1574

Cushing, Harvey 1869–1939

Cuvier, Georges 1769–1832

Cuzzi, Alessandro 1849–1895

Daddi, G. aa 1897

Da Fano, Corrado 1879–1927

D'Agata, Giuseppe 1884–1951

D'Alessio, Francesco aa 1926

Danilewsky, Vasili Iakovlevich aa 1886

D'Annunzio, Gabriele 1863–1938

Darwin, Charles 1809–1882

Davaine, Casimir Joseph 1812–1882

De Amicis, Edmondo 1846–1908

Debierre, Charles Marie 1853–1932

De Dominicis, Vincenzo aa 1904

De Filippi Filippo 1814–1867

De Giovanni, Achille 1838–1916

De Gubernatis, Angelo aa 1880

Deiters, Otto Friedrich Karl 1834–1863

Del Giudice, Pasquale 1842–1924

Della Torre, Marcantonio 1478–1511

De Sanctis, Francesco 1817–1883

Descartes, René 1506–1650

d'Eternod, Auguste François aa 1900

Devoto, Luigi 1864–1936

Di Vestea, Alfonso 1854–1938

Dogiel, Alexander Stanislavovich 1852–1922

Dohrn, Anton 1840–1909

Donaggio, Arturo 1868–1942

Donaldson, Henry Herbert 1857–1939

Doniselli, Ulderico aa 1859

Donizetti, Gaetano 1797–1848

du Bois-Reymond, Emil 1818–1896

Duse, Eleonora 1858–1924

Dutrochet, René Joachim-Henri 1776–1847

Ebner, Victor von 1842–1925

Eccles, John 1903–1997

Edgren, Johan Gustaf aa 1906

Edinger, Ludwig 1855–1918

Edison, Thomas Alva 1847–1931

Eggeling, H. aa 1900

Ehrenberg, Christian Gottfried 1795–1876

Ehrlich, Paul 1854–1915

Einstein, Albert 1879–1955

Einstein, Hermann aa 1895

Einstein, Jakob aa 1895

Eismond, Joseph aa 1900

Emery, Carlo 1848–1925

Erba, Prospero aa 1900

Eulenburg, Albert 1840–1917

Falchi, Francesco 1848–1946

Fallopius, Gabriel 1523–1562

Falzacappa, Ernesto aa 1889

Feletti, Raimondo aa 1900

Fermi, Enrico 1901–1954

Ferrata, Adolfo 1880–1946

Ferrier, David 1843–1928

Fick, Adolf 1829–1901

Fieschi, Davide aa 1895

Filippini, Attilio aa 1900

Fiorito, Giuseppe aa 1908

Flemming, Walther 1843–1905

Flourens, Pierre 1794–1867

Flügge, Carl 1847–1923

Foà, Pio 1848–1923

Fontana, Felice 1730–1805

Forel, August-Henri 1848–1931

Forlanini, Carlo 1847–1918

Formenti, Carlo 1841–1918

Foscolo, Ugo 1778–1827

Foster, Michael 1836–1907

Francis Ferdinand of Austria-Este 1863–1914

Frerichs, Friederich Theodor 1818–1885

Fritsch, Theodor 1838–1927

Frohse, Fritz aa 1900

Frugoni, Cesare 1881–1978

Fürst, Carl Magnus aa 1905

Fusari, Romeo 1857–1919

Gadelius, Bror aa 1906

Galen 129–da 200

Galilei, Galileo 1564–1642

Gall, Franz Joseph 1758–1828

Galvani, Luigi 1737–1798

Garibaldi, Giuseppe 1807–1882

Garino, Elia aa 1895

Garovaglio, Santo 1805–1882

Gasbaroni, Antonio (Gasparone) 1794–1882

Gasbarrini, Antonio 1882–1963

Gasparrini, Guglielmo 1804–1866

Gemelli, Edoardo 1878–1959

Gentile, Giovanni 1875–1945

Gerlach, Joseph von 1820–1896

Germanò, Domenico 1856–1941

Ghinaglia, Ferruccio 1899–1921

Ghisio (Veterinarian) aa 1882

Giacommini, Carlo 1840–1898

Giacomini, Ercole 1864–1946

Giacosa, Piero 1853–1928

Gilardoni, Arturo aa 1895

Gilardoni, Enrico aa 1895

Giolitti, Giovanni 1842–1928

Golgi Camillo (grandfather) aa 1813

Golgi, Alessandro (Sandro) (nephew) ba 1888–sa 1926

Golgi, Alessandro Antonio Nicola (father) 1814–1896

Golgi, Angelica Nicolletti (grandmother) aa 1814

Golgi, Bartolomeo Camillo Emilio 1843–1926

Luys, Jules Bernard 1828–1897
Luzzani, Lina 1881–1963
Maccabruni, Francesco aa 1910
Macchi, Alfredo aa 1905
Màcola, Ferruccio aa 1898
Maffi, Fabrizio 1868–1955
Maggi, Leopoldo 1840–1905
Maggiora, Romano aa 1900
Magini, Giuseppe 1851–1916
Magnaghi, Luigi aa 1920
Maj, Angelo aa 1900
Majno, Luigi 1852–1915
Malfitano, Giovanni 1872–1941
Malpighi, Marcello 1628–1694
Manfredi, Nicolò 1836–1916
Mangiagalli, Luigi 1849–1928
Mangini, Carlo ap 1890s
Mann, Gustav 1864–1921
Manson, Patrick 1844–1922
Mantegazza, Paolo 1831–1910
Mantovani, Giuseppe 1860–1916
Manzoni, Alessandro 1785–1873
Maragliano, Edoardo 1849–1940
Marcacci, Arturo 1855–1915
Marchand, Felix 1846–1928
Marchi, Vittorio 1851–1908
Marchiafava, Ettore 1847–1935
Marcora, Ferruccio ap 1906–1912
Marenghi, Giovanni 1868–1903
Maria Theresa of Austria (Empress)
    1717–1780
Marinesco, Georges 1864–1938
Mariotti, Ugo aa 1884
Mariottini, Antonio aa 1898
Martinotti, Carlo 1859–1918
Matteucci, Carlo 1811–1868
Mayer, Heinrich aa 1900
Mazzini, Giuseppe 1805–1872
Mazzoni, Nino aa 1907
Mazzoni, Vittorio aa 1891
Medea, Eugenio 1873–1967
Melland, B. aa 1885
Merkel, Friedrich Siegmund 1845–1919
Metschnikoff, Elie 1845–1916
Metternich, Klemens Wenzel 1773–1859
Meynert, Theodor 1833–1892
Mingazzini, Giovanni 1859–1929

Minot, Charles Sedgwick 1852–1914
Moissan, Ferdinand Frédéric Henri
    1832–1907
Moleschott, Jakob 1822–1893
Monakow, Constantin von 1853–1930
Mondino, Casimiro 1859–1924
Mongardi, Romeo aa 1890
Montaigne, Michel Eyquem de 1533–1592
Montemartini, Luigi 1869–1952
Montemezzani aa 1920
Monti, Achille 1863–1937
Monti, Rina 1861–1937
Monti, Vincenzo 1754–1828
Morelli Eugenio 1881–1960
Moreschi, Carlo 1866–1921
Morgagni, Giovan Battista 1682–1771
Moriani, Giuseppe 1879–1951
Mörner, Karl Axel Hampus aa 1906
Morpurgo, Benedetto 1861–1944
Morselli, Enrico 1852–1929
Moruzzi, Giuseppe 1910–1986
Moscati, Pietro 1739–1824
Moschini, A. aa 1890
Mosso, Angelo 1846–1910
Motti, Francesco aa 1900
Mottinelli, Stefano aa 1843
Müller Erik ap 1893–1926
Müller Heinrich 1820–1864
Müller, Johannes 1801–1858
Mussi, Giuseppe 1836–1904
Mussi, Muzio d 1898
Mussolini, Benito 1883–1945
Nansen, Fritjof 1861–1930
Nasi, Nunzio 1850–1935
Nazari, A. aa 1911
Necchi, Ambrogio 1860–1916
Negri, Adelchi 1876–1912
Nicolas aa 1900
Nissl, Franz 1860–1919
Nosotti, Innocente aa 1882
Nothnagel, Hermann 1841–1905
Nusbaum, Jósef aa 1913
Oberdan, Guglielmo 1858–1882
Obersteiner, Heinrich 1847–1922
Oddo, Giuseppe 1865–1954
Oehl, Eusebio 1827–1903
Oppenheim, Hermann 1858–1919

Orlando, Vittorio Emanuele 1860–1952

Orsi, Francesco 1828–1900

Osler, William 1849–1919

Ostwald, Wilhelm 1853–1932

Owsjannikov, Philip aa 1860

Pacini, Filippo 1812–1883

Pane, Domenico aa 1905

Panizza, Bartolomeo 1785–1867

Paracelso (Hohenheim, Aureolus
    Theophrastus Bombastus von) 1493–1541

Parona, Emilio aa 1882

Parona, Ernesto 1849–1902

Pascal, Blaise 1623–1662

Pasteur, Louis 1822–1895

Pavesi, Pietro 1844–1907

Pavlov, Ivan Petrovich 1849–1936

Pelloux, Luigi 1839–1924

Pensa, Antonio 1874–1970

Perini, Egidio aa 1897

Perroncito, Aldo 1882–1929

Perroncito, Edoardo 1847–1936

Pertick, Otto aa 1881

Petrone, Angelo ap 1889–1899

Pettenkofer, Max Joseph 1818–1901

Pieraccini, Gaetano aa 1907

Pizzocaro, (Colonel) aa 1860

Planck, Max 1858–1947

Podwyssozki, Wladimir 1857–1913

Ponfick, Emil Clemens 1844–1913

Popper, Karl 1902–1994

Porro, Edoardo 1842–1902

Porta, Luigi 1800–1875

Pott, Percivall 1714–1788

Pouchet, Georges ap 1887–1900

Priestley, Joseph 1733–1804

Pupilli, Giulio Cesare 1893–1973

Purkinje, Jan Evangelista 1787–1869

Purpura, Francesco

Putelli, Romolo ap 1909–1923

Quaglino, Antonio 1817–1894

Radaeli, Francesco 1870–1936

Raggi, Antigono ap 1880–1898

Ramón y Cajal, Santiago see Cajal

Rampoldi, Roberto 1850–1926

Ranelletti, Oreste 1868–1956

Ranvier, Louis Antoine 1835–1922

Rasori, Giovanni 1766–1837

Ratti, Achille (Pope Pius XI) 1857–1939

Recklinghausen, Friedrich Daniel von
    1833–1910

Regaud, Claude aa 1900

Remak, Robert 1815–1865

Renaut, J. aa 1880s

Resinelli, Giuseppe 1865–1915

Retzius, Gustaf Magnus 1842–1919

Reysch Gregor 1467–1525

Rezia, Giacomo 1745–1825

Rezzonico, Giulio aa 1880

Riberi, Alessandro 1794–1861

Ricasoli, Bettino 1809–1880

Richard, Eugène aa 1881

Richiardi, Salvatore 1834–1904

Rindfleisch, Georg Eduard 1836–1885

Rinekcer, Franz 1811–1883

Riquier, Giuseppe Carlo 1886–1962

Ris, F. aa 1900

Rivella aa 1868

Rizzi, Giuseppe ap 1870s

Robecchi-Bricchetti, Luigi 1855–1926

Robolini Del Majno, Luigia ap 1865–1873

Rodondi, Giuseppe aa 1907

Rokitansky, Karl 1804–1878

Romiti, Guglielmo 1850–1036

Röntgen, Wilhelm Konrad 1845–1923

Rosa (student) aa 1901

Rosenstein, Moisey aa 1854

Rosenthal, Joseph F. 1817–1887

Ross, Ronald 1857–1932

Rossbach, M. J. aa 1888

Rossi, Ottorino 1877–1936

Rossignoli, Giovanni aa 1906

Rossini, Giovanni Battista aa 1900

Rossoni (internist) aa 1893

Roussy, Gustave 1874–1948

Rudinì Starabba, Antonio di 1839–1908

Ruffini, Angelo 1864–1929

Rusconi, Mauro 1776–1849

Sabbia, (student) aa 1901

Saccheri, Gerolamo 1667–1733

Sacconaghi, Giulio Luigi 1875–1933

Saccozzi, A. aa 1885

Sacerdotti, Cesare 1868–1953

Sala, Guido 1887–1939

Sala, Luigi 1863–1930

Salandra, Antonio 1853–1931

Sangalli, Giacomo 1821–1897

Savoia Luigi Amedeo, Duke of
   Abruzzi 1873–1933

Scarenzio, Angelo 1831–1904

Scarpa, Antonio 1752–1832

Schenk, Samuel Leopold 1840–1902

Schiavuzzi, Bernardo aa 1888

Schiefferdecker, Paul 1849–1931

Schiff, Moritz 1823–1896

Schleiden, Matthias Jacob 1804–1881

Schultze, Maximilian 1825–1874

Schwalbe, Gustav 1844–1916

Schwann, Theodor 1810–1882

Scola (dog catcher) ap 1890s

Sehrwald, E. aa 1888

Semmelweis, Ignaz Philipp 1818–1865

Seppilli, Giuseppe aa 1880

Sertoli, Enrico 1842–1910

Sherrington, Charles Scott 1857–1952

Silva, Bernardino 1855–1905

Simarro Lacabra, Luis 1851–1921

Simon, Theodor 1841–1874

Sinigaglia, Giorgio aa 1910

Skoda, Joseph 1805–1881

Sonnino, Sidney Giorgio 1847–1922

Sormani, Giuseppe 1844–1923

Soukhanoff, Serge 1867–1916

Soury, Jules 1842–1915

Spallanzani, Lazzaro 1729–1799

Spurzheim, Johann Caspar 1776–1832

Stahl, Georg Ernst 1660–1734

Staurenghi, Cesare 1858–1912

Stefanini, Antonio 1857–1945

Stefanini, Domenico 1841–1901

Stefanini, Giovan Battista 1894–1964

Sternberg, George Miller 1837–1918

Stilling, Benedict 1810–1879

Stöhr, Philipp 1849–1911

Strambio, Gaetano 1820–1905

Stricker, Salomon 1834–1898

Stropeni, Luigi 1885–1962

Studnicka, F. K. aa 1900

Sundberg, Carl aa 1906

Sydenham, Thomas 1624–1689

Tamassia, Arrigo 1849–1916

Tamburini, Augusto 1848–1919

Tandler, Julius 1869–1936

Tanzi, Eugenio 1856–1934

Tartagli, Augusto aa 1900

Tartuferi, Ferruccio aa 1890

Taussig, (internist) aa 1893

Tenchini, Lorenzo 1852–1906

Tertullian ba 160– da 220

Teuscher, R. aa 1894

Thanhoffer, Ludwig 1843–1909

Thomson, Joseph John 1865–1940

Tirelli, Vitige 1866–1941

Tissot, Samuel August 1728–1797

Todaro Francesco 1839–1918

Toldt, Karl 1840–1920

Tolstoy, Lev 1828–1910

Tommasi, Salvatore 1813–1888

Tommasi-Crudeli, Corrado 1834–1900

Tovini, Livio aa 1909

Tragella, Pio aa 1872

Tricomi Allegra, Giuseppe aa 1895

Turati, Filippo 1853–1932

Umberto I (King) 1844–1900

Unna, Paul Gerson 1850–1929

Vaccari, Pietro aa 1926

Valentin, Gabriel Gustav 1810–1883

Valerio, Siro d 1893

Valla, Lorenzo 1407–1457

van Gehuchten, Arthur 1861–1914

Vanlair, C. ap 1882–1888

Vant'Hoff, Jacobus Hendricus 1852–1911

Varro, Marcus Terentius 117–27 BC

Vecchi, Arnaldo aa 1910

Veratti, Emilio 1872–1967

Verdi, Giuseppe 1813–1901

Verga, Andrea 1811–1895

Verga, Giovanni ap 1904–1919

Verson, Saverio aa 1905

Vicq d'Azyr, Feliz 1748–1794

Villa, Luigi 1867–1896

Vincenzi, Livio 1860–1915

Violini, Luigi ap 1890s

Virchow, Rudolf 1821–1902

Visconti, Achille 1836–1911

Vittadini, Angelo ap 1859–1866

Vittadini, Carlo 1800–1865

Vittorio Emanuele III (King) 1869–1947

Vivante, Raffaele aa 1892

Vogt, Karl 1817–1895

Volta, Alessandro 1745–1827

Voltaire (Arouet), Fraçois Marie 1694–1778

Volterra, Vito 1860–1940

von Lenhossék, Joseph 1818–1888

von Lenhossék, Michael 1863–1936

Voronoff, Serge 1866–1951

Vulpian, Alfred 1826–18878

Wagner, Richard Wilhelm 1813–1883

Wagner, Rudolph 1805–1864

Waldeyer, Wilhelm 1836–1921

Waldstein, L. aa 1882

Weber, E. ap 1870s

Weichselbaum, Anton 1845–1920

Weigert, Carl 1845–1904

Weismann, August 1834–1914

Welch, Henry William 1850–1934

Wernicke, Carl 1848–1904

William the Conqueror 1027–1087

Willis, Thomas 1621–1675

Wöhler, Friedrich 1800–1882

Wyler, Giulio aa 1910

Zacconi, Ermete 1857–1948

Zaina, Barolomeo aa 1843

Zeiss, Carl 1816–1888

Zenker, Konrad aa 1894

Ziemann, Hans Richard Paul aa 1900

Ziemssen, Hugo Wilheim von 1829–1902

Zoja, Alfonso 1877–1896

Zoja, Giovanni 1832–1899

Zoja, Raffaello 1869–1896

Zucchi, Carlo aa 1880

References

Aarli J. A. (1989). Fritjof Nansen and the neuron theory. In *Neuroscience across the century* (ed. F. Clifford Rose). Smith-Gordon, London, pp. 73–7.

Addis Saba M. (1993). *Anna Kuliscioff. Vita privata e passione politica*. Arnoldo Mondadori Editore. Milano.

Afzelius B. (1980). Gustaf Retzius, Camillo Golgi and Santiago Ramon y Cajal. The early days of neurobiology. *Atti Accademia dei Fisiocritici di Siena*. Serie 14ª, **12**, pp. 681–93.

Akert K. (1993). August Forel—Cofounder of the neuron theory. *Brain Pathology*, **3**, pp. 425–30.

Albertotti G. (1917). Brevi note sulla vita e sull'opera scientifica del professore emerito Comm. Nicolò Manfredi. *Memorie della R. Accademia di Scienze, Lettere ed Arti in Modena*. Serie 3ª, **13** (sezione scienze), pp. 1–22 **of the reprint**.

Alfieri A. (1916). Nicola Manfredi. *Archivio di Ottalmologia*, 23, pp. 405–10.

Apáthy I. (1897). Das leitende Element des Nervensystems und seine topographischen Beziehungen zu den Zellen. *Mittheilungen aus der zoologischen Station zu Neapel*, **12**, pp. 495–748.

Arcieri G. P. (1952). *Figure della medicina contemporanea italiana*. Bocca, Milano.

Armocida G. and Zanobio B. (1994). Le trasformazioni della medicina nell'epoca di Camillo Golgi (1843–1926). *Bollettino della Società Medico-Chirurgica di Pavia*, **108** (Suppl.1), pp. 61–79.

Assagioli A. and Bonvecchiato E. (1878). Contributo alla patogenesi della corea sintomatica di lesione cerebrale. *Rivista Sperimentale di Freniatria e Medicina Legale*, **4**, pp. 362–75.

Baima Bollone P. L. (1992). *Cesare Lombroso*. Sei, Torino.

Beach F. A., Hebb D. O., Morgan C. T., and Nissen H. W. (ed.) (1960). *The neuropsychology of Lashley*. New York. McGraw Hill.

Beccari N. (1944–45). *Il problema del neurone*. I, La Nuova Italia, Firenze.

Belfanti S. (1926). Commemorazione di Camillo Golgi. *Rendiconti del R. Istituto Lombardo di Scienze Lettere ed Arti*. **59** d. S., pp. 765–75.

Bellonci G. (1880). Ricerche comparative sulla struttura dei centri nervosi dei vertebrati. *Atti della R. Accademia dei Lincei. Memorie della Classe di Scienze Fisiche, Matematiche e Naturali*, **5**, pp. 157–82.

Bellonci G. (1881). Contribuzione all'istologia del cervelletto. *Atti della R. Accademia dei Lincei. Memorie della Classe di Scienze Fisiche, Matematiche e Naturali*, **9**, pp. 45–8.

Belloni L. (1951). Una ricerca del contagio vivo agli albori dell'Ottocento. *Gesnerus*, **8**, pp. 15–31.

Belloni L. (1961). Echi del 'Discorso accademico' di P. Moscati sull'uomo quadrupede. La recensione di Kant. *Physis*, **3**, pp. 167–72.

Belloni L. (1974). Vittorio Marchi. In *Dictionary of scientific biography* (ed. C. Gillispie). Scribner, New York, Vol. 9, pp. 93–4.

Belloni L. (1975). L'epistolario di Albert Kölliker a Camillo Golgi al Museo per la Storia della Università di Pavia. *Memorie dell'Istituto Lombardo—Accademia di Scienze e Lettere. Classe di Scienze Matematiche e Naturali (Memoria 4)*, **26**, pp. 135–243.

Belloni L. (1978). Allievi minori di Camillo Golgi: Anna Kuliscioff e il suo contributo alla etiologia della febbre puerperale. *Istituto Lombardo (Rend. Sc.). B*, **112**, pp. 111–17.

Belloni L. (1978a). Anna Kuliscioff allieva del Cantani e del Golgi, e le sue ricerche sulla etiologia della febbre puerperale. *Physis*, **20**, pp. 337–48.

Belloni L. (1978b). Contributi della Università di Pavia (Grassi—Golgi—Negri) alla diagnosi microscopica dell'anchilostomiasi della malaria e della rabbia. *Memorie dell'Istituto Lombardo-Accademia di Scienze Lettere Classe di Scienze Matematiche e Naturali (Memoria 2)*, **27**, pp. 29–48.

Belloni L. (1980). Franz Boll, scopritore della porpora retinica. *Memorie dell'Istituto Lombardo-Accademia di Scienze Lettere Classe di Scienze Matematiche e Naturali (Memoria 6)*, **27**, pp. 315–437.

Belmondo E. (1888). Sulla teoria della colorazione nera del Golgi. *Rivista Sperimentale di Freniatria e di Medicina Legale*, **14**, pp. 349–59.

Bentivoglio M. and Mazzarello P. (1999). The history of radial glia. *Brain Res. Bull.* in press.

Bentivoglio M., Pannese E., and Mazzarello, P. (1997). The first Golgi impregnation of the developing cerebral cortex. *Society for Neuroscience*, **23**, p. 278.

Berlucchi G. (1999). Some aspects of the history of the law of dynamic polarization of the neuron, from William James to Sherrington, from Cajal and van Gehuchten to Golgi. *Journal of the History of the Neurosciences*. In press.

Bernardi A. (1967). I quattro secoli del Ghislieri. In *Collegio Ghislieri (1567–1967)*. Alfieri & Lacroix, Milano, pp. 23–208.

Bernardini C. (1888). Sulla reazione nera del Golgi in cervelli di paralitici ed epilettici. *Atti del XII congresso della Associazione Medica Italiana*. Tipografia Fratelli Fusi, Pavia, Vol. 2, pp. 139–40. Excerpted in *Rivista Sperimentale di Freniatria e di Medicina Legale* (1887), **13**, pp. 207–8.

Bertarelli E. (1950). *Camillo Golgi ed il suo tempo*. Istituto Sieroterapico Milanese S. Belfanti, Milano.

Bianchi G. (1956). I Golgi a Corteno. *Giornale di Brescia*, 15 febbraio.

Bianchi G. (1973). Personaggi di ceppo cortenese. *Editrice Pavoniana*, Brescia, pp. 11–35.

Bizzozero G. (1868). Di alcune alterazioni dei linfatici del cervello e della pia madre. *Rivista Clinica*. Anno 7°, pp. 33–7.

Bizzozero G. (1872). Del rapporto che sta fra la struttura dei tumori e la natura del tessuto da cui prendono origine. *Giornale della R. Accademia di Medicina di Torino*. Anno 35°, Serie 3ª, **12**, pp. 129–49.

Bizzozero G. (1873). *Prelezione al corso di Patologia Generale nella Università di Torino*. Tip. Lit. Camilla e Bertolero—Editori, Torino.

Bizzozero G. (1877). Sullo stroma dei sarcomi. *Archivio per le Scienze Mediche*, **2**, pp. 465–78.

Bizzozero G. and Golgi C. (1873). Ueber die Veranderungen des Muskelgewebes nach Nervendurchschneidung. *Wiener Medizinische Jahrbucher* **3**, pp. 125–7. *Opera Omnia*, pp. 851–3.

Bizzozero G. and Golgi C. (1879). Über die Einwirkung der Bluttransfusion in das Peritoneum auf den Hämoglobingehalt des kreisenden Blutes. *Centralblatt für die Medizinischen Wissenschaften*, **17**, pp. 917–18.

Bizzozero G. and Golgi C. (1880). Della trasfusione di sangue nel peritoneo e della sua influenza sulla ricchezza globulare del sangue circolante. *Archivio per le Scienze Mediche* (1880) **4**, pp. 67–77. *Gazzetta delle Cliniche di Torino (Com. Prev.)*, **XV**, N° 44, 4 novembre (1879). *Opera Omnia*, pp. 923–32.

Boll F. (1873). Die Histiologie und Histiogenese der Nervosen Centralorgane. *Archiv für Psychiatrie und Nervenkrankheiten*, **IV**, pp. 1–138.

Bonomelli G. M. (1975). I Grandi Camuni. Camillo Golgi. *l'Ogliolo*. Anno 1°, N° 3, marzo.

Bonuzzi L. (1990). Novità editoriali oltramontane e rinnovamento della neurologia in Italia nel secondo '700. In *Lo sviluppo storico della neurologia italiana: lo studio delle fonti* (ed. G. Zanchin and L. Premuda). La Garangola, Padova, pp. 127–32.

Bovero A. (1926). Camillo Golgi (un gigante delle scienze mediche italiane). *Ars Medica*. Anno 3°, N° 5 Casa Mayenca. S. Paulo, pp. 1–15 **of the reprint**.

Bracegirdle B. (1978). *A history of microtechnique: the evolution of the microtome and the development of tissue preparation*. Heinemann, London.

Brazier M. A. B. (1958). The evolution of concepts relating to the electrical activity of the nervous system. In *The brain and its functions*. Blackwell Scientific, Oxford, pp. 191–222.

Bruni A. C. (1919). Romeo Fusari. *Monitore Zoologico Italiano*, **30**, pp. 78–80.

Buchholz R. (1863). Bemerkungen über den histologischen Bau des Centralnervensystems der Süsswassermollusken. *Archiv für Anatomie, Physiologie und wissenschaftliche Medicin*. Jahrgang 1863, pp. 234–4, 265–309.

Buchtel H. A. and Berlucchi G. (1977). Learning and memory and the nervous system. In *The encyclopaedia of ignorance* (ed. R. Duncan and M. Weston-Smith). Pergamon Press, Oxford, pp. 283–97.

Bulferetti L. (1975). *Lombroso*. Utet, Torino.

Butzke V. (1872). Studien über den feineren Bau der Grosshirnrinde. *Archiv für Psychiatrie und Nervenkrank-heiten*, **3**, pp. 575–600.

Cajal S. R. (1888). Estructura de los centros nerviosos de las aves. *Revista Trimestral de Histologia normal y patologica*, **1**, pp. 1–10.

Cajal S. R. (1888a). Sobre las fibras nerviosas de la capa molecular del cerebelo. *Revista Trimestral de Histologia normal y patologica*, **1**, pp. 33–49.

Cajal S. R. (1889). Conexion general de los elementos nerviosos. *La Medicina Practica*, **2**, pp. 341–6.

Cajal S. R. (1889a). Sur la morphologie et les connexions des éléments de la rétine des oiseaux. *Anatomischer Anzeiger*, **4**, pp. 111–21.

Cajal S. R. (1890). Sur l'origine et les ramifications des fibres nerveuses de la moelle embryonnaire. *Anatomischer Anzeiger*, **5**, pp. 85–95, 111–19.

Cajal S. R. (1890a). Résponse à Mr. Golgi à propos des fibrilles collatérales de la moëlle épinière, et de la structure générale de la substance grise. *Anatomischer Anzeiger*, **5**, pp. 579–87.

Cajal S. R. (1891). Significación fisiológica de las expansiones protoplasmáticas y nerviosas de las células de la substancia gris. *Revista de Ciencias médicas de Barcelona*, **27**, pp. 1–15.

Cajal S. R. (1895). Algunas conjeturas sobre el mecanismo anatomico de la ideacion, asociation, y atencion. *Revista de Medicina y Cirurgía Practicás*, **36**, pp. 497–508.

Cajal S. R. (1909). *Histologie du système nerveux de l'homme et de vertébrés*, Vol. 1, Maloine, Paris.

Cajal S. R. (1917). *Recuerdos de mi vida: historia de mi labor científica*. Imprenta y libreria de Nicolas Moya, Madrid. Engl. trans. E. H. Craigie, with the assistance of J. Cano. *Recollections of my life*. American Philosophical Society, Philadelphia (1937). Reprinted (1966, 1989) MIT Press, Cambridge, Mass. Quotations in the text are from the Alianza Universidad edition, Madrid (4th edn, 1984).

Calligaro A. (1994). Camillo Golgi e Santiago Ramón y Cajal. *Bollettino della Società Medico-Chirurgica di Pavia*, **108** (Suppl.1), pp. 61–79.

Cannon D. F. (1949). *Explorer of the human brain. The life of Santiago Ramón y Cajal*. Schuman, New York.

Cappelletti V. (1968). Giulio Bizzozero. In *Dizionario biografico degli Italiani*, Vol. 10. Ist. Enciclopedia Ital. Roma, pp. 747–51.

Castellani C. (1990). Lazzaro Spallanzani nelle sue lettere e nei suoi giornali. *Bollettino della Società Pavese di Storia Patria*, **42**, pp. 235–49.

Castiglioni A. (1948). *Storia della medicina*. Vol. 2. Arnoldo Mondadori Editore, Verona.

Cattaneo A. (1886). Sugli organi nervosi terminali muscolo-tendinei in condizioni normali e sul loro modo di comportarsi in seguito al taglio delle radici nervose. *Gazzetta degli Ospedali*. Anno 7°, pp. 586–7.

Cattaneo A. and Monti A. (1887). Degenerazione dei corpuscoli rossi del sangue (secondo Mosso) e supposta sua corrispondenza nelle alterazioni malariche degli stessi elementi. *Bollettino della Società Medico-Chirurgica di Pavia*. Anno 2°, pp. 39–40.

Cattaneo A. and Monti A. (1888). Alterazioni degenerative dei corpuscoli rossi del sangue e alterazioni malariche dei medesimi. Diagnosi differenziale. *Archivio per le Scienze Mediche*, **12**, pp. 99–116.

Cattaneo A. and Monti A. (1888a). Altérations dégénératives des corpuscules rouges du sang et leurs altérations malariques. Diagnose différentielle. *Archives Italiennes de Biologie*, **9**, pp. 408–22.

Ceci A. (1881). Contribuzione allo studio della fibra nervosa midollata ed osservazioni sui corpuscoli amilacei dell'encefalo e midollo spinale. *Atti della R. Accademia dei Lincei. Memorie della Classe di Scienze Fisiche, Matematiche e Naturali*, **9**, pp. 81–101.

Céline L. F. (1952). *Semmelweis (1818–1865)*. Gallimard, Paris.

Changeux J. P. (1983). *L'homme neuronal*. Librairie Arthème Fayard, Paris.

Chorobski J. (1936). Camillo Golgi. In *Neurological biographies and addresses* (ed. W. Penfield). Oxford University Press, London, pp. 121–7.

Cimino G. (1984). La mente e il suo substratum. Studi sul pensiero neurofisiologico dell'Ottocento. *Domus Galilaeana, Quaderni di storia e critica della scienza*. Tipografia Ambrosini, Roma.

Cimino G. (1995). *Camillo Golgi. L'istologia del sistema nervoso*. Edizioni Teknos, Roma.

Clarke E. and O'Malley C. D. (ed.) (1968). *The human brain and the spinal cord. A historical study illustrated by writings from antiquity to the twentieth century*. University of California Press, Berkeley.

Conklin E. G. (1939). Henry Herbert Donaldson. *Biographical Memoirs*. National Academy of Sciences (USA), Vol. 20, pp. 229–43.

Corradi A. (1877–78). *Memorie e documenti per la storia dell'Università di Pavia e degli uomini più illustri che vi insegnarono*. Parte I e II. Tip. Bizzoni, Pavia.

Corsi P. (1986). *Camillo Golgi. Morfologia e neuroanatomia*. Fidia Biomedical Information. Anno 3°, N° 4.

Corti A. (1956). Nel centenario della nascita di Battista Grassi. *Studia Ghisleriana*. Serie 3ª, **II**, pp. 1–41.

Corti A. (1961). Battista Grassi e la trasmissione della malaria. Studia Ghisleriana. *Coll. monografica*, **1**, pp. 5–73.

Cosmacini G. (1982). *Scienza medica e giacobinismo. L'impresa politico-culturale di Giovanni Rasori (1796–1799)*. Angeli, Milano.

Cosmacini G. (1985). *Gemelli. Il Machiavelli di Dio*. Rizzoli, Milano.

Cosmacini G. (1988). *Storia della medicina e della sanità in Italia*. Laterza, Bari.

Cosmacini G. (1989). *Medicina e sanità in Italia nel ventesimo secolo*. Laterza, Bari.

Cuboni G. and Marchiafava E. (1881). Nuovi studi sulla natura della malaria. *Atti della R. Accademia dei Lincei. Memorie della Classe di Scienze Fisiche, Matematiche e Naturali*, **9**, pp. 31–44.

Curti E. (1928). Pubblicazioni di Camillo Golgi. *Bollettino della Società Medico-Chirurgica Bresciana*. Anno 2°, N° 1, pp. 25–8.

Daddi G. (1897). Contributo alla anatomia patologica della rabbia nell'uomo. *Bollettino della Società Medico-Chirurgica di Pavia*. Anno 12°, pp. 79–86.

Da Fano C. (1926). Camillo Golgi, 1843–1926. *Journal of Pathology and Bacteriology*, **29**, pp. 500–14.

Debove N. (1873). Note sur l'histologie pathologique de sclérose en plaques. *Archives de Physiologie normale et pathologique*, **5**, pp. 745–7.

de Candolle A. (1873). *Histoire des sciences et des savants depuis deux siècles*. Bale e Lyon, Georg, Genève.

De Castro F. (1952). Santiago Ramón y Cajal. *Atti del Primo Congresso Internazionale di Istopatologia del Sistema Nervoso—Proceedings of the first International Congress of Neuropathology*. Casa Editrice Libraria Rosenberg and Sellier, Torino, pp. 33–49.

DeFelipe J. and Jones E. G. (1988). *Cajal on the cerebral cortex. An annotated translation of the complete writings*. Oxford University Press, New York.

DeFelipe J. and Jones E. G. (1991). *Cajal's degeneration & regeneration of the nervous system*. Oxford University Press, New York.

De Gubernatis A. (1879). *Dizionario biografico degli scrittori contemporanei*. Le Monnier, Firenze.

Deiters O. F. K. (1865). *Untersuchungen über Gehirn und Ruckenmark des Menschen und der Saugethiere*. F. Vieweg und Sohn, Brunschweig.

DeJong R. N. (1953). George Sumner Huntington. In *The founders of neurology* (ed. W. Haymaker). C. Thomas, Springfield, pp. 305–8.

Delle Piane G. M. (1966). Nel cinquantenario della morte di Nicolò Manfredi. *La Provincia di Alessandria*. Anno 13°, N° 7–8, pp. 21–3.

Detti T. (1987). *Fabrizio Maffi. Vita di un medico socialista*. Franco Angeli, Milano.

Dianzani M. U. (1989). Dopo Bizzozero: le sue scuole. In *Giulio Bizzozero* (ed. E. Gravela). U. Allemandi & C. Torino, pp. 187–96.

Dogiel A. S. (1908). *Der Bau der Spinalganglien des Menschen und der Säugetiere*. G. Fischer, Jena.

Donaggio A. (1926). Camillo Golgi. *Rivista Sperimentale di Freniatria e Medicina Legale*, **51**, pp. V–XVI.

du Bois-Reymond E. (1891). *Über die Grenzen des Naturerkennens. Die sieben Welträthsel*. Verlag (3rd edn), Leipzig.

Edinger L. (1887). Vergleichend-entwicklungsgeschichtliche Studien im Bereich der Gehirn-Anatomie. *Anatomischer Anzeiger*, **2**, pp. 145–53.

Edinger L. (1889). *Zwölf Vorlesungen über den Bau der nervösen Centralorgane*. Vogel (2nd edn), Leipzig. Engl. trans. W. H. Vittum *Twelve lectures on the structure of the central nervous system* (ed. C. E. Riggs). Davis, Philadelphia (1891).

Erba L. (1976). *Guida storico-artistica dell'Università di Pavia*. Università di Pavia, Pavia.

Falzacappa E. (1889). Ricerche istologiche sul midollo spinale. *Rendiconti della R. Accademia dei Lincei*, **5** (1° semestre), pp. 696–704.

Fantini B. (1992). Biologie, médecine et politique de santé publique: l'exemple historique du paludisme en Italie.Thèse pour le Doctorat Nouveau Régime. **École Pratique des Hautes Étude, Sorbonne, Paris**.

Fappani A. (1974–93). *Enciclopedia Bresciana*, Vol. 6. Edizioni Voce del Popolo, Brescia.

Ferraro A. (1953). Camillo Golgi, 1843–1926. In *The founders of neurology* (ed. W. Haymaker). C. Thomas, Springfield, pp. 41–4.

Finger S. (1994). *Origins of neuroscience*. Oxford University Press, New York.

Foà P. (1901). Commemorazione del socio Giulio Bizzozero. *Rendiconti della R. Accademia dei Lincei*, **10**, pp. 375–87.

Forel A. (1887). Einige hirnananatomische Betrachtungen und Ergebnisse. *Archiv für Psychiatrie und Nervenkrankheiten*, **18**, pp. 162–98.

Forel A. (1937). *Out of my life and work*. Norton, New York.

Forel A. (1968). *Briefe—correspondence 1864–1927*. H. H. Walser, Bern und Stuttgart.

Fraccaro P. (1950). L'Università di Pavia. Fritz Lindner Editore, Küssnacht Am Rigi.

Franklin K. J. (1968). A short history of the international congresses of physiologists. In *History of the international congresses of physiological sciences* (ed. W. O. Fenn). The American Physiological Society, Waverly Press, Baltimore, pp. 258–62.

Freud S. (1893). Quelques considérations pour une étude comparative des paralysies organiques et hystériques. Archives de Neurologie, **26**, pp. 29–43.

Fusari R. (1898). Carlo Giacomini. *Annuario della R. Università di Torino*, Anno 1898–99. Stamperia Reale della ditta G. B. Paravia e C.,Torino, pp. 5–19 **of the reprint**.

Fuxe K. and Agnati L. F. (1991).*Volume transmission in the brain*. Raven Press, New York.

Garovaglio S. (1872). Laboratorio di botanica crittogamica. *Il Patriota*, N° 9, 20 gennaio.

Garrison F. H. (1929). *An introduction to the history of medicine*. **Fourth edition, reprinted.** W. B. Saunders, Philadelphia.

Gehuchten A. van (1891). La structure des centres nerveux: La moelle épinère et le cervelet. *La Cellule*, **7**, pp. 79–122.

Gerlach J. von (1872). Über die Struktur der grauen Substanz des menschlichen Grosshirns. *Centralblatt für die medicinischen Wissenschaften*, **10**, pp. 273–5. **English translation in Shepherd (1991). Partially translated in Clarke and O'Malley (1968).**

Gigli Berzolari A. (1993). *Alessandro Volta e la cultura scientifica e tecnologica tra '700 e '800*. Cisalpino Istituto Editoriale Universitario, Milano.

Goldaniga G. and Marchetti G. (1993).*Vita e opera dello scienziato e senatore camuno Camillo Golgi*.Tipo-Litografia Lineagrafica, Boario Terme. Second edition 1994.

Golgi C. (1868). Storia di pellagra non maniaca. *Gazzetta Medica Italiana-Provincie Venete*. Anno 11°, N° 49, pp. 389–90. *Opera Omnia*, pp. 737–9.

Golgi C. (1869). Sull'eziologia delle alienazioni mentali in rapporto alla prognosi ed alla cura. Studio condotto col metodo sperimentale nella Clinica Psichiatrica di Pavia dal dott. Camillo Golgi. *Annali Universali di Medicina* (1869), **207**, pp. 564–632.**With the title** Eziologia delle malattie mentali in rapporto alla prognosi e cura **in** *Rivista Clinica* (1869), Anno 8°, pp. 145–6 **(summary) and** *Archivio Italiano per le Malatie Nervose* (1869), Anno 6°, pp. 305–8 **(summary). Part of the conclusions of the work was communicated by Lombroso to the** Regio Istituto Lombardo di Scienze e Lettere; see *Rendiconti del R. Istituto Lombardo di Scienze e Lettere* (1869), Serie 2ª, **2**, pp. 307–9.**With the title** Sull'eziologia delle alienazioni mentali in *Opera Omnia*, pp. 741–95.

Golgi C. (1869a). Sulla struttura e sullo sviluppo degli psammomi. *Morgagni* (1869), Anno 11°, pp. 874–86; *Rendiconti R. Istituto Lombardo di Scienze e Lettere* (1869), Serie 2ª, **2**, pp. 918–20; *Opera Omnia*, pp. 797–810.

Golgi C. (1870). Sulle alterazioni dei vasi linfatici del cervello. *Rivista Clinica* (1870), Anno 9°, pp. 324–43; *Archivio per le Malatie Nervose* (1871), Anno 8°, pp. 172–6 **(summary); part of the work with the title** Alterazioni dei linfatici del cervello **in** *Gazzeta Medica Italiana, Lombardia* (1870), Serie 6ª, **30**, tomo 3°, pp. 157–8. **A summary with the title** Delle alterazioni dei vasi linfatici del cervello **was published in** *Rivista di Medicina, di Chirurgia e Terapeutica*, Anno 2°, Fasc. 4, pp. 101–6.**With the title** Sulle alterazioni dei vasi linfatici del cervello in *Opera Omnia*, pp. 811–49.

Golgi C. (1870a). Sulla sostanza connettiva del cervello. *Rendiconti del R. Istituto Lombardo di Scienze e Lettere* (1870), Serie 2ª, **3**, pp. 275–7; *Gazzetta Medica Italiana* (1870), **30**, pp. 145–6. *Opera Omnia*, pp. 1–4.

Golgi C. (1870b). Un caso di eterotopia della sostanza grigia del cervello. Studio di Hoffmann. *Archivio Italiano per le Malatie Nervose*, Anno 7°, pp. 103–9.

Golgi C. (1871–72). Contribuzione alla fina anatomia degli organi centrali del sistema nervoso. *Rivista Clinica* (1871), Anno 1°, N 11° (novembre), pp. 338–50; (1871) N 12° (dicembre), pp. 371–380; (1872) Anno 2°, N 2° (febbraio), pp. 38–46. *Opera Omnia*, pp. 5–70.

Golgi C. (1873). Sulle alterazioni del midollo delle ossa nel vaiuolo. *Rivista Clinica*. Serie 2ª, Anno 3°, pp. 238–44. *Gazzetta delle Cliniche di Torino*, Vol. XI, martedì 17 marzo. The final section of the work with the title Sul sangue dei vajuolosi was also published in *Gazzetta Medica Italiana, Lombardia*, **33**, pp. 339–40. *Opera Omnia*, pp. 855–66.

Golgi C. (1873a). Sulla struttura della sostanza grigia del cervello (Comunicazione preventiva). *Gazzetta Medica Italiana, Lombardia* (1873), **33**, pp. 244–6. Part of the work also in *Rivista di Medicina Chirurgia e Terapeutica* (1873), 2° semestre, pp. 465–8. German translation in Golgi (1894c) No II, pp. 35–8. English translation in Santini (1975), pp. 647–50 and Shepherd (1991), pp. 84–8. With the title Sulla sostanza grigia del cervello in *Opera Omnia*, pp. 91–8 and in Cimino (1995), pp. 1–9.

Golgi C. (1873–75). Rivista di istologia normale e patologica del sistema nervoso centrale. *Rivista di Medicina Chirurgia e Terapeutica* (1873), 1° semestre, pp. 413–40; (1873), 2° semestre, pp. 464–90; (1874), 1° semestre, pp. 501–30; (1874), 2° semestre, pp. 309–46; (1875), 1° semestre, pp. 567–92. See also *Annali Universali di Medicina e Chirurgia* (1875), **232**, pp. 519–47.

Golgi C. (1874). Sulle alterazioni degli organi centrali nervosi in un caso di corea gesticolatoria associata ad alienazione mentale. *Rivista Clinica*, Serie 2ª, Anno 4°, pp. 361–77. *Opera Omnia*, pp. 867–99.

Golgi C. (1874a). Sulla fina anatomia del cervelletto umano. *Rendiconti del R. Istituto Lombardo di Scienze e Lettere* (1874), Serie 2ª, **7**, pp. 69–72. *Archivio Italiano per le Malatie Nervose* (1874), Anno 11°, pp. 90–107. *Opera Omnia*, pp. 99–111.

Golgi C. (1875). Sui gliomi del cervello. *Rivista Sperimentale di Freniatria e Medicina Legale*, **1**, pp. 66–78. *Opera Omnia*, pp. 901–11.

Golgi C. (1875a). I recenti studi sull'istologia del sistema nervoso centrale. Rivista critica. *Rivista Sperimentale di Freniatria e Medicina Legale*, **1**, pp. 121–30 (first part); pp. 260–74 (second part).

Golgi C. (1875b). Sulla fina struttura dei bulbi olfattori. *Rivista Sperimentale di Freniatria e Medicina Legale*, **1**, pp. 403–25. *Opera Omnia*, pp. 113–32.

Golgi C. (1876). Sulla degenerazione calcarea delle cellule nervose centrali. *Archivio per le Scienze Mediche*, **1**, Fasc. 4, pp. 442–53. *Opera Omnia*, pp. 913–22.

Golgi C. (1878). Intorno alla distribuzione e terminazione dei nervi nei tendini dell'uomo e di altri vertebrati. *Gazzetta Medica Italiana, Lombardia* (1878), **38**, pp. 221–4. *Rendiconti del R. Istituto Lombardo di Scienze e Lettere* (1878), Serie 2ª, **11**, pp. 445–53. *Opera Omnia*, pp. 133–42.

Golgi C. (1878a). Della terminazione dei nervi nei tendini e di un nuovo apparato nervoso terminale muscolo-tendineo. *Atti della settima riunione straordinaria della Società Italiana di Scienze Naturali in Varese*. Tipografia di Giuseppe Bernardoni, Milano, pp. 272–5.

Golgi C. (1878–79). Di una nuova reazione apparentemente nera delle cellule nervose cerebrali ottenuta col bicloruro di mercurio. *Archivio per le Scienze Mediche* (1878–79), **3**, Fasc. 2, memoria N° 11, pp. 1–7. With the title Un nuovo processo di tecnica microscopica **in** *Rendiconti del R. Istituto Lombardo di Scienze e Lettere* (1879), Serie 2ª, **12**, pp. 206–10. *Opera Omnia*, pp. 143–8.

Golgi C. (1879). Sulla struttura delle fibre nervose midollate periferiche e centrali. *Rendiconti del R. Istituto Lombardo di Scienze e Lettere* (1879), Serie 2ª, **12**, pp. 926–34. *Archivio per le Scienze Mediche* (1880), **4**, N° 10, pp. 221–46. *Archivio Italiano per le Malattie Nervose* (1880), Anno 17°, pp. 137–43. *Opera Omnia*, pp. 149–70.

Golgi C. (1880). Sui nervi dei tendini dell'uomo e di altri vertebrati e di un nuovo organo nervoso terminale muscolo-tendineo. *Memorie della R. Accademia delle Scienze di Torino*, Serie 2ª, **32**, pp. 359–86. *Opera Omnia*, pp. 171–98.

Golgi C. (1880–81). Sulla origine centrale dei nervi. Communication to the Medical Congress of Genova (1880). Proceedings quoted in *Opera Omnia*, p. 578 (not verified). *Giornale Internazionale delle Scienze*

Mediche (1881), **3**, pp. 225–34. *Opera Omnia*, pp. 243–9. **See also** Golgi (1885 e 1886), pp. 33–50 **and** *Opera Omnia*, pp. 324–39.

Golgi C. (1880–81a). Studii istologici sul midollo spinale. **Communication to the 3° Congress of the** Società Freniatrica Italiana. Reggio Emilia (1880). *Rendiconti del Congresso* (**not verified**). *Archivio Italiano per le Malattie Nervose* (1881), Anno 18°, pp. 155–65. *Gazzetta delle Cliniche di Torino*, **XVIII**, 1 febbraio. **With the title** Ricerche istologiche sul midollo spinale in *Rivista Sperimentale di Freniatria e Medicina Legale* (1880), **6**, pp. 376–9 (**summary**) e sulla *Gazzetta Medica Italiana, Lombardia* (1881), **41**, pp. 88–9 (summary). *Opera Omnia*, pp. 235–42.

Golgi C. (1881). Annotazioni intorno all'istologia normale e patologica dei muscoli volontari. *Archivio per le Scienze Mediche* (1881), **5**, Fasc. 3, N° 11, pp. 194–236. **Parts of this work were communicated to the** Reale Istituto Lombardo di Scienze e Lettere, **see** *Rendiconti R. Istituto Lombardo di Scienze e lettere*: Contribuzione all'istologia dei muscoli volontari (1880), Serie 2ª, **13**, pp. 25–31; Contribuzione alla patologia dei muscoli volontari (1881), Serie 2ª, **14**, pp. 9–18; Alterazioni delle fibre muscolari in un caso di atassia locomotoria (1881), Serie 2ª, **14**, pp. 495–500. **Part of the work with the title** Contribuzione all'istologia dei muscoli volontarj **in** *Annali Universali di Medicina* (1880), **251**, pp. 250–61. **With the title** Contribuzione alla istologia normale e patologica dei muscoli volontari **in** *Opera Omnia*, pp. 199–234.

Golgi C. (1881a). Relazione sull'atlante di fotomicrografie mandato dal Dott. Gray di Utica. *Archivio Italiano per le Malattie Nervose*, Anno 18°, pp. 245–6.

Golgi C. (1882). Origine del tractus olfactorius e struttura dei lobi olfattorii dell'uomo e di altri mammiferi. *Rendiconti del R. Istituto Lombardo di Scienze e Lettere* (1882), Serie 2ª, **15**, pp. 216–24; *Gazzetta degli Ospitali* (1882), **3**, pp. 210–12, 218–19; *Archivio Italiano per le Malattie Nervose* (1882), Anno 9°, pp. 112–18 (**summary**). *Opera Omnia*, pp. 251–60. **Slightly modified also in** Golgi (1885, 1886), pp. 120–8. **See also** (Golgi 1882a).

Golgi C. (1882a). Origine du tractus olfactorius et structure des lobes olfactifs de l'homme et d'autres mammifères. *Archives Italiennes de Biologie*, **1**, pp. 454–62.

Golgi C. (1882b). Una parola dell'anatomia a proposito di una questione di Fisiologia e di Clinica. *Gazzetta degli Ospitali*, Anno 3°, pp. 481–2, 489–90, 497–9, 505–7, 529–30, 545–6, 553–5, 561–3, 569–70. **With the title** Considerazioni anatomiche sulla dottrina delle localizzazioni cerebrali **in** *Opera Omnia*, pp. 261–93.

Golgi C. (1882c). Considérations anatomiques sur la doctrine des localisations cérébrales. *Archives Italiennes de Biologie*, **2**, pp. 237–53, 255–68.

Golgi C. (1882d). Nervoso (sistema). *Enciclopedia Medica Vallardi* (inizio serie 1878), Milano. Serie 2ª, **3**, Parte 1ª, pp. 93–122. **Slightly modified also in** Il sistema nervoso centrale, *Biblioteca medica contemporanea* (1883), Vallardi, Milano, pp. 1–47.

Golgi C. (1882e). Nevroglia. *Enciclopedia Medica Vallardi* (inizio serie 1878), Milano. Serie 2ª, Vol. 3, Parte 1ª, pp. 263–79. **Slightly modified also in** Il sistema nervoso centrale, *Biblioteca Medica Contemporanea* (1883), Vallardi, Milano, pp. 47–82.

Golgi C. (1882f). La pneumonite infettiva. *Gazzetta degli Ospitali*, Anno 3°, pp. 17–20, 25–8.

Golgi C. (1882g). Osservazioni al lavoro di G. Sangalli 'Bacterj del carbonchio nel feto di giovenca morta per questa malattia. *Rendiconti del R. Istituto Lombardo di Scienze e Lettere*, Serie 2ª, **15**, pp. 672–4.

Golgi C. (1882h). Sulla ipertrofia compensatoria dei reni. *Rendiconti del R. Istituto Lombardo di Scienze e Lettere*, Serie 2ª, **15**, pp. 591–8. *Archivio per le Scienze Mediche* (1882), **6**, pp. 346–56. *Gazzetta degli Ospitali* (1882), Anno 3°, pp. 779–81. *Opera Omnia*, pp. 951–9.

Golgi C. (1882i). Sur l'hypertrophie compensative des reins. *Archives Italiennes de Biologie*, **2**, pp. 268–73.

Golgi C. (1882–85). Sulla fina anatomia degli organi centrali del sistema nervoso. *Rivista Sperimentale di Freniatria e Medicina Legale* (1882), **8**, pp. 165–95, 361–91; (1883), **9**, pp. 1–17, 161–92, 385–402; (1885), **11**, pp. 72–123, 193–220. *Opera Omnia*, pp. 295–394, 397–536. **See also** Golgi (1885, 1886).

Golgi C. (1883). Recherches sur l'histologie des centres nerveux. *Archives Italiennes de Biologie*, **3**, pp. 285–317; **4**, pp. 92–123. **Excerpted and translated in Clarke and O'Malley (1968), pp. 92–6.**

Golgi C. (1883a). II. Continuation of the study of the minute anatomy of the central nervous system. III. Morphology and disposition of the nervous cells in the anterior, central, and superior-occipital convolutions. *Alienist and Neurologist*, **4**, pp. 236–69, 383–416.

Golgi C. (1883–84). La cellula nervosa motrice. **Communication to the 4th Congress of the** Società Freniatrica Italiana. Voghera (1883). Atti congressuali, pp. 3–6 **of the reprints**, Tipografia Fratelli Rechiedei, Milano (1884). *Archivio Italiano per le Malattie Nervose* (1884), quoted in *Opera Omnia*, p. 578, Anno 21° (**not verified**). *Rivista Sperimentale di Freniatria e Medicina Legale* (1883), **9**, p. 210 (**summary**). **See also** Golgi (1885, 1886). *Opera Omnia*, pp. 537–42.

Golgi C. (1884). Lo sperimentalismo nella medicina. *Annuario Università di Pavia, Anno scolastico 1883–84*. Tipografia successori Bizzoni, Pavia, pp. 15–66.

Golgi C. (1884a). Neoformazione dell'epitelio de' canalicoli oriniferi nella malattia di Bright. *Rendiconti del R. Istituto Lombardo di Scienze e Lettere*, Serie 2ª, **17**, pp. 345–8. *Archivio per le Scienze Mediche* (1884), **8**, pp. 105–16. *Opera Omnia*, pp. 961–9.

Golgi C. (1884b). *Sulla fina anatomia degli organi centrali del sistema nervoso. Studi di Camillo Golgi Professore di Patologia Generale e Istologia nell'Università di Pavia (con 24 tavole)*. Tip. S. Calderini e Figlio, Reggio Emilia.

Golgi C. (1885). *Sulla fina anatomia degli organi centrali del sistema nervoso. Studi di Camillo Golgi Professore di Patologia Generale e Istologia nell'Università di Pavia (con 24 tavole)*. Tip. S. Calderini e Figlio, Reggio Emilia.

Golgi C. (1885a). Continuation of the study of the minute anatomy of the central nervous system. V. On the minute anatomy of the great foot of the hippocampus. *Alienist and Neurologist*, **6**, pp. 307–24.

Golgi C. (1886). *Sulla fina anatomia degli organi centrali del sistema nervoso. Studi di Camillo Golgi Professore di Patologia Generale e Istologia nell'Università di Pavia (con 24 tavole)*. U. Hoepli, Milano.

Golgi C. (1886a). Sur l'anatomie microscopique des organes centraux du système nerveux. Méthodes de Recherche. *Archives Italiennes de Biologie*, **7**, pp. 15–47.

Golgi C. (1886b). Sull'infezione malarica. *Archivio per le Scienze Mediche*, **10**, pp. 109–35. **With the title** Sulla infezione malarica in *Opera Omnia*, pp. 989–1012. **Also in** *Studi di Camillo Golgi sulla malaria, raccolti e ordinati dal Prof. Aldo Perroncito*. L. Pozzi, Roma (1929), pp. 1–22.

Golgi C. (1886c). Sull'infezione malarica. *Bollettino della Società Medico-Chirurgica di Pavia*, Anno 1°, N° 1, pp. 29–33. *Gazzetta degli Ospitali*, **7**, pp. 373–5.

Golgi C. (1886d). Rivista bibliografica del libro di Alessandro Tafani 'L'organo dell'udito'. *Gazzetta degli Ospitali*, **7**, pp. 591–2.

Golgi C. (1886e). Ancora sulla infezione malarica. *Gazzetta degli Ospitali*, **7**, pp. 419–22. *Opera Omnia*, pp. 1013–21. **Also in** *Studi di Camillo Golgi sulla malaria, raccolti e ordinati dal Prof. Aldo Perroncito*. L. Pozzi, Roma (1929), pp. 23–32.

Golgi C. (1886f). Ancora sulla infezione malarica. *Bollettino della Società Medico-Chirurgica di Pavia*, Anno 1°, N° 2, pp. 51–3.

Golgi C. (1886g). Professor Golgi's method of black coloring of the central nervous organs. *Alienist and Neurologist*, **7**, pp. 127–31.

Golgi C. (1887). Sur l'infection malarique. *Archives Italiennes de Biologie*, **8**, pp. 154–75.

Golgi C. (1887a). Contribuzione allo studio delle alterazioni istologiche del sistema nervoso centrale nella rabbia sperimentale. *Gazzetta degli Ospitali*, **8**, p. 101.

Golgi C. (1887b). Contribution à l'étude des altérations histologiques du système nerveux central dans la rage expérimentale. *Archives Italiennes de Biologie*, **8**, pp. 192–3.

Golgi C. (1888). Discorso pronunciato per la solenne apertura del XII congresso medico. *Atti del dodicesimo congresso della Associazione Medica Italiana*. Tipografia Fratelli Fusi, Pavia, Vol. 1, pp. 4–11.

Golgi C. (1888a). Annotazioni intorno all'istologia dei reni. *Bollettino della Società Medico-Chirurgica di Pavia*, Anno 3°, N° 1, pp. 19–23. *Gazzetta degli Ospitali*, **9**, pp. 259–60.

Golgi C. (1888b). A qual punto del ciclo evolutivo dei parassiti malarici la somministrazione della chinina, arrestandone lo sviluppo, valga ad impedire il più vicino accesso febbrile. *Bollettino della Società Medico-Chirurgica di Pavia*, Anno 3°, N° 1, pp. 39–42. *Gazzetta degli Ospitali*, **9**, p. 349.

Golgi C. (1888c). Il fagocitismo nella infezione malarica. *Bollettino della Società Medico-Chirurgica di Pavia*, Anno 3°, N° 2, pp. 14–17. *Gazzetta degli Ospitali*, **9**, pp. 436–7. *La Riforma Medica*, **4**, pp. 734–5, 740, 746–7. *Opera Omnia*, pp. 1023–32. **Also in** *Studi di Camillo Golgi sulla malaria, raccolti e ordinati dal Prof. Aldo Perroncito*. L. Pozzi, Roma (1929), pp. 33–42.

Golgi C. (1888d). Intorno all'istogenesi dei canalicoli uriniferi dell'uomo e di altri mammiferi. *Bollettino della Società Medico-Chirurgica di Pavia*, Anno 3°, N° 2, pp. 43–9. *Gazzetta degli Ospitali*, **9**, pp. 524–5.

Golgi C. (1889). Sul ciclo evolutivo dei parassiti malarici nella febbre terzana. Diagnosi differenziale tra i parassiti endoglobulari malarici della terzana e quelli della quartana. *Archivio per le Scienze Mediche*, **13**, pp. 173–96. *Gazzetta degli Ospitali*, **10**, pp. 220–1. *Opera Omnia*, pp. 1063–83. **Also in** *Studi di Camillo Golgi sulla malaria, raccolti e ordinati dal Prof. Aldo Perroncito*. L. Pozzi, Roma (1929), pp. 75–94.

Golgi C. (1889a). Intorno al preteso 'Bacillus malariae' di Klebs, Tommasi-Crudeli e Schiavuzzi. *Archivio per le Scienze Mediche*, **13**, pp. 93–128. *Opera Omnia*, pp. 1033–61. **Also in** *Studi di Camillo Golgi sulla malaria, raccolti e ordinati dal Prof. Aldo Perroncito*. L. Pozzi, Roma (1929), pp. 43–74.

Golgi C. (1889b). Annotazioni intorno all'Istologia dei reni dell'uomo e di altri mammiferi e sull'Istogenesi dei canalicoli oriniferi. *Atti della R. Accademia dei Lincei. Rendiconti*, Serie 4ª, **5** (1° semestre), pp. 334–42. *Opera Omnia*, pp. 543–53.

Golgi C. (1889c). Le phagocytisme dans l'infection malarique. *Archives Italiennes de Biologie*, **11**, pp. 95–103.

Golgi C. (1889d). Ueber den angeblichen Bacillus malariae von Klebs, Tommasi-Crudeli und Schiavuzzi. *Beiträge zur pathologischen Anatomie und zur allgemeinen Pathologie*, **4**, pp. 419–52.

Golgi C. (1889e). Sul ciclo evolutivo dei parassiti malarici nella febbre terzana. (Diagnosi differenziale tra i parassiti malarici endoglobulari della febbre terzana e quelli della quartana). *Bollettino della Società Medico-Chirurgica di Pavia*, Anno 4°, N° 1, pp. 26–31. *Gazzetta degli Ospitali*, **10**, pp. 220–1.

Golgi C. (1889f). Ueber den Entwickelungskreislauf der Malariaparasiten bei der Febris tertiana (Differentialdiagnose zwischen den endoglobulären Parasiten des tertianen und denen des quartanen Fiebers). *Fortschritte der Medizin*, **7**, pp. 81–100.

Golgi C. (1889g). Sulle febbri intermittenti malariche a lunghi intervalli. Criteri fondamentali di classificazione delle febbri malariche. *Bollettino della Società Medico-Chirurgica di Pavia*, Anno 4°, N° 2, pp. 5–8. *Gazzetta degli Ospitali*, **10**, p. 516. Sur les fièvres intermittentes à long intervalles. Fondaments de la classification des fièvres malariques. *Archives Italiennes de Biologie*, **11**, pp. XLIX–LI.

Golgi C. (1890). Sulle febbri intermittenti malariche a lunghi intervalli. Criterii fondamentali di classificazione delle febbri malariche. *Archivio per le Scienze Mediche*, **14**, pp. 293–313. **With the title** Sulle febbri intermittenti malariche a lunghi intervalli in *Opera Omnia*, pp. 1085–103. **Also in** *Studi di Camillo Golgi sulla malaria, raccolti e ordinati dal Prof. Aldo Perroncito*. L. Pozzi, Roma (1929), pp. 95–115.

Golgi C. (1890a). Ueber intermittirende Fieberformen der Malaria mit langen Intervallen. Hauptunterscheidungsmerkmale für die Gruppirung der Fieberformen der Malaria. *Beiträge zur pathologischen Anatomie und zur allgemeinen Pathologie*, **7**, pp. 647–67.

Golgi C. (1890b). Sull'attuale epidemia di influenza. *Bollettino della Società Medico-Chirurgica di Pavia*, Anno 5°, pp. 13–25. *Gazzetta degli Ospitali*, **11**, pp. 92–4, 101–3, 109–10. *Opera Omnia*, pp. 1105–18.

Golgi C. (1890c). Dimostrazione fotografica dello sviluppo dei parassiti della malaria (1ª serie, febbre quartana). *Bollettino della Società Medico-Chirurgica di Pavia*, Anno 5°, pp. 35–7. *Gazzetta degli Ospitali*, **11**, pp. 692–3. **Also in** *Studi di Camillo Golgi sulla malaria, raccolti e ordinati dal Prof. Aldo Perroncito*. L. Pozzi, Roma (1929), pp. 115–18.

Golgi C. (1890d). Dimostrazione fotografica dello sviluppo dei parassiti della malaria (2ª serie, febbre terzana). *Bollettino della Società Medico-Chirurgica di Pavia*, Anno 5°, pp. 92–6. *Opera Omnia*, pp. 1131–35. *Giornale della R. Accademia di Medicina di Torino*, **38**, pp. 747–54. **Also in** *Studi di Camillo Golgi sulla malaria, raccolti e ordinati dal Prof. Aldo Perroncito*. L. Pozzi, Roma (1929), pp. 119–24.

Golgi C. (1890e). Di nuovo sulle alterazioni degli organi centrali del sistema nervoso nella rabbia sperimentale. *Bollettino della Società Medico-Chirurgica di Pavia*, Anno 5°, pp. 41–3. *Gazzetta degli Ospitali*, **11**, pp. 701–2.

Golgi C. (1890f). Sulla fina anatomia del midollo spinale. *Atti della R. Accademia dei Lincei. Memorie della Classe di Scienze Fisiche, Matematiche e Naturali*, **7** (Serie quarta), pp. 123–48. *Opera Omnia*, pp. 555–78.

Golgi C. (1890g). Über den feineren Bau des Rückenmarkes. *Anatomischer Anzeiger*, **5**, pp. 372–96, 423–35.

Golgi C. (1891). Modificazione del metodo di colorazione degli elementi nervosi col cloruro di mercurio. *Riforma Medica Anno 7°*, **2**, N° 142, pp. 793–4. **With the title** Una modificazione alla reazione del bicloruro di mercurio sugli elementi nervosi. *Bollettino della Società Medico-Chirurgica di Pavia* (1891). Anno 6°, N° 2, p. 29 (**presented to the Society but not published**). *Opera Omnia*, pp. 607–11.

Golgi C. (1891a). Sur le cycle évolutif des parasites malariques dans la fièvre tierce. Diagnose différentielle entre les parasites endoglobulaires malariques de la fièvre tierce et ceux de la fièvre quarte. *Archives Italiennes de Biologie*, **14**, pp. 81–100.

Golgi C. (1891b). Sur les fièvres intermittentes à longues intervalles. Fondements de la classification des fièvres malariques. *Archives Italiennes de Biologie*, **14**, pp. 113–32.

Golgi C. (1891c). Représentation photographique du développement des parasites de l'infection paludéenne. *Verhandlungen des X Internationalen Medicinischen Congresses*. Dritte Abtheilung, Berlin, Band II, Abtheilung III, pp. 200–5.

Golgi C. (1891d). Demonstration der Entwickelung der Malariaparasiten durch Photographien. Erste Reihe: Entwickelung der Amoeba malariae febris quartanae. *Zeitschrift für Hygiene*, **10**, pp. 136–44. *Opera Omnia*, pp. 1119–29.

Golgi C. (1891e). La rete nervosa diffusa degli organi centrali del sistema nervoso. Suo significato fisiologico. *Rendiconti del R. Istituto Lombardo di Scienze e Lettere*, Serie 2ª, **24**, pp. 594–603, 656–73. *Opera Omnia*, pp. 579–605.

Golgi C. (1891f). La rete nervosa diffusa degli organi centrali del sistema nervoso. Suo significato fisiologico. *Bollettino della Società Medico-Chirurgica di Pavia*, Anno 6°, N° 2, pp. 21–3.

Golgi C. (1891g). Les reseaux nerveux diffus. Ses attributes physiologiques. Methode suvie dans le recherches histologique. *Archives Italiennes de Biologie*, **15**, pp. 434–63.

Golgi C. (1891h). Sulla cura antitubercolare col metodo Koch. *Bollettino della Società Medico-Chirurgica di Pavia*, Anno 6°, N° 1, pp. 20–5. *Riforma Medica* (1891), N° 70 marzo (**not verified**).

Golgi C. (1891i). Zur feineren Anatomie des grossen Seepferdefusses. *Zeitschrift für wissenschaftliche Zoologie*, **52**, pp. 18–45.

Golgi C. (1891j). *Nervensystem. Ergebnisse der Anatomie und Entwickelungsgeschichte (für 1891)*. Verlagsbuchandlung, J. Bergmann, Wiesbaden, Vol. 1, pp. 256–63 (**not verified**).

Golgi C. (1892). Azione della chinina sui parassiti malarici e sui corrispondenti accessi febbrili. *Gazzetta Medica di Pavia* (1892), **1**, pp. 11–19, 34–41, 79–91, 106–17. *Rendiconti del R. Istituto Lombardo di Scienze e Lettere* (1892), **25**, pp. 163–84, 335–61. *Gazzetta delle Cliniche di Torino*, N° 38, settembre. *Opera Omnia*, pp. 1143–83. **Also in** *Studi di Camillo Golgi sulla malaria, raccolti e ordinati dal Prof. Aldo Perroncito*. L. Pozzi, Roma (1929), pp. 133–69.

Golgi C. (1892a). Action de la quinine sur les parasites malariques et sur les accès fébriles qu'ils déterminent. *Archives Italiennes de Biologie*, **17**, pp. 456–71.

Golgi C. (1892b). Ueber die Wirkung des Chinins auf die Malariaparasiten und die diesen entsprechenden Fieberanfälle. *Deutsche Medicinische Wochenschrift*, **18**, pp. 663–7, 685–9, 707–9, 729–32.

Golgi C. (1892c). Il cloridrato di fenocolla nelle febbri intermittenti malariche. *Bollettino della Società Medico-Chirurgica di Pavia*, Anno 7°, pp. 25–9. *Gazzetta Medica di Pavia*, **1**, pp. 159–63. *Opera Omnia*, pp. 1137–42.

Golgi C. (1892d). Ancora una nota a contribuzione delle conoscenze sull'anatomia patologica della rabbia sperimentale. *Bollettino della Società Medico-Chirurgica di Pavia*, Anno 7°, pp. 32–5. *Gazzetta Medica di Pavia*, **1**, pp. 180–3.

Golgi C. (1892e). *Nervensystem. Ergebnisse der Anatomie und Entwickelungsgeschichte (für 1891)*. Verlagsbuchandlung, J. Bergmann, Wiesbaden, Vol. 1, pp. 288–377.

Golgi C. (1893). Sulla fina organizzazione delle ghiandole peptiche dei mammiferi. *Bollettino della Società Medico-Chirurgica di Pavia*, Anno 8°, pp. 16–21. *Gazzetta Medica di Pavia*, **2**, pp. 241–7. *Opera Omnia*, pp. 612–23.

Golgi C. (1893a). Sur la fine organisation des glandes peptiques des mammifères. *Archives Italiennes de Biologie*, **19**, pp. 448–53.

Golgi C. (1893b). Intorno all'origine del quarto nervo cerebrale (patetico o trocleare) e di una questione di Isto-fisiologia generale che a questo argomento si collega. *Bollettino della Società Medico-Chirurgica di Pavia*, Anno 8°, pp. 37–46.

Golgi C. (1893c). Intorno all'origine del quarto nervo cerebrale (patetico o trocleare) e di una questione di Isto-fisiologia generale che a questo argomento si collega. *Rendiconti della R. Accademia dei Lincei*, Serie 5ª, **2** (1° semestre), pp. 379–89, 443–50. *Gazzetta Medica di Pavia*, **2**, pp. 457–68. *Opera Omnia*, pp. 624–42.

Golgi C. (1893d). Sur l'origine du quatrième nerf cérébral (pathétique) et sur un point d'Histo-physiologie générale qui se rattache à cette question. *Archives Italiennes de Biologie*, **19**, pp. 454–74.

Golgi C. (1893e). Sulle febbri malariche estivo-autunnali di Roma. Lettera al Prof. Guido Baccelli. *Gazzetta Medica di Pavia*, **2**, pp. 481–93, 505–20, 529–44, 553–9. *Gazzetta delle Cliniche di Torino* (1894), 18 febbraio.

Opera Omnia, pp. 1185–235. **Also in** *Studi di Camillo Golgi sulla malaria, raccolti e ordinati dal Prof. Aldo Perroncito*. L. Pozzi, Roma (1929), pp. 173–217.

Golgi C. (1893f). *Nervensystem. Ergebnisse der Anatomie und Entwickelungsgeschichte (für 1892)*. Verlagsbuchandlung, J. Bergmann, Wiesbaden, pp. 288–402.

Golgi C. (1894). Sur les fièvres malariques estivo-automnales de Rome. *Archives Italiennes de Biologie*, **20**, pp. 288–333.

Golgi C. (1894a). Ueber die römischen Sommer-Herbst-Malariafieber. *Deutsche Medicinische Wochenschrift*, **20**, pp. 291–2, 316–18.

Golgi (1894b). Parole del rettore Camillo Golgi nella solenne inaugurazione dell'anno accademico 1893–94. *Annuario Università di Pavia, Anno scolastico 1893–94*. Tipografia successori Bizzoni, Pavia, pp. 5–20.

Golgi C. (1894c). *Untersuchungen über den feineren Bau des centralen und peripheren Nervensystems*. G. Fischer, Jena.

Golgi C. (1894d). Sull'istologia patologica della rabbia sperimentale. *Atti XI Congresso Internazionale di Medicina. Sezione di Patologia Generale ed Anatomia Patologica*, pp. 250–4.

Golgi C. (1894e). Ueber die pathologische Histologie der Rabies experimentalis. *Berliner Klinische Wochenschrift*, **31**, pp. 325–31. *Opera Omnia*, pp. 1237–53.

Golgi C. (1894f). Midollo spinale. *Enciclopedia Medica Vallardi* (inizio serie 1878), Milano. Serie 2ª, **4**, Parte 2ª, pp. 180–214.

Golgi C. (1894g). *Nervensystem. Ergebnisse der Anatomie und Entwickelungsgeschichte (für 1893)*. Verlagsbuchandlung, J. Bergmann, Wiesbaden (**not verified**).

Golgi C. (1895). Per la solenne inaugurazione dell'anno accademico 1894–95. *Annuario Università di Pavia. Anno scolastico 1894–95*. Tipografia successori Bizzoni, Pavia, pp. 5–31.

Golgi C. (1896). Per la solenne inaugurazione dell'anno accademico 1895–96. *Annuario Università di Pavia. Anno scolastico 1895–96*. Tipografia successori Bizzoni, Pavia, pp. 5–25.

Golgi C (1896a). Commemorazione del Dott. Luigi Villa. *Bollettino della Società Medico-Chirurgica di Pavia*, Anno 11°, pp. 152–5.

Golgi C. (1898). Intorno alla struttura delle cellule nervose. *Bollettino della Società Medico-Chirurgica di Pavia*, Anno 13, N° 1, pp. 3–16. **Partially translated by N. Geller Lipsky: On the structure of nerve cells,** *Journal of Microscopy*, 155, pp. 3–7. *Opera Omnia*, pp. 643–53.

Golgi C. (1898a). Appunti intorno alla struttura delle cellule nervose. *Rendiconti del R. Istituto Lombardo di Scienze e Lettere*, **31**, pp. 930–41. *Gazzetta Medica Lombarda*, pp. 269, 279. *Riforma Medica*, **14**, p. 329.

Golgi C. (1898b). Sur la structure des cellules nerveuses. *Archives Italiennes de Biologie*, **30**, pp. 60–71.

Golgi C. (1898c). Sulla struttura delle cellule nervose dei gangli spinali. *Bollettino della Società Medico-Chirurgica di Pavia*, Anno 13°, N° 2, pp. 5–15. *Opera Omnia*, pp. 655–63.

Golgi C. (1898d). Sur la structure des cellules nerveuses des ganglions spinaux. *Archives Italiennes de Biologie*, **30**, pp. 278–86.

Golgi C. (1899). Di nuovo sulla struttura delle cellule nervose dei gangli spinali. *Bollettino della Società Medico-Chirurgica di Pavia*, Anno 14°, pp. 1–12. *Opera Omnia*, pp. 667–75.

Golgi C. (1899a). De nouveau sur la structure des cellules nerveuses des ganglions spinaux. *Archives Italiennes de Biologie*, **31**, pp. 273–80.

Golgi C. (1899b). Sur la structure des cellules nerveuses de la moelle épinière. *Volume Jubilaire publié par la Société de Biologie*. Masson & C. Editeurs, Paris, pp. 507–30.

Golgi C. (1899c). Nell'inaugurazione dei congressi medici ed apertura del 1° congresso italiano di elettro-biologia. *L'Avvenire*, pp. 3–10 **of the reprint**.

Golgi C. (1899d). Nell'inaugurazione dei congressi medici ed apertura dei congressi di igiene e medicina veterinaria. *L'Avvenire*, pp. 3–10 **of the reprint**.

Golgi C. (1900). Sulla struttura delle cellule nervose del midollo spinale. *Bollettino della Società Medico-Chirurgica di Pavia*, Anno 15°, pp. 1–32. *Opera Omnia*, pp. 677–705.

Golgi C. (1900a). Intorno alla struttura delle cellule nervose della corteccia cerebrale. *Verhandlungen der Anatomischen Gesellschaft*, **14**, pp. 164–76. *Opera Omnia*, pp. 707–19.

Golgi C. (1900b). Le reticulum intracellulaire et la structure fibrillaire peripherique de la cellule nerveuse. *Comptes rendus de la section de neurologie*, pp. 582–6. XIII Congrés internationelle de médicine, Paris.

Golgi C. (1901). Giulio Bizzozero. *Archivio per le Scienze Mediche*, **25**, pp. 205–34. **See also** *In memoria di Giulio Bizzozero nel primo anniversario della sua morte. La famiglia*. Stab. Fratelli Pozzo, Torino (1902), pp. 368–91.

Golgi C. (1901a). *Discorso del Senatore Golgi, Rappresentante dell'Università di Pavia*. 11 aprile 1901. **See also** *In memoria di Giulio Bizzozero nel primo anniversario della sua morte. La famiglia*. Stab. Fratelli Pozzo, Torino (1902), pp. 41–5.

Golgi C. (1901b). Commemorazione del S. C. Giulio Bizzozero. *Rendiconti del R. Istituto Lombardo di Scienze e Lettere*, Serie 2ª, **34**, pp. 533–8. **See also** *In memoria di Giulio Bizzozero nel primo anniversario della sua morte. La famiglia*. Stab. Fratelli Pozzo, Torino (1902), pp. 171–7.

Golgi C. (1901c). Per la solenne inaugurazione dell'anno scolastico 1901–902. *Annuario Università di Pavia. Anno scolastico 1901–902*. Tipografia successori Bizzoni, Pavia, pp. 5–18.

Golgi C. (1903). Parole in onore del M. E. Eusebio Oehl. *Rendiconti del R. Istituto Lombardo di Scienze e Lettere*, Serie 2ª, **36**, pp. 491–4.

Golgi C. (1903a). Per la solenne inaugurazione dell'anno scolastico 1902–903. *Annuario Università di Pavia. Anno scolastico 1902–903*. Tipografia successori Bizzoni, Pavia, pp. 5–41.

Golgi C. (1903b). Sulla fina organizzazione del sistema nervoso (lettera al Prof. Luigi Luciani). *Opera Omnia*, pp. 721–33.

Golgi C. (1903c). *Relazione letta nella seduta del consiglio del Consorzio. Relazione prima*. Tipografia e legatoria cooperativa, Pavia, pp. 3–22.

Golgi C. (1903d). *Opera Omnia*, Volumes I–III. R. Fusari, G. Marenghi, and L. Sala (ed.). Hoepli Editore, Milano.

Golgi C. (1903e). *Relazione letta nella seduta del consiglio del Consorzio. Relazione seconda*. Tipografia e legatoria cooperativa, Pavia, pp. 3–19.

Golgi C. (1904). Per la solenne inaugurazione dell'anno scolastico 1903–904. *Annuario Università di Pavia. Anno scolastico 1903–904*. Tipografia successori Bizzoni, Pavia, pp. 5–43.

Golgi C. (1904a). L'opera scientifica di Giovanni Marenghi. *Bollettino della Società Medico-Chirurgica di Pavia*, Anno 19°, pp. 1–21.

Golgi (1904b). Per la solenne inaugurazione dell'anno scolastico 1904–905. *Annuario Università di Pavia. Anno scolastico 1904–905*. Tipografia successori Bizzoni, Pavia, pp. 5–30.

Golgi C. (1905). *Le opere scientifiche di Giulio Bizzozero*. Introduzione all'Opera Omnia di Giulio Bizzozero. Hoepli, Milano, pp. XI–XXVIII.

Golgi C. (1905a). *VIII congresso interuniversitario italiano*. Parole d'apertura. Atti congressuali (**not verified**). **Typewritten copy kept at the** Biblioteca dell'Università di Pavia, pp. 1–8 (Misc. in 4° T 1473, N° 7).

Golgi C. (1906). La doctrine du neurone, théorie et faits. In *Les Prix Nobel 1904–1906*. Norstedt & Söner, Imprimerie Royale, Stockholm (1908). Neuronen. Teori oct Fakta. *Allmänno Sventka Läkartihningen* (1906), N° 51. *Nordiskt Mediciniskt Arkiv* (1907). **1**, pp. 1–26. La dottrina del neurone. Teoria e fatti. *Archivio di Fisiologia*. (1907), **IV**, pp. 187–215. The neuron doctrine. Theory and facts. In *Nobel lectures Physiology or Medicine 1901–1921*. Elsevier, New York (1967), pp. 189–217. **Excerpted and translated in Clarke and O'Malley (1968), p. 96**. **Also published** in Cimino (1995), pp. 11–45, **and** in Goldaniga e Marchetti (1993), pp. 153–62. *Opera Omnia*, pp. 1259–91.

Golgi C. (1906a). Per la solenne inaugurazione dell'anno scolastico 1905–906. *Annuario Università di Pavia. Anno scolastico 1905–906*. Tipografia successori Bizzoni, Pavia, pp. 5–29, I–V.

Golgi C. (1906b). Per l'apertura della IVª riunione della Società Italiana di Patologia. Parole pronunziate dal presidente del comitato ordinatore. *Atti della Società Italiana di Patologia* (Supplemento al *Bollettino della Società Medico-Chirurgica di Pavia*), Tipografia e legatoria cooperativa, Pavia, pp. 1–6.

Golgi C. (1907). Per la solenne inaugurazione dell'anno scolastico 1906–907. *Annuario dell'Università di Pavia. Anno scolastico 1906–907*. Tipografia successori Bizzoni, Pavia, pp. 5–19.

Golgi C. (1907a). Le condizioni fisiche dei contadini nelle zone risicole. *Atti del terzo Congresso Risicolo Internazionale*. Stab. Lito-Tipografico Giuseppe Abbiati, Milano, pp. 3–46 **of the reprint**.

Golgi C. (1908). Di un metodo per la facile e pronta dimostrazione dell'apparato reticolare interno delle cellule nervose. *Bollettino della Società Medico-Chirurgica di Pavia*, Anno 23°, pp. 81–7. *Gazzetta Medica Lombarda*, pp. 419–21. *Opera Omnia*, pp. 1293–8.

Golgi C. (1908a). Une méthode pour la prompte et facile démonstration de l'appareil rèticulaire interne des cellules nerveuses. *Archives Italiennes de Biologie*, **59**, pp. 269–74.

Golgi C. (1908b). Per la solenne inaugurazione dell'anno scolastico 1907–908. *Annuario Università di Pavia. Anno scolastico 1907–908.* Tipografia successori Bizzoni, Pavia, pp. 5–24.

Golgi C. (1909). Di una minuta particolarità di struttura dell'epitelio della mucosa gastrica ed intestinale di alcuni vertebrati. *Bollettino della Società Medico-Chirurgica di Pavia*, Anno 24°, pp. 1–22. *Archivio per le Scienze Mediche*, **33**, pp. 1–37. *Pathologica*, Anno 1°, N° 10, pp. 229–33. *Monitore Zoologico Italiano*, Anno 20°, pp. 50–2 (**summary**). *Opera Omnia*, pp. 1299–333.

Golgi C. (1909a). Sur une fine particularité de structure de l'épithélium de la muqueuse gastrique et intestinale de quelques vertébrés. *Archives Italiennes de Biologie*, **51**, pp. 213–45.

Golgi C. (1909b). Per la solenne inaugurazione dell'anno scolastico 1908–909. *Annuario Università di Pavia. Anno scolastico 1908–909.* Tipografia successori Bizzoni, Pavia, pp. 5–21.

Golgi C. (1909c). Discorso del Senatore Prof. Camillo Golgi. Fondazione 'Camillo Golgi'. *Annuario Università di Pavia. Anno scolastico 1908–909.* Tipografia successori Bizzoni, Pavia, pp. 373–80.

Golgi C. (1909d). Sulla struttura delle cellule nervose della corteccia del cervello. *Bollettino della Società Medico-Chirurgica di Pavia*, Anno 24°, pp. 341–8. *Opera Omnia*, pp. 1335–40.

Golgi C. (1909e). *Discorso di apertura del congresso per la fondazione di una Lega Nazionale contro la malaria.* Stab. Tipo-Litografico Romeo Longatti, Como, pp. 5–15 **of the reprint**. *Gazzetta Medica Lombarda*, Anno 68°, N° 42, pp. 417–19.

Golgi C. (1910). Evoluzione delle dottrine e delle conoscenze intorno al substrato anatomico delle funzioni psichiche e sensitive. *Atti della Società Italiana per il Progresso delle Scienze.* Tipografia Nazionale G. Bertero, Roma, pp. 3–74 **of the reprint. Also published** in Cimino (1995), pp. 47–122. *Opera Omnia*, pp. 1341–419.

Golgi C. (1910a). Le substratum anatomique de fonctions psychique et sensorielles. *Nederlandsch Tijdschrift vorr Genesskunden*, **45**, N° 17 (10 aprile), pp. 1196–232. Vereeniging Secties Voor Wetenschappelijken Arbeid. *Voordrachten Gehouden Voor de Medische en Natuurphilosophische Studenten der Universiteit Van Amsterdam*, N° 13, C. Golgi, pp. 3–40 **of the reprint**.

Golgi C. (1911). Breve cenno necrologico del Dott. Achille Visconti. *Rendiconti del R. Istituto Lombardo di Scienze e Lettere*, **44**, pp. 884–8.

Golgi C. (1912). L'opera scientifica di Adelchi Negri. *Bollettino della Società Medico-Chirurgica di Pavia*, Anno 27°, pp. 87–124.

Golgi C. (1912a). Bonifica umana o profilassi chimnica nelle regioni risicole. *Atti del quarto congresso risicolo internazionale.* Vercelli, pp. 3–56 **of the reprint. Also published** in Goldaniga e Marchetti (1993), pp. 174–92. *Opera Omnia*, pp. 1469–518.

Golgi C. (1913). *Per l'apertura dell'acquario-incubatorio a Pavia.* Pro Pavia Edizioni, Pavia.

Golgi C. (1913a). Parole pronunziate dal Senatore prof. Camillo Golgi nella seduta inaugurale del convegno nazionale di pesca lacuale e fluviale. *Atti del convegno nazionale di pesca lacuale e fluviale tenutosi in Pavia il 25–27 maggio*, pp. 1–3 **of the reprint. (No indication of the publisher and place of publication.)**

Golgi C. (1914). La moderna evoluzione delle dottrine e delle conoscenze sulla vita. *Rendiconti del R. Istituto Lombardo di Scienze e Lettere*, Serie 2ª, **47**, pp. 53–104. *Scientia, Rivista di Scienze*, **16**, pp. 199–224 (I parte); 1–20 **of the reprint (second part). Also published** in Cimino (1995), pp. 123–64. *Opera Omnia*, pp. 1421–67.

Golgi C. (1915). *Inaugurazione del secondo anno di vita autonoma della clinica neuropatologica. Discorso del Prof. Camillo Golgi.* Tipografia e legatoria cooperativa, Pavia, pp. 50–61.

Golgi C. (1916). La missione della Società Italiana per il progresso delle scienze nell'ora presente e nel prossimo avvenire. *Atti della Società Italiana per il Progresso delle Scienze.* Roma, pp. 3–16 **of the reprint. Also published** in Goldaniga e Marchetti (1993), pp. 225–31.

Golgi C. (1916a). *Note commemorative del presidente Prof. Camillo Golgi sul socio fondatore Prof. Architetto Ing. Angelo Savoldi.* 'Pro Pavia'. Associazione per gli interessi di Pavia. Successori Marelli, Pavia.

Golgi C. (1917). *Il Reparto Neuropatologico specializzato presso l'Ospedale Militare di riserva 'Collegio Borromeo' di Pavia.* Comitato Provinciale 'Pro Mutilati ed Invalidi' Tipografia A. Ponzio, Pavia. *Bollettino della Società Medico-Chirurgica di Pavia*, Anno 32°, pp. 2–59. **Also published** in Goldaniga e Marchetti (1993), pp. 233–49.

Golgi C. (1918). *A ricordo dell'Avv. Comm. Gaspare Emilio Brugnatelli.* Tipografia e legatoria cooperativa, Pavia.

Golgi C. (1918a). Carlo Forlanini. *Rendiconti R. Istituto Lombardo,* Serie 2ª, **51**, pp. 654–8.

Golgi C. (1918b). The neurological centres in Italy. *Inter-Allied Conference of After Care Disabled Men.* London, **2**, pp. 251–4.

Golgi C. (1919). Sulla struttura dei globuli rossi dell'uomo e di altri mammiferi. *Bollettino della Società Medico-Chirurgica di Pavia,* Anno 34°, pp. 197–214. *Haematologica* (1920), **1**, pp. 1–16. *Il Policlinico,* **26**, p. 858. *Opera Omnia,* pp. 1519–32.

Golgi C. (1920). Il centrosoma dei globuli rossi del sangue circolante dell'uomo e di altri mammiferi. *Rendiconti del R. Istituto Lombardo di Scienze e Lettere,* Serie 2ª, **53**, pp. 344–52. *Haematologica,* **1**, pp. 333–59. *Opera Omnia,* pp. 1533–42.

Golgi C. (1923). Intorno alla struttura ed alla biologia dei così detti globuli o piastrine del tuorlo. *Memorie del R. Istituto Lombardo di Scienze e Lettere,* **22** (13° della serie 3), pp. 161–74. *Opera Omnia,* pp. 1543–63.

Golgi C. (1925). *Opere di Agostino Bassi. Presentazione.* Tipografia cooperativa, Pavia, pp. 9–10.

Golgi C. (1929). *Opera Omnia,* Vol. IV. L. Sala, E. Veratti, and G. Sala (ed.). Hoepli Editore, Milano.

Golgi C. and Fusari R. (1895). *Nervensystem. Ergebnisse der Anatomie und Entwickelungsgeschichte (für 1894).* Verlagsbuchhandlung, J. Bergmann, Wiesbaden, pp. 205–307.

Golgi C. and Manfredi N. (1872). Annotazioni istologiche sulla retina del cavallo. *Giornale della R. Accademia di Medicina di Torino,* Anno 35°, Serie 3ª, **12**, pp. 289–307, 351–6. *Opera Omnia,* pp. 71–89.

Golgi C. and Monti A. (1884). Intorno ad una questione elmintologica. *Rendiconti del R. Istituto Lombardo di Scienze e Lettere.* Serie 2ª, **17**, pp. 285–8. *Gazzetta degli Ospitali,* **5**, p. 218.

Golgi C. and Monti A. (1885–86). Su la storia naturale e sul significato clinico patologico delle così dette anguillule intestinali e stercorali. *Atti della R. Accademia delle Scienze di Torino,* **21**, pp. 55–9.

Golgi C. and Monti A. (1886). Sulla storia naturale e sul significato clinico-patologico delle anguillule stercorali e intestinali. *Archivio per le Scienze Mediche,* **10**, pp. 93–108. *Opera Omnia,* pp. 973–88.

Golgi C. and Pensa A. (1900). Capsule surrenali e loro affezioni (morbo di Addison). *Trattato italiano di Chirurgia.* Vallardi, Milano, Vol. 5, Parte I (Organi genito-orinari maschili), pp. 185–208.

Golgi C. and Raggi A. (1880). Trasfusione di sangue nel peritoneo in un alienato oligocitemico. Effetti sul sangue circolante e sullo stato generale del paziente. *Rendiconti del R. Istituto Lombardo di Scienze e Lettere,* Serie 2ª, **13**, pp. 86–90. *Gazzetta Medica Italiana, Lombardia,* **40**, pp. 61–2. *Annali di Chimica applicati alla Medicina cioè alla Farmacia, alla Tossicologia, all'Igiene, alla Fisiologia, alla Patologia, ed alla Terapeutica,* **71**, pp. 37–41. *Gazzetta delle Cliniche di Torino,* **XVI**, N° 8, 24 febbraio. *Opera Omnia,* pp. 933–7.

Golgi C. and Raggi A. (1880a). Secondo caso di trasfusione peritoneale con esito felice in alienato oligocitemico. *Rendiconti del R. Istituto Lombardo di Scienze e Lettere.* Serie 2ª, **13**, pp. 206–9. *Opera Omnia,* pp. 939–42.

Golgi C. and Raggi A. (1880b). Primo caso di trasfusione peritoneale ripetuta, con un nuovo successo felice in alienato oligocitemico. *Rendiconti del R. Istituto Lombardo di Scienze e Lettere,* Serie 2ª, **13**, pp. 544–8. *Gazzetta delle Cliniche di Torino,* **XVI**, N° 28, 13 luglio. *Opera Omnia,* pp. 945–9.

Golgi C. and Silva B. (1891). Relazione sommaria sulla cura della tubercolosi con la linfa di Koch dopo otto mesi di esperienze in Pavia. *Riforma Medica,* N° 173, 174, luglio–agosto, pp. 3–45 **of the reprint**.

Gombault M. (1873). Études récentes relatives à l'anatomie normale de la néuroglie. *Archives de Physiologie normale et pathologique,* **5**, pp. 458–66.

Grant G. (1999). Golgi and Gustaf Retzius. *Journal of the History of the Neurosciences.* In press.

Grassi G. B. (1888). Su alcuni parassiti dell'uomo. *Atti del 12° congresso della Associazione Medica Italiana.* Tipografia Fratelli Fusi, Pavia, Vol. 1, pp. 136–45.

Grassi G. B. (1911). I progressi della Biologia e delle sue applicazioni pratiche conseguiti in Italia nell'ultimo cinquantennio. In *Cinquanta anni di storia Italiana.* Pubbl. della R. Accademia dei Lincei, Vol. 3, parte 1ª. Hoepli, Milano, pp. 1–416.

Gravela E. (1989). *Giulio Bizzozero.* U. Allemandi & C., Torino.

Greppin L. (1888). Weiterer Beitrag zur Kenntniss der Golgischen Untersuchungsmethode des centralen Nervensystems. *Archiv für Anatomie und Physiologie.* Suppl., pp. 55–78.

Greppin L. (1889). Beitrag zur Golgi'schen Färbungsmethode der nervösen Centralorgane. *Archiv für Psychiatrie und Nervenkrankheiten,* **20**, pp. 222–9.

Griffini L. (1882). Sull'immunità contro il Carbonchio. *Rendiconti del R. Istituto Lombardo di Scienze e Lettere*, Serie 2ª, **15**, pp. 546–7.

Gualino L. (1936). L'oculista Nicolò Manfredi da Boscomarengo (1836–1916). *Alexandria*, Anno 4°, N° 4–5, aprile-maggio.

Guderzo G. (1982). La riforma dell'Università di Pavia. In *Economia, Istituzione, Cultura in Lombardia nell'età di Maria Teresa* (ed. G. Barbarini, A. De Maddalena, and E. Rotelli). Vol. III, Il Mulino, Bologna.

Guthrie D. (1958). *A History of medicine.* Thomas Nelson and Sons, London. **It. trans.** L. Dann Treves, *Storia della Medicina.* Feltrinelli (1967, 1977).

Hayden M. R. (1981). *Huntington's chorea.* Springer-Verlag, Berlin, pp. 1–12.

Hebb D. O. (1949). *The organization of behaviour.* Wiley, New York.

His W. (1886). Zur Geschichte des menschlichen Rückenmarkes und der Nervenwurzeln. Abhandlungen der mathematisch-physischen Classe der Königl. *Sächsischen Gesellschaft der Wissenschaften*, **13**, pp. 147–209, 477–514.

Huxley A. F. (1977). Looking back on muscle. In T*he pursuit of nature: informal essays on the history of physiology.* Cambridge University Press, New York, pp. 23–64.

Introzzi P. (1961). Figure illustri della clinica medica e della ematologia dell'Università di Pavia. In *Discipline e Maestri dell'Ateneo Pavese.* Arnoldo Mondadori editore, Verona, pp. 321–35.

Jacobson M. (1975). Development and evolution of type II Neurons: Conjectures a century after Golgi. In *Golgi centennial symposium* (ed. M. Santini). Proceedings. Raven Press, New York, pp. 147–51.

Jacobson M. (1993). *Foundations of neuroscience.* Plenum Press, New York and London.

James W. (1890). *The Principles of psychology,* Vol. II. Holt, New York.

Klebs E. and Tommasi-Crudeli C. (1879). Studi sulla natura della malaria. *Atti della R. Accademia dei Lincei. Memoria della Classe di Scienze Fisiche, Matematiche e Naturali*, **4**, pp. 172–235.

Klebs E. and Tommasi-Crudeli C. (1879a). Studien über die Ursache des Wechselfiebers und über die Natur der Malaria. *Archiv für experimentelle Pathologie und Pharmakologie*, **11**, pp. 311–98.

Klein E. (1885). *Nouveaux éléments d'histologie.* O. Doin, Paris.

Kölliker A. von (1856). *Manuale di istologia umana pei medici e studenti di A. Kölliker Professore di Anatomia e Fisiologia in Wurzburg.* Versione compendiata sulla seconda edizione tedesca del Dott. E. Oehl, Società per la Pubblicazione degli Annali Universali delle Scienze e dell'Industria, Milano.

Kölliker A. von (1867). *Handbuch der Gewebelehre des Menschen.* Engelmann, Leipzig.

Kölliker A. von (1887). Ueber Golgi's Untersuchungen, den feineren Bau des centralen Nervensystems betreffend. *Sitzungsberichte der Physikalisch-Medicinischen Gesellschaft zu Würzburg*, pp. 56–62, 68.

Kölliker A. von (1887a). Die Untersuchungen von Golgi über den feineren Bau des zentralen Nervensystems. *Anatomischer Anzeiger*, **2**, pp. 480–3.

Kölliker A. von (1890). Ueber den feineren Bau des Rückenmarks. *Sitzungsberichte der Physikalisch-Medicinischen Gesellschaft zu Würzburg*, pp. 44–56.

Kölliker A. von (1890a). Zur feineren Anatomie des centralen Nervensystems. Zweiter Beitrag. Das Rückenmark. *Zeitschrift für wissenschaftliche Zoologie*, **51**, pp. 1–54.

Kölliker A. von (1899). *Erinnerungen aus meinem Leben.* Engelmann, Leipzig.

Kölliker A. von (1900). Kurzer Bericht über den Anatomischen Kongress zu Pavia 1900. *Verhandlungen der Physikalisch-Medicinischen Gesellschaft zu Würzburg*, 34, d. N. F., N° 1, pp. 1–29.

Kölliker A. von (1902). Die Golgifeier in Pavia. *Anatomischer Anzeiger*, **22**, pp. 325–8.

Kopsch F. (1902). Die Darstellung des Binnennetzes in spinalen Ganglienzellen und anderen Körperzellen mittels Osmiumsäure. *Sitzungsberichte der K. Preussischen Akademie der Wissenschaften*, **2**, pp. 929–932.

Koulischioff A. (1886). Sui microrganismi dei lochj normali. *Bollettino della Società Medico-Chirurgica di Pavia*, Anno 1°, pp. 62–4. *Gazzetta degli Ospitali* (1886), Anno 7°, pp. 612–13. **The number of the page quoted in the text refers to** *Gazzetta degli Ospitali*.

Kronthal P. (1887). Zur patologischen Anatomie der progressiven Paralyse der Irren. *Neurologisches Central-blatt*, **6**, pp. 313–18.

Kuhn T. S. (1962). *The structure of scientific revolutions.* University of Chicago Press, Chicago.

Kuhn T. S. (1970). *The structure of scientific revolutions.* Second (enlarged) edition. University of Chicago Press, Chicago.

Lain Entralgo P. (1949). *Dos Biologos: Claudio Bernard y Ramón y Cajal*. Espasa Calpe, Buenos Aires.

Lambertini G. (1990). Le scoperte del Ruffini sui recettori nervosi e il suo carteggio con lo Sherrington. In *Lo sviluppo storico della neurologia italiana: lo studio delle fonti* (ed. G. Zanchin and L. Premuda). La Garangola, Padova, pp. 133–40.

Lashley K. S. (1929). *Brain mechanisms and intelligence: a quantitative study of injuries to the brain*. University of Chicago Press, Chicago.

Laveran C. L. A. (1880). Note sur un nouveau parasite trouvé dans le sang de plusieurs malades atteints de fièvre palustre. *Bullettin de l'Académie de Médecine*, 2nd series, **9** p. 1235.

Laveran C. L. A. (1880a). Deuxième note relative à un nouveau parasite trouvé dans le sang des malades atteints de la fièvre palustre. *Bullettin de l'Académie de Médecine*, 2nd series, **9**, pp. 1346–7.

Laveran C. L. A. (1884). *Traité des fièvres palustres avec la description des microbes du paludisme*. Octave Doin, Paris.

Laveran C. L. A. (1887). Des hématozoaires du paludisme. *Annales de l'Institut Pasteur*, **1**, pp. 266–88.

Legée G. (1982). Evolution de l'histologie du système nerveux au XIXe siècle; l'impulsion donnée par Camillo Golgi (1844–1926). *Clio Medica*, **17**, pp. 15–32.

Linskens H. F. and Cresti M. (1996). Golgi in Siena. *Atti Accademia Fisiocritici*. Serie 15ᵃ, **15**, pp. 45–53.

Liberini P. and Spano P. (1995). Science, medicine and Golgi. *Nature Medicine*, **1** p. 386.

Locatelli P. (1961). Patologia generale e istituzione del primo gabinetto di patologia sperimentale cento anni or sono a Pavia. *Atti della Società Italiana di Patologia*, **7**, Parte 2ᵃ, Milano, pp. 451–64.

Locatelli P. (1961a). Camillo Golgi e l'indirizzo di studio nella scuola di Patologia Generale all'Università di Pavia. *Archivio per le Scienze Mediche*, **112**, pp. 407–19.

Lombroso C. (1865). *La medicina legale delle alienazioni mentali studiata con il metodo esperimentale*. Prosperini, Padova.

Lombroso C. (1867). Le pigmentazioni e l'erpetismo nelle alienazioni mentali. *Giornale Italiano delle malattie veneree e delle malattie della pelle*, Anno 2°, **4**, pp. 17–29.

Lombroso C. (1868). Sulla pellagra maniaca e sua cura. Lettera del prof. Cesare Lombroso al prof. Griesinger. *Giornale Italiano delle malattie veneree e delle malattie della pelle*, Anno 3°, **5**, pp. 83–97.

Lombroso C. (1868a). Apoplessia e rammollimento del cervello seguita da mania epilettica e da ematomi intermuscolari e sottoperiostei. *Rivista Clinica*, Anno 7°, pp. 205–6.

Lombroso C. (1868b). Pseudomelanosi ed infiammazione corticale del cervello e mania per causa morale. *Rivista Clinica*. Anno 7°, pp. 301–2.

Lombroso C. and Golgi C. (1873). Diagnosi medico-legali eseguite col metodo antropologico e sperimentale. *Annali Universali di Medicina*, **223**, Fasc. 668, pp. 225–85. **Parts of this article were also published** in *Archivio Italiano per le Malattie Nervose e Mentali* **and** in *Gazzetta Medica Italiana, Provincie Venete*.

Lombroso C. (1882). Gasparone. *Archivio di Psichiatria, Antropologia Criminale e Scienze Penali per servire allo studio dell'uomo alienato e delinquente*, **3**, pp. 269–80. **Also published** in C. Lombroso (1995). Delitto, Genio, Follia. *Scritti scelti* (ed. D. Frigessi, F. Giacanelli, and L. Mangoni). Bollati Boringhieri, Torino, pp. 261–7.

Lombroso C. (1887). Le nuove conquiste della Psichiatria. *Rivista di Filosofia Scientifica*, **6**, pp. 641–59. **Part of the article also** in C. Lombroso (1995). Delitto, Genio, Follia. *Scritti scelti* (ed. D. Frigessi, F. Giacanelli, and L. Mangoni). Bollati Boringhieri, Torino, pp. 212–14.

Lombroso P. and Lombroso G. (1906). *Cesare Lombroso. Appunti sulla vita. Le opere*. Bocca, Torino.

Lombroso Ferrero G. (1915). *Cesare Lombroso. Storia della vita e delle opere narrata dalla figlia*. Bocca, Torino.

Lovejoy A. O. (1959). Kant and evolution. In *Forerunners of Darwin 1745–1859* (ed. B. Glass, O. Temkin, and W. L. Strauss). Johns Hopkins University Press, Baltimore, pp. 173–206.

Luciani, L. (1884) On the sensorial localizations in the cortex cerebri. *Brain*, 7, 145–60.

Luciani L. (1905). *Fisiologia dell'uomo*. Vol. 2. Società Editrice Libraria, Milano.

Luciani L. and Tamburini A. (1878–79). Ricerche sperimentali sulle funzioni del cervello. *Rivista Sperimentale di Freniatria e Medicina Legale* (1878), **4**, pp. 69–89; (1879), **5**, pp. 1–76.

Lugaro E. (1895). Sulla struttura del nucleo dentato del cervello nell'uomo. *Monitore zoologico Italiano*, **6**, pp. 5–12.

Lugaro E. (1898). A proposito di un presunto rivestimento isolatore della cellula nervosa. *Rivista di Patologia Nervosa e Mentale*, **3**, pp. 265–71.

Maggi L. (1895). *Su la sottrazione di locali al nuovo Istituto di Anatomia e Fisiologia comparate della R. Università di Pavia nell'ex palazzo Botta. Protesta presentata il 24 febbraio 1895 all'onorevole presidente della deputazione provinciale di Pavia.* Tipografia e legatoria cooperativa, Pavia.

Maggi L. (1899). L'Istituto di Anatomia e Fisiologia comparate e di Protistologia della R. Università di Pavia. *Bollettino Scientifico di Pavia*, Anno 21°, N° 4, pp. 1–8 **of the reprint**.

Magini G. (1888). Nevroglia e cellule nervose cerebrali nei feti. *Atti del 12° congresso della Associazione Medica Italiana.* Tipografia Fratelli Fusi, Pavia, Vol. 1, pp. 281–91.

Magini (G.) J. (1888a). Nouvelles recherches histologiques sur le cerveau du foetus. *Archives Italiennes de Biologie*, **10**, pp. 384–7.

Majno E. (1984). La fondazione della Clinica del Lavoro di Milano attraverso il carteggio Luigi Devoto—Ersilia Majno Bronzini. *Memorie dell'Istituto Lombardo—Accademia di Scienze Lettere Classe di Scienze Matematiche e Naturali*, **XXVIII**, pp. 223–310.

Majno E. (1994). La diffusione all'estero delle scoperte di Camillo Golgi. In *La storia della medicina e della scienza tra archivio e laboratorio* (ed. G. Cimino and C. Maccagni). Olschki, Firenze, pp. 129–38.

Mangiagalli L. (1907). *Il presente e l'avvenire dell'insegnamento medico di perfezionamento in Milano.* Stab. Tipografico Enrico Reggiani, Milano, pp. 1–25.

Mann G. (1894). Ueber die Behandlung der Nervenzellen für experimentellhistologische Untersuchungen. *Zeitschrift für wissenschaftliche Mikroskopie und für mikroskopische Technik*, **11**, pp. 479–94.

Mantegazza P. (1859). Sulle virtù igieniche e medicinali della coca e sugli alimenti nervosi in generale. *Annali Universali di Medicina*, Serie 4ª, **31**, pp. 449–519.

Marcacci A. (1909). *Discorso del Presidente del Comitato, Prof. Arturo Marcacci.* Fondazione Camillo Golgi. Annuario Università di Pavia. Anno scolastico 1908–909. Tipografia successori Bizzoni, Pavia, pp. 355–63.

Marchi V. (1880–81). Sugli organi terminali nervosi nei tendini dei muscoli motori dell'occhio. *Atti della R. Accademia delle Scienze di Torino*, **16**, pp. 206–7.

Marchi V. (1881). Sugli organi terminali nervosi (corpi di Golgi) nei tendini dei muscoli motori del bulbo oculare. *Archivio per le Scienze Mediche*, **5**, pp. 273–82.

Marchi V. (1882). Ueber Terminalorgane der Nerven (Golgi's Nervenkörperchen) in den Sehnen der Augenmuskeln. *Albrecht v. Graefes Archiv für Ophthalmologie*, **28**, pp. 203–13.

Marchi V. (1883). Sulla fina anatomia dei corpi striati. *Rivista Sperimentale di Freniatria e Medicina Legale*, **9**, pp. 331–4.

Marchi V. (1883a). Sull'istologia patologica della paralisi progressiva. *Rivista Sperimentale di Freniatria e Medicina Legale*, **9**, pp. 220–1.

Marchi V. and Algeri G. (1885). Sulle degenerazioni discendenti consecutive a lesioni della corteccia cerebrale. *Rivista Sperimentale di Freniatria e Medicina Legale*, **11**, pp. 492–4.

Marchiafava E. (1894). Sulle febbri estivo-autunnali in genere, in ispecie sulla perniciosa con localizzazione gastro-intestinale. *Atti XI Congresso Internazionale di Medicina. Sezione di Patologia Generale ed Anatomia Patologica*, pp. 226–30.

Marchiafava E. and Celli A. (1884). Sulle alterazioni dei globuli rossi nella infezione da malaria e sulla genesi della melanemia. *Atti della R. Accademia dei Lincei. Memoria della Classe di Scienze Fisiche, Matematiche e Naturali*, **18**, pp. 381–402.

Marchiafava E. and Celli A. (1885). Nuove ricerche sulla infezione malarica. *Archivio per le Scienze Mediche*, **9**, pp. 311–40.

Marchiafava E. and Celli A. (1885a). Neue Untersuchungen über die Malaria-Infection. *Fortschritte der Medizin*, **3**, pp. 339–54.

Marchiafava E. and Celli A. (1885b). Weitere Untersuchungen über die Malariainfection. *Fortschritte der Medizin*, **3**, pp. 787–806.

Marchiafava E. and Celli A. (1886). Studi ulteriori sulla infezione malarica. *Archivio per le Scienze Mediche*, **10**, pp. 185–211.

Marcora F. (1927). Camillo Golgi. *Rivista di Biologia*, **9**, pp. 117–27.

Mariani M. (1900). Cenni storici intorno all'Università. *Annuario Università di Pavia, anno scolastico 1899–900.* Tipografia successori Bizzoni, Pavia, pp. 5–19.

Marinesco G. (1909). *La cellule nerveuse*. Octave Doin et Fils, Paris.

Mariotti U. and Ciarrocchi G. (1884). Sulla trasmissibilità dell'infezione da Malaria. *Lo Sperimentale*, Anno 38°, pp. 623–30.

Martinotti C. (1889). Contributo allo studio della corteccia cerebrale e dell'origine centrale dei nervi. *Bollettino della Società Medico-Chirurgica di Pavia*, Anno 4°, N° 2, pp. 36–9.

Martinotti C. (1890). Beitrag zum Studium der Hirnrinde und dem Centralursprung der Nerven. Internationale Monatsschrift für Anatomie und Physiologie. *Journal International d'Anatomie et de Physiologie*, **7**, pp. 69–90.

Martinotti C. (1897). Su alcune particolarità delle cellule nervose del midollo spinale messe in evidenza colla reazione nera del Golgi. *Giornale della R. Accademia di Medicina di Torino*, Serie 4ª, **40**, pp. 103–4.

Mayer S. (1879). Specielle Nervenphysiologie. In *Handbuch der Physiologie* (ed. L. Hermann). F. C. W. Vogel, Leipzig, pp. 199–288.

Mazzarello P. (1993). Un inedito autobiografico di Camillo Golgi. *Istituto Lombardo (Rend. Sc.) B.*, **127**, pp. 327–41.

Mazzarello P. and Della Sala S. (1993). The demonstration of the visual area by means of the atrophic degeneration method in the work of Bartolomeo Panizza (1855). *Journal of History of Neuroscience*, **2**, pp. 315–22.

Medea E. (1918). Camillo Golgi. *Rivista d'Italia*, Anno 21°, **3**, pp. 447–55.

Medea E. (1966). *Come, quando, dove li ho conosciuti. Profili di grandi medici*. Edizioni Minerva Medica, Torino.

Metschnikoff E. (1887). Sur la lutte des cellules de l'organisme contre l'invasion des microbes. *Annales de l'Institut Pasteur*, **1**, pp. 321–36.

Milani M. (1985). *Storia di Pavia*. Camunia Editrice, Brescia.

Mondino C. (1884). Sulla struttura delle fibre nervose midollate periferiche. *Archivio per le Scienze Mediche*, **8**, pp. 45–66.

Mondino C. (1885). Sull'uso del bicloruro di mercurio nello studio degli organi centrali del sistema nervoso. *Giornale della R. Accademia di Medicina di Torino*, Anno 48°, **33**, pp. 38–47.

Mondino C. (1885a). Ricerche sull'antimuro e sul nucleo amigdaleo. *Archivio per le Scienze Mediche*, **9**, pp. 117–30.

Monti A. (1890). Una nuova reazione degli elementi del sistema nervoso centrale. *Rendiconti della R. Accademia dei Lincei*, **5** (1° semestre), pp. 705–9.

Monti A. (1895). *Sulla fina anatomia del bulbo olfattorio. Fatti vecchi e nuovi che contraddicono alla teoria dei neuroni*. Tip. Fratelli Fusi, Pavia.

Monti A. (1926). Per la storia dell'anatomia patologica in Pavia. *Bollettino della Società Medico-Chirurgica di Pavia*, **40**, pp. 777–95.

Monti A. (1927). *La figura di Antonio Scarpa nella storia della scienza e nelle fortune dell'università di Pavia*. Istituto Pavese di Arti Grafiche, Pavia. **Engl. trans.** F. L. Loria. *Antonio Scarpa in scientific history and his role in the fortunes of the University of Pavia*. Vigo Press, New York (1957).

Monti A. (1935). *Congedo*. Hoepli, Milano.

Morpurgo B. (1926). Camillo Golgi (1843–1926). Commemorazione fatta dal Prof. Morpurgo alla R. Accademia di Medicina di Torino. *Giornale della R. Accademia di Medicina di Torino*, Anno 89°, Serie 4ª, **32**, pp. 31–52; *Note e Riviste di Psichiatria* (1926), Serie 3ª, **14**, N° 1, pp. 199–218. Il testo con il titolo 'Commemorazione del socio nazionale prof. Camillo Golgi letta dal socio Benedetto Morpurgo nella seduta del 2 maggio 1926'e l'aggiunta di una frase finale si trova anche *nelle Memorie della R. Accademia Nazionale dei Lincei. Classe di Scienze Fisiche, Matematiche e Naturali* (1927), **2**, pp. I–XVIII. **The number of the page quoted in the text refers to** *Giornale della R. Accademia di Medicina di Torino*.

Morselli E. (1875). **Review of Golgi's article** Sulle alterazioni degli organi centrali nervosi in un caso di corea gesticolatoria associata ad alienazione mentale. *Rivista Sperimentale Freniatria e Medicina Legale*, **1**, pp. 132–4.

Moruzzi G. (1973). L'opera elettrofisiologica di Carlo Matteucci. *Quaderni di storia della scienza e della medicina*, **12**, pp. 1–53.

Mosso A. (1887). Degenerazione dei corpuscoli rossi del sangue. *Atti della R. Accademia dei Lincei. Rendiconti*, Serie 4ª, **3** (1° semestre), pp. 334–9.

Mosso A. (1897). *Fisiologia dell'uomo sulle alpi*. Fratelli Treves Editori, Milano.

Mountcastle V. B. (1995). The evolution of ideas concerning the function of the neocortex. *Cerebral Cortex*, **5**, pp. 289–95.

Nansen F. (1887). *The structure and combination of the histological elements of the central nervous system*. Bergens Museums Aarsberetning 1886. John Griegs Bogtrykkeri, Bergen.

Nansen F. (1887a). Les éléments nerveux, leur structure et leurs réunions dans le système nerveux central. *Nordiskt Medicinskt Arkiv*, **19**, N° 27, pp. 3–6.

Negri A. (1900). Di una fina particolarità di struttura delle cellule di alcune ghiandole dei mammiferi. *Bollettino della Società Medico-Chirurgica di Pavia*, Anno 15°, pp. 61–70.

Negri A. (1903). Contributo allo studio della eziologia della rabbia. *Bollettino della Società Medico-Chirurgica di Pavia*, Anno 18°, pp. 88–114.

Negri A. (1903a). Beitrag zum Studium der Aetiologie der Tollwuth. *Zeitschrift für Hygiene und Infectionskrankheiten*, **43**, pp. 507–28.

Obersteiner H. (1883). Ursprung und centrale Verbindungen der Riechnerven. *Biologisches Centralblatt*, **3**, pp. 464–8.

Obersteiner H. (1888). *Anleitung beim Studium des Baues der Nervösen Centralorgane im gesunden und kranken Zustande*. Toeplitz & Deuticke, Leipzig und Wien.

Obregia A. (1890). Fixierungsmethode der Golgi'chen Präparate des centralen Nervensystems. *Virchow Archiv*, **122**, pp. 387–8.

Orsi F. (1881). Episodio nella storia del bacillus malariae. Curiosità cliniche. *Gazzetta Medica Italiana, Lombardia*, **41**, pp. 91–2.

Orsi F. (1881a). La portata scientifica del 1°. articolo delle mie curiosità cliniche. *Gazzetta Medica Italiana, Lombardia*, **41**, pp. 211–12.

Pagel J. (1901). *Biographisches Lexikon hervorragender Ärzte des neunzehnten Jahrhunderts*. Urban & Schwarzenberg, Berlin.

Pancaldi G. (1983). *Darwin in Italia*. Società Editrice il Mulino, Bologna.

Panizza B. (1855). Osservazioni sul nervo ottico. *Giornale dell'I. R. Istituto Lombardo di Scienze Lettere ed Arti*, **7**, pp. 237–52. *Memorie dell'I. R. Istituto Lombardo di Scienze Lettere ed Arti (1856)*, **5**, pp. 375–90.

Papez J. W. (1953). Theodor Meynert (1833–1892). In *The founders of neurology* (ed. W. Haymaker). C. Thomas, Springfield, pp. 64–7.

Papez J. W. (1953a). Bernhard Aloys von Gudden (1824–1886). In *The founders of neurology* (ed. W. Haymaker). C. Thomas, Springfield, pp. 45–8.

Pasi Testa A. (1981). Il colera a Pavia nell'Ottocento. Annali di Storia Pavese. N° 6–7, pp. 39–56.

Pensa A. (1926). Commemorazione di Camillo Golgi nel trigesimo della morte detta alla Società Medico-Chirurgica di Parma il 24 febbraio 1926 dal socio A. P. *Bollettino della Società Medica di Parma*, 19, d. S. II, pp. 33–50; *Giornale di Clinica Medica* (1926), **7**, pp. 121–35. **Engl. trans. in** *Journal of American Association for Medico-Physical Research* (1927), **4**, pp. 187–95. **The number of the page quoted in the text refers to** *Bollettino della Società Medica di Parma*.

Pensa A. (1961). Pietro Moscati, Antonio Scarpa, Bartolomeo Panizza, Agostino Bassi, Giulio Bizzozero e Camillo Golgi. In *Discipline e Maestri dell'Ateneo Pavese*. Arnoldo Mondadori editore, Verona, pp. 235–82.

Pensa A. (1961a). *Trattato di istologia generale*. Ristampa della 5ª edizione con appendice. Società Editrice Libraria, Milano.

Pensa A. (1961b). *Visita al Museo della storia dell'Università di Pavia*. Alfieri & Lacroix, Milano.

Pensa A. (1991). *Ricordi di vita universitaria*. B. Zanobio ed. Cisalpino Istituto Editoriale Universitario Milano.

Pera M. (1982). *Apologia del metodo*. Laterza, Bari.

Pera M. (1986). *La rana ambigua*. Einaudi, Torino (reprinted 1994).

Perls M. (1877). *Lehrbuch der Allgemeinen Pathologischen Anatomie und Pathogenese*. Verlag von Ferdinand Enke, Stuttgart.

Perroncito A. (1926). Commemorazione di Camillo Golgi. *Bollettino della Società Medico-Chirurgica di Pavia*, **40** (Suppl), pp. 11–48; *Il Policlinico, Sezione pratica*, **33**, pp. 387–91. **The number of the page quoted in the text refers to** *Bollettino della Società Medico-Chirurgica di Pavia*.

Perroncito E. (1883). Sulla trasmissibilità del carbonchio dalle madri ai feti. *Atti della R. Accademia dei Lincei. Memoria della Classe di Scienze Fisiche, Matematiche e Naturali*, **14**, pp. 201–10.

Pertik O. (1881). Untersuchungen über Nervenfasern. *Archiv für Mikroskopische Anatomie*, **19**, pp. 183–239.

Piccolino M. (1988). Cajal and the retina: a 100-year retrospective. *Trends in Neuroscience*, **11**, pp. 521–5.

Piccolino M., Laurenzi E., and Strettoi E. (1988). Un secolo dopo l'anno della fortuna: teoria del neurone, reti nervose e retina nell'opera di Santiago Ramón y Cajal. *Fidia Biomedical Information*, N° 9–10, pp. 18–29.

Pilleri G. (1984). *Camillo Golgi (1843–1926); Santiago Ramón y Cajal (1852–1934); Adelchi Negri (1876–1912)*. Biographical sketches published for the 50th anniversary of the Bern University Brain Anatomy Institute. Vammalan Kirjapaino Oy, Vammala (Finland).

Podwyssozki W. (1886). Experimentelle Untersuchungen über die Regeneration der Drüsengewebe. Erster thei. Untersuchungen über die Regeneration des Lebergewebes. *Beiträge zur pathologischen Anatomie und zur allgemeinen Pathologie*, **1**, pp. 259–360.

Pogliano C. (1985). Bizzozero. In *Dizionario Biografico della Storia della Medicina e delle Scienze Naturali*. Franco Maria Ricci editore, Milano, pp. 111–12.

Putelli R. (1913). *La fulgidissima gloria camuna: il senatore Camillo Golgi da Corteno*. Illustrazione Camuna e Sebina, settembre.

Putelli R. (1923). *Il senatore Prof. Camillo Golgi da Corteno*. Illustrazione Camuna, 6 giugno. **See also** *Dal Tonale al Sebino*, anno 2°, numero 1 (1953).

Raggi A. (1898). Commemorazione del M. E. Andrea Verga. Rendiconti del R. Istituto Lombardo di Scienze e Lettere, **31**, pp. 75–110.

Raimondi C. (1880). Degli avvelenamenti lenti di arsenico mercurio e piombo con ispeciale riguardo alle alterazioni del midollo delle ossa. *Annali Universali di Medicina*, **251**, pp. 52–92.

Ranvier M. L. (1873). Sur les éléments conjonctifs de la moelle épinière. *Comptes Rendus hebdomadaires des séances de l'Académie des sciences*, Juillet-Décembre, pp. 1299–302.

Ranvier M. L. (1875–1886). *Traité Technique d'Histologie*. F. Savy, Paris.

Ranvier M. L. (1882). De la Névroglie. *Comptes Rendus hebdomadaires des séances de l'Académie des sciences*, Janvier-Juin, pp. 1536–9.

Raviola E. and Gilula N. B. (1973). Gap junctions between photoreceptor cells in the vertebrate retina. *Proceedings of the National Academy of Sciences (USA)*, **70**, pp. 1677–81.

Renaut J. (1882). Recherches sur les centres nerveux amyéliniques. *Archives de Physiologie normale et pathologique*, **9**, 1er semestre, pp. 593–638.

Retzius G. (1890). *Zur Kenntnis des Nervensystems der Crustaceen*. Biologisches Untersuchungen, Neue Folge, Samson & Wallin, Vol. 1, pp. 1–50.

Retzius G. (1908). The principles of the minute structure of the nervous system as revealed by recent investigations. *Proceedings of the Royal Society of London. Series B*, **80**, pp. 414–43.

Retzius G. (1948). *Biografiska Anteckningar och Minnen*. Vol. 2. Almqvist & Wiksell AB, Uppsala.

Rezzonico G. (1880). Sulla struttura delle fibre nervose del midollo spinale. *Archivio per le Scienze Mediche*, 4, N° 4, pp. 78–88.

Richard M. (1882). Sur le parasite de la malaria. *Comptes Rendus hebdomadaires des séances de l'Académie des sciences*, Janvier-Juin, pp. 496–9.

Rindfleisch E. (1872). Zur Kenntniss der Nervenendigung in der Hirnrinde. *Archiv für Mikroskopische Anatomie*, **8**, pp. 453–4.

Riquier G. C. (1952). Camillo Golgi e la sua polemica con S. Ramón Y Cajal. *Atti del Primo Congresso Internazionale di Istopatologia del Sistema Nervoso—Proceedings of the first International Congress of Neuropathology*. Casa Editrice Libraria Rosenberg and Sellier, Torino, pp. 51–7.

Rizzoli A. A. (1990). Vittorio Marchi, neurologo ed istologo. In *Lo sviluppo storico della neurologia italiana: lo studio delle fonti* (ed. G. Zanchin and L. Premuda). La Garangola, Padova, pp. 219–24.

Roizin L. (1953). Vittorio Marchi (1851–1908). In *The founders of neurology* (ed. W. Haymaker). C. Thomas, Springfield, pp. 61–3.

Rondoni P. (1943). Commemorazione di Camillo Golgi (1843–1926). *Atti R. Accademia d'Italia. Rendiconti della Classe di Scienze Fisiche, Matematiche e Naturali*, **4**, d. s. VII, pp. 536–46.

Rondoni P. (1943a). Camillo Golgi (1843–1926). *Bollettino dell'Istituto Sieroterapico Milanese*, **22**, pp. 223–6.

Rossbach M. J. and Sehrwald E. (1888). *Ueber die Lymphwege des Gehirns*. Centralblatt für die medicinischen Wissenschaften, pp. 498–501.

Rossi O. (1927). *Camillo Golgi. Conferenza commemorativa tenuta dal Prof. O. R. Rettore Magnifico della R. Università di Pavia, Ordinario di Neuropatologia nel Salone del Palazzo Municipale di Varese il giorno 11 novembre 1927*. Arti grafiche Gaviratesi, Varese.

Rostand J. (1951). *Les origines de la biologie expérimentale et l'Abbé Spallanzani*. Fasquelle Editeurs, Paris. **It. trans.** G. Barberis, *Lazzaro Spallanzani e le origini della biologia sperimentale*. Picc. Bibl. Einaudi, Torino (1963), second edition (1967).

Sacerdotti C. (1926). Camillo Golgi. *Pathologica*, **18**, pp. 53–6.

Sacerdotti C. (1947). Due grandi maestri visti da un allievo. *L'illustrazione del Medico*, pp. 1–4.

Saffron M. H. (1980). Donaldson, Henry Herbert. In *Dictionary of scientific biography* (ed. C. Gillispie). Scribner, New York, pp. 160–1.

Sala L. (1925). Camillo Golgi. In *Universitatis Ticinensis Saecularia Undecima* (ed. G. Rossi, P. Fraccaro, and L. Montemartini). Tipografia Soc. An. Bruni Marelli, Pavia, pp. 41–2.

Salvatorelli L. (1971). *Storia del Novecento*. Oscar Mondadori, Milano.

Sangalli G. (1882). Bacterj del carbonchio nel feto di giovenca morta per questa malattia. *Rendiconti del R. Istituto Lombardo di Scienze e Lettere*, Serie 2ª, **15**, pp. 668–72; Controsservazioni. Ibid., pp. 674–80.

Sanquirico C. (1882). Sulla trasfusione del sangue. *Gazzetta degli Ospitali*, Anno 3°, pp. 241–2.

Santamaria L. (1994). Camillo Golgi patologo clinico. *Bollettino della Società Medico-Chirurgica di Pavia*, **108** (Suppl.1), pp. 25–45.

Santini M. (ed.) (1975). *Golgi centennial symposium*. Proceedings. Raven Press, New York.

Savoldi F. (1990). Guido Sala neurologo. *Bollettino della Società Pavese di Storia Patria*, **42**, pp. 263–70.

Scarpa A. (1938). *Epistolario* (ed. G. Sala). Tipografia B. Bianchi, Pavia.

Schiavuzzi B. (1888). Untersuchungen über die Malaria in Pola. *Beiträge zur Biologie der Pflanzen*, **5**, pp. 245–89.

Schiefferdecker P. (1886). Studien zur vergleichenden Histologie der Retina. *Archiv für Mikroskopische Anatomie*, **28**, pp. 305–96.

Schultze M. (1868). *Observationes de structura cellularum fibrarumque nervearum*. Bonner Universitats-programm.

Schultze M. (1871). Allgemeiner uber die Structurelemente des Nervensystems. In *Handbuch der lehre von den geweben des menschen und thiere* (ed. S. Stricker). Leipzig, pp. 108–36.

Schwalbe G. (1881). *Lehrbuch der Neurologie*. Verlag von Eduard Besold, Erlangen.

Sehrwald E. (1889). Zur Technik der Golgischen Färbung. *Zeitschrift für wissenschaftliche Mikroskopie*, **6**, pp. 443–56.

Senise T. (1926). Camillo Golgi. *Il cervello*, **5**, pp. 60–4.

Seppilli G. (1877). Golgi. Degenerazione calcarea delle cellule nervose. *Rivista Sperimentale di Freniatria e Medicina Legale*, **3**, pp. 491–2.

Seppilli G. (1880). Recensione del lavoro di Golgi (1879). Sulla struttura delle fibre nervose midollate periferiche e centrali. *Rivista Sperimentale di Freniatria e Medicina Legale*, **6**, pp. 226–7.

Seppilli G. (1881). **On the communication of** Caselli, Golgi Raggi, Trasfusioni peritoneali in alienati oligoemici **to the Congress of Reggio Emilia (23–29 September 1880)**. *Archivio Italiano per le Malattie Nervose*, Anno 18°, pp. 17–21.

Shepherd G. M. (1991). *Foundations of the neuron doctrine*. Oxford University Press, New York.

Sherrington C. S. (1935). Santiago Ramón y Cajal 1852–1934. *Obituary Notice of the Royal Society of London*, N° 4, pp. 425–41.

Shryock R. H. (1936). *The development of modern medicine, an interpretation of the social and scientific factors involved*. Hafner Publishing, New York, succ. ediz. 1947, 1969. **It. trans.** *Storia della medicina nella società moderna*. Isedi, Milano (1977).

Signori E. (1993). L'Università in uniforme. Momenti e aspetti di vita universitaria a Pavia tra regime e guerra mondiale. *Storia in Lombardia*, N° 1–2, pp. 191–247.

Simon T. (1874). Das Spinnenzellen und Pinselzellen—Gliom. *Archiv für pathologische Anatomie und Physiologie und für Klinische medicin*, **61**, pp. 90–100.

Soury J. (1892). *Les fonctions du cerveau*. Babé, Paris.

Soury J. (1899). *Système nerveux central. Structure & fonctions. Histoire critique des théories et des doctrines*. Carré & Naud, Paris.

Spadoni D. (1925). Cenno storico della università di Pavia. In *Universitatis Ticinensis Saecularia Undecima* (ed. G. Rossi, P. Fraccaro, and L. Montemartini). Tipografia Soc. An. Bruni Marelli, Pavia, pp. 1–3.

Stefanini D. (1877). Caso d'atrofia progressiva con alterazione de' gangli simpatici. *Archivio per le Scienze Mediche*, **2**, pp. 387–91.

Stricker S. (1869–72). *Handbuch der lehre von den geweben des menschen und thiere.* Verlag von Wilhelm Engelmann, Leipzig.

Tamburini A. and Marchi V. (1883). Contributo allo studio delle localizzazioni e dei gliomi cerebrali. *Archivio per le Scienze Mediche*, **7**, pp. 413–14.

Tanzi E. (1893). I fatti e le induzioni nell'odierna istologia del sistema nervoso. *Rivista Sperimentale di Freniatria e Medicina Legale*, **19**, pp. 419–72.

Tartuferi F. (1888). Sulla anatomia della retina. *Archivio per le Scienze Mediche*, **12**, pp. 335–58.

Terni C. (1925). *Università di Pavia e Università di Milano nel pensiero della maggioranza dei medici lombardi. Spunti critici e polemici.* Tipo-Litografia Prata, Milano.

Tesoro M. (1981). Democrazia e amministrazione: la prima giunta 'popolare' a Pavia (1899–1902). *Annali di Storia Pavese.* N° 6–7, pp. 119–28.

Thanhoffer L. (1882). Beiträge zur Histologie und Nervenendigung der quergestreiften Muskelfasern. *Archiv für Mikroskopische Anatomie*, **21**, pp. 26–44.

Tirelli V. (1918). Per Carlo Martinotti. *Giornale della R. Accademia di Medicina di Torino*, Anno 81°, Serie 4ª, **24**, pp. 185–92.

Toldt C. (1888). *Lehrbuch der Gewebelehre mit vorzugsweiser Berücksichtigung des menschlichen Hörpers: Mit einer topographischen Darstellung des Faserverlaufes im Centralnervensystem von Prof. O. Kahler.* 3ª edizione, Enke, Stuttgart.

Tommasi-Crudeli C. (1879). Della distribuzione delle acque nel sottosuolo dell'Agro romano e della sua influenza nella produzione della malaria. *Atti della R. Accademia dei Lincei. Memoria della Classe di Scienze Fisiche, Matematiche e Naturali*, **3**, pp. 183–97.

Tommasi-Crudeli C. (1886). Sopra un bacillo rinvenuto nelle atmosfere malariche dei dintorni di Pola (Istria). *Atti della R. Accademia dei Lincei. Rendiconti*, Serie 4ª, **2** (1° semestre), pp. 223–7.

Tommasi-Crudeli C. (1886a). Sul Plasmodium Malariae di Marchiafava, Celli e Golgi. *Atti della R. Accademia dei Lincei. Rendiconti*, Serie 4ª, **2** (1° semestre), pp. 313–19.

Tommasi-Crudeli C. (1886b). Ricerche sulla natura della malaria, eseguite dal dott. Bernardo Schiavuzzi in Pola (Istria). *Atti della R. Accademia dei Lincei. Rendiconti*, Serie 4ª, **2** (2° semestre), pp. 329–31.

Tommasi-Crudeli C. (1887). Stato attuale delle nostre conoscenze sulla natura della malaria, e sulla bonifica dei paesi malarici. *Atti della R. Accademia dei Lincei. Rendiconti*, Serie 4ª, **3** (1° semestre), pp. 355–65.

Tommasi-Crudeli C. (1888). Il bacillo della malaria. *Atti della R. Accademia dei Lincei. Rendiconti*, Serie 4ª, **4** (1° semestre), pp. 305–8.

Trautmann J. C. (1988). Camillo Golgi (1843–1926) und die Entdeckung des 'apparato reticolare interno'. Dissertation, Medizinischen Universität Lübeck, Lübeck.

Vaccari P. (1957). *Storia dell'Università di Pavia.* Università di Pavia editrice, Pavia.

Vanzetti F. (1926). Commemorazione del socio Prof. Sen. Pio Foà. *Giornale della R. Accademia di Medicina di Torino*, Anno 89°, Serie 4ª, **32**, pp. 57–77.

Vasari G. (1568). *Le vite de' più eccellenti pittori scultori e architettori.* Firenze. **Quotations in the text are from the edition edited by** G. Milanesi, Tomo IV. G. C. Sansoni Editore, Firenze (1879).

Veratti E. (1902). Ricerche sulla fine struttura della fibra muscolare striata. *Memorie dell'Istituto Lombardo Classe di Scienze Matematiche e Naturali*, **19**, pp. 87–133. **Engl. trans.** Investigations on the fine structure of the striated muscle fiber. *Journal of Biophysical and Biochemical Cytology* (1961), **10** (4), Suppl. 3–59.

Veratti E. (1926). Camillo Golgi e la sua opera scientifica. *Bollettino dell'Istituto Sieroterapico Milanese*, **5**, pp. 1–14.

Veratti E. (1929). La vita e l'opera scientifica di Aldo Perroncito. *Bollettino della Società Medico-Chirurgica di Pavia*, **44**, pp. 149–69.

Veratti E. (1942–43). A cento anni dalla nascita di Camillo Golgi. *Rendiconti R. Istituto Lombardo di Scienze e Lettere*, **76** (7° della serie 3ª), Fasc. 2, pp. 97–102.

Veratti E. (1953). L'interpretazione dei corpi del Negri cinquant'anni dopo la scoperta. *Bollettino della Società Medico-Chirurgica di Pavia*, **67**, pp. 1–13.

Verga A. (1869). *Sulla vita e sugli scritti di Bartolomeo Panizza*. Tipografia di Giuseppe Bernardoni, Milano.

Verga A. (1872). Recensione del lavoro di Golgi (1871–72). Contribuzione alla fina anatomia degli organi centrali del sistema nervoso. *Archivio Italiano per le Malatie Nervose*, Anno 9°, pp. 356–7.

Verga A. (1875). Recensione del lavoro di Golgi (1874). Sulle alterazioni degli organi centrali nervosi in un caso di corea gesticolatoria associata ad alienazione mentale. *Archivio Italiano per le Malatie Nervose*, Anno 12°, pp. 196–201.

Vialli M. (1961). Mauro Rusconi. In *Discipline e Maestri dell'Ateneo Pavese*. Arnoldo Mondadori editore, Verona, pp. 285–90.

Villa L. (1984). Camillo Golgi e la istologia (Alcuni documenti). *Memorie dell'Istituto Lombardo—Accademia di Scienze e Lettere. Classe di Scienze Matematiche e Naturali (Memoria 11)*, **28**, pp. 313–16.

Vincenzi L. (1883). Note istologiche sull'origine reale di alcuni nervi cerebrali. *Archivio per le Scienze Mediche*, **7**, pp. 319–48.

Viviano B. (1985). La Pia Casa di Abbiategrasso. In *Pia Casa di Abbiategrasso, Istituto Geriatrico Camillo Golgi*. Officina Grafica Piero Arrara & F., Abbiategrasso, pp. 13–77.

Volta Z. (1900). Saggio di bibliografia storica e descrittiva dell'Università di Pavia. *Annuario Università di Pavia, Anno scolastico 1899–900*. Tipografia successori Bizzoni, Pavia, pp. 20–6.

Waldeyer W. (1891). Über einige neuere Forschungen im Gebiete der Anatomie des Centralnervensystems. *Deutsche medicinische Wochenschrift*, **17**, pp. 1213–18, 1244–6, 1267–9, 1287–9, 1331–2, 1352–6.

Waldstein L. and Weber E. (1882). Etudes histochimiques sur les tubes nerveux a myéline. *Archives de Physiologie normale et pathologique*, **10**, 2e semestre, pp. 1–27.

Weiskrantz, L. (1997). *Consciousness lost and found*. Oxford University Press, Oxford.

Williams H. (1954). *Don Quixote of the microscope. An interpretation of the Spanish savant Santiago Ramón y Cajal (1852–1934)*. Jonathan Cape, London.

Zanobio B. (1959). Le osservazioni microscopiche di Felice Fontana sulla struttura dei nervi. *Physis*, **1**, pp. 307–20.

Zanobio B. (1960). L'immagine filamentoso-reticolare nell'anatomia microscopica dal XVII al XIX secolo. *Physis*, **2**, pp. 299–317.

Zanobio B. (1963). The work of Camillo Golgi in Neurology. In *Essays on the history of Italian neurology* (ed. L. Belloni). Instituto di Storia della Medicina di Milano, Milano, pp. 179–93.

Zanobio B. (1971). Micrographie illusoire et théories sur la structure de la matière vivante. *Clio Medica*, **6**, pp. 25–40.

Zanobio B. (1973). Campagne antimalariche di 'bonifica umana' nella Bassa Lombardia e loro significato medico-sociale. *Annales Cisalpines d'Histoire Sociale*, Série I, N° 4, pp. 255–65.

Zanobio B. (1978). *La morfologia dell'olfatto e l'università di Pavia*. Tipografia Fusi, Pavia.

Zanobio B. (1978a). Il soggiorno di Camillo Golgi 'premio Nobel 1906' a Stoccolma, attraverso lettere familiari. *Istituto Lombardo (Rend. Lett.)*, **112**, pp. 143–58.

Zanobio B. (1986). La società medico-chirurgica di Pavia nella storia della medicina. *Inaugurazione Anno Acc. 1985–86 Università di Pavia*. Meroni tip.-lit., Albese con Cassano, pp. 47–58.

Zanobio B. (1986a). Sul conferimento del premio Nobel a Camillo Golgi e Santiago Ramón y Cajal. Qualche notizia nell'ottantesimo anniversario. *Istituto Lombardo (Rend. Sc.) B*, 120, pp. 45–8.

Zanobio B. (1992). Fondazione, nascita, primi passi della clinica del lavoro di Milano. Suoi contesti storico e sociali. *La Medicina del Lavoro*, **83**, pp. 18–32.

Zanobio B. and Armocida G. (1994). Some aspects of Camillo Golgi's parliamentary activity. *Medicina nei Secoli. Arte e Scienza*, **6**, pp. 609–20.

Zanobio B., Belloni L., Lesky E., Wandruszka A., Milani F., Grignani E., and Repossi C. (1980). *Giovanni Alessandro Brambilla nella cultura medica del Settecento europeo*. Cisalpino Istituto Editoriale Universitario. Milano.

Zenker K. (1894). Chromkali-Sublimat-Eisessig als Fixirungsmittel. *Münchener Medizinische Wochenschrift*, **41**, pp. 532–4.

Zerbi D. and Trabattoni G. R. (1988). *Serafino Biffi un neurologue milanais*. Fondation Marcel Merieux, Lyon, pp. 115–20.

Ziemssen H. W. von (1877). Chorea. *Handbuch der Krankheiten des Nervensystems*. F. C. W. Vogel, Leipzig, pp. 433–88.

Index

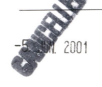